Understanding the

AUSTRALIAN HEALTH CARE SYSTEM

FIFTH EDITION

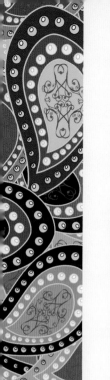

Understanding the

AUSTRALIAN HEALTH CARE SYSTEM

FIFTH EDITION

Louise Reynolds, RP, PhD, BHSc(PHC), GradCertEd, MPH, FACPara
Chief Paramedic Officer, Safer Care Victoria
Associate Professor in Paramedicine, College of Sport, Health & Engineering
Victoria University, Melbourne, Victoria, Australia

Deborah Debono, PhD, GC HEdT&L, BA (Psych Hons), RN
Associate Professor Health Services Management,
School of Public Health, Faculty of Health
University of Technology Sydney, Sydney, New South Wales, Australia

Joanne Travaglia, PhD, BSocStuds (Hons), MEd
Head of School, Professor Public Health and Social Work
Queensland University of Technology, Brisbane, Queensland, Australia;
Honorary Professor, School of Public Health
University of Technology Sydney, Sydney, New South Wales, Australia

ELSEVIER

Elsevier Australia. ACN 001 002 357
(a division of Reed International Books Australia Pty Ltd)
Tower 2, 475 Victoria Avenue, Chatswood, NSW 2067

ISBN: 978-0-7295-4429-0

Notice

This publication has been carefully reviewed and checked to ensure that the content is as accurate and current as possible at time of publication. We would recommend, however, that the reader verify any procedures, treatments, drug dosages or legal content described in this book. Neither the author, the contributors nor the publisher assume any liability for injury and/or damage to persons or property arising from any error in or omission from this publication.

National Library of Australia Cataloguing-in-Publication Data

A catalogue record for this book is available from the National Library of Australia

Content Strategist: Melinda McEvoy
Content Project Manager: Abdus Salam Mazumder
Edited by Laura Davies
Proofread by Tim Learner
Copyrights Coordinator: Vengatesh Thirunavukkarasu
Cover Designer: Gopalakrishnan Venkatraman
Index by Innodata
Typeset by GW Tech
Printed in China by 1010 Printing International Ltd.

Last digit is the print number: 9   8   7   6   5   4   3   2   1

CONTENTS

Video Table of Contents, vii
Dedication, viii
Acknowledgements, ix
Contributors, x
Reviewers, xv

1 **Understanding the Australian Health Care System: How to Use this Book,** 1
Louise Reynolds, Deborah Debono and Joanne Travaglia

SECTION ONE   System Overview

2 **The Public Health Sector and Medicare,** 14
Kees van Gool and Jane Hall

3 **The Private Health Sector and Private Health Insurance,** 30
Nathan Kettlewell

4 **International Health Care Systems,** 41
Judith Daire, Delia Hendrie and Suzanne Robinson

5 **Public Health in Australia,** 55
Helen Keleher

6 **Primary Health Care in Australia,** 64
Paresh Dawda and Angelene True

7 **The Pharmaceutical Benefits Scheme,** 79
Lisa Pont

8 **The Aged Care Sector: Residential and Community Care,** 89
Hamish Robertson and David Smith

9 **Equity and Access: A Spotlight on Rural Health,** 100
Bernadette Ward and Pam Harvey

10 **Indigenous Health Systems and Services,** 114
Colleen Hayes and Kerry Taylor

11 **Mental Health and Recovery-Oriented Mental Health Services,** 125
Fiona Orr

12 **People Living with Disability: Navigating Support and Health Systems,** 138
Caroline Ellison

13 **Australian Workers' Compensation Systems,** 150
Alex Collie and Tyler Lane

14 **The Complementary and Alternative Health Care System in Australia,** 163
Julia Twohig

15 **Oral Health and Dental Services,** 175
Julie Satur

16 **Digital Health and the Divide,** 191
Sandeep Reddy

SECTION TWO   Health Professionals

17 **Australia's Health Workforce,** 201
Susan Waller, Keith Sutton and Tony Smith

18 **Clinical Exercise Physiology in the Australian Health Care System,** 214
Steve Selig, Melainie Cameron and Kirsty Rawlings

19 **Nutrition and Dietetics: Promoting Health for All Australians,** 225
Louisa Matwiejczyk, Adeline Lau and Marian McAllister

20 **Health Services Managers in the Australian Health Care System,** 237
Joanne Travaglia and Deborah Debono

21 **The Medical Profession in Australia,** 248
E Michael Shanahan

22 **Midwifery in Australia,** 258
Kathleen Baird, Vanessa Scarf and Melanie Briggs

23 **Nursing in Australia,** 271
Sarah Wise and Christine Duffield

24 **Occupational Therapy,** 282
Sandra Mortimer and Ellice Willcourt

25 **Paramedicine and the Health Care System,** 292
Alan Morrison and Louise Reynolds

26 **The Pharmacist's Unique Contribution to Australia's Health System,** 303
Stephen Carter

27 **Health Profession Regulation: The Case of Physiotherapy,** 313
Matthew Sutton

28 **Speech Pathology and Audiology: Assessment and Intervention for Communication Impairment,** 323
Jane Bickford, Lisa Callahan, Giriraj Singh Shekhawat and Lauren Sullivan

29 **The Social Work Profession in the Australian Health Care System,** 336
Joanne Travaglia, Angel Carrasco, Bobbi Henao Urrego

Glossary, 345
Abbreviations, 356
Index, 358

VIDEO TABLE OF CONTENTS

A suite of video interviews with practitioners and thought leaders have been created for this edition and are available on the Evolve site: http://evolve.elsevier.com/AU/Reynolds/understanding/

The videos further explore the themes and content within the chapters, as well as outlining challenges of the profession and advice for new graduates.

- Public health in Australia (Chapter 5)
- People living with disability: navigating support and health systems (Chapter 12)
- The complementary and alternative health care system in Australia (Chapter 14)
- Oral health and dental services (Chapter 15)
- Health profession regulation: the case of physiotherapy (Chapter 27)
- Occupational therapy (Chapter 24)
- Clinical exercise physiology in the Australian health care system (Chapter 18)
- Speech pathology: assessment and intervention for communication impairment (Chapter 28)
- Audiology: assessment and intervention for communication impairment (Chapter 28)
- Health care managers in a changing system (Chapter 20)

This edition is dedicated to our esteemed colleague, co-editor and friend Professor Joanne Travaglia who passed away before the final publication of this edition. Her passion to improve equity, access and delivery of health and social services, particularly to those whom the system and society make vulnerable, knew no bounds. Jo was an excellent teacher, researcher, advocate and mentor, and, importantly, a wonderful human being. She will be proud of her legacy that lives on in this edition for her past, current and future health and social care professional students.

ACKNOWLEDGEMENTS

Understanding the Australian Health Care System is the fifth edition of this book. It has involved collaborative effort, plus the skills, knowledge and resources of many people to whom we offer our gratitude.

We are again indebted to our contributors, those who are new and those who have stayed with us for this fifth edition. We thank them for sharing their expert knowledge from their fields of practice and the special insights that they bring to their chapters. The manuscript is enhanced by the thoughtful comments provided by anonymous reviewers whom we also thank and acknowledge.

We thank and are indebted as always to the Elsevier team – Melinda McEvoy, Kritika Kaushik, Abdus Salam Mazumder, Laura Davies and others behind the scenes. Their continued interest in this book and its development, along with their skills and patience, helped us meet deadlines amid the busy lives of both editors and contributors, and are much appreciated.

We wish to acknowledge with special thanks Emeritus Professor Eileen Willis who was co-editor for the first four editions and Professor Trudy Rudge, co-editor for the fourth edition. A warm welcome to Professor Joanne Travaglia and Associate Professor Deborah Debono as co-editors.

We also thank those nearest and dearest to us for their forbearance, especially on long evenings and weekends when we were distracted by the manuscript. We deeply appreciate your support and encouragement.

We have again enjoyed working together on this book, and we trust that readers enjoy the book as much as we have enjoyed our collaborations during its preparation and production.

CONTRIBUTORS

Kathleen Baird, PhD, RM, MA Ed. Pg Dip HE,
BSc(Hons), HDE, SFHEA
Professor, Head of School,
Nursing and Midwifery,
Faculty of Health,
University of Technology Sydney,
Sydney, New South Wales

Jane Bickford, PhD, BAppSc(SpPath)
Academic Lead,
Speech Pathology,
College of Nursing and Health Sciences,
Flinders University,
Adelaide, South Australia

Melanie Briggs, BMid, Master of Primary Maternity
Care, AdvDip Leadership and Management
Senior Koori Leadership,
South Coast Women's Health and Wellbeing Aboriginal
Corporation Waminda;
Minga Gudjaga and Birthing on Country Manager,
Minga Gudjaga, Maternity,
Nowra, New South Wales

Lisa Callahan, MPH, MAud, GradCert Educ
(Higher Educ), B Beh Sci (Psych)
Audiology,
College of Nursing and Health Sciences,
Flinders University,
Adelaide, South Australia

Melainie Cameron, PhD, MHSc, BAppSc (Ost)
Associate Professor,
School of Health and Wellbeing,
University of Southern Queensland;
Extraordinary Professor,
Research entity for Physical Activity,
Sport, and Recreation (PhASRec),
North-West University,
Potchefstroom, South Africa

Angel Carrasco, BSW, MMH(Psychotherapy),
GradCert (DisMgt)
Director of Social Work and Support Services,
Directorate of Emergency and Specialist Services,
Gold Coast Hospital and Health Service,
Southport, Queensland;
Adjunct Senior Lecturer,
School of Health Sciences and Social Work,
Griffith University,
Queensland

Stephen Carter, PhD, BPharm, MSc
Senior Lecturer,
School of Pharmacy,
University of Sydney,
Sydney, New South Wales

Alex Collie, PhD, BA, BAppSc(Hons)
Professor and ARC Future Fellow,
School of Public Health and Preventive Medicine,
Monash University,
Melbourne, Victoria

Judith Daire, PhD, MSc Health Management, Planning
and Policy, BSc
Nursing and Midwifery,
School of Population Health,
Curtin University,
Perth, Western Australia

Paresh Dawda, MB BS, DRCOG, DFRSH, FRACGP,
FRCGP
Director and Principal,
Prestantia Health,
Canberra, Australian Capital Territory

Christine Duffield, PhD, BScN, MHP, FACN, FAAN, FAICD, FACHSM
Emeritus Professor,
Nursing,
University of Technology Sydney,
Sydney, New South Wales;
Emeritus Professor,
Edith Cowan University,
Perth, Western Australia

Caroline Ellison, PhD, BappSc (Dis Stud)(Hons)
Associate Professor,
Justice and Society,
University of South Australia,
Adelaide, South Australia

Kees van Gool, PhD, MEc, BEc, BA
Professor,
Menzies Centre for Health Policy and Economics,
University of Sydney,
Sydney, New South Wales

Jane Hall, PhD, BA, FASSA, FAHMS
Distinguished Professor,
Centre for Health Economics Research and Evaluation,
University of Technology Sydney,
Sydney, New South Wales

Pam Harvey, PhD, BAppSci(Physio), MEd,
School of Rural Health,
Monash University,
Bendigo, Victoria

Colleen Hayes, PostGradCert Remote Health Practice
Research Fellow,
Community and Public Health,
Flinders University,
Alice Springs, Northern Territory

Bobbi Henao Urrego, BSW, MSW, MPH, MHM, AFCHSM, CHM
Director,
Allied Health,
Sydney Children's Hospitals Network,
New South Wales;
Adjunct Fellow,
School of Public Health,
University Technology Sydney,
Sydney, New South Wales

Delia Hendrie, PhD
Associate Professor,
Curtin School of Population Health,
Curtin University,
Perth, Western Australia

Helen Marie Keleher, PhD, MA, BA
Professor (Adj),
School of Rural Health,
Monash University,
Melbourne, Victoria;
Australia Director,
Keleher Consulting

Nathan Kettlewell, PhD (Econ), MEcon, BCom(Hons)
Chancellor's Senior Research Fellow,
Economics Discipline Group,
University of Technology Sydney,
Sydney, New South Wales

Tyler Lane, DPhil, MSc, BA
Department of Epidemiology and Preventive Medicine,
Monash University,
Melbourne, Victoria

Adeline Lau, BNutDiet(Hons), MSc Applied
Gerontology
Nutrition and Dietetics,
Flinders University,
Adelaide, South Australia

Marian McAllister, APD, BSc, BSc(Hons), MND
Lecturer,
Flinders University,
Adelaide, South Australia

Louisa Matwiejczyk, PhD, BArts(Hons), PostGradDip
(Nutr&Diet), AdvAPD
Nutrition and Dietetics,
College of Nursing and Health Sciences,
Flinders University,
Adelaide, South Australia

Alan Morrison, ASM, MPET, GradDipPAdmin,
GradDipEd, BParaPrac, BAppSc(Biomedical), FACPara
Adjunct Associate Professor,
School of Paramedicine,
University of Tasmania,
Australia;
Adjunct Fellow,
Western Sydney University,
Australia

Sandra Mortimer, Doctor of Public Health,
BAppSc (OT)
Senior Lecturer,
Occupational Therapy,
Flinders University,
Bedford Park, South Australia

Fiona Orr, PhD, BHSc(Nursing), MLitt
Senior Lecturer,
School of Nursing and Midwifery,
University of Notre Dame Australia,
Sydney, New South Wales;
Adjunct Fellow,
School of Nursing and Midwifery,
University of Technology,
Sydney, New South Wales

Lisa Pont, PhD, BPharm, MSc(Epi)
Professor,
Discipline of Pharmacy,
Graduate School of Health,
University of Technology Sydney,
Sydney, New South Wales

Kirsty Rawlings, BAppExSpSc, BEdStudies (Hons)
HMS, ESSAM, GAICD
Lecturer,
Allied Health and Human Performance,
University of South Australia,
Adelaide, South Australia

Sandeep Reddy, PhD, MBBS, MSc, MMgmt, CHIA
Associate Professor,
School of Medicine,
Deakin University,
Geelong, Victoria

Hamish Robertson, PhD
Senior Lecturer,
Faculty of Health, Queensland University of
Technology,
Brisbane, Queensland

Suzanne Robinson, PhD
Chair,
Health Economics,
Deakin University,
Melbourne, Victoria;
Adjunct Professor,
Curtin University,
Perth, Western Australia

Julie Satur, PhD, DipApplSci (DTher), MHSci
(H Prom)
Professor Oral Health,
Melbourne Dental School,
University of Melbourne,
Melbourne, Victoria

Vanessa Scarf, PhD, GDMid, GC Child and Family Health Nursing, GCClinEpi
Faculty of Health,
University of Technology Sydney,
Sydney, New South Wales

Steve Selig, PhD, BSc(Hons)
Chair,
Clinical Exercise Science,
School of Exercise and Nutrition Sciences,
Deakin University,
Melbourne, Victoria

E Michael Shanahan, PhD, BMBS, MPH, MHPE, FAFOEM, FRACP
Head of Rheumatology,
Southern Adelaide Local Health Network,
South Australia;
Professor,
College of Medicine and Public Health,
Flinders University,
Adelaide, South Australia

Giriraj Singh Shekhawat, PhD, FHERDSA, SFHEA, CMALT, MAICD, PGCertAP, TEDx Speaker
Dean of Research,
College of Education, Psychology, and Social Work,
Flinders University,
Adelaide, South Australia;
Honorary Professor Audiology,
Ear Institute,
University College London,
London, United Kingdom;
Public Relations Manager,
Tinnitus Research Initiative,
Regensburg, Germany

David Smith,
Director at Community and Aged Care Consulting Services
Hurstville, New South wales

Tony Smith, PhD, MSc, BSc, DipAppSci(MedRad), FASMIRT
Associate Professor (retired),
Department of Rural Health,
University of Newcastle,
Newcastle, New South Wales;
Sessional Academic,
Department of Medical Imaging and Radiation Sciences,
Monash University,
Victoria

Lauren Sullivan, BAppScSP(Hons)
Flinders University,
Speech Pathology,
College of Nursing and Health Sciences,
Adelaide, South Australia

Keith Sutton, PhD, BN
Lecturer,
Rural Mental Health,
Monash Rural Health (Warragul),
Monash University,
Warragul, Victoria

Matthew Sutton, MMusc&SportPhty, BPhty
College of Nursing and Health Sciences,
Flinders University,
Adelaide, South Australia

Kerry Taylor, PhD, MPHC, BNg, GradDip Hlth Ed, DipTch
Associate Professor,
College of Medicine and Public Health,
Flinders University,
Adelaide, South Australia

Julia Twohig, PhD, BAdult&VocEduc(Hons)
Education Futures,
University of South Australia,
Adelaide, South Australia

Angelene True, MBA
Principal Consultant,
Prestantia Health,
Canberra, Australian Capital Territory

Susan Waller, PhD, MPhty, GradCertPhty, BPhty
Adjunct Senior Research Fellow,
Monash Rural Health,
Monash University,
Bendigo, Victoria;
Assistant Professor,
Department of Medical Education,
College of Medicine and Health Sciences,
United Arab Emirates University,
Al Ain,
Abu Dhabi, United Arab Emirates

Bernadette Ward, PhD, BN, MPH&TM, MHSci
Associate Professor,
School of Rural Health,
Monash University,
Bendigo, Victoria

Ellice Willcourt, BOT
Senior Lecturer,
Occupational Therapy,
Flinders University,
Adelaide, South Australia

Sarah Wise, PhD, LLB, MSc
Senior Lecturer,
School of Public Health,
University of Technology Sydney,
Sydney, New South Wales

REVIEWERS

Judith Anderson, PhD, MN, MHSM, BN, RN
Associate Professor,
Charles Sturt University,
Bathurst, New South Wales

Sally Bristow, PhD, MNurs, Grad Dip Mid, RM,
Cert Adv Nephrology, BN, RN
Nursing Academic University of New England,
Armidale, New South Wales

Sue Gledhill, PhD, SFHEA, Grad. Cert. (Higher Ed.)
(ACU), MHA (UNSW), B. Bus (QUT), RN, RM
Academic,
School of Nursing, Midwifery and Paramedicine,
Australian Catholic University (ACU),
Brisbane, Queensland

Peta Harbour
Deputy Head of School,
Nursing, Midwifery and Paramedicine,
Australian Catholic University (ACU),
Canberra, Australian Capital Territory

Clare Mangoyana, GradDipDHDT, MPH, DPH,
AFHEA
Adjunct Lecturer/Research Fellow,
School of Dentistry,
University of Queensland,
Brisbane, Queensland

Pen Roe, PhD
Lecturer,
College of Nursing and Health Sciences,
Flinders University,
Bedford Park, South Australia

Patricia Taylor, PhD
Lecturer,
School of Health and Social Development,
Deakin University,
Burwood, Victoria

Understanding the Australian Health Care System: How to Use this Book

Louise Reynolds, Deborah Debono and Joanne Travaglia[a]

KEY LEARNING OUTCOMES

When you finish this chapter you should be able to:
- understand the structure of this book
- identify the main drivers for health system reform and key conceptual ideas that underpin those drivers
- be familiar with the three main types of health care systems across the developed world
- recognise major ideas impacting on health care reform arising from economic rationalism and neoliberalism
- have an idea of the outcomes of any health reform using Tuohy's theories of institutional mix and structural power
- understand the key questions to ask using Bacchi's framework of 'What's the problem represented to be?'
- understood what is meant by 'interprofessional practice'
- consider the impact of the SARS-CoV-2 pandemic on health care system delivery and workforce.

KEY TERMS AND ABBREVIATIONS

activity-based funding (ABF)
acute care
adverse events
Australian Health Practitioner Regulation Agency (Ahpra)
Australian Institute of Health and Welfare (AIHW)
Australian Medical Association (AMA)
autonomy of practice
casemix
COVID-19
Diagnosis Related Groups (DRG)
economic rationalism
effectiveness
efficiency

evidence-based medicine (EBM)
general practice/general practitioner (GP)
global financial crisis (GFC)
Independent Hospital Pricing Authority (IHPA)
institutional mix
interprofessional education (IPE)
interprofessional education/practice (IPE/IPP)
interprofessional practice (IPP)
medical dominance
Medicare
mixed system
neoliberalism
new public management (NPM)

Organisation for Economic Co-operation and Development (OECD)
Pharmaceutical Benefits Scheme (PBS)
private for-profit
productivity
professional monopoly
public–private partnership (PPP)
regulation
risk management
SARS-CoV-2 pandemic
self-regulate
sentinel event
structural balance
systematic literature review (SLR)

[a]We acknowledge previous contributors Eileen Willis and Trudy Rudge in the preparation of this chapter.

the State
theory
United Kingdom (UK)

universal health coverage
welfare state

What's the problem represented
to be? (WPR)

INTRODUCTION TO THE STRUCTURE OF THIS BOOK

Welcome to the fifth edition of *Understanding the Australian Health Care System*. This book introduces you to some of the core issues and theoretical concepts that provide insight into the way various Australian health care systems are organised. All health professionals work within these systems, so having a grasp of how they are organised will ease your pathway in your future health-related professional life. The contributing authors have all been selected for their grasp of interprofessional health practice, their first-hand knowledge of these systems, and their experience in teaching undergraduate and postgraduate health professionals.

How the Book Works

Section One

The book is divided into two sections. Section One includes 16 chapters in which we introduce you to the range of Australian health care systems. These include mental health, workers' compensation, Indigenous, complementary and private health care systems, along with the organisation of social services for those with a disability or chronic illness. This section also touches on the role of **Medicare**, the **Pharmaceutical Benefits Scheme (PBS)**, and concepts such as public health, primary health care, digital health and rural health. Many of these systems continue to change, as a result of government attempts to make them more efficient and productive. We also consider the impact of the **SARS-CoV-2 pandemic** on the way in which Australian health care systems are organised and care delivered.

Section Two

Section Two of the book has 13 chapters covering Australia's health workforce and a range of health professions. The authors of these chapters were tasked with writing about their profession and the work that is performed by professionals from the fields of: nursing, midwifery, speech pathology and audiology, health services management, paramedics, social work, pharmacy, exercise physiology, nutrition and diet, medicine, occupational therapy and physiotherapy. In our brief to the authors of these chapters we asked them to:

- outline the impact that various health reforms have had on key quality and safety issues of relevance to their professional practice
- explore how their profession works interprofessionally, particularly with people who have chronic conditions
- outline the effects, if any, of the global SARS-CoV-2 pandemic on patient care practices.

THINKING ABOUT PROFESSIONALS

Not all occupations call themselves professionals. So, what do we mean when we talk about the health professions? When sociologists answer this question, they invariably draw on the ideas of an American sociologist, Eliot Freidson (1923–2005), who framed the answer by asking 'Who controls the work?' He argued that work in capitalist societies could be controlled by the market (for-profit sector), or by **the State** (governments), or by a specialised highly skilled group of workers or professionals. He suggested that where the knowledge and skills required to do a task is highly specialised, control is in the hands of a profession.

In Freidson's (1970a, 1970b) classic study of the professions, he positioned medicine as the most ideal typical profession and in doing so outlined the key characteristics that all professions aspire to. These are:

- a strong service ethic with set standards and ideals that sets it apart from other occupations
- specialised training and a science orientation that forms a unique body of knowledge that gives it a **professional monopoly** in this area. This monopoly is often achieved through accreditation of its educational course, and formal registration that restricts access so

that other occupational groups cannot perform many of the procedures, such as prescribing drugs. This is called professional closure. In some instances the use of the title will be protected, such as 'nurse' or 'midwife'
• **autonomy of practice** over this work, with the capacity to set their own price and **self-regulate** (Freidson 1970a, p. 2).

The power of particular health professions (such as medicine) comes from the fact that illness and disease are so unique and full of uncertainty that only this expert group has the specialist skills and knowledge to cure. Both the State and the individual patient put their trust in the professional's capacity to use their discretionary judgement to determine what is the best treatment for the patient. This trust is given to professionals by the State and the patient because it is assumed that they work in the best interest of their patients with a high level of skill underpinned by a high level of education (Freidson 1970a, 1970b). This gives the profession considerable esteem in the eyes of patients and in some instances power over the work of other health professionals. This power over other professions is described as **medical dominance** (Kenny 2004; Willis 1983).

As governments have increasingly strived to control costs through imposing health care reforms, they have moved to negotiate with the health professions, particularly medicine. Ultimately, these negotiations are over the control that the medical profession has within the health care system and attempts to curb that power through reforms, as well as control of costs.

One way that governments impose control over the health professions is through **regulation**. To this end, in 2009, the Australian federal government established the National Registration and Accreditation Scheme (NRAS), inclusive of creating the **Australian Health Practitioner Regulation Agency (Ahpra)**. This was in response to concerns with the maldistribution of health professionals, the lack of flexibility in gaining registration across state borders and the limited access to services for some population groups. The primary purpose of the NRAS is 'to provide for the protection of the public by ensuring that only health practitioners who are suitably trained and qualified to practise in a competent and ethical manner are registered' (Health Practitioner Regulation National Law (NSW) 2009). Ahpra supports the national regulatory functions of 15 national boards covering 16 health professions. This includes student registration. The functions of the national boards include:

• registering health professionals and students
• developing standards, codes and guidelines for their profession
• handling notifications, complaints, investigations and disciplinary hearings (except in NSW and Queensland where this is undertaken by co-regulatory arrangements for these states)
• assessing overseas-trained practitioners who wish to practise in Australia
• approving accreditation standards and accredited programs of study.

Pause *for* Reflection ...
As a student in a health care study program, have you noticed a hierarchy or difference in status and prestige within the various health degree programs at your university? If so, how would you organise this hierarchy of professional health degrees? Is it based on a student's score? Is it based on the number of years students must study to gain accreditation, or is it based on some other factors?

The establishment of the NRAS extends government control into the management of professions and their associations.

Another control mechanism is the attempt to contain rising costs. Examples include the introduction of **Diagnosis Related Groups (DRG)** or **casemix** and **activity-based funding (ABF)** in the late 1990s and more recently the announcement by the **Independent Hospital Pricing Authority (IHPA)** to change the funding for **sentinel** and **adverse events** (IHPA 2017a, 2017b). These government-directed processes impact on the way health professionals, particularly doctors and nurses, organise care and as a consequence challenge professional autonomy (see Chapter 3).

So far, we have suggested that there are three major players in health care: the professions, the government (which we sometimes refer to as 'the State') and the **private for-profit** sector (which we will sometimes refer to as 'the market'). Of course, there is also the consumer movement representing patients (sometimes called clients, or consumers), but there is debate and, indeed, uncertainty about how powerful they actually are in the business of health care reform (Tuohy 1999).

In the next section we provide a theoretical discussion on the factors behind health care reform. We have taken two approaches to this. Firstly, we outline what we find theoretically helpful and what we think is happening in the health care sector here in Australia, but also in many other developed nations. Secondly, we provide you with some questions for tackling health reform and health policy wherever you see it, in the hospital, in residential aged care or in your profession's registration board.

Tuohy's Theory of Health Care Systems Change

Our own theory is based on the work of Tuohy, a Canadian political scientist and her book *Accidental Logics*. Before you read our interpretation of her work, bear in mind that it is a **theory**, which is a way of explaining a concept or idea. You should read this definition as a way of interpreting a political or sociological idea, rather than as a 'fact' or evidence-base. Theories help us to shape both what we see and how we understand the world, they can help us predict what might happen in particular contexts, but they are not the truth, just a theory, just as Tuohy uses case studies to support her theory. Secondly, we suggest that health care reform is driven by a series of economic philosophies and practices. They are also driven by values-based arguments about equity and the costs of inaction on equity and effectiveness. **Efficiency**, **effectiveness** and **equity** are core drivers for health system performance, so the theorists we have selected address these outputs in some way.

Fundamental to any theory of health care reform is the question of who pays for the services that are provided. Tuohy (1999) argues that health care reform has been high on the policy agenda in most developed nations since the early 1980s and that in all cases the debate has been couched in the following way – *given that health is central to the well-being of a nation, what role should the state play, and what role should the market play in providing health care* (Tuohy 1999, p. 3)? Behind Tuohy's question is the tension between three types of systems (Docteur & Oxley 2003). These are the public-integrated model, the public-contracted model (see Chapter 2) and the private insurance model (see Chapter 3). In the *public-integrated model*, hospitals and health services are funded directly by the government as part of the **welfare state** through levies and taxation. In Australia, **Medicare** funding for public hospitals fits this model (public-integrated model). Medicare funds are also used to fund **general practice** and medical specialist services. This is an example of a *public-contracted*

service delivery model provided by private providers (Docteur & Oxley 2003). The third model, the *private insurance model*, is a system where citizens pay for their health care directly to an insurer, or the professional such as you do when you go to your physiotherapist who is in private practice.

As you'll read, Australian health care is a **mixed system** of all three models of service provision. We can summarise the first two models as welfare state–based or public systems (with some patient co-payments), while the third model is a market-driven system.

You can see from this three-cornered model that there are three players: the government or State, the professionals and the private for-profit sector (insurance companies, private hospitals, private professionals, medical device and pharmaceutical industries, consultants). Tuohy's theory helps us understand that health reform rises or falls on who has the power between these three players. The group that holds the balance of power holds the **structural balance** (Tuohy 1999). For example, power might reside in the government with its authority to freeze Medicare reimbursements for **general practitioners (GPs)** (Australian Government 2018) (Case study 1.1), or in the professions (particularly medicine) with their highly sophisticated skills, or in the private sector with its wealth and political capacity to influence decisions. As a consequence, the patient is either portrayed in health policy as a citizen of the State with the right to free health care, or as a patient to whom the doctor provides the best possible care, or a consumer purchasing a health product in a competitive market.

What's New in the 21st century?

In the past, these three groups (professions, the State and the private sector) were presumed to use very different tactics. However, this is no longer so. Over the last 30 years all three groups have moved to use similar tactics and strategies to deliver patient-centred care (Tuohy 1999). The State may employ market mechanisms, or take control of the collegial system, or the private system might enter into arrangements with the State to the point that these systems are now radically changed. The classic example of this is the way in which the State has introduced market measures into the welfare state forms of health care provision. This is called **new public management (NPM)** and it is driven by a philosophy called **neoliberalism** and the practices of **economic rationalism** (Stanton et al. 2003).

CASE STUDY 1.1   Shifts in the Balance of Power: The Medicare Rebate Freeze 2014–20

In the 2016 federal election the Australian Labor Party announced it would lift the freeze on GP rebates if it won the election. The irony of this was not lost of the federal Coalition Government, given it was the Labor Party that introduced this freeze on GP rebates in 2013 in order to reel the budget back in. In 2014 in the May budget the Coalition Government attempted to deal with the cost blow-outs in Medicare in other ways; one proposal was a (AU)$7 co-payment made by the patient for GP consultations, and pathology and imaging services that would be offset by a $5 reduction in the Medicare rebate the doctor received. The government quickly retracted this proposal, given the strong campaign by the **Australian Medical Association (AMA)**, the Labor Party, the Greens, the Independents and other health groups and also because the freeze proposed till 2020 on GP rebates saved more money than the $7 co-payment. However, at the 2016 election the Coalition agreed to review the medical benefits schedule, and to introduce a Practice Incentive Program (Caruso et al. 2008). It also established the Health Care Homes Program (Department of Health 2018). Health Care Homes funds GP services independently of Medicare reimbursement and is not based on the time spent with a patient (as Medicare rebates currently are), but on the quality of the outcome.

As Tuohy reminds us, the political party in power must have the will to bring about particular changes, but it must also be able to mobilise support across government, the private sector and the professions to bring about change. In the case of the $7 co-payment, the Coalition Government lacked political support from within its own party and from the cross-bench members[a] whom it needed to support the legislation. It was also opposed by the medical profession and a number of health advocacy groups who ran very successful campaigns focusing on the high cost to vulnerable patients. Opposition also came from private providers of pathology services such as Sonic Health Care claiming they had had a drop in services even though the legislation was not passed. In their case, this would also have led to a drop in share price.

Tuohy (1999) refers to the idea that all the conditions for change must be right before it can be achieved as the **institutional mix** and this case study demonstrates that the medical profession was able to mobilise **structural power**.

[a]These are members of parliament who come from minor parties or are independent.

Philosophies, Practices and Pandemics Driving Change

Economic rationalism, or microeconomic reform, is a philosophical approach, emerging from neoliberalism, to inform government economic management known as the welfare state or the range of services it provides for citizens. The use of the word 'rationalism' suggests that all economic decisions should first focus on **productivity**, profits and efficiency of practices, over questions of equity and social justice. However, it is important to note that governments do not outrightly reject equity and social justice in providing welfare services such as health and education to its citizens; however, they do prioritise productivity and efficiency while arguing for strategies to justify spending tax payers' money.

Proponents of economic rationalism also argue that the best way to ensure a robust economy and prosperity for the majority of people in any society is for the economy to be under the control of the private sector, rather than governments. Behind this philosophy is the idea that freedom in the economic sphere of society will generate wealth, productivity and efficiency across society (Stanton et al. 2005). Neoliberals also hold the view that individuals tend to act in their own self-interest. As a consequence, they believe that, in a robust democracy, there should be maximum freedom of choice for the individual and limited interference by governments in citizens' lives or in their business dealings, in the belief that individuals will strive to achieve the best outcomes for themselves.

New Public Management (NPM)

NPM suggests that the public service and the welfare state, funded by government through tax payers' money, can be made more efficient and productive if it is run like a private company operating through competitive practices. Examples include paying public hospitals bonuses if they see more patients, or keeping back a percentage of the budget until a service meets a target. Activity-based funding is another example. NPM can also include outsourcing non-essential services in the public sector such as cleaning and catering to a private company, or turning a public hospital pathology and radiology service into a business that must make a profit. It also means that when governments want a particular task done they must put it out to competitive tender allowing private companies to compete for the job, and in some cases the government and a private company may run a service such as a hospital together in what is known as a **public–private partnership (PPP)**.

As a set of practices, NPM is not limited to health care or to Australia. NPM practices can be found in many other parts of the welfare state such as education, Indigenous affairs and provisions for the unemployed (outsourcing of funds to private companies to help the unemployed find work), and in many other countries. For example, following the **global financial crisis (GFC)** the International Monetary Fund and World Bank insisted that countries that needed to borrow funds to bail out their economies introduce the practices of NPM into their health care systems (van Gool & Pearson 2014).

Is New Public Management Dead?

Some political scientists argue that new public management is dead (Crouch 2011). We would argue that it is alive and well, and takes new forms with each decade. One new approach deals with patient quality, safety and risk. Throughout this book, various authors will discuss the impact of the Australian Commission for Safety and Quality in Health Care on their profession (Australian Commission for Safety and Quality in Health Care (ACSQHC) 2017). The Commission publishes a number of standards that clinicians, hospitals and health organisations need to meet in order to be accredited. This brings the control down to the level of the professional doctor, nurse or manager. Accreditation of hospitals is linked to the capacity to abide by the national standards. While it is important to keep Australian patients safe and to provide them with quality health care, many clinical standards and practices are now set by regulatory agencies such as the ACSQHC. You may like to return to an earlier section of this chapter where we discussed the key characteristics of professions and the role of the Ahpra, another regulatory agency. If the Commission sets standards that must be met by hospitals, and Ahpra accredits the professions, do health professions continue to have autonomy of practice?

The Impact of SARS-CoV-2 on Health Care

There is no doubt that **SARS-CoV-2 (COVID-19)** has profoundly changed the health sector around the world, even in Australia where the pandemic's impact has not been as severe as in other countries such as the USA or those in Europe. It has shifted the focus of governments and health systems towards population level strategies for the containment and management of disease, while at the same time highlighting many of the issues included in this book, such as health inequalities, the effects of the social determinants of health (Shadmi et al. 2020) and the poor integration of services (Blecher et al. 2020). As Duckett wrote at the start of the pandemic, 'The coronavirus pandemic transformed Australia's health system as new ways of working were implemented with unbelievable speed. Faced with a national catastrophe at the start of March as infections grew exponentially, it was clear that "business as normal" wouldn't be enough: without dramatic action, hospitals would have been overwhelmed by mid-April' (Duckett 2020, p. 335).

Andrew et al. (2022) reiterated the sentiment of a 'dramatic impact' on the Australian health care system. Their study focused on the ambulance service in Victoria and identified '... deteriorating ambulance response times, extended case times and hospital delays' (p. 23). Delays and disruptions to cancer care were also notable (Edge et al. 2021), as were missed, delayed and avoided health care in everything from primary care consultations, breast screening, visits to emergency departments and public hospital surgeries (Follent et al. 2021; Sutherland et al. 2020).

The Australian Institute of Health and Welfare (AIHW) (2022b, p. 20) summed up the impact of COVID on the use of health services in Australia in the following way: 'COVID-19 changed the way Australians used health services. Some services were suspended, some services changed, extra demands were put on hospitals when COVID-19 admissions were higher, and some people were hesitant to seek health care for fear of contracting COVID-19.' Cormack (2022, p. 256) argued that while the Australian health care system 'demonstrated strong resilience, capacity, and responsiveness in its financing and payment functions' and in vaccine, therapeutics and workforce regulation it highlighted '... simultaneously chasmic shortcomings in the regulation of service delivery to the most vulnerable i.e. residential aged care and services for people with disability'.

The impact on health care staff was equally dramatic. Willis and Smallwood (2021, p. 169) describe the situation for health care workers in Melbourne as the second wave of the pandemic hit that city: '... the combination of increased stress and anxiety, changed work conditions and changes in social arrangements appear to have overwhelmed many frontline health professionals. Personal risk of catching the coronavirus was only one of their fears'. These findings are consistent with international reports of stress, anxiety and depressive symptoms in health care workers as a result of COVID (Shreffler et al. 2020) and other Australian studies of the health workforce (Holton et al. 2020).

The pandemic also brought to the fore a number of societal inequities and inequalities, particularly for those vulnerable populations who experience issues with accessing health care (Australian Bureau of Statistics (ABS) 2022), highlighting the inequity of health care service delivery. Internationally, the rationing of health care services highlighted both the existing assumptions and existing inequities in health care, as people with disability and the elderly were 'triaged' out of potentially life-saving interventions (Farrell et al. 2020). In the UK, for example, '60 per cent of those who died from COVID-19 in the first year of the pandemic were disabled' (The King's Fund 2022, n.p.). Case study 1.2 explores this in further detail.

Pause *for* Reflection …

According to Chen and McNamara (2020), in relation to the SARS-CoV-2 pandemic:

> The current public health crisis has exposed deep cracks in social equality and justice for marginalised and vulnerable communities around the world. The reported rise in the number of 'do not resuscitate' orders being imposed on people with disabilities has caused particular concerns from a human rights perspective.
>
> (Chen & McNamara 2020, p. 511)

What dilemma can you see now facing the health care system as a result of this shift?

CASE STUDY 1.2   The Australian Health Care System and the Impact of SARS-CoV-2

As noted previously in this chapter, the SARS-CoV-2 pandemic brought to the fore existing challenges in the delivery of health care. For example, in Australia prior to 2020, access to publicly funded dental, psychological and other allied health services such as physiotherapy was challenging. Long waiting lists and delays added to the burden of illness for those who could not afford to pay for health services. Restrictions enforced to reduce the spread of SARS-CoV-2 exacerbated delays to access to publicly funded services and further compounded health issues. For those people waiting for publicly funded health services, pre-existing inequities were exacerbated. As you read through the following case study, consider the impact of SARS-CoV-2 pandemic-related restrictions on the health of individuals, on health services staff and on the health care system.

Sally is a 48-year-old female living in Sydney. Prior to marrying John 23 years ago, Sally had a permanent job as a primary school teacher in one of the inner city public primary schools. Following the birth of her second child, Chris, 20 years ago, Sally took on the role of full-time mum, although she occasionally did some casual teaching shifts just to keep her skills up. Not long after both children moved into their own houses, the first SARS-CoV-2 pandemic lockdown in 2020 required John to work from home. John's behaviour towards Sally changed dramatically and when he hit her one evening, breaking her front tooth, Sally contacted Domestic and Family Violence services and ultimately moved out of the family home and away from John.

Sadly, Sally knew that more and more women were in her situation. During the first three months of the pandemic, two-thirds of women surveyed who reported domestic abuse indicated that it had either escalated or started during the SARS-CoV-2 pandemic and because of concerns about safety due to SARS-CoV-2 pandemic restrictions, more than one-third of these women felt unable to seek help (Boxall et al. 2020). Sally had heard that while the number of women experiencing domestic abuse had increased during SARS-CoV-2 pandemic restrictions, there was a significant reduction in the services provided (Carrington et al. 2021). This was partly because of a reduction in the availability of public meeting places, less space at women's refuges due to distancing requirements and a shift to online service delivery, which introduced new barriers for some clients (e.g. people with disabilities and other health issues, those from Indigenous and culturally and linguistically diverse communities). These changes also impacted frontline staff working in the Domestic and Family Violence sector who reported increased work pressures, isolation and feelings of insufficient capacity to meet demand (Carrington et al. 2021). Sally wondered about the ongoing impacts on women's health, the staff and the health care system. Were the situation not improved, the need for women impacted by ongoing domestic abuse to access the health care system would increase. Staff facing ongoing work-related stress would also be more likely to need to access health services.

Continued

CASE STUDY 1.2   The Australian Health Care System and the Impact of SARS-CoV-2—cont'd

Finding work was difficult for Sally. Permanent teaching positions are rare and having only worked intermittently since Chris was born, Sally found it hard to get regular casual work. In addition, the front tooth that John had broken when he hit her was now also discoloured. Sally knew that because of her teeth, people looked at her differently and it affected how she interacted with them. She was sure that this did not help the job situation. Without regular work, Sally could not secure a lease and could not afford Sydney rent and so lived in her car. With irregular work, Sally could not afford to pay for the dentist. Even if she could have borrowed money to pay for dental services (not possible without a consistent income), there were long waiting lists. Public health orders requiring cancellation of non-urgent dental care appointments had led to long waiting lists, postponed treatment and, once restrictions were lifted, increased workload for dental staff (Nahidi et al. 2022). However, the waiting lists for public dental treatment were much longer with around 100,000 people on the waiting list and a wait time of around 15 months.

Sally knew that poor dental health could lead to heart disease, cancers, diabetes, pneumonia and mental health issues. Knowing that in 2019–20, 'about 67,000 hospitalisations for dental conditions may have been prevented with earlier treatment' (AIHW 2022a, n.p.),

Sally pondered how much higher the number of preventable hospitalisations were currently and into the future given the even longer waiting lists since 2020 related to SARS-CoV-2 pandemic restrictions. In some locations across Australia, waiting lists can be up to five years. In NSW alone, in December 2021 there were over 140,000 (51,121 children and 94,051 adults) on the waiting list for treatment and over 40,000 (11,490 children and 32,322 adults) on the waiting list for assessment (NSW Health 2022).

Case Study Questions

1. What are some of the potential social, economic and health impacts of increased demand on services to support people experiencing domestic abuse because of SARS-CoV-2 pandemic restrictions?
2. What are some of the potential social, economic and health impacts of Sally needing to wait such a long time to see a dentist because of SARS-CoV-2 pandemic restrictions?
3. What is the 'catch-up effect' as a result of the lag in provision of dental care because of SARS-CoV-2 pandemic restrictions on the health care system as a whole?
4. How will the Australian health care system respond to a potential increase in dental-related hospitalisations?

How to Ask Questions About Health Care Reform

As you progress through your studies it will be useful to have a set of strategies for examining all health care reforms. There will certainly be many over the life of your career. Tuohy (1999) asks who has the balance of power at that particular time. Another approach is to examine the policy problem and to ask questions about how the problem is described. A political scientist who has done much work in this area is Carol Bacchi. She has developed a set of questions and bundled them together under the heading '*What's the problem represented to be?*' (Bacchi 2012, 2016). **What's the problem represented to be (WPR)** argues that, when governments (or private companies) decide on a particular policy action, what is proposed tells us what they think the problem is. WPR provides six questions you can use when reading each chapter for your program of study. These six questions are presented in Table 1.1, along with Tuohy's question as no. 7. We have taken the proposed $7 co-payment as

an example of how to use the questions to analyse a policy. We suggest you use this framework when you come to each chapter and consider the issues raised by the authors.

Interprofessional Practice or Navigator

Many attempts at health reform have been efforts to overcome fragmentation and duplication of health service delivery. Dealing with the fragmentation of how health professionals work has given rise to the concept of **interprofessional practice (IPP)**, which is the intended outcome from **interprofessional education (IPE)**. If you are studying health systems with students from a range of other professions, this is the first step in understanding their practice, in order that you might eventually work together. To summarise: 'interprofessional education is defined as an intervention where the members of more than one health or social care profession, or both, learn interactively together, for the explicit purpose of improving interprofessional collaboration

TABLE 1.1   Bacchi and Tuohy Policy Key Questions

1 What's the 'problem' represented to be in a specific policy proposal?	In the example of the $7 co-payment, it would appear the government saw the problem as a blow-out of the Medicare budget.
2 What presuppositions or assumptions underpin this representation of the 'problem'?	A co-payment would send a price signal to patients that each visit is costly. Behind this is the assumption that Australian citizens go to the doctor too often, and at times these visits are unnecessary. If we were aware of the costs we would go less often.
	There is an assumption that health expenditure must 'fit' within the current budget.
	An alternative policy direction could have been to increase the Medicare levy (taxing everyone, not just those who go to the doctor).
3 How has this representation of the 'problem' come about?	There is an assumption that citizens will abuse anything that is free, and be more careful when they have to pay for a service.
4 What is left unproblematic in this problem representation? Where are the silences? Can the problem be thought about differently?	The problem with this assumption is that we do not know whether or not people go to the doctor unnecessarily. There are no data to suggest this either way. But it is clear that this behaviour is what the policy set out to change.
5 What effects are produced by this representation of the 'problem'?	Well before the legislation was dropped by the Coalition Government many people stopped going to the doctor, and went to Accident and Emergency Departments instead. Private providers of pathology services claimed there was a drop in services even though the legislation had not been passed.
6 How/where has this represen-tation of the 'problem' been produced, disseminated and defended? How has it been (or could it be) questioned, disrupted and replaced? (Bacchi 2012).	Another way of defining the problem might be to suggest that paying doctors by the quantity of patients they treat, rather than the quality or effectiveness of their treatment, might be a fundamental flaw of Medicare.
	While it is true that health care costs have spiralled, it is also true that there has been little debate within the political arena about how much money we could spend, or want to spend, on health care, or where such escalation of costs comes from within the system. The co-payment focuses only on the user component rather than many aspects of demand in the system that could be considered as part of 'the problem'.
7 What do the three interest groups say about this problem, and what assumptions do they make?	The medical profession argued that it was inequitable and would mean poorer people would go without health care. They successfully lobbied for the policy to be dropped. Other consumer-led groups such as Save Our Medicare and GetUp had local campaigns and rallies, petition signing, phone calling and pamphlet campaigns to voice consumer concerns. Even within the government, politicians on the cross-bench argued against the co-payment.

Source: Bacchi C (2012) Introducing the 'What's the problem represented to be?' approach. In: Bletsas A, Beasely C (Eds.) Engaging with Carol Bacchi: Strategic Interventions and Exchanges, University of Adelaide Press, Adelaide, pp. 21–24, https://www.adelaide.edu.au/carst/docs/wpr/wpr-summary.pdf.

or the health/well-being of patients/clients, or both' (Reeves et al. 2013, p. 2).

The champions of IPP suggest it is required because it promotes efficiencies through teamwork and collaboration. IPP is seen as a strategy to help ameliorate the worldwide shortage of health professionals, estimated to be around 4.3 million (**World Health Organization**

(WHO) 2010). Given the high costs associated with health care, including the cost of educating professionals, there is an argument for stronger team and collaborative approaches to patient care. This argument extends across the health spectrum from community and public health to **acute care** and from the developed world with its highly technological health systems to countries with low levels of health infrastructure. A genuine team approach provides opportunities for quality time spent in patient assessment and referrals, and may even reduce the number of tests ordered. IPE that leads to IPP is also seen to reduce adverse events and to have higher patient satisfaction (WHO 2010).

If, as professionals, our work is based on the best scientific evidence it is important to test the evidence of those who champion IPP given its claims that it can improve the way professionals work. This can be done through examining **evidence-based medicine (EBM)**, particularly what is provided through the Cochrane database for **systematic literature review (SLR).** A Cochrane SLR published in 2013 by Reeves et al., which updated their previous study (Laurant et al. 2005), examined IPP research published between 2006 and 2011. All these studies asked whether IPP had a positive impact on patient outcomes.

Reeves et al. (2013, p. 16) note that in 1999 when they did their first review they could find no eligible studies. However, they agree IPP is a growing area of health care reform that focuses on the very way health professionals work. This puts you and your profession smack in the middle of exciting and dynamic reform processes that promise to improve treatment for patients, to make work more interesting for clinicians and to provide a service that saves money. However, they write that what is still required are 'studies that assess the effectiveness of IPP interventions compared to separate, profession-specific interventions; second, RCT, CBA or ITS studies with qualitative strands examining processes relating to the IPP and practice changes; third, cost-benefit analyses' (p. 2). In support of this they did a further review in 2017 (Reeves et al. 2017), where once again they were

cautiously in support of IPP, grading the evidence as low. This is a strange outcome, given the difficulties health professionals (and patients) experience in communicating and that many adverse events are thought to originate in poor communication.

Another approach being taken in some Australian states, given the poor communication between health professionals, is the appointment of nurse navigators, midwife navigators or patient navigators (Queensland Government 2015). These health professionals take a patient focus, rather than a professional focus, and navigate the system for the person with a chronic illness, or a woman who is vulnerable following the birth of a child (Dick 2017).

WHAT ELSE HAVE WE PROVIDED?

To assist you in thinking about these questions, this book provides a number of resources. These include cross-references to other chapters that refer to similar topics, **Further Reading** lists useful for following up the issues, a **Glossary** of concepts and acronyms, and a list of **Abbreviations**. Remembering these terms is one strategy for coming to grips with all the complex systems. All chapters provide a list of **Review Questions** and **Online Resources.** If you are doing a tutorial these questions and the additional readings will be a useful guide. The chapters also provide you with **Case Studies** that illustrate some of the issues pertinent to the topic. These are mainly patient or consumer focused. The **Pause for Reflection** boxes provide you with the opportunity to reflect on the material. Throughout the book, the term 'patient' is generally used to refer to someone in an acute setting, and 'client' as someone in a community setting.

▌ S U M M A R Y

In this introductory chapter we have provided background on the following:
- The book is organised into two sections, with the first section covering a number of Australian health care systems and the second section dealing with 12 health professional groups.
- Key theoretical ideas proposed by Tuohy (1999) suggest that serious health reform occurs only at particular moments in history when all the necessary factors are in place for the group/s with the balance of power. These groups are the State, the market and the professions.
- We also suggested that you apply the questions raised by Bacchi (2012) to any health policy reform you encounter.

- The reform process of new public management was also discussed. We suggested it is still in use.
- Among new directions for clinical reform are interprofessional education and interprofessional practice. While these are being enthusiastically supported, to date there is insufficient evidence to suggest that they will revolutionise health care. An alternative approach is to use navigators.
- Consideration is given to the SARS-CoV-2 pandemic that impacted the way health care services have been delivered. These changes have impacted patient care with delays, and stress and burnout to health professionals.

REVIEW QUESTIONS

1. What three groups have the balance of power in any health care system?
2. If a country has a national health service, what group would you presume has the balance of power?
3. Besides the balance of power, Tuohy (1999) suggests reform is shaped by a particular institutional mix. Can you identify particular political, historical or cultural factors that might influence the kinds of reforms introduced in Australia in the next few years?
4. Given that the federal government has established a number of regulatory agencies to oversee health care such as the Independent Hospital Pricing Authority (which sets the price paid for care) and the Australian Commission for Safety and Quality in Health Care, how much autonomy do health professionals have when they work within a hospital or GP clinic?
5. In our view, nurses, midwives and allied health professionals have more to gain from IPP than doctors. Do you agree with this statement and, if so, why?
6. The SARS-CoV-2 pandemic required a rapid shift in delivery of various health care services as well as patient care practices. How well do you think Australia's health care system adapted to these changes?

REFERENCES

Andrew, E., Nehme, Z., Stephenson, M., et al., 2022. The impact of the COVID-19 pandemic on demand for emergency ambulances in Victoria, Australia. Prehosp Emerg Care 26 (1), 23–29.

Australian Bureau of Statistics (ABS), 2022. COVID-19 Mortality in Australia, deaths registered to 31 January 2022. ABS, Canberra. https://www.abs.gov.au/articles/covid-19-mortality-australia-deaths-registered-31-january-2022#death-due-to-covid-19-country-of-birth.

Australian Commission for Safety and Quality in Health Care (ACSQHC), 2017. Australian safety and quality framework for health care: putting the framework into action. ACSQHC, Sydney. https://www.safetyandquality.gov.au/wp-content/uploads/2011/01/ASQFHC-Guide-Healthcare-team.pdf.

Australian Commission for Safety and Quality in Health Care (ACSQHC), 2018. Antimicrobial stewardship in Australian health care 2018. ACSQHC, Sydney.

Australian Government, 2018. Medicare indexation schedule. https://www.humanservices.gov.au/individuals/services/medicare/medicare-safety-net.

Australian Health Practitioner Regulation Agency (Ahpra), 2018. Home page. https://www.ahpra.gov.au/.

Australian Institute of Health and Welfare (AIHW), 2022a. Oral health and dental care in Australia. AIHW, Canberra. https://www.aihw.gov.au/reports/dental-oral-health/oral-health-and-dental-care-in-australia/contents/about.

Australian Institute of Health and Welfare (AIHW), 2022b. Australia's health 2022: in brief. Canberra: A AIHW, Canberra.

Bacchi, C., 2012. Introducing the 'What's the problem represented to be?' approach. In: Bletsas, A., Beasley, C. (Eds.), Engaging With Carol Bacchi: Strategic Interventions and Exchanges. University of Adelaide Press, Adelaide, pp. 21–24. https://www.adelaide.edu.au/carst/docs/wpr/wpr-summary.pdf.

Bacchi, C., 2016. Problematizations in health policy: questioning how "problems" are constituted in policies. Paper presented at the ASSA (Academy of the Social Sciences)-funded Workshop on Understanding Australian Policies on Public Health, Flinders University.

Blecher, G., Blashki, G. A., Judkins, S., 2020. Crisis as opportunity: How COVID-19 will reshape the Australian health system. Med J Aust 213 (5), 196–198.e1. doi:10.5694/mja2.50730.

Boxall, H., Morgan, A., Brown, R., 2020. The prevalence of domestic violence among women during the COVID-19 pandemic. Australasian Policing 12 (3), 38–46.

Braithwaite, J., Hindle, D., 1998. Casemix funding in Australia. Med J Aust 168 (11), 558–560.

Carrington, K., Morley, C., Warren, S., et al., 2021. The impact of COVID-19 pandemic on Australian domestic and family violence services and their clients. Aust J Soc Issues 56 (4), 539–558.

Caruso, E., Cisar, N., Pipe, T., 2008. Creating a healing environment: an innovative educational approach for adopting Jean Watson's theory of human caring. Nurs Adm Q 32 (2), 126–132.

Chen, B., & McNamara, D. M., 2020. Disability discrimination, medical rationing and COVID-19. Asian Bioeth Rev 12 (4), 511–518.

Cormack, M., 2022. Federated health system governance in the post-COVID-19 era. Aust Health Rev 46 (3), 256–257.

Crouch, C., 2011. The Strange Non-Death of Neo-Liberalism. Polity Press, Cambridge.

Department of Health (DOH), 2018. Health Care Homes' updates and factsheets. http://www.health.gov.au/internet/main/publishing.nsf/Content/health-care-homes-information.

Dick, C., 2017. Vulnerable women to receive specialised midwifery care. http://statements.qld.gov.au/Statement/2017/8/2/vulnerable-women-to-receive-specialised-midwifery-care.

Docteur, E., Oxley, H., 2003. Health-care systems: lessons from the reform experience. OECD, Paris. www.oecd.org/dataoecd/5/53/22364122.pdf.

Duckett, S., 2020. Governance lessons from COVID-19. Aust Health Rev 44 (3), 335–335.

Edge, R., Meyers, J., Tiernan, G., et al., 2021. Cancer care disruption and reorganisation during the COVID-19 pandemic in Australia: A patient, carer and healthcare worker perspective. PLOS ONE 16 (9), e0257420.

Farrell, T. W., Francis, L., Brown, T., et al., 2020. Rationing limited healthcare resources in the COVID-19 era and beyond: ethical considerations regarding older adults. J Am Geriatr Soc 68 (6), 1143–1149.

Follent, D., Paulson, C., Orcher, P., et al., 2021. The indirect impacts of COVID-19 on Aboriginal communities across New South Wales. Med J Aust 214 (5), 199.

Freidson, E., 1970a. Professional Dominance. Atherton Press, New York.

Freidson, E., 1970b. Profession of Medicine: A Study of the Sociology of Applied Knowledge. University of Chicago Press, Chicago.

Health Practitioner Regulation National Law (NSW) No 86a of 2009. https://legislation.nsw.gov.au/view/html/inforce/current/act-2009-86a#pt.1.

Holton, S., Wynter, K., Trueman, M., et al., 2020. Psychological well-being of Australian hospital clinical staff during the COVID-19 pandemic. Aust Health Rev 45 (3), 297–305.

Independent Hospital Pricing Authority (IHPA), 2017a. Pricing framework for Australian public hospital services 2017–2018. IHPA, Sydney. https://www.ihpa.gov.au/consultation/pricing-framework-australian-public-hospital-services-2017-18.

Independent Hospital Pricing Authority (IHPA), 2017b. Risk adjustment model for hospital acquired complications: technical specifications – version 1.0. IHPA, Sydney. https://www.ihpa.gov.au/sites/g/files/net636/f/risk_adjustment_model_for_hospital_acquired_complications_-_technical_specifications_v1.0_july_2017_pdf.pdf.

Kenny, A., 2004. Medical dominance and power: a rural perspective. Health Sociol Rev 13, 158–165.

Laurant, M., Reeves, D., Hermanns, R., et al., 2005. Substitution of doctors by nurses in primary care. Cochrane Database Syst Rev (2), CD001271.

Mazurek Melnyk, B., Fineout-Overholt, E., Giggleman, M., 2017. A test of the ARCC C model improves implementation of evidence-based practice, healthcare culture, and patient outcomes. Worldviews Evid Based Nurs, 14 (1), 5–9.

National Health Ministers' Benchmarketing Commonwealth of Australia, 1996. First National Report on the health sector performance indicators: public hositals-state of play. https://www.aihw.gov.au/getmedia/a6bff00a-d7d8-45d6-8dd0-42ace859d4b8/fnrhspi-c00.pdf.aspx.

NSW Health, 2022. NSW public dental waiting lists: by financial quarter. https://www.health.nsw.gov.au/oral-health/Pages/waiting.aspx.

Queensland Government, 2015. Nurse navigators. https://www.health.qld.gov.au/ocnmo/nursing/nurse-navigators.

Reeves, S., Peline, F., Harrison, R., et al., 2017. Interprofessional collaboration to improve professional practice and healthcare outcomes (reveiw). Cochrane Database Syst Rev (6), CD000072.

Reeves, S., Perrier, L., Goldman, J., et al., 2013. Interprofessional education: effects on professional practice and healthcare outcomes (update). Cochrane Database Syst Rev (3), CD002213.

Shadmi, E., Chen, Y., Dourado, I., et al., 2020. Health equity and COVID-19: global perspectives. Int J Equity Health 19 (1), 1–16.

Shreffler, J., Petrey, J., Huecker, M., 2020. The impact of COVID-19 on healthcare worker wellness: a scoping review. West J Emerg Med 21 (5), 1059.

Stanton, P., Willis, E., White, S., 2005. Workplace Reform in the Healthcare Sector: The Australian Experience. Palgrave Macmillan, London.

Stanton, P., Young, S., Willis, E. M., 2003. Financial restraint, budget cuts and outsourcing: impact of the new public management of health care in Victoria. Contemp Nurse 14 (2), 115–122.

Sutherland, K., Chessman, J., Zhao, J., et al., 2020. Impact of COVID-19 on healthcare activity in NSW, Australia. Public Health Res Pract 30 (4). doi:10.17061/phrp 3042030.

The King's Fund, 2022. Towards a new partnership between disabled people and health and care services: getting our voices heard. https://www.kingsfund.org.uk/publications/partnership-disabled-people-health-care-services.

Tuohy, C., 1999. Accidental Logics: The Dynamics of Change in the Health Care Arena in the United States, Britain and Canada. OUP, New York.

van Gool, K., Pearson, M., 2014. Health, austerity and economic crisis: assessing the short-term impact in OECD countries. OECD working paper 76. OECD, Paris. https://www.oecd-ilibrary.org/docserver/5jxx71lt1zg6-en.pdf?expires=1556038444&id=id&accname=guest&checksum=B51ED36DA7B4FAC4D7F6B2395926F786.

Willis, E., 1983. Medical Dominance: the division of labour in Australian health care. Allan and Unwin, Sydney.

Willis, K., & Smallwood, N., 2021. Risky Work: Providing healthcare in the age of COVID-19. In: Lupton, D.,

Willis, K. (Eds.), The COVID-19 Crisis -Social Perspectives. Routledge, London, pp. 168–180.

World Bank, 2014. Public-private partnerships: reference guide version 2.0. http://documents.worldbank.org/curated/en/2014/01/20182310/public-private-partnerships-reference-guide-version-20.

World Health Organization (WHO), 2010. Framework for action on interprofessional education and collaborative practice (WHO/HRH/HPN/10.3). https://apps.who.int/iris/bitstream/handle/10665/70185/WHO_HRH_HPN_10.3_eng.pdf;jsessionid=A6E1F14B1A6E48045764A7505BBF87F9?sequence=1.

World Health Organization (WHO), 2018. Universal health coverage and health financing. http://www.who.int/health_financing/universal_coverage_definition/en/.

FURTHER READING

Alford, R., 1975. Health Care Politics: Ideological and Interest Group Barriers to Reform. University of Chicago Press, Chicago.

Mody, L., Meddings, J., Edson, B., et al., 2015. Enhancing resident safety by preventing healthcare-associated infection: a national initiative to reduce catheter-associated urinary tract infections in nursing homes. Clin. Infect. Dis. 1 (61), 86–94.

Tuohy, C., 1999. Accidental Logics: The Dynamics of Change in the Health Care Arena in the United States, Britain and Canada. OUP, New York.

Willis, E., 1989. Medical Dominance. Allen and Unwin, Sydney.

ONLINE RESOURCES

Keep up with all the major reforms in Australian Health at: https://www.health.gov.au/.

Keep up with the latest digital health innovations at: https://www.pulseit.news/.

Learn what is happening in your professions at: https://www.ahpra.gov.au/.

2

The Public Health Sector and Medicare

Kees van Gool and Jane Hall

KEY LEARNING OUTCOMES

When you finish this chapter you should be able to:
- understand how the public health care sector in Australia is organised, funded and delivered
- describe the purpose and function of Medicare and its role in the Australian health care system
- evaluate health systems against the objective of universal health coverage

- assess the function and objectives of Medicare against the aims of universal health coverage
- identify the role of funding policy in driving health care delivery and access
- recognise the role of public hospitals within the Australian health care system, and how they are funded.

KEY TERMS AND ABBREVIATIONS

activity-based funding (ABF)
blame game
bulk-billing
casemix
compulsory health insurance
concession card
cost-shifting
Department of Veterans' Affairs (DVA)
Extended Medicare Safety Net (EMSN)
Family Tax Benefit Part A (FTB(A))
financial protection
gross domestic product (GDP)

health care financing
Independent Health and Aged Care Pricing Authority (IHACPA)
Local Hospital Network (LHN)
inpatient
market pressure
MBS fee
MBS benefit
Medicare
Medicare Benefits Schedule (MBS)
Medicare levy
Medicare rebate
National Disability Insurance Scheme (NDIS)

National Health Reform Agreement (NHRA)
Organisation for Economic Co-operation and Development (OECD)
out-of-hospital service
out-of-pocket (OOP) cost
Pharmaceutical Benefits Scheme (PBS)
provider fee
public health insurance
universal health coverage (UHC)
World Health Organization (WHO)

INTRODUCTION TO AUSTRALIA'S MEDICARE PROGRAM

This chapter examines two major components of **Medicare**, Australia's publicly funded health care system: medical services funded through the **Medicare Benefits Schedule (MBS)** program and public hospital services funded by federal, state and territory governments through the **National Health Reform Agreement (NHRA)**. A third major component of Medicare is the Pharmaceutical Benefit Scheme (PBS), which is discussed in Chapter 7.

Before turning to these aspects of **health care financing**, this chapter outlines the reasons why many countries have developed and implemented publicly funded programs that provide **financial protection** against the costs of health care for those who are ill. Without such publicly funded programs, health care would essentially be paid through private financing channels such as private health insurance or **out-of-pocket (OOP)** costs that are paid directly by patients. The chapter then presents recent trends in Australia's health care expenditure as well as examining who pays for Australia's health care.

There are numerous other government programs and policies that directly impact the health and wellbeing of Australians but these are usually not regarded as being part of Medicare. Examples of such programs are: cancer screening, health promotion and public health measures, the **National Disability Insurance Scheme (NDIS)**, the Indigenous Australians' Health Programme, the private health insurance rebate, the Commonwealth Home Care Package and residential aged-care support. While these programs are not the direct focus of this chapter, it is acknowledged that these programs interact with patients' access to health care.

WHY MEDICARE?

Medicare, in its current form, was introduced in 1984 but its foundations can be traced back to the late 1960s when two academics, John Deeble and Richard Scotton, wrote a paper entitled '**Compulsory health insurance for Australia**' that helped to convince the then opposition leader Gough Whitlam to adopt a policy to introduce universal health care (Scotton & Deeble 1968; Whitlam 1997). Medicare (or Medibank as it was originally known) was introduced in 1974, dismantled between 1976 and 1983, and then re-introduced in 1984 by the Hawke Government.

Scotton and Deeble describe their proposed scheme as evolutionary rather revolutionary. The scheme was intentionally designed to introduce universal coverage within the context of the existing health care system and Australia's constitution. In doing so, it was hoped that the proposal would least disturb existing arrangements, yet still achieve universal coverage. This meant that the proposal placed a strong emphasis on publicly financed health care and privately provided medical practice paid for on a fee-for-service basis. Medicare also maintained the clinical autonomy to medical providers within the confines of a tax-financed health care program (Scotton & Deeble 1968). Furthermore, it has supplemented, rather than replaced, Australia's existing private health insurance arrangements for hospital treatments (private health insurance is covered further in Chapter 3).

Medicare is based on the principles of **universal health coverage (UHC)**. UHC seeks to ensure that all individuals and communities have access to health care. Achieving UHC is one of the United Nations' (UN) Sustainable Development Goals and this commitment was reaffirmed at the UN's General Assembly High Level Meeting on UHC in 2019.

The goal of UHC is to protect people from the financial consequences of paying for health services out of their own pockets. This will prevent patients and their families from potential financial hardship and poverty due to unexpected illness. Without proper coverage, people who suffer illness are at risk of poverty. This risk arises because the high cost of health care may require patients and their family to use up their life savings, sell assets or borrow at a time when, due to illness, their ability to earn income may be severely limited.

UHC is also essential in providing patients with financial access to care. UHC raises the purchasing power of those who are sick and in need of care. People who do not have coverage will be severely limited by their income and wealth in terms of the amount and type of care they can afford. Without coverage many people simply cannot afford the care they need and go without. It is perhaps not surprising that in health systems without widespread insurance coverage, health care is disproportionally allocated to those who can afford care (i.e. typically wealthier and more powerful sections of the community). This is even true in wealthy countries like Australia; particularly in health care sectors where there are high OOP costs or there is a lack of private or **public health insurance**. Hence, UHC is an essential element towards achieving equity of access to health care.

The **World Health Organization (WHO)** describes the goal of UHC along three dimensions:

- **The extent to which the overall population of a country is covered by insurance**. This dimension focuses on whether there are groups of people in a population who are not covered by health care. On this dimension, Medicare is quite comprehensive because it covers most citizens and permanent residents. Humanitarian visa class holders are also covered by Medicare but many other types of visa class holders are not.
- **The extent to which different health services and products are covered by insurance.** Medicare covers a wide range of services and health care products but does not cover everything. Most over-the-counter medicines, for example, are not covered. In order for new medical services and pharmaceutical products to be covered, they must go through rigorous evaluations to assess their safety, effectiveness and cost-effectiveness before the government decides whether they will be covered (see Chapter 7 on the PBS for the process for listing new items).
- **The extent of private financing required to pay for health care services and products.** In some instances, Medicare covers the full costs of health care (e.g. public hospital episodes), in other instances it partially covers the costs (e.g. PBS-listed medications) and in other instances it depends on the fees and charges of the health care provider (e.g. a doctor may choose to bulk-bill their patient in which case the government covers the entire cost of the services; in other instances they incur an OOP cost if the doctor decides not to bulk-bill). So in terms of this dimension, the extent of UHC in Australia very much depends on the health care sector in question.

FINANCING AUSTRALIA'S HEALTH SYSTEM

The Australian health system comprises a mix of public and private financing sources. In total, it amounts to $203 billion per year, or around 10.2% of Australia's **gross domestic product (GDP)** – a measure of the value of Australia's entire economy (AIHW 2021). Fig. 2.1 shows per capita health expenditure between 2009–10 and 2019–20. In the most recent year available, Australians spent $7926 per person on health. Over the last ten years, this amount has grown by over 30%. This comprises money spent on health care by all levels of government, private health insurance funds and individuals.

Who Pays?

Ultimately, all health care is paid for by individuals in the economy. What varies are the channels by which individuals' financial contributions reach the providers of health care. Broadly, there are three main channels:

- Direct payments from individual patient to providers through co-payments or OOP costs.

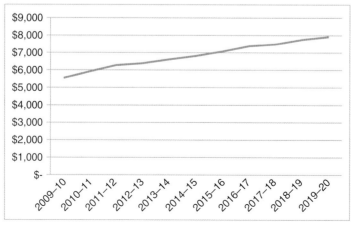

Figure 2.1 Per capita health care spending, current dollars, 2009–10 to 2019–20. *Source*: The data in this figure are taken from AIHW (2021) report.

- Taxes paid to government which then uses tax revenue to pay health care providers.
- Premiums paid to private health insurance funds who then use those funds to pay providers.

Further to these main channels, there are small amounts that are funded through charities and insurance companies besides health insurance (e.g. workers' compensation, third-party motor vehicle).

In Australia (Fig. 2.2), around 72% of total health care expenditure is funded through government (and therefore paid for by taxes). Out of this, the federal government (also referred to as the Commonwealth Government) finances around two-thirds and the state, territory and local governments contribute the other one-third. These proportions have been reasonably steady over time. Around 9% is funded through private health insurance funds and 16% by individuals through direct OOP costs.

The taxes that pay for Medicare are financed through general taxation measures and are not hypothecated to health care spending. This means that the federal government does not have a dedicated source of taxation revenue that is devoted to health care. Health care spending therefore has to compete with other government spending priorities. Even the **Medicare levy**, which is a 2% additional tax on income paid by most Australian wage earners, contributes to general revenue and does not need to be spent on health care.

The source of funding varies considerably depending on the type of health care sector. As noted in Chapter 15, for example, a substantial proportion of the population is not insured for, and do not have ready access to,

dental care. Fig. 2.2 shows that, as a result of this, the majority of dental health expenditure (58%) is sourced directly from patients (individuals) through OOP costs. This compares to only 2% for public hospitals and 16% overall. Further, 20% of dental services are funded through private health insurance (compared to 8% for all other health care expenditure).

It is perhaps not surprising that many studies find that wealthier sections of the population are greater users of dental services in Australia compared to those with lower wealth. This is despite the fact that lower socio-economic groups typically have greater oral health care needs than their higher socio-economic counterparts (Do et al. 2010; Ju et al. 2021; Ju et al. 2022; Meija et al. 2018; Singh et al. 2018).

Pause *for* Reflection ...

According to Williams and Maynard (1984), health care systems reflect prevailing ideologies. At one extreme, libertarian views posit that health care should be accessible to those willing and able to pay; and that user payments should be the main approach to funding. This implies that health care will only be purchased by those willing and able to pay for it. At the other end, egalitarian approaches support a system where health service use is not limited by income and wealth; and health care is financed through taxes. Would you describe the financing of public hospitals in Australia as egalitarian or libertarian? Would you apply the same description to dental care? What could explain the very different approaches to financing public hospitals and dental care within the same health care system?

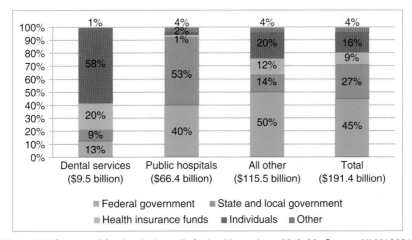

Figure 2.2 Sources of funding in Australia for health services, 2019–20. *Source*: AIHW 2021.

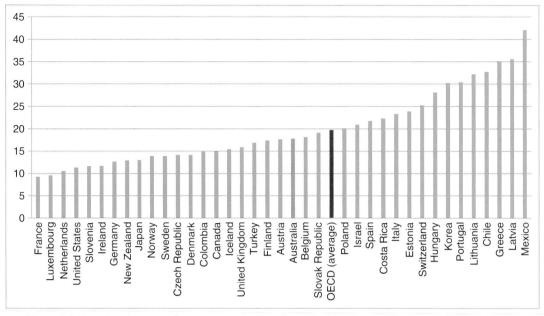

Figure 2.3 Out-of-pocket expenditure as a percentage of total health care spending across OECD countries, 2019 or most recent year. *Source*: OECD Health Statistics 2021.

In terms of the share of health expenditure paid through OOP costs, Australia is close to the OECD average. Fig. 2.3 shows the extent to which patients are responsible for paying for health care in terms of the percentage of total health care expenditure in a country that is paid through out-of-pocket costs (rather than, say, public or private insurance). Across all OECD countries, patients contribute, on average, 20% of total health expenditure through OOP costs. In Australia, the corresponding figure is 18%.[1] In countries where this percentage is substantially higher, UHC is still very much under development.

How Does the Medicare Benefits Schedule Work?

All citizens, permanent residents and those with some other classes of visas are eligible for benefits under Medicare. Each adult in a household is issued with a Medicare card (usually listing all members of the household) which proves eligibility for the program. Virtually all Australians are enrolled in the program, although there are some notable exceptions like people who are incarcerated.

As part of the MBS, Australians receive a fixed rate benefit (more commonly referred to as a Medicare benefit) for each eligible medical service they use. Under the Medicare program, the public benefit (often referred to as the 'Medicare benefit') for each item is directly related to the **MBS fee**. The Medicare benefit for **out-of-hospital services** is usually 85% of the MBS fee, with two exceptions:

- Since January 2005, patients have received a Medicare benefit worth 100% of the MBS fee for all GP and other non-referred attendance items for out-of-hospital services.
- There is a maximum gap between the Medicare benefit and the MBS fee of $87.90 (as at November 2021). This essentially implies that for items with an MBS fee of over $586.20 the Medicare benefit is equal to the MBS fee minus $87.90 (rather than Medicare benefit = 0.85 × MBS fee).

---

[1]Note that the OECD and AIHW have slightly different methods and definitions that explain why the percentage of health care expenditure in Figs 2.2 and 2.3 is different.

Medicare services are generally provided by independent private practitioners and are delivered to patients in the out-of-hospital setting or to private **inpatients**. Providers are paid on a fee-for-service basis.

For a medical service to be eligible for Medicare benefits, it has to be listed on the MBS. The Schedule lists over 5700 different medical services and for each of these there is an MBS item number which describes the service and also sets out the eligibility rules for both providers and patients (see www.mbsonline.gov.au for details). Importantly, each item number has an MBS fee associated with it. This government-determined MBS fee is the basis for calculating the Medicare benefit that patients are entitled to. For services that are provided out of hospital, Medicare is the only form of insurance available. In other words, private health insurance cannot cover out-of-hospital services where an MBS claim has been made. Note that this is not true for private inpatient services where both the MBS and private health insurance contribute to the cost of medical services (see Chapter 3).

For out-of-hospital services patients pay (from their own pockets) the component of the provider charge that is above the Medicare benefit. Importantly, providers are not restricted by the MBS fee. Providers can determine the charge they set for patients to pay.

When a doctor's charge is equivalent to the Medicare benefit, the provider accepts this benefit as full payment for the service, and there is no OOP cost for the patient. This is often referred to as a 'bulk-billed' service. The percentage of services that are bulk-billed varies considerably by service type (Fig. 2.4). For example, in 2020–21, nearly 90% of all general practice attendances and almost all pathology services were bulk-billed. However, in that same year only 46% of specialists' consultations were bulk-billed. Unlike for GPs, there is no MBS incentive for specialists to bulk-bill their **concession card** patients however many specialists reduce their fees for lower income groups (Johar et al. 2017). Until recently, the **bulk-billing** trend for most services has been upwards, however the bulk-billing rate for allied health services has been trending downwards and the most recent data are showing a drop in bulk-billing rates among some medical providers like GPs and radiation oncologists.

Overall expenditure on out-of-hospital MBS claims has grown over time. Fig. 2.5 shows that Australians spend around $28 billion dollars on these services alone. Of that amount, the federal government contributes around $24 billion (or 87%) through **MBS benefits**; leaving around $3.7 billion for patient OOP costs. The patient OOP costs amount is represented by the gap between the fees charged and MBS benefits paid by the federal government in Fig. 2.5. In the years between 2009 and 2021, overall MBS expenditure has increased by 82%, federal government expenditure by 80% and patient OOP costs have increased by 92%.

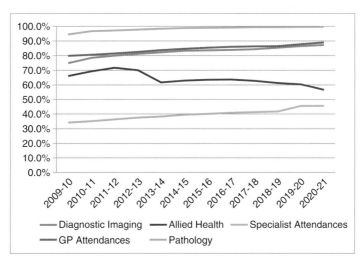

Figure 2.4 Bulk-billing rate as a percentage of service claims, by broad type of service, 2009–10 to 2021–22. Data from Medicare annual statistics – State and territory (2009–10 to 2021–22), Australian Government, Department of Health and Aged Care.

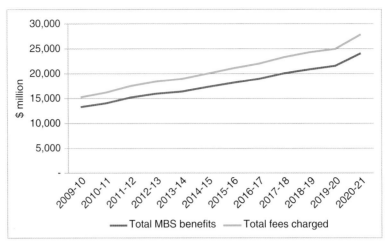

Figure 2.5 Total MBS expenditure for out-of-hospital, current dollars, 2009–10 to 2020–21. Data from Medicare annual statistics – State and territory (2009–10 to 2021–22), Australian Government, Department of Health and Aged Care.

Pause *for* Reflection ...
Consider Figs 2.4 and 2.5. If OOP costs are rising, should that be a concern? Does your answer reflect a libertarian or egalitarian view? Would your answer be different if you took the other perspective?

The MBS funding arrangements give considerable flexibility to providers on what they charge and to whom they charge. As a result, while Medicare services are subsidised through tax-financed funding, OOP costs will vary depending on how much the fee charged by the doctor is above the benefit amount. In the case of general practitioners, for example, the fee charged in 89% of consultations is equivalent to the Medicare benefit, leaving patients who use those services with zero OOP costs.

These various financing rules mean that the decisions taken by both patients and providers will impact on who ends up paying the bill for many types of health care services and products. How patients navigate (or are navigated through) the health care system can potentially alter the contribution of each of the main financing channels. It is, for example, possible for patients to protect themselves from OOP costs depending not only on whether they use the system but also on how they use the system.

Within the MBS rules, patients are allowed to choose their doctor, particularly GPs, and can switch at any time. In most places, it is feasible for them to seek out GPs with low charges and therefore low (or zero) OOP costs. In practice, the ability of patients to switch varies by location. Some metropolitan, rural and remote areas have a low proportion of GPs who bulk-bill, making it more difficult for patients to reduce their OOP costs. For specialist providers, patients also have choice but are typically more reliant on the advice and referral given to them by their GP. Furthermore, choice of specialists is more limited – especially in rural and remote areas of Australia – where there are far fewer medical practitioners. The lack of access to some types of providers in some locations is associated with higher fees and higher OOP costs for patients.

As noted, the MBS lists over 5700 different medical services and covers a wide range of consultations, pathology and diagnostic imaging services and procedures. The list is dynamic with the possibility of adding new items and also removing old and obsolete items. For example, the MBS Taskforce and its various subcommittees reviewed the MBS between 2015 and 2020 identifying items that could be amended, updated or removed. The review made recommendations to the Australian Government to remove services that were obsolete, outdated or potentially unsafe.

In addition, it is possible to add new items on the MBS to reflect changes in medical practice and new technology. The Medical Services Advisory Committee makes recommendations to the Australian Government about updating the MBS. In doing so, it reviews the evidence on the safety, effectiveness, cost-effectiveness and affordability of any proposed new service.

At the beginning of the COVID-19 pandemic, the Australian Government was able to utilise the dynamic aspect of the MBS by adding a wide range of telehealth services for general practice and specialist consultations as well as a range of other COVID-related items. This enabled MBS reimbursement for GP and specialist consultations conducted over the phone or video-link. Prior to the listing of these items, reimbursement was mostly restricted to face-to-face consultations between the patient and the GP. Telehealth proved to be an important tool for patient access to health care and at the same time enabled them to maintain social distancing during a pandemic.

Additional Financial Protection from OOP Costs

The federal government has put in place additional measures to protect vulnerable groups in society from high OOP costs. One of the primary policy instruments used to provide additional protection to vulnerable groups is the Australian Government's concession card program. Around 1 in 4 Australians qualify for a concession card, which brings additional MBS and PBS entitlements to reduce the financial burden of health care on patients. The Australian Government spends around $10 billion per year on these entitlements.

Table 2.1 provides details on the range of concession cards available and their eligibility criteria and the additional protection that each card provides. Eligibility for a pensioner, health care or seniors' health care card is primarily linked to whether an individual or household is a recipient of qualifying government benefits such as the age pension or a specified government allowance, or has sufficiently low income.

In addition to the concession cards listed in Table 2.1, veterans of Australia's defence forces who have qualifying service may be eligible for a **Department of Veterans' Affairs (DVA)** card. DVA cardholders are also entitled to a wider range of subsidies depending on the type of card they qualify for.

TABLE 2.1   Concession Card Types and Eligibility Criteria

Concession Card Type	Main Eligibility Criteria	No. of Recipients	% of CC Recipients
Pensioner Concession Card	Individuals qualify if they receive the full or partial aged pension. That is, they (i) have reached the qualifying age; (ii) satisfy residency requirements; and (iii) satisfy income and assets tests (e.g. a couple can earn up to $82k per annum and have up to $876k in assets excluding the principal home).	4,372,544	61%
Commonwealth Seniors Health Card	Individuals who have reached the pension age but do not qualify for an aged pension. There is no asset test for this card, but there is an income test (e.g. a couple can earn up $89k per year).	405,586	6%
Health Care Card	This card is issued to recipients of certain social security benefits or allowance payments including, but not limited to, youth allowance, job seeking allowance and widow allowance.	2,228,572	31%
Low Income Health Care Card	This card can be claimed by low-income earners (e.g. a couple can earn up to $51k to qualify). There is no asset test.	195,248	3%
	Total	7,201,950	100%

Data from A guide to Australian Government payments, Australian Government. https://www.servicesaustralia.gov.au/sites/default/files/co029-2101.pdf and DSS Benefit and Payment Recipient Demographics – quarterly data https://data.gov.au/dataset/ds-dga-cff2ae8a-55e4-47db-a66d-e177fe0ac6a0/details.

Concession cardholders are entitled to a range of additional subsidies and reduced prices for health care services and products. Table 2.2 shows the additional entitlements that concession cardholders qualify for.

Importantly, the holders of concession cards are not automatically entitled to reduced doctor charges. The decision to charge reduced fees to cardholders remains with the doctor. However, it is clear that in many cases, providers choose to lower their charges for concession cardholders (Johar et al. 2014; Johar et al. 2017; Jones et al. 2008).

A number of the entitlements listed in Table 2.2 were part of the *Strengthening Medicare* package introduced and implemented between 2004 and 2005. The package provides a higher payment to GPs for every bulk-billed consultation provided to children under the age of 16 or to concession cardholders. This incentive is higher in selected locations of Australia (typically rural and remote regions as well as some outer metropolitan areas). In addition, the reforms effectively increased the Medicare benefit for a GP visit by 17.6% by reimbursing 100%, rather than 85%, of the MBS fee. The *Strengthening Medicare* reforms also introduced the **Extended Medicare Safety Net (EMSN)**, which provided additional Medicare benefits for those households who incurred high OOP costs during a calendar year – see Table 2.2 for details.

Prior to the introduction of the EMSN, patients faced the burden of paying any provider charges above the Medicare benefit through OOP costs. In this way providers face **market pressures** to contain their charges and this aspect of the Medicare program is widely regarded as a major factor in keeping medical fee inflation – and therefore OOP costs – in check (Scotton 1998). At the time of its introduction, the government stated that the purpose of the EMSN was to protect all Australians from high OOP costs for medical services that are provided out of hospital.

The EMSN takes effect once a family or single person has reached a given threshold in OOP costs. Once the threshold is reached, the EMSN pays additional benefits

TABLE 2.2   MBS and PBS Entitlements for Concession Cardholders and the General Population

	Concession Cardholders	General Population
MBS		
MBS entitlement (introduced 1984)	Fixed rebate for each eligible medical service rendered by providers in accordance with the MBS fee	Fixed rebate for each eligible medical service rendered by providers in accordance with the MBS fee
Bulk-billing incentive payment to GPs per consultation (introduced 2004)	$6.40 per GP consultation in metropolitan areas; $9.60 in selected rural and regional areas	No incentive
Extended Medicare Safety Net – EMSN (introduced 2004)	CC households qualify for the EMSN once they incur $697 in out-of-pocket costs within a calendar year for MBS-related out-of-hospital services. The EMSN reduces patient co-payments by (up to) 80% of the gap between provider fees and the MBS rebate.	General households qualify for the EMSN once they incur $2184 in out-of-pocket costs within a calendar year for MBS-related out-of-hospital services. EMSN reduces patient co-payments by (up to) 80% of the gap between provider fees and the MBS rebate.
PBS		
Co-payment (introduced 1960)	$6.60 per script	$41 per script
Co-payment after qualifying for the PBS Safety Net (introduced 1960)	$0 per script if the household has incurred $316.80 in out-of-pocket PBS-related costs	$6.60 per script if the household has incurred $1486.80 in out-of-pocket PBS-related costs

Data from Health care and Medicare, https://www.servicesaustralia.gov.au/health-care-and-medicare?context=60092 and benefits and thresholds of MBS, EMSN and PBS: https://www.servicesaustralia.gov.au/what-are-medicare-safety-nets-thresholds?context=22001, https://www.servicesaustralia.gov.au/education-guide-claiming-bulk-bill-incentive-items?context=20#a2.

to help cover OOP costs for Medicare-related services for the rest of the calendar year. The EMSN covers all out-of-hospital services that are listed in the MBS. Importantly, the EMSN does not cover private inpatient care even though the MBS subsidises both out-of-hospital and private inpatient health services.

Before households qualify for the EMSN, they must reach one of two OOP cost thresholds:

- Commonwealth concession cardholders and/or recipients of **Family Tax Benefit Part A (FTB(A))** qualify once they reach the lower OOP cost threshold, which was $300 when the policy commenced in March 2004.
- All other members of the public qualify once they reach the general OOP cost threshold, which was $700 when the policy commenced.

The OOP cost thresholds operate on a calendar year basis and the threshold count starts afresh on 1 January of each year. This means that in each calendar year, a family has to incur sufficient OOP costs to reach the threshold and qualify for EMSN benefits. Family members can combine their individual OOP costs to reach a threshold sooner but the thresholds do not vary by family size.

As at January 2023, the lower and higher EMSN thresholds were $770.30 and $2414 respectively. Thresholds are indexed to the Consumer Price Index and adjusted at the start of each calendar year and experienced additional one-off increases in 2005 and 2015.

Once a family reaches their EMSN threshold, subsequent OOP costs will be reimbursed up to 80% for most MBS items – although some items have a cap which restricts the amount of EMSN benefits that can be paid. Let's run through two examples of how EMSN benefits are calculated. The first example is for an uncapped item and the second example is for a capped item.

Let's look at the example of an uncapped item, say a radiotherapy planning item (MBS item: 15500). The MBS rebate for this item is $214.65. Let's say that the doctor charges $350 for this item. If the patient had not yet reached the EMSN threshold, the OOP costs for this service would be $135.35 ($350 − $214.65). If the patient *had* reached the EMSN threshold, the EMSN would cover 80% of the OOP costs which is equal to $108.28 (0.8 × $135.35). This would imply that the OOP cost for the radiotherapy item would be $27.07 ($350 − 214.65 − $108.28). It is easy to see that OOP costs reduce substantially for patients who qualify for the EMSN benefits.

Since 2010, the federal government has introduced caps on EMSN benefits for selected MBS items. In the first instance, the capped items were assisted reproductive services (ART), private obstetric services and a select number of procedures. The reason for this selection was due to the high growth in EMSN expenditure for these clinical services and evidence of higher **provider fees** caused by the EMSN. Since then, all consultation items have also been capped.

Caps place a maximum limit on the amount of EMSN benefits. Let's look at MBS item 13209, which is a planning and management item for fertility services. The MBS rebate for this item is $74.95 and the EMSN cap is $11.50. This means that the maximum EMSN benefit payable is $11.50 for this item – noting that each capped MBS item has its own unique EMSN cap amount. Let's see what happens if the provider charges $85 for the item and the patient is eligible for EMSN benefits. In this instance, the EMSN benefit is $8.04 (80% of the OOP costs which is $85 − $74.95). As $8.04 is less that the capped amount of $11.50, the patient will receive their entitlement and so the OOP cost for the service will be $2.01 ($85 − $74.95 − $8.04). Now let's imagine the patient sees a provider who charges $100 for the same service. In this instance, 80% of the OOP costs is greater than the cap (0.8 × $25.05 = $20.04) and therefore the cap becomes effective and will only pay the patient $11.50. Hence, the OOP costs now will be $13.55 ($100 − $74.95 − $11.50). From this example, it becomes clear that if a patient goes to see doctors who charge fees that will exceed the EMSN cap, the patient is responsible for paying it again. It puts the onus back on the patient to find lower charging doctors if they want to avoid high OOP costs for MBS items that are capped.

Case study 2.1 provides another example of Medicare and Extended Medicare Safety Net entitlements.

Pause *for* Reflection ...

Visit the Medicare Benefits Schedule website (www.mbsonline.gov.au) and explore some of the several thousand services funded under the MBS and the rebates provided for these services. Can you find an EMSN capped and uncapped item?

PUBLIC HOSPITALS

Australian hospitals reflect the intricacies of federal–state financial relationships and responsibilities. State

CASE STUDY 2.1   Medicare and Extended Medicare Safety Net Entitlements

The Li family comprises two adults and one child. Their household income is $95,000 a year and they are eligible for Family Tax Benefits (Part A) – FTB(A). As they are recipients of the FTB(A), they can qualify for the lower EMSN threshold of $770.30. This is the lower EMSN threshold in 2023 and it gets indexed with the rate of inflation each year. The family will receive EMSN benefits to cover OOP costs once they accumulate $770.30 in OOP costs. They will receive EMSN benefits to cover out-of-hospital MBS-related OOP costs from the moment they reach the threshold to the end of the calendar year.

In this case study, we follow the Li family over the course of a year and record their health care use and costs to examine their entitlements under Medicare and the EMSN. The table below is a record of the health care use, fees and charges incurred by the Li family as well as the benefits received from Medicare and the resulting OOP costs. The EMSN works on a household basis. As such, the OOP costs of all three members of the Li family contribute to the EMSN threshold count, and once the threshold is reached all members qualify to receive additional benefits.

Ms Vivienne Li has been feeling tired lately and also has a pain in her hip. She visits her GP where she has a 15-minute consultation after which she has a blood test. Her GP charges her $45 and the MBS rebate is $39.75. This means that her OOP cost for the GP consultation is $5.25. The pathology company bulk-bills her for the services. This means that the fee charged by pathology is equal to the **Medicare rebate** of $8.50. As Ms Li does not have to pay anything for the pathology test, the cumulative OOP costs do not change at this point. To investigate her hip pain, the GP refers Vivienne to a specialist. She makes an appointment for 15 February. The fee charged by the specialist for this initial consultation is $200 but the Medicare rebate is

$78.05. This implies that the OOP cost for this claim is $121.95 ($200 – $78.05). During the appointment, the specialist writes out a referral for an MRI scan of Vivienne's hip.

The MRI provider charges $432.60 for the scan and the Medicare rebate is $348.25, implying an OOP cost of $84.35 for this service. Vivienne has two follow-up consultations with her specialist and the OOP costs incurred for those visits are added to the family's cumulative OOP cost for the year.

On 1 June, Mr Jason Li visits his GP seeking help for some anxiety he's been suffering lately. The GP charges $45 and also refers Jason to a psychologist. As part of a GP management plan, Medicare will contribute towards the cost of up to 10 psychologist consultations in a calendar year. For each psychologist service (MBS item 10968), the provider charges Jason $150 and the MBS rebate is $56 – leaving Jason with OOP costs of $94 for the first, second and third consultation. However, after the third consultation, the cumulative OOP cost for the Li family hits $770.30. This is equal to the EMSN threshold and means that, from here on in, the Li family is eligible for EMSN benefits for the remainder of the calendar year.

Having qualified for the EMSN, Jason's fourth visit to his psychologist will result in additional benefits. The psychologist still charges $150, the MBS rebate is still $56 but the EMSN now provides Jason with additional support of $75.20 which is equal to 80% of $94. Instead of incurring an OOP cost of $94 for the psychology service prior to qualifying for EMSN benefits, Jason now only has to pay $18.80.

The EMSN will provide additional benefits for all three members of the Li household for the remainder of the calendar year for any Medicare-covered service provided in the out-of-hospital setting. As the EMSN operates on a calendar year basis, the claim incurred on 2 January the following year will not be covered by the EMSN but will count towards the threshold for the next calendar year.

Date of Service	MBS Item	Fee Charged	MBS Rebate	EMSN Benefit	EMSN Capped Item	OOP cost	Cumulative OOP cost
1/02/2023	23	45.00	39.75	-	Y	5.25	5.25
1/02/2023	73527	8.50	8.50	-	N	0.00	5.25
15/02/2023	104	200.00	78.05		Y	121.95	127.20
22/02/2023	63322	432.60	348.25		N	84.35	211.55
28/02/2023	105	175.00	39.25		Y	135.75	347.30
28/03/2023	105	175.00	39.25		Y	135.75	483.05
1/06/2023	23	45.00	39.75		Y	5.25	488.30
15/06/2023	10968	150.00	56.00		Y	94.00	582.30
29/06/2023	10968	150.00	56.00		Y	94.00	676.30
13/07/2023	10968	150.00	56.00		Y	94.00	770.30
27/07/2023	10968	150.00	56.00	75.20	Y	18.80	789.10
10/08/2023	10968	150.00	56.00	75.20	Y	18.80	807.90
29/08/2023	23	45.00	39.75	4.20	Y	1.05	808.95
2/01/2024	23	45.00	39.75		Y	5.25	5.25

CASE STUDY 2.1   Medicare and Extended Medicare Safety Net Entitlements—cont'd

The table also shows which of the Medicare items, claimed by the Li family during the year, are capped. As noted above, some MBS items have EMSN caps which implies that there is a maximum benefit paid by the EMSN. In the case of the Li family's expenses, the caps did not come into play. This is because they visited medical providers whose fees were sufficiently low for the caps not to take effect.

Let's examine a scenario where the cap did take effect. Imagine that for the GP visit on 29 August, the GP charged a fee of $200. The EMSN cap for item 23 is $119.25 (as at March 2023). If item 23 was uncapped, the EMSN benefit for that consultation would have been 128.20 (i.e. 0.8×($200 – $39.75)) and Jason would have incurred an OOP cost of $32.05 ($200 – $39.75 – 128.20). However, because this item does have an EMSN cap, the maximum EMSN benefit paid will be $119.25. This means that the OOP cost for this consultation will be $41.00 ($200 – $39.75 – $119.25). Now that the EMSN cap has been reached, if the GP increased their fees for this consultation, the increase would be borne entirely by the patient. For example, if the GP charged $205 instead of $200, the OOP cost for the patient would increase by $5.

and territory governments own and operate public hospitals but are reliant on financial transfers from the federal government, which has the greater tax-raising powers. The funding of public hospitals has been a highly politicised area of federal–state relationships (Duckett 1999; Duckett & Wilcox 2015). So much so, that a major promise of the incoming Rudd Government in 2007 was to 'end the blame game', referring to the constant arguing between the state and territory first ministers and the prime minister of the day about public hospitals. This section first focuses on public hospital funding arrangements prior to 2011 and then on the National Health Reform Agreement (NHRA).

Pre-National Health Reform Arrangements

Specific bilateral agreements between the federal government and each of the state and territory governments have underpinned public hospital funding and been negotiated on a five-yearly basis since the 1940s. The introduction of Medicare in 1984 gave every Australian the right to treatment in a public hospital free of charge. This required a higher level of financial compensation from the federal government, which has been around 50% of total public hospital expenditure (Deeble 2008). But this share was not fixed and was influenced by the timing of elections and the cycle of each five-year agreement, reaching a low of 38% in 2007 (AIHW 2012). This funding was provided to state treasuries, which then determined how to channel it to hospitals and other services. Increasing budgetary pressures for all governments, increasing hospital costs and growing demands, and public concern about their access to public hospital care provided the perfect environment for each level of government to blame the other for not providing sufficient funds and ineffective management.

One issue that was a frequent point of contention was the fact that the federal government contribution is divorced from the volume of hospital activity. Each five-year agreement typically set out the federal government's annual contribution, which was indexed on a range of measures including expected population growth. However, over the five-year period, state and territory governments typically had to absorb the additional costs of hospital activity growth. This meant that the federal government's contribution to public hospitals may have increased in absolute terms but decreased as a proportion of overall public hospital expenditure.

Another point of contention and common aspect of the '**blame game**' were accusations of **cost-shifting** between levels of governments. This occurs when a government takes an action that reduces the costs of financing health from their own budget and adds it to the budget of another level of government. Here are some examples:

- State governments may attempt to shift services away from hospital care (which they largely fund and are responsible for) towards out-of-hospital care funded through the MBS. As MBS funding for GP and specialist services comes from the federal government, this shifts the costs to that level of government.
- Public hospitals are responsible for paying for medications to inpatients during their stay as part of their package of care. If hospitals only supply a minimal amount of medication upon discharge, the patient then has to go and see their GP and/or a community pharmacy, which then shifts the costs to the federal government-funded **Pharmaceutical Benefits Scheme (PBS)**.

- In 2012, the Chronic Disease Dental Scheme, which was funded by the federal government, was shut down. This meant that more patients in need of dental services, particularly those without private health insurance, were shifted to public dental clinics funded (in part) by state and territory governments.
- Between 1996 and 2004, OOP costs for GP consultations increased markedly with many GPs reducing the number of services they bulk-billed. This led to assertions that patients were substituting away from GP care and were instead attending the Emergency Department, which was paid for by state and territory governments.

From a resource perspective, cost-shifting behaviours do not necessarily introduce waste into the system per se. After all, all publicly financed health care is paid for by taxpayers regardless of which level of government ends up paying the bill. The real problem with cost-shifting is when the behaviours add additional costs and inefficiency to the patient (including inconvenience) or the system overall. Take the PBS example listed above. In that instance, patients may face the additional burden of going to see their GP and visiting their community pharmacy for their medication at a time when they have just been discharged from hospital. This inconvenience is an additional cost to the overall system (and patient) as is the additional visit to the GP.

Cost-shifting behaviours also introduce managerial waste – where effort and resources are expended to partake in cost-shifting behaviours rather than seeking to make the system more efficient.

From both a policy and a political perspective, the health care blame game became a major issue at the 2007 federal election. Following on from the election of the Rudd Government, the National Health and Hospitals Reform Commission was established to make recommendations on how to improve the health system and end the blame game. One of its major recommendations for hospitals was to introduce **activity-based funding** (**ABF**) throughout the country (National Health and Hospitals Reform Commission 2009). This recommendation was implemented as part of the NHRA – signed by all state and territory governments as well as the federal government.

The 2011 National Health Reform Agreement

The NHRA of 2011 introduced a basis for shared hospital funding between the state, territory and federal governments. The new arrangements provided increased federal funding determined by the growth in public hospital activity and hospital costs. Activity was measured by DRG (Diagnosis Related Groups) weights. Hospital costs were set by determining a national efficient price. Federal funding was paid directly to **Local Hospital Networks** (**LHNs**), regionally based groupings of hospitals. States and territories were designated the system managers with responsibility for managing volume growth; as their treasuries provide the balance of funds this was expected to ensure a constraint on volume growth.

This initiated the establishment of national activity-based funding (ABF) for the public hospital sector. Australia has had a long history of collecting national **casemix** data on activity and costs. This included its own version of the Diagnosis Related Groups, now AR-DRGs. The state of Victoria was the first jurisdiction in the world to introduce casemix funding (Duckett 1995). Over time, most but not all states and territories had moved to this form of funding in whole or in part. So although the introduction of national ABF represented a significant change, considerable infrastructure around casemix classification, activity measurement and costing was already in place.

The 2011 Agreement established a new body, the Independent Hospital Pricing Authority (which has since been renamed the **Independent Health and Aged Care Pricing Authority** (**IHACPA**)), to determine the national efficient price for public hospital services. IHACPA has responsibility for the ongoing development of the component parts required by ABF: a classification system (AR-DRGs and for sub-acute and non-acute services the Australian National Subacute and Non-Acute Patient (SNAP) classification), data collection on activity (the National Hospital Data Collection) and calculating costs (with a standard framework for costing activities, the Australian Hospital Patient Costing Standards). Expenditure is split across five types of service: admitted acute, emergency, non-admitted, sub-acute and non-acute, and 'other'.[2]

The national efficient price is based on the average cost of an admission (IHPA 2017). Casemix is adjusted by the National Weighted Activity Unit (NWAU); more

---

[2]SNAP is applied to admissions for rehabilitation care, palliative care, geriatric evaluation and management, or maintenance care.

complex cases have a NWAU of greater than one. NWAUs are a common metric across admitted, sub-acute, emergency and outpatient services. Prices are also adjusted 'to reflect legitimate and unavoidable variations in the cost of delivering health services' (NHRA 2011), including indigeneity, remoteness of patients' residential area, and remoteness of the treating hospital. Prices are updated annually.

There are some other adjustments. Where the federal government makes direct payments under special programs (i.e. highly specialised drugs, supply of blood), these are deducted from the calculation of the national efficient price. Public hospitals can also treat private inpatients, in which case private insurers and the federal government (through reimbursement of fees for private medical practitioners) make payments to hospitals; the national efficient price is adjusted to allow for this (IHPA 2017). Adjustments are made for outliers, with long-stays receiving a per diem rate.

Australian geography is such that there are a number (approximately 400) of small hospitals serving small and often rural-remote population groups where ABF is not viable. IHACPA determines a national efficient price based on size, location and type of services. A national efficient price is also determined for services that are not yet able to be described in terms of activity. A key difference is that the block funding amounts are directed to states and territories to allocate to the hospitals.

Consultation and stakeholder feedback is an integral part of the price-setting processes. IHACPA works with a Jurisdictional Advisory Committee and a Clinical Advisory Committee in developing its systems and analysing data. Its pricing framework establishes various principles, including transparency, and the framework itself is reviewed annually in consultation with the federal, state and territory governments; there is also a period of public consultation. Its work is published via the IHACPA website. This includes full details of pricing frameworks and the list of prices.

One important provision of the NHRA is that where changes are made to the classification systems or costing methods, these should not result in unwarranted payments (either due to apparently more or less activity). IHACPA has developed a back-casting policy for the purpose of calculating federal funding, remembering that this contribution is based on a share of growth in both prices and activity (IHPA 2018a). The National Hospital Cost Data Collection is independently reviewed to assess quality (IHPA 2018b). As states and territories and the federal governments are scrutinising IHACPA's determinations, there is considerable scope for review.

There have been several developments over time, reflecting improved data collection, changes in practice and new technologies. From June 2017, pricing was required not just to recognise efficiency but also to address safety and quality. IHACPA worked with another independent body, the Australian Commission on Health Care Safety and Quality, to develop its approach. Hospital admissions which include a sentinel event (never events) attract no payment. Hospital-acquired complications attract a lower payment, which is risk adjusted for patient characteristics. Avoidable hospital admissions have been investigated but as yet not included in pricing or funding (IHPA 2017).

Finally IHACPA's responsibility is the price determination. The actual payment of monies is the province of the National Funding Administrator, who recommends payments to the Treasurer after reconciliation of activity data.

SUMMARY

This chapter has introduced you to some of the main publicly financed components of the Australian health care system. Major issues discussed include the following:

- Medicare provides universal access to free public hospital care for all Australian citizens and subsidised access to other medical services.
- Medicare is Australia's version of universal health coverage (UHC). It seeks to deliver equity of access to health care without leading to financial stress for patients.

- Health expenditure in Australia has been rising year on year, which presents concerns and challenges for health policy-makers.
- Australian health care system responsibilities is shared across federal, state and local governments, with each sector of government responsible for different aspects in isolation or through shared ventures.
- A range of policies have been explored that look at restricting growth and dealing with the governance of health care.

REVIEW QUESTIONS

1. List some reasons why health expenditures may be rising.
2. Why are patients vulnerable to OOP costs under current MBS arrangements?
3. What is cost-shifting and under what circumstances is cost-shifting a concern?
4. Describe how cost-shifting might impact on public hospitals. Do you think that the NHRA of 2011 has resolved cost-shifting?
5. Given the overlap in funding and responsibility for the management of various parts of the Australian health care system, what do you see as the potential problems arising from this arrangement?

REFERENCES

Australian Institute of Health and Welfare (AIHW), 2012. Health expenditure Australia 2010–11. Health and welfare expenditure series no. 47. Cat. no. HWE 56. AIHW, Canberra.

Australian Institute of Health and Welfare (AIHW), 2021. Health expenditure in Australia 2019–20. AIHW, Canberra. https://www.aihw.gov.au/reports/health-welfare-expenditure/health-expenditure-australia-2019-20/contents/overview-of-data-sources-and-methodology/the-australian-national-health-account.

Deeble, J.S., 2008. Medicare: where have we been? Where are we going? Aust N Z J Public Health 23,1–7.

Department of Health and Aged Care, 2022. Medicare statistics, 2022. https://www.health.gov.au/resources/publications/medicare-annual-statistics-state-and-territory-2009-10-to-2021-22?language=en

Do, L.G., Spencer, A.J., Slade, G.D., et al., 2010. Trend of income-related inequality of child oral health in Australia. J Dent Res 89 (9), 959–964.

Duckett, S.J., 1995. Hospital payment arrangements to encourage efficiency: the case of Victoria, Australia. Health Policy 34, 113–134.

Duckett, S., 1999. Commonwealth / state relations in health. In: Hancock, L. (Ed.), Health Policy in the Market State. Allen & Unwin, Sydney.

Duckett, S., Willcox, S., 2015. The Australian Health Care System, fifth ed. OUP, Victoria.

Independent Hospital Pricing Authority (IHPA), 2017. Risk adjustment model for hospital acquired complications – technical specifications version 1.0. IHPA, Sydney. https://www.ihpa.gov.au/sites/g/files/net636/f/risk_adjustment_model_for_hospital_acquired_complications_-_technical_specifications_v1.0_july_2017_pdf.pdf.

Independent Hospital Pricing Authority (IHPA), 2018a. Back-casting policy. IHPA, Sydney. https://www.ihacpa.gov.au.

Independent Hospital Pricing Authority (IHPA), 2018b. National hospital cost data collection, independent financial review, round 20 (financial year 2015–16). IHPA, Sydney. https://www.ihacpa.gov.au.

Johar, M., Jones, G., Savage, E., 2014. What explains the quality and price of GP services? An investigation using linked survey and administrative data. Health Econ 23 (9), 1115–1133.

Johar, M., Mu, C., Van Gool, K., et al., 2017. Bleeding hearts, profiteers, or both: specialist physician fees in an unregulated market. Health Econ 26 (4), 528–535.

Jones, G., Savage, E., Van Gool, K., 2008. The distribution of household health expenditures in Australia. Econ Rec 84, S99–S114.

Ju, X., Mejia, G.C., Wu, Q., et al., 2021. Use of oral health care services in the United States: unequal, inequitable—a cross-sectional study. BMC Oral Health 21 (1), 1–9.

Ju, X., Do, L.G., Brennan, D.S., et al., 2022. Inequality and inequity in the use of oral health services in Australian adults. JDR Clin Trans Res 7 (4), 389–397.

Mejia, G.C., Elani, H.W., Harper, S., et al., 2018. Socioeconomic status, oral health and dental disease in Australia, Canada, New Zealand and the United States. BMC Oral Health, 18 (1), 1–9.

National Health and Hospitals Reform Commission, 2009. A healthier future for all Australians – final report of the National Health and Hospitals Reform Commission June 2009. COAG, Canberra. http://www.federalfinancialrelations.gov.au/content/npa/health/_archive/national-agreement.pdf.

Organisation for Economic Co-operation and Development (OECD), 2021. Health statistics, 2021. https://www.oecd.org/els/health-systems/health-data.htm.

Scotton, R.B., 1998. The doctor business. In: Mooney, G., & Scotton, R. B. (Eds), Economics and Australian Health Policy. Allen & Unwin, Sydney.

Scotton, R.B., Deeble, J.S., 1968. Compulsory health insurance for Australia. Aust Econ Rev, 4 (4), 9–16.

Singh, A., Harford, J., Antunes, J.L.F., et al., 2018. Area-level income inequality and oral health among Australian adults—a population-based multilevel study. PLOS ONE 13 (1), e0191438.

Whitlam, G., 1997. Abiding interests. University of Queensland Press, Brisbane.

Williams, A., Maynard, A., 1984. Privatisation and the NHS. In: Le Grand, J., Robinson, R. (Eds), Privatisation and the Welfare State. Allen & Unwin, London.

FURTHER READING

Australian Institute of Health and Welfare, 2018. Australia's health 2018. Australia's health series no. 16. AUS221. AIHW, Canberra. https://www.aihw.gov.au/getmedia/7c42913d-295f-4bc9-9c24-4e44eff4a04a/aihw-aus-221.pdf.aspx?inline=true.

Bartlett, C., Butler, S., Haines, L., 2016. Reimagining health reform in Australia: taking a systems approach to health and wellness. https://www.strategyand.pwc.com/media/file/Reimagining-health-reform-in-Australia.pdf.

Department of Health, 2017. History of the Department. http://www.health.gov.au/internet/main/publishing.nsf/Content/health-history.htm.

Duckett, S., Willcox, S., 2015. The Australian Health Care System, fifth ed. OUP, Victoria.

Hall, J., Viney, R., 2000. The political economy of health sector reform. In: Bloom, A. (Ed.), Health Reform in Australia and New Zealand. OUP, South Melbourne.

National Health Reform Agreement, 2011. Council of Australian Governments. http://www.federalfinancialrelations.gov.au/content/npa/health/_archive/national-agreement.pdf.

Palmer, G., Short, S., 2014. Health Care and Public Policy: An Australian Analysis, fifth ed. Palgrave Macmillan, South Yarra.

ONLINE RESOURCES

Australian Institute of Health and Welfare – provides comprehensive information, publications and statistics about most aspects of the Australian health care system, population groups and specific diseases: https://www.aihw.gov.au.

Department of Human Services – administers Medicare Australia: https://ww.humanservices.gov.au.

Medicare Benefits Schedule: https://www.mbsonline.gov.au.

MyHospitals – search for any hospital and review the waiting times for surgery. You can also compare hospitals, download data and review additional measures such as length of stay, emergency department attendances and safety and quality performance: https://www.aihw.gov.au/reports-data/myhospitals.

National Health Funding Pool Administrator: https://www.publichospitalfunding.gov.au/.

Independent Health and Aged Care Pricing Authority: https://www.ihacpa.gov.au.

3

The Private Health Sector and Private Health Insurance

Nathan Kettlewell

KEY LEARNING OUTCOMES

When you finish this chapter you should be able to:
- explain the scope of the private health sector within the Australian health care system and how it is organised, funded and delivered
- discuss current debates about private health insurance in Australia and implications for equity and access
- describe the tensions between advocates for universal access via Medicare and advocates for a strong private sector.

KEY TERMS AND ABBREVIATIONS

Australian Institute of Health
  and Welfare (AIHW)
day hospital
moral hazard
price elasticity

private health insurance (PHI)
privatisation
private health insurance rebate
Private Hospital Data Bureau
  (PHDB)

private hospital
public–private partnerships
  (PPPs)
sentinel event

INTRODUCTION

This chapter is about the private health care sector in Australia. As noted earlier in this book, Australia has a hybrid, public–private health system. This offers many challenges to government and to patients navigating services. This chapter will focus primarily on **private health insurance (PHI)** and **private hospitals**, as these are the two most prominent and influential aspects of the private health care system in Australia. The provision of public medical services and the funding of the universal health insurance system, Medicare, are discussed in Chapter 2, while other aspects of Australian health care with a significant private component, such as the aged care sector, complementary health care

and dental care, are discussed in Chapters 8, 14 and 15 respectively. We will see that since the late 1990s, Australians have been strongly encouraged to contribute to the financing of their health needs by purchasing PHI, in addition to the universal tax-based insurance coverage provided by Medicare. This has greatly influenced the health care system in Australia.

BRIEF HISTORY OF PRIVATE HEALTH INSURANCE (PHI)

The earliest form of PHI in Australia dates back to the Friendly and Mutual societies of the 19th century. Members of these societies would receive access to subsidised medical and other social services in exchange for membership fees, with members typically belonging to the same industry group. Many of the functions of the Friendly Societies were displaced by the establishment of the modern welfare state in the 20th century. However, the private market for health insurance has endured, even after the establishment of universal public insurance.

Collyer et al. (2015) discuss how Australia's public–private insurance system developed throughout the 20th century. Historically, professional medical bodies (such as the Australian Medical Association) opposed efforts to expand the public provision of medical care, and conservative parties (such as the Liberal and National parties) favoured policies that supported private provision of medical services. Of particular importance was the passage of the *National Health Act 1953* by the Menzies Coalition Government, which laid the foundation for the modern structure of PHI (Shamsullah 2011). This established a system of private voluntary health insurance as the preferred means for funding medical care, with a public safety net available only for the most vulnerable. It also employed various subsidies and regulations to support PHI, a legacy that continues to this day. A key regulation was community rating, which is still a feature of PHI. Community rating requires insurers to charge the same premium to everyone (regardless of underlying risk), which is facilitated through risk equalisation arrangements, whereby funds with favourable membership pools (i.e. lower risk members) effectively cross-subsidise funds with less favourable pools.

The Contemporary PHI Environment

The model of voluntary health insurance that operated under the Menzies Coalition Government was significantly disrupted by the introduction of universal public insurance, beginning with Medibank in the 1970s and later Medicare in 1984. Under Medicare, all Australians can access free medical care through the public hospital system. Medicare dramatically decreased the value of PHI and unsurprisingly membership rates dropped. In June 1983, 63.6% of Australians were covered by PHI. By 1997 this had dropped to 32.1% (APRA 2022a).

The decline in PHI membership was a political issue in the 1990s, with insurers raising concerns about the sustainability of the market. In response, the Keating Labor Government made some regulatory changes to promote greater efficiency and cost reductions, the most significant being to allow insurance funds to negotiate

'preferred provider' contracts with doctors and hospitals in the hope of lower costs for patients (Duckett et al. 2019). Those reforms did little to arrest the decline in membership, and in the late 1990s the Howard Liberal-Coalition Government embarked on a much more substantial set of policy reforms. Specifically, a set of incentives to purchase PHI ('carrots' and 'sticks') were introduced including:

- the **private health insurance rebate**: a consumer subsidy for the cost of PHI, which was originally only available to lower income earners, but from 1 July 1999 was set at 30% for everyone, regardless of income. Today, the rebate is means tested with different rates based on age and income
- the Medicare Levy Surcharge: a tax penalty for people over a certain income without PHI
- Lifetime Health Cover Loading: a 2% penalty loading on top of the PHI premium for every year individuals aged over 30 delay buying PHI for hospital cover (with the loading removed after 10 years of continuous cover).

These reforms coincided with a large increase in the number of people covered by PHI. In 1999, around 31% of Australians had PHI that covered hospital care. By 2021 approximately 45% of Australians were covered for hospital care with 54% holding general treatment or extras insurance (covering dental, optical and other non-hospital related benefits).

PHI in Australia is fundamentally different to other types of insurance. Insurance is generally associated with financial protection from catastrophic events. Medicare already provides this protection. The value of PHI for consumers is that it provides them with the option of using the private hospital system without paying out-of-pocket, which can mean shorter waiting times (particularly for elective procedures), choice of physician and potentially a more pleasant care experience (e.g. access to a non-shared room). PHI can also cover out-of-hospital expenses not covered by Medicare (like dental and optical). However, benefits for such 'extras' are typically capped and therefore PHI offers limited financial protection for these services.

As of 6 June 2022, there were 34 private health insurers listed with the government regulator, the **Australian Prudential Regulation Authority (APRA)** (APRA 2022b), including for-profit and not-for-profit funds. This also includes 11 smaller funds with restricted membership (similar to the Friendly Societies of yesteryear). The five largest funds account for 80.3% of policies with the two largest, Medibank and Bupa, accounting for 26.2% and 25.6% respectively (ACCC 2021). Since the **privatisation** of Medibank in 2014, most Australians belong to a for-profit fund. Whether profit motives are harmful to consumers in the PHI market is a contentious issue, but it is worth bearing in mind that the behaviour of all funds is heavily regulated, including with respect to the minimum level of cover provided and premium setting.

Case study 3.1 highlights the experience of Australians with and without PHI. While in the past, PHI could be regarded merely as an additional 'choice' for Australians, the 'sticks and carrots' policy mechanisms have altered the landscape, increasing the number of people with PHI, shifting people's perceptions and practices about how best to meet their health needs, and expanding the number of private-sector services as new opportunities open up for health professionals to work in the private sector.

CASE STUDY 3.1   'Choosing' to Go Private

Given that Australia offers free public hospital treatment to all citizens, which citizens contribute to through the taxation system, why do so many people buy PHI? A representative survey of 1200 Australians (Zhang & Prakash 2021) found the main reasons for buying PHI are:

- security and peace of mind (44%)
- shorter waiting time and choice of doctor (44%)
- better off financially (e.g. because of policy incentives) (30%)
- need it for a current health condition (26%).

It is noteworthy that the main reason for buying PHI is security and peace of mind, which implies that many people see the private health care sector as providing something not offered by Medicare alone. The fourth reason is indicative of adverse selection, the tendency for higher risk people to purchase insurance. This can drive up premiums and is sometimes used as an argument in favour of premium subsidies. However, in Australia people who purchase PHI actually tend to have lower hospitalisation risk than those without PHI (Buchmueller et al. 2013).

The following examples from interviews with 78 people conducted by Professor Karen Willis and colleagues (Willis et al. 2016) illustrate the dominance of positive views about the private sector, as well as the challenges people have in navigating between public and private.

Consider the cases of Penny, Ahn and Jin, and Paul. As you read through these examples, make a list of what you believe their story highlights about health care:

- Does the system work in the ways they discuss?
- Are their experiences indicative of a health policy problem?
- What does their experience tell us about the health care system in Australia?

Penny is aged 21 years and has two children, both with multiple, ongoing health problems. Penny is on a low income and does not have private health insurance. She wishes she could afford it:

> If I knew my children and I were going to be so sick, I would've got private health insurance

> because we would've been well a lot quicker, I think.

With no experience of the private system, Penny believes the private system would be better than the public:

> I think in the private system they might get more choice than in the public ... With private you're paying for your own health instead of public so you should get more when you pay for it. You might get looked after quicker and there might be a waiting time still but not as long, more comfortable – if you have surgery or something more comfortable, maybe more space in a room. I'm not 100% sure but maybe those are the things that are better.

Ahn (aged 65) and **Jin** (aged 61) migrated to Australia from China 30 years ago. They have two adult daughters. Ahn is a hospital porter and Jin works in a supermarket. They purchased PHI in 2000:

> ... because that year I think the government push the people to join the Medibank Private. That's why we joined the private. They're talking about when you're old you will pay more money. That's why we go to join.

Additionally, they worry about waiting lists for surgery in the public system:

> I think they told me if you go to private it's faster. If not, you need to wait long periods, maybe two months, three months. If you go to private, maybe couple of weeks.

As PHI has become more expensive, the pair have contemplated dropping their cover and relying on the public system. However, as they are ageing, they worry about doing this:

> You see when you get older your problem will come up you see. You need more health care. Maybe now we don't need to go to the

CASE STUDY 3.1   'Choosing' to Go Private—cont'd

hospital, or maybe later you need to go to the hospital to do the operation or do something, so I think if no, I don't have the private fund I think it's not secure.

Ahn and Jin draw on their experience from a time when their daughter needed surgery, and how the specialist persuaded them they should use the private system:

Then the doctor say, 'If you go to public I only watch. You see, my assistant do the opera-tion' ... But on that occasion, my daughter is different. He has to do it. So he told me that I'm doing the operation and then we'll change to private. I think, oh you are good doctor, so I better rely on you to do it.

Paul, aged 34, is university educated and has a manage-rial position in local government. Married with two chil-dren, his family has had many encounters with the health care system. He discusses how important PHI is to him, and how he has navigated between public and private health care systems.

When discussing the decision to 'go private' Paul says:

I've been a private patient for having diagnos-tic scopes done. And I did those as a private patient obviously, because as a private patient I can get in and get them done, which is the absolute benefit of having private cover, I can choose my treating specialist and I can say I'm available on these days, how does that work for you, rather than sitting on the waitlist.

Paul says that the private system:

Is nicer, not so much that the staff are nicer, but the staff are under a lot less pressure is the perception of it. Because you are going into the private hospital to have very specific treatments, they are not dealing with the emergency cases and the ambulances and that sort of dynamic workflow. They have a roster of what's on for the day and they work to that roster and they leave, and it's done so there's a lot less stress in that environment and as a result they are nicer about it ... Even though some of the procedures that people are going for can be reasonably heavy, they have spoken

to their specialist they've chosen, and they have chosen this date, everything is a lot more planned for and structured. It's just that more 'nicer' environment to be in.

Paul discusses his use of the public system:

In emergency situations I have to go to the public hospital, but I definitely notify them that I am a private patient and use whatever perks and privileges that might bring with them, because I have paid for them I suppose. For elective surgery I will always go private where I can afford the opportunity to do so.

Paul highly values having PHI:

There have been times in our life where you know, we have thought of dropping the private health insurance because the bills were tight and you know the family had to come first, but we always managed to find a way to keep the private health cover, because if something happened to go wrong for us and touch wood nothing's gone too wrong for us ... But had anything come up we could get to the top of the waitlist, we could pick our specialist, pick our hospital, basically pick from a choice of treatment dates. Which is always preferable to going on the waitlist.

This brief case study of PHI tells us quite a bit about people's views. One strong theme emerging from these interviews is that people feel they 'get something extra' if they have PHI, though they are not always sure of what this might be. Another is the level of concern raised about not being treated quickly if they have to rely on the public system. Quite notable is that very few participants sug-gest their choices are drawn from lived experience of differences between public and private forms of care. This raises questions about the extent to which their choices are 'free', or perhaps have been shaped by the higher premiums that will be imposed if they fail to join by a certain age, or by prevailing discourses in the media and elsewhere that systematically encourage them to be fear-ful about the public system and which emphasise the benefits of the private system (Lewis et al. 2018).

One controversial topic is the use of public hospitals by privately insured patients. The Commonwealth and states have an agreement that people can choose to be a private patient in a public hospital, and that the public hospitals can charge for these private patients at a fee set by each state. Importantly, however, there is no requirement for people to declare their PHI status (Seah et al. 2013). Some argue that this compromises one of the objectives of subsidising PHI in the first place, which was to 'take the pressure off the public system'. However, patients with PHI are also paying for access to the public system through the tax-funded Medicare.

There is also some dispute about whether patients should be using their PHI at public hospitals at all. On the one hand, this provides public hospitals with additional revenue and takes pressure off Medicare. However, patients may also feel pressured (or be actively pressured) to provide this information, even though being admitted as a private patient could leave them with OOP costs. While many people are happy to use their PHI for the benefit of the public hospital, the personal benefits from being a private patient are often unclear to people (Lewis et al. 2019). Benefits can include greater choice of specialist and access to a private room, but such privileges are not guaranteed. By law, PHI should not be a factor in the quality or timing of treatment in public hospitals, which is important for the equity of the public health care system. However, there is some evidence that privately admitted patients in public hospitals may be preferentially treated, with shorter waiting times compared to observationally similar public patients (Shmueli & Savage 2014).

THE PRIVATE HEALTH CARE SECTOR IN AUSTRALIA

The private sector comprises private hospitals, most medical, dental and allied health services, pharmacies, much of the aged care sector, most radiology and pathology services, PHI and companies engaged in the manufacturing or sale of medical devices and e-health technologies.

Private Hospitals in Australia

Private hospitals in Australia are those that are owned and operated by non-government agents, which can include charity and religious groups, offering user-paid accommodation and health care services. This definition captures a broad range of facilities, including acute, psychiatric and free-standing **day hospitals**. As of 31 December 2021, there were 637 registered private hospitals across the country and 680 public hospitals. However, the composition of these hospitals is different, resulting in very different casemixes (see Figure 3.1). More than half of private hospitals (348) are day hospitals, which carry out specialised procedures that do not require overnight stays, such as endoscopies, colonoscopies, ophthalmic procedures and cosmetic procedures. Private hospitals only provide a small fraction of emergency care (8% of separations in 2019–20), but are responsible for a large fraction of surgery, particularly elective surgeries. While private hospitals only account for 40% of separations overall, they account for 57% of all elective surgeries.

In addition to ownership, another key difference between public and private hospitals is source of funding. About 93% of public hospital funding comes from the Australian and state and territory governments (AIHW 2021a). Private insurers are primarily responsible for the remaining 9% through reimbursements for privately admitted patients in public hospitals. In contrast, PHI is the single most important source of funding for private hospitals, accounting for 50% of funding. As such, demand for private hospital care is strongly tied to the PHI market. Private hospitals also receive some reimbursements from the Australian and state and territory governments, accounting for 23% and 6% of funding respectively. Private OOP costs account for a further 13%.

The strong connection between PHI and private hospital utilisation is demonstrated by recent trends. The private sector grew significantly in the 2000s (Collyer et al. 2015), with a large rise in the proportion of people with PHI over this period. However, between 2015 and 2020, participation in PHI declined from 47.4% to 43.6% and during the same period growth in private hospital separations also declined (Bai et al. 2020). The SARS-CoV-2 pandemic has seen a slight

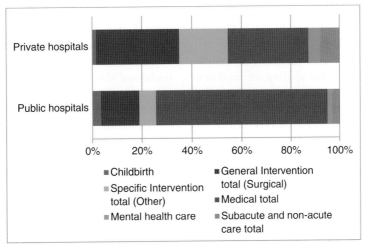

Figure 3.1 Casemixes in Public and Private Hospitals. *Source*: Author's calculations based on AIHW (2021a).

rebound in PHI ownership, but it is unclear what this means for private hospital utilisation as the pandemic has also disrupted hospital service delivery, with resources being redirected to managing the pandemic.

Both private and public hospitals are subject to National Safety and Quality Health Service Standards of care. The states and territories also have their own legislation to regulate private health facilities and enforce licensing standards. State and territory licensing provisions for private hospitals mandate compliance with a range of operational and quality requirements. Private and public hospitals are required by legislation to submit episode-level data to state and territory governments as well as to report **sentinel events** and adverse outcomes data. The collection of such data contributes to the transparency of consumer information about the two sectors, although in reality most consumers are unlikely to know how to access this information.

Data on private hospitals is published online by the **Australian Institute of Health and Welfare (AIHW)** and by the Australian Government Department of Health through the **Private Hospital Data Bureau (PHDB)**. The AIHW publishes a range of aggregated annual statistics for both public and private hospitals on admissions, safety, expenditure and workforce on its MyHospitals portal. However, because public and private hospitals have different classification levels, it is difficult to compare their relative performance, and some statistics are only available for public hospitals. A person who wants to know about the health and safety records of a particular hospital (e.g. because they are considering receiving care there) can search for this information on MyHospitals. However, presently most private hospitals report very little information, which impedes the ability of people to make informed choices. Prospective patients also face significant uncertainty about fees they will incur. The Department of Health's online Medical Costs Finder tool partly addresses this, but only provides general pricing guides for procedures, and not for specific hospitals.

Pause *for* Reflection …
Do you think people usually have enough information to make an informed choice between public versus private hospital treatment?

Ownership of Private Hospitals

Private hospitals vary in terms of categories of ownership and funding, and in size from small facilities with a few beds to major facilities with several hundred beds. Unlike the United States, with its multiple, privately owned, large teaching and research hospitals, private hospitals in Australia primarily offer little in the way of emergency medicine, play a relatively small role in research or teaching and conduct only elective (planned) surgical services. Industry ownership of private hospitals ranges from for-profit hospitals through religious/charitable hospitals to not-for-profit hospitals. In 2016–17, 62% of private overnight hospitals were for-profit (ABS 2018). The largest provider of private hospitals is Ramsay Health Care, who currently operate 72 for-profit private acute and day hospitals throughout

Australia, and account for 27.6% of industry revenue (Richardson 2021). The next largest player is Healthscope (14.4% market share).

Many private hospitals are co-located with public hospitals, which 'allows for the sharing of facilities, equipment and staff, provides greater convenience for doctors, and enhances patient choice, allowing them access to a wider range of services' (AIHW 2014). In 2016–17 approximately 10% of private hospitals were co-located (ABS 2018). Co-location provides hospital owners with multiple business opportunities, as it 'funnels' patients into the private hospital from the nearby emergency departments, enables specialists, nurses and other health care workers to work in both environments and allows the private hospital operator to focus on the most profitable areas of medicine. Brown and Barnett (2004, p. 429) identify four variants of co-located public–private hospitals in Australia:

(1) *the traditional model of locating a for-profit hospital in close proximity to a public hospital;*
(2) *a shared campus where a private and a public hospital occupy the same site;*
(3) *a shared building with the two hospitals occupying different space within the building; and*
(4) *where the public hospital, under contract to a state government, is operated and owned by the corporate hospital chain in return for patient payments from the state concerned.*

PUBLIC–PRIVATE PARTNERSHIPS

Since the 1990s, private-sector financing has increasingly been sought for the construction and operation of health care facilities for treating public patients (Collyer & White 2001; Collyer et al. 2001). Under such arrangements, the private sector builds and finances new hospital facilities, and may also enter into a contract to manage the facility (Productivity Commission 1999). Duckett (2013) explains that under some of these **public–private partnerships (PPPs)** a private company will take responsibility for both building the new hospital and providing the maintenance on the building for a 20- or 50-year period – known as a design, build, finance and maintain arrangement. The costs of the building and the maintenance are paid for through regular facility payments over the life of the building. This means that the state government does not have to pay the full capital costs

up front and the immediate debt burden for governments is thereby reduced.

There is some evidence that PPPs are a cost-effective way of delivering care to public patients compared to traditional state-run facilities (Forbes et al. 2010). However, there is also need for caution regarding such arrangements, and they should not be viewed as a panacea for administration and governance. Duckett (2013) cites the many hospitals around Australia built under such arrangements that have been returned to the public sector at considerable cost to governments and the public purse. Collyer et al. (2001) analyse the case of the Port Macquarie Base Hospital, a PPP, which cost government 30% more than equivalent publicly funded hospitals. At present, PPPs comprise a small but non-trivial fraction of hospitals in Australia. In 2019–20, there were 13 privately owned and/or operated hospitals providing public hospital services which were predominantly or substantially funded by state governments (AIHW 2021c).

Private Hospitals and the SARS-CoV-2 Pandemic

The SARS-CoV-2 pandemic and associated public health restrictions have had a profound effect on hospital activity since the beginning of 2020. One of the early effects of the pandemic was a reduction in overall hospital admissions, driven in part by the temporary suspension of non-urgent elective surgeries as the first wave of the pandemic took hold. This drop in admissions was sharpest in private hospitals – admissions to private hospitals dropped by 4.5% in 2019–20 compared to 1.7% for public hospitals (AIHW 2021b). Temporary suspensions of non-urgent elective surgery have continued to be utilised whenever confirmed SARS-CoV-2 cases have spiked in different states and territories.

The public sector has primarily dealt with the direct impacts of SARS-CoV-2. However, the private hospital sector has also been called on during acute phases of the pandemic. The ACCC relaxed anti-competition rules around cooperation between public and private hospitals during the pandemic to allow for coordinated action (ACCC 2020). The federal government further supported a cooperative response; on 31 March 2020, a deal with private hospitals was announced that would guarantee their financial viability in return for the availability of infrastructure, equipment, supplies, workforce and other resources, should the public sector become overwhelmed (Hunt 2020). This agreement was largely unused until the delta and omicron outbreaks in mid-2021 and the summer of 2021–22. The omicron outbreak in particular saw health care staff being furloughed to the public sector in many regions (ABC News 2022).

Tensions in the Public–Private Health Space

If we wish to understand the Australian health care system, questions need to be asked about whether the public and private systems in Australia are successfully complementary or in competition, whether the private sector actually creates capacity in the public sector, and how PHI membership levels might have an effect on public hospital waiting lists (and whether this is a positive or negative effect).

The usual argument for privatisation is that the profit motive creates incentives for cost-efficiency that are absent when services are publicly provided. However, profit motives can create other perverse incentives. For example, the fact that private hospitals typically charge on a per service basis, rather than outcome basis, can lead to some over-servicing and provision of low value care (Duckett & Nemet 2019). Private hospitals are also more likely to transfer out complex payments, a practice known as 'cream skimming' (Yang et al. 2020). Ultimately, the degree to which public and private hospitals are more or less cost efficient is an empirical one, and unfortunately not straightforward to resolve. One reason is that the mix of patients and procedures are very different between public and private hospitals, with public hospitals more likely to take on complex patients. Another issue is inconsistent accounting practices across sectors and incomplete data on private hospitals (Productivity Commission 2009). With these caveats in mind, a Productivity Commission report found that 'public and private hospitals had broadly similar costs per casemix-adjusted separation' (Productivity Commission, p. 112), although there were some differences in the composition of costs. Medical, prosthesis and diagnostic costs were found to be higher in the private sector, while nursing and other salaries, allied health, operating rooms and specialist suites, critical care, hotel costs, supplies, on-costs and capital costs were found to be higher in the public sector. A follow-up study (Forbes et al. 2010) found evidence that for-profit private hospitals were slightly more cost efficient than public hospitals. However, this conclusion was sensitive to how efficiency was defined, and the sample only included a subset of private acute hospitals. Overall, the limited evidence suggests public and private hospitals are similarly cost efficient.

Does the private hospital system take pressure off the public system? When patients use the private hospital system, this in theory frees up resources in the public sector, which should lead to benefits like shorter waiting times for surgeries. However, in practice longer waiting times are associated with a greater share of private hospital activity (Duckett et al. 2017). There are many potential explanations for this. For example, hospitals compete for a limited number of surgeons and medical staff (at least in the short-run), and an expanded private sector may attract staff away from the public sector. The association might also be related to **moral hazard**. Moral hazard occurs when a person has an incentive to increase an activity beyond its personal benefits because they do not bear the full cost. Studies have shown that PHI induces people to have more hospital admissions than they otherwise would (Kettlewell & Doiron 2018). The association may also be reverse-causal – people might seek out private care in regions with long waiting times precisely because of the long waiting times.

The key message is that it is highly uncertain whether additional private-sector care improves outcomes in the public sector. Moreover, any policy around public–private mix should be cognisant of both efficiency and *equity* concerns. People with PHI, or the means to pay for private care, have an expanded choice set compared to patients who rely solely on the public system. This is not inherently bad – it is reasonable that people should be allowed to use their income to invest in their own health. But it is also reasonable to question how much government policy should influence such a two-tiered system of care.

To finish this chapter, let us consider the policy question of government support for PHI. Government support for PHI is controversial. As Duckett et al. (2019) discuss, the case for government intervention is related to its purpose, which is a contested issue. On one side is the argument that PHI is merely a complement to public insurance. According to this view, PHI provides mostly private benefits to members as a kind of 'top up' to the public system. This is clearly true for general treatment cover. The other view is that PHI is a substitute for public insurance. This argument purports that PHI takes pressure off the public hospital system because people either use their PHI to receive treatment in a private hospital, rather than public, or they receive treatment in a public hospital as a private patient, so the insurer pays the bill.

In reality, PHI has elements of both a complement and substitute. When it comes to government support, the important question, from a purely economic efficiency perspective, is whether the substitution effect is large enough to justify the cost. The PHI rebate, for example, cost taxpayers $6.5 billion in 2020–21; approximately 7.3% of the federal government's health outlays. If the rebate were removed, this money could be redirected to the public hospital system. Key to whether the subsidy is self-financing is the degree to which people's demand for PHI is 'price sensitive'. Studies suggest people are not very sensitive to price (Duckett et al. 2019), which implies the rebate largely goes to people who would have purchased insurance anyway.

> **Pause *for* Reflection …**
> 1. Given the cost of the PHI subsidy, and its effects on the health care system, why do you think governments on both sides of politics continue to support it?
> 2. What effects might there be on the health system if the PHI rebate is removed and funds reallocated to public **hospitals**?

SUMMARY

This chapter has provided an overview of the private health care sector in Australia and some of the tensions between its growth and issues of cost, quality of health care, access and equity. Despite the existence of Medicare, a universal health insurance scheme that provides free public-hospital care, there continues to be strong demand for PHI in Australia, and private hospitals play a significant role in the provision of health care. However, prior to the SARS-CoV-2 pandemic participation in PHI had been declining and, with it, growth in the utilisation of private care. How these trends evolve in the future, and whether and how policy-makers will respond, is uncertain. Based on recent history, governments on both sides would appear reluctant to allow the private sector to lose share completely unchecked.

REVIEW QUESTIONS

1. What are some of the benefits, and the drawbacks, of a hybrid private–public health care system?
2. Does private health insurance provide meaningful choice?
3. Why do you think governments intervene in the private health insurance market?
4. Consider the arguments in Chapter 2 about the viability of Medicare. What do you think would be the effect on Medicare if people with private health insurance were able to opt out of paying the Medicare levy on condition that they used private health insurance or self-financed their care in public hospitals?
5. What role has the private hospital sector played in managing the SARS-CoV-2 pandemic? Has the pandemic influenced your views on the appropriate balance between public and private health care in Australia?

REFERENCES

ABC News, 2022. Private hospitals on standby to take patients as Omicron COVID-19 wave puts pressure on health system. 18 January 2022.

Australian Bureau of Statistics (ABS), 2018. Private hospitals, Australia. ABS, Canberra. https://www.abs.gov.au/statistics/health/health-services/private-hospitals-australia/2016-17.

Australian Competition and Consumer Commission (ACCC), 2020. Private and public hospitals can continue cooperating on COVID-19. ACCC Media Release No. 141/20, 9 July 2020.

Australian Competition and Consumer Commission (ACCC), 2021. Report to the Australian Senate on anti-competitive and other practices by health insurers and providers in relation to private health insurance. https://www.accc.gov.au/system/files/Private%20health%20insurance%20report%202020-21.pdf

Australian Institute of Health and Welfare (AIHW), 2014. Australia's health 2014. Australia's health series no. 14. Cat. no. AUS 178. AIHW, Canberra.

Australian Institute of Health and Welfare (AIHW), 2021a. Health expenditure Australia 2019–20. https://www.aihw.gov.au/reports/health-welfare-expenditure/health-expenditure-australia-2019-20.

Australian Institute of Health and Welfare (AIHW), 2021b. Hospital activity low during early months of COVID-19 pandemic. AIHW Media Release, 3 June 2021.

Australian Institute of Health and Welfare (AIHW), 2021c. Hospital resources 2019–20 tables. https://www.aihw.gov.au/getmedia/be85db73-a207-4291-8aa4-7149be9fd862/Hospital-resources-2019-20-data-tables-17-August-2021.xlsx.aspx.

Australian Prudential Regulation Authority (APRA), 2022a. Quarterly private health insurance statistics. https://www.apra.gov.au/quarterly-private-health-insurance-statistics.

Australian Prudential Regulation Authority (APRA), 2022b. Register of private health insurers. https://www.apra.gov.au/register-of-private-health-insurers.

Bai, T., Méndez, S., Scott, A., et al., 2020. The falling growth in the use of private hospitals in Australia. Melbourne Institute Working Paper No. 18/20/.

Brown, L., Barnett, J.R., 2004. Is the corporate transformation of hospitals creating a new hybrid health care space? A case study of the impact of co-location of public and private hospitals in Australia. Soc Sci Med 58, 427–444.

Buchmueller T.C., Fiebig, D., Jones, G., et al., 2013. Preference heterogeneity and selection in private health insurance: The case of Australia. J Health Econ 32, 757–767.

Collyer, F.M., McMaster, J., Wettenhall, R.W., 2001. Public enterprise divestment: Australian case studies. University of South Pacific Press, Fiji.

Collyer, F.M., White, K.N., 2001. Corporate control of healthcare in Australia. Discussion paper no. 42, Australia Institute, Australian National University, Canberra.

Collyer, F.M., Harley, K., Short, S.D., 2015. Money and markets in Australia's healthcare system. In: Meagher, G., Goodwin, S. (Eds.), Markets, Rights and Power in Australian Social Policy. Sydney University Press, Sydney, pp. 257–291.

Doiron, D., Kettlewell, N., 2018. The effect of health insurance on the substitution between public and private hospital care. The Economic Record, 94 (305), 135–154.

Duckett, S., 2013. Public–private hospital partnerships are risky business. The Conversation, 30 July. https://theconversation.com/public-private-hospital-partnerships-are-risky-business-16421.

Duckett, S., Moran, G., Danks, L., 2017. Making health care more affordable and effective for both taxpayers and patients. Grattan Institute submission to the Senate Community Affairs References Committee inquiry into the value and affordability of private health insurance and out-of-pocket medical costs.

Duckett, S., Cowgill, M., Nemet, K., 2019. Saving private health 2: Making private health insurance viable. Grattan Institute.

Duckett, S., Nemet, K., 2019. Saving private health 1: reining in hospital costs and specialist bills. Grattan Institute.

Forbes, M., Harslett, P., Mastoris, I., Risse, L., 2010. Measuring the technical efficiency of public and private hospitals in Australia. Paper presented at the Australian Conference of Economists, Sydney, September 27–29 2010.

Hunt, G., 2020. Australian Government partnership with private health sector secures 30,000 hospital beds and 105,000 nurses and staff, to help fight COVID-19 pandemic. Minister for Health Media Release, 1 April 2020.

Lewis, S., Collyer, F., Willis, K., et al., 2018. Healthcare in the news media: The privileging of private over public. J Sociol 54 (4), 574–590.

Lewis, S., Willis, K., Olsen, R.E., 2019. If you've got private health insurance, the choice to use it in a public hospital is your own. The Conversation, 15 March. https://theconversation.com/if-youve-got-private-health-insurance-the-choice-to-use-it-in-a-public-hospital-is-your-own-113367.

Productivity Commission, 1999. Private hospitals in Australia, Commission research paper. AusInfo, Canberra. https://www.pc.gov.au/research/completed/private-hospitals/privatehospitals.pdf.

Productivity Commission, 2009. Public and private hospitals, research report. Canberra.

Richardson, A., 2021. Private general hospitals in Australia. IBISWorld AU Industry (ANZSIC) Report Q8401b.

Seah, D., Cheong, T., Anstey, M., 2013. The hidden cost of private health insurance in Australia. Aust Health Rev 37 (1), 1–3.

Shamsulla A., 2011. Australia's private health insurance industry: structure, competition, regulation and role in a less than 'ideal world'. Aust Health Rev 35 (1), 23–31.

Shmuelli. A., Savage, E., 2014. Private and public patients in public hospitals in Australia. Health Policy. 115, 189–195.

Willis, K., Collyer, F., Lewis, S., et al., 2016. Knowledge matters: producing and using knowledge to navigate healthcare systems. Health Sociol Rev 25 (2), 202–216.

Yang, O., Chan, M.K., Cheng, T.C., et al., 2020. Cream skimming: Theory and evidence from hospital transfers and capacity utilization. J Econ Behav Org 173, 68–87.

Zhang, Y., Prakash, K., 2021. Why do Australians buy private hospital insurance? Melbourne Institute: Research Highlights No. 06/21.

FURTHER READING

Australian Institute of Health and Welfare (AIHW), 2022. Australia's health 2022: in brief. Canberra: AIHW.

Duckett, S., Stobart, A., 2021. 4 ways to fix private health insurance so it can sustain a growing, ageing population. The Conversation, 19 May. https://theconversation.com/4-ways-to-fix-private-health-insurance-so-it-can-sustain-a-growing-ageing-population-161171.

ONLINE RESOURCES

Australian Institute of Health and Welfare (AIHW) – collects data on hospital funding and separations for both public and private hospitals: https://www.aihw.gov.au/reports-data/myhospitals.

Australian Prudential Regulation Authority (APRA; formerly Private Health Insurance Administration Council, PHIAC) – regulates (from July 2015) the private health insurance industry in Australia; the site includes reports and statistics on PHI in Australia: https://ww.apra.gov.au.

Private Hospital Data Bureau (PHDB) – collects data on all private hospital separations; the site includes reports and data tables on private hospitals: https://www1.health.gov.au/internet/main/publishing.nsf/Content/health-casemix-data-collections-about-PHDB.

4

International Health Care Systems

Judith Daire, Delia Hendrie and Suzanne Robinson

KEY LEARNING OUTCOMES

When you finish this chapter you should be able to:
- define the key concepts related to international health care systems
- discuss how health care systems are organised, how they operate and what they aim to achieve
- distinguish and compare types and performance of health care system models

- examine key driving factors for the current health system strengthening efforts to improve health system performance and outcomes
- understand future challenges for health care systems.

KEY TERMS AND ABBREVIATIONS

activity-based funding (ABF)
bipartisan agreement
electronic health record (EHR)
Health Care Home (HCH)
health care system
health care system performance
health financing
health security
health system
health system strengthening (HSS)

market-driven health care system
Millennium Development Goals (MDGs)
national health insurance (NHI) model
Patient Centered Medical Home (PCMH)
payment for performance (P4P)
private health insurance (PHI) model

public health insurance
resilience
Sustainable Development Goals (SDGs)
social health insurance (SHI)
universal health coverage (UHC)
welfare health care system
World Health Organization (WHO)

INTRODUCTION

This chapter considers **health care systems** around the world. It aims to compare international health care systems. First, the chapter applies the World Health Organization (WHO) Health System Building Block Framework to describe how international health care systems are generally organised, how they function and what they aim to achieve. The chapter will then discuss the types of health system models, the international health system strengthening efforts and the driving factors. Finally, the chapter will compare the performance of health systems in different countries and examine implications for future policy directions to improve health care systems in Australia and beyond.

Definition of the Key Concepts

The terms 'health system, healthcare system, healthcare delivery system, health service delivery system, medical care system, health sector, and health services organisations' are used interchangeably (Papanicolas et al. 2022, p. 13). Although they all define characteristics of a system, they differ in that some have more inclusive, or wider, connotations than others. A system generally refers to a collection of parts that interact together and function as a whole (Scanlon 2021). In a narrower sense, a **health system** is seen as an institution of 'health care', where *health care* refers to organised social actions in response to the occurrence of disease and disability, and for averting the risks to health (Jarvis et al. 2020). In a broader sense, the health system is viewed as including more than just health services, encompassing activities falling beyond the general scope of the health sector (sanitation, nutrition, housing, transport, education, etc.), which affect the health of the population (WHO 2019). It is this more inclusive definition that will be used in this chapter, adopted from the health system

definition used by the **World Health Organization (WHO)**. This broad definition includes efforts to influence determinants of health as well as more direct health-improving activities. For a more detailed definition of related concepts, see Box 4.1. What all definitions have in common is that health care systems are complex and involve a number of different institutions, organisations and professions (Shaw et al. 2018).

ORGANISATION, FUNCTIONS AND GOALS OF HEALTH CARE SYSTEMS

Health systems have multiple goals and to achieve their goals, all health systems carry out some basic functions, regardless of how they are organised and where they operate. They provide services; develop health workers and other key resources; mobilise and allocate finances and ensure health system leadership and governance

---

BOX 4.1 Definition of a Health System and the Related Concepts

Health care system: an organised plan of health services. The term is usually used to refer to the system or program by which health care is made available to the population and financed by government, private enterprise, or both.

Health care system performance: includes the three dimensions of accessibility, quality and efficiency. Together these determine the extent to which the achievable in health care can be attained. Health system performance refers to how far health systems achieve each of these goals relative to the country's overall context.

Health financing: refers to how financial resources are mobilised, allocated and used to ensure that the health system can adequately cover the collective health needs of every person.

Health security: the existence of strong and resilient public health systems that can prevent, detect and respond to infectious disease threats, wherever they occur in the world.

Health system: consists of all organisations, people and actions whose primary intent is to promote, restore or maintain health. This includes efforts to influence determinants of health as well as more direct health-improving activities (WHO 2007).

Public Health Insurance: (in the USA) a program run by US federal, state, or local governments in which people

have some or all of their healthcare costs paid for by the government. The two main types of public health insurance are Medicare and Medicaid.

Resilience (of the health system): the capacity of health actors, institutions and populations to prepare for and effectively respond to crises; maintain core functions when a crisis hits; and, informed by lessons learned during the crisis, reorganise if conditions require it. Health systems are resilient if they protect human life and produce good health outcomes for all during a crisis and in its aftermath.

Social health insurance: a scheme initiated by the government to serve as a source of revenue for health financing to decrease the out-of-pocket burden on the people.

Universal health coverage (UHC): Universal health coverage means that all people have access to the health services they need, when and where they need them, without financial hardship. It includes the full range of essential health services, from health promotion to prevention, treatment, rehabilitation and palliative care.

Welfare health care systems: The provision of services for the whole population that highlight the ability of the health system to reach the entire population with the available health care services.

Source: World Health Organization (WHO) (2007). Everybody's business – strengthening health systems to improve health outcomes: WHO's framework for action. https://apps.who.int/iris/handle/10665/43918.

(also known as stewardship, which is about oversight and guidance of the whole system). The functions of health systems are broken down into a set of six essential 'building blocks' (Sacks et al. 2019). All are needed to improve outcomes, as outlined by the WHO's health system framework shown in Fig. 4.1.

1. *Leadership and governance* involve ensuring strategic policy frameworks exist and are combined with effective oversight, coalition building, the provision of appropriate regulations and incentives, attention to system-design and accountability.

2. *A good health financing system* raises adequate funds for health, in ways that ensure people can use needed services, and are protected from financial catastrophe or impoverishment associated with having to pay for them.

3. *A well-performing health workforce* refers to the sufficient numbers and mix of staff, fairly distributed; they are competent, responsive and productive.

4. *A well-functioning health system* ensures equitable access to essential medical products, vaccines and technologies of assured quality, safety, efficacy and cost-effectiveness, and their scientifically sound and cost-effective use.

5. *A well-functioning health information system* is one that ensures the production, analysis, dissemination, and use of reliable and timely information on health determinants, health systems performance and health status.

6. *Good health services* are those which deliver effective, safe, quality personal and non-personal health interventions available for those who need them, when and where needed, with minimum waste of resources.

The building blocks provide a useful way of clarifying essential health system elements and their functions, but how well they function hinges on the interdependence of each building block and integrated action towards achieving the overall outcomes and goals. Health systems have multiple goals; improving population health remains the ultimate goal but it is not enough in itself. There is an expectation that the overall goal of a health system is to improve population health by being responsive to the needs of its citizens, while being financially fair in the delivery of the best, or most efficient, care (Kumah et al. 2020).

As the foundation of health care delivery system, there is a growing commitment over the years to achieve health for all through **universal health coverage (UHC)** (Ghebreyesus 2020). UHC means that all people have access to the health services they need, when and where they need them, without financial hardship (Tumusiime et al. 2020, p. 2). UHC has gained political commitment at an international level in view of health as both a right and an important factor for sustainable development

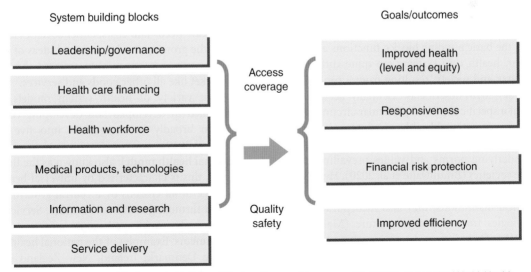

Figure 4.1 The Health System Building Blocks. *Source:* Manyazewal T. (2017). Using the World Health Organization health system building blocks through survey of healthcare professionals to determine the performance of public healthcare facilities. Arch Public Health 75 (50), 2.

(Chapman 2016). The focus on UHC represents governments' efforts to maintain the health gains achieved during the **Millennium Development Goals (MDGs)** era and accelerate progress towards the long-term health system goals embodied by **Sustainable Development Goals (SDGs)** (Tumusiime et al. 2020).

The progress to operationalise and attain UHC at country level has been slowed down by challenges posed by the SARS-CoV-2 pandemic, hence testing the resilience of health systems to external shocks and threatening health security. The view of UHC and health security as two sides of one coin (Ghebreyesus 2020) underpins the renewed call for strong and resilient health systems as the vehicle through which countries can best prepare for, respond to and recover from the negative impacts of health emergencies (Wenham et al. 2019; Ibeneme et al. 2020).

Pause *for* Reflection ...

Consider how well the Australian health system performs in relation to the WHO building blocks. Which health system elements that are not included in these building blocks have been key in determining health system performance in Australia? Why do you think they are not included in the WHO building blocks? How has COVID-19 affected the health system in Australia?

NATIONAL HEALTH CARE SYSTEM MODELS OR TYPOLOGIES

Although the basic building blocks, functions and goals are similar, health care systems are quite different in each country and society, resulting from a process that Klinga et al. (2018) describe as essentially 'accidental', a product of a specific time and particular circumstances. The variation in national health care systems is strongly influenced by the economic and political systems as well as the underlying norms and values prevailing in the respective societies (Braithwaite et al. 2020). Health care systems are not only organised around social structures and political institutions; they also incorporate values and ideologies from the larger culture (Mannion & Davies 2018). These factors determine what constitutes health problems worthy of government attention in specific country contexts; the type of health care service packages to address the identified health problems (Bacchi 2016). At the same time, the design of the health

system as a solution to the prevailing health problems in a country can also perpetuate problems such as inequalities in access to health care, poverty resulting from catastrophic health expenditure, infections due to poor infection prevention practices or treatment errors, just to mention a few. Consequently, the state of national health systems in terms of what they constitute, what they do and what they achieve often reflects political institutions, prevailing power imbalances and dominant perspectives. Understandings of what health is and how it should be improved are deeply rooted in social values, ideologies from larger society and cultural norms, and expectations of the citizenry.

The contextual differences also explain why health care systems vary considerably in how they are funded and administered and in how medical services are distributed. Generally, health care systems may be thought of as being either:

- **welfare based** – a public system where the government provides the health care system for all citizens, or
- **market-driven** – a private system where the services are run by private providers, and citizens pay for their own health care.

Welfare-based health care systems are predominantly underpinned by the principles of solidarity, where the cost of care in a country is subsidised across population age groups and levels of income. In welfare-based health care systems, health care is primarily viewed as a social or collective good, and all citizens benefit, irrespective of health care needs and costs. Other societies are influenced by the growing market-oriented ideas of perceiving health care as a commodity accessed through the open market like all other goods and services.

A great variety of health system models can be distinguished in developed and developing countries. These can broadly be categorised into five models (Hasanovna 2019):

- **National health model:** also known as the Beveridge model, this is characterised by universal health care coverage of all citizens by a central government, financed through general tax revenues. Service distribution and provider payments are controlled by governments. Examples of the national health model include Denmark, Ireland, New Zealand and the United Kingdom.
- **Social insurance model:** also known as the Bismarck model, this is characterised by compulsory coverage

that is funded by employer, individual and private insurance funds. Factors of production are controlled and owned by government or private entities. It is also referred to as tax-based insurance. Funding is derived from employment taxes and held in separate funds specifically for the national health program. Examples of the social insurance model include Austria, Belgium, France, Germany, Luxemburg and the Netherlands.

- **National health insurance (NHI) model**: this system has elements of both Beveridge and Bismarck. It uses private-sector providers, but payment comes from a government-run insurance program that every citizen pays into. The classic NHI system is found in Canada, but some newly industrialised countries – Taiwan and South Korea, for example – have also adopted the NHI model.
- **Private health insurance (PHI) model**: this model is characterised by employment-based or individual purchase of private health insurance financed by individual and employer contributions. Service delivery and financing are owned and managed by the private entities operating in an open market economy. Examples of the private insurance model include Switzerland and the United States.
- **Out-of-pocket model**: though not formally recognised, this model is prevalent in countries which are still developing their national health care systems towards an organised mass medical care health care system. For example, in many developing countries, consumers tend to pay for services out of pocket, which is associated with catastrophic health expenditure. If they cannot pay, they do not get medical care.

No country has a pure form of one health system model; instead, most countries have mixed models where two or more models may coexist. National health systems are therefore characterised by the dominant model at one time. The way health care system models are funded determines the pathway to universal health coverage (Hasanovna 2019). Countries with national health insurance (i.e. the UK) that's fully funded by the government (single payer) are generally better able to provide universal access to health care. Some countries, such as Germany, France and Japan, employ a multi-payer system to achieve UHC. In countries with a multiple-payer system and without national health insurance, not everyone has coverage. A lack of health coverage also exists in countries where national health

care infrastructure is not well established and/or funding for health care is predominantly out of pocket. Thus, no government options exist to offer people coverage and access to services is limited. See Fig. 4.2 for an infographic summarising health care system models and how well they offer universal coverage for the population.

Pause *for* Reflection ...

Considering the different health care system models, how do you think each of these impacts on health care access for disadvantaged population groups? What might this mean for their health care outcomes? What new funding models can countries explore to complement the existing ones to achieve universal health coverage?

HEALTH SYSTEM STRENGTHENING AND THE DRIVING FACTORS

More recently, governments have deliberately implemented changes to strengthen performance of their health care systems and improve population health outcomes as a response to prevailing organisational and contextual changes (Ghebreyesus 2020). Advocated as a means for progressing towards UHC, **health system strengthening (HSS)** refers to significant and purposeful effort to improve the system's performance. It includes any initiatives that aim to improve one or more of the health system's building blocks and that leads to better health through improvements in health system performance (Papanicolas 2022). In line with the global vison of resilient health systems for UHC, countries are addressing the attributes of high-performing health systems – quality, efficiency, equity, accountability, sustainability and resilience – in their national policies and plans of ongoing HSS efforts (see Fig. 4.3).

Emerging lessons from different countries propose future HSS efforts that take a whole-of-systems approach with more integrated primary health care service delivery that places individuals, families and communities at the centre of HSS efforts (Witter et al. 2019). Literature on country experiences also shows the urgent need to accelerate progress in strengthening health systems, through reforms that improve security and resilience to current and future health system challenges and threats like the SARS-CoV-2 pandemic (WHO 2021).

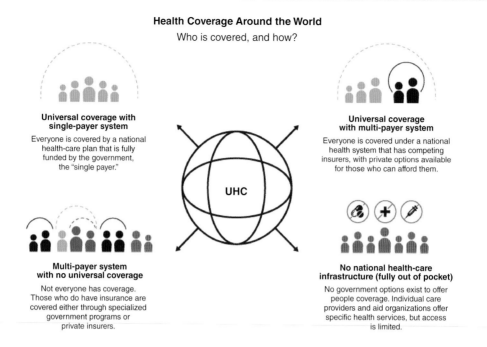

Health Coverage Around the World

Who is covered, and how?

Universal coverage with single-payer system

Everyone is covered by a national health-care plan that is fully funded by the government, the "single payer."

Universal coverage with multi-payer system

Everyone is covered under a national health system that has competing insurers, with private options available for those who can afford them.

UHC

Multi-payer system with no universal coverage

Not everyone has coverage. Those who do have insurance are covered either through specialized government programs or private insurers.

No national health-care infrastructure (fully out of pocket)

No government options exist to offer people coverage. Individual care providers and aid organizations offer specific health services, but access is limited.

Figure 4.2 Models of Health Care Systems and Health Coverage Around the World. *Source*: Health Economic Forum (2020). Healthcare system models and how they work. https://www.weforum.org/agenda/2020/10/covid-19-healthcare-health-service-vaccine-health-insurance-pandemic/.

Besides the SARS-CoV-2 pandemic, several driving factors have led to governments' commitment to implement reforms that aim to strengthen their health systems for improved performance and health outcomes. They include changing and growing health service demands driven by population mobility and population growth; environmental pressures from natural and human-induced disasters; emergence of new diseases and re-emergence of previously controlled diseases; growth of non-communicable diseases (NCDs); and higher populations' expectations and/or preferences for quality health services. Along with new medical technologies and inadequate preventive measures, these pressures contribute to the rising cost of health care. The impact of these driving factors and corresponding HSS strategies by governments is dependent on context. Case study 4.1 discusses driving factors for HSS from countries in the Western Pacific region.

Pause *for* Reflection ...

Consider the mixed health care system model in Australia as outlined in Chapters 2 and 3. How is the government strengthening the health system to achieve UHC? Think about the health system changes that have happened over the last 20 years to address health needs of at-risk populations. Identify the main driving factors that led to the changes.

HEALTH CARE SYSTEM PERFORMANCE

A key concern of governments and others who invest in health systems is how to tell whether and when the desired improvements in **health care system performance** and population health outcomes are being achieved. It is not easy to compare health system performance due to different processes, structures, institutions and organisation of health care systems. Nevertheless, agencies have developed standardised ways of comparing health system performance across countries and regions. For example, the Commonwealth Fund accesses and compares performance of health care systems across 11 Organisation for Economic Co-operation and Development (OECD) countries (Schneider et al. 2021). The key performance areas of interest relate to quality, access,

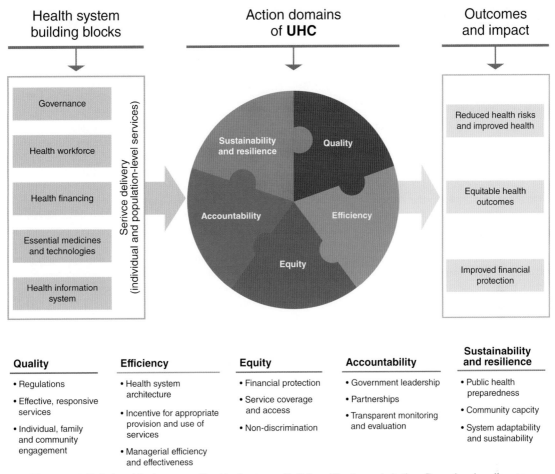

Figure 4.3 Relationship between Health Systems Building Blocks and Action Domains Leading to UHC. *Source*: WHO (2016). Universal health coverage: moving towards better health: action framework for the Western Pacific Region. World Health Organization Regional Office for the Western Pacific, Manila, Philippines, p. 2.

efficiency, equity and healthy lives. See Table 4.1 for the 2021 health care system performance rankings in OECD countries.

Overall, Norway, the Netherlands and Australia are the top performing countries with the United Sates ranking last. The US ranks last on access to care, administrative efficiency, equity and health care outcomes, but second on measures of care process. The next three countries in the ranking are the UK, Germany and New Zealand. Though both sets of countries are ranked similarly in their categories, they perform differently as shown by scores for each indicator. Health systems perform differently because, over time, countries have unique mixes of policies, service delivery systems and financing models in

line with political governance and available resources for health (Schneider et al. 2021). Approaches vary significantly even among high-income countries that have options to spend more on health care. These choices affect health system performance in terms of access to care, patients' experiences with health care and people's health outcomes. Four features that distinguish top-performing countries from those not performing well include: (1) provision of universal coverage and removal of cost barriers, (2) investment in primary health care systems to ensure availability and equitable distribution of essential health care services to all people, (3) reduced administrative burdens that divert time, efforts and spending from health improvement efforts, and (4) investment in social

CASE STUDY 4.1   Driving Factors for HSS from Countries in Western Pacific Region

The Western Pacific Region, a home to one-quarter of the world's population, is undergoing economic transition, which is creating tremendous change in health. Globalisation, urbanisation, technological innovation, environmental change and shifting demographics are creating opportunities that make better health possible. But these same forces are also increasing the complexity of health problems and complicating the process of developing and implementing solutions. There has been significant progress made in reaching the Millennium Development Goals (MDGs) for child health and communicable diseases. Many countries and areas in the Western Pacific Region expected to achieve their 2015 targets. For example, HIV incidence decreased in Cambodia, Malaysia, Papua New Guinea and Vietnam, and tuberculosis targets were also reached. Compared to other regions, the Western Pacific Region was on track to achieve nearly all of the health-related MDGs (WHO 2014a).

Sustaining the gains made and addressing new challenges, such as non-communicable diseases (NCDs), viral hepatitis, antimicrobial resistance and ageing populations, have been shown to be equally important in recent years. For example, the major NCDs represent more than 80% of all deaths in the Region, while the top 10 countries with the highest rate of diabetes globally are in the Pacific

(WHO 2014b). In addition, over 100 million people suffer from mental disorders in the Region, with 500 suicides occurring per day in the Region (WHO 2014b). Health systems in the Region are increasingly challenged to provide all people with access to quality health services that do not leave anyone vulnerable to financial hardship from personally paying for needed health care.

In the Asia-Pacific region, an estimated 105 million people suffer financial catastrophe, and more than 70 million are impoverished, because of health care costs (WHO 2009). Many countries are still heavily reliant on out-of-pocket payments to finance their health systems. Moreover, 900 million people in the Western Pacific live on less than US$ 2 a day (Asian Development Bank and World Trade Organization 2011). These individuals and families have no or little access to health care. For many countries in the Region, per capita government allocations for health remain low. This situation can push large numbers of households into poverty due to ill health and out-of-pocket spending for health care. In addition, these factors threaten to impede economic progress and may even reverse recent gains in development status. In the Pacific, countries face economic volatility with significant portions of their funding coming from donors.

Source: WHO (2016). Universal health coverage: moving towards better health: action framework for the Western Pacific Region. World Health Organization Regional Office for the Western Pacific, Manila, Philippines, pp. 3–5. https://apps.who.int/iris/handle/10665/246420.

TABLE 4.1   Health System Performance Rankings in OECD Countries

	AUS	CAN	FRA	GER	NETH	NZ	NOR	SWE	SWIZ	UK	US
Overall ranking	**3**	**10**	**8**	**5**	**2**	**6**	**1**	**7**	**9**	**4**	**11**
Access to care	8	9	7	3	1	5	2	6	10	4	11
Care process	6	4	10	9	3	1	8	11	7	5	2
Administrative efficiency	2	7	6	9	8	3	1	5	10	4	11
Equity	1	10	7	2	5	9	8	6	3	4	11
Health care outcomes	1	10	6	7	4	8	2	5	3	9	11

Source: Schneider, E.C., Shah, A., Doty, M.M., et al. (2021). Mirror, mirror 2021 — reflecting poorly: health care in the US compared to other high-income countries. Commonwealth Fund, New York, p. 3. https://www.commonwealthfund.org/publications/fund-reports/2021/aug/mirror-mirror-2021-reflecting-poorly.

services, especially for children and working-age adults (Schneider et al. 2021, p. 3).

Comparing international health system performance offers learning opportunities to understand principles that underpin performing health care systems. For example, the main difference between the US and UK systems relates to the differences around market-driven and welfare health care systems (Glover & Woods 2020). That is, the US system is founded on market-driven values and a culture that has been characterised by a respect for individualism and entrepreneurship (Health Economic Forum 2020). The UK health care system was shaped by notions of equality and equity – quite different values to those that underpinned the US health care system. However, in recent times the UK system has moved towards more market-based principles around competition and incentive-driven provision of care in line with the ideas of new public management outlined in Chapter 1. The UK system remains underpinned by the principle of universal access to health care with a mixture of market-based approaches to ensure efficient administrative health system performance.

Described as a complex 'web' of services, providers, recipients and organisational structures, Australia's health care system falls somewhere in the middle, combining features similar to the US and the UK health care systems. For example, when Australia introduced a universal health insurance system in the 1970s, it followed the same principles that underpinned the UK NHS, but funded practitioners on a fee-for-service basis and allowed people the freedom to select their provider without needing to register with any particular gatekeeper (Tikkanen et al. 2020). It appears, however, that the UK and the US are now taking on a number of elements from the Australian health care system. Both countries are moving towards health care systems characterised by a public–private mix such as that of Australia. The question then becomes: how public or how private should the system be?

Comparing countries' health care system performance using standardised performance data also offers benchmarks and useful insights about alternative approaches to delivering health care and building better health systems that yield better health outcomes (Tikkanen et al. 2020). For example, lessons from the three top-performing country health systems outlined – Norway, the Netherlands and Australia – can inform the USA and other countries seeking to improve their health system performance and population health outcomes. As the SARS-CoV-2 pandemic has sufficiently shown, no nation has the perfect health system. Health care is a work in progress; the science continues to advance, creating new opportunities and challenges. But by learning from what has and has not worked elsewhere in the world, all countries can try out new policies and practices that may move them closer to the ideal of a health system that achieves optimal health for all its people at a price the nation can afford (Schneider et al. 2021).

> **Pause _for_ Reflection …**
> Consider the following:
> - What do you consider to be the major contributing factors to health system performance?
> - In comparing the UK and the USA to Australia, what are the key differences in both funding and government involvement?
> - What relationship does health expenditure in the UK, USA and Australia have on health status and outcomes?
> - How well do the health systems of these countries perform in terms of life expectancy or morbidity or mortality rates?
> - What organisations portray these statistics and why do we need to know this information?
> - How should health expenditure be controlled?

Health System Performance and the Influencing Factors

The performance of health systems is affected by several aspects relating to the _hardware_ and _software_ of the system as an organisation. The hardware relates to organisational and structural aspects (legal, financing structures) as well as clinical and service delivery aspects (Shatrov et al. 2021). The software includes the norms, values, culture and traditions of institutions (Scanlon 2021). As noted above, the US health system has a much more individualistic and market-based perspective on health care than the UK – the NHS encompasses a more egalitarian perspective that provides universal access and a notion that health care should be available to all regardless of wealth (Health Economic Forum 2020). These different perspectives underpin both the hardware and the software elements of the US and UK health systems and are interlinked (Hasanovna 2019). Whereas the UK system is funded by taxation, the funding distribution mechanisms have taken on a more market-based approach and have moved from block funding (which tends to be based on historical patterns of funding) to **activity-based funding (ABF)** (which focuses on **payment for performance (P4P)**).

This approach has been adopted by a number of countries and is aimed at increasing efficiencies in the health system (Valentelyte et al. 2021). However, evidence for its effectiveness relating to efficiency and other aspects is mixed. What we do know is that ABF, along with other efficiency measures, seems to have increased awareness of the cost of health interventions.

However, ABF can limit system reform, especially when such reform means that services may need to change or reduce activity. The limiting factor of payment for performance is that it rewards activity without consideration for equity and effectiveness (Islam 2019). In Australia, we have seen a shift in focus to include ABF in the hospital setting; although this could go some way to increasing the awareness of costs and potential efficiency savings, it does need to be considered alongside other policies that reward effectiveness and equity considerations (Global Access Partners 2019).

Another difference between Australia and the UK is in the government structure. The UK has a single, centralised government system while Australia has two tiers of government concerned with health: the Commonwealth and state governments. In Australia, the health services (hospitals) are the business of state governments, with different hardware and software dimensions existing across them, while the business of primary care, such as GP services, tends to sit with the Commonwealth Government (Glover & Woods 2020). This adds even more complexity to the system and can make system integration even more problematic. (See Chapter 2 for an example of this problem, sometimes referred to as the 'blame game'.) Internationally, evidence shows that it is very difficult to change the organisation and mechanism of health systems once established. In terms of Australia, it is unlikely that changes to the tiers of government will be made any sooner, rendering health system reform problematic. Lessons from other countries demonstrate a need for **bipartisan agreement** across different governments (state and national) and with opposition parties, so that more joined-up approaches to the design, development and implementation of health system reform can be undertaken.

FUTURE DIRECTIONS AND CHALLENGES FOR HEALTH CARE SYSTEMS

Globally health systems face similar issues and challenges – including changing demographics with an ageing population that has more chronic and complex health needs, a rise in technological advances that are costly to implement, a rise in resistance to antibiotics and the spread of infectious diseases. These challenges are complex, requiring responses that involve a number of different stakeholder groups who often have very different values and cultures and different interests and perspectives.

Ageing and Non-Communicable Diseases (NCDs)

The increasing prevalence of chronic conditions is placing unprecedented demand on health care systems globally and is a priority for action (Kämpfen et al. 2018). How we manage chronic disease has seen a push to provide services outside of the hospital settings and out into primary care, the focus being a better understanding of health determinants, risk factors and multiple morbidities combined with a reorientation of current health funding and delivering services through better design. For example, derived from the Chronic Care Model, the concept of patients having a Medical Home to manage their primary health care needs has been widely supported across the United States through the **Patient Centered Medical Home (PCMH)** model (Metusela et al. 2020). Australia's **Health Care Home (HCH)** model has been adapted from the PCMH to address the complex health care needs of people living with chronic conditions within a different fiscal environment (Department of Health 2020). The concept of medical homes links to the principles of patient-centred, comprehensive and coordinated care through integrated services. Its prime focus is to reduce spending while simultaneously improving quality as there is strong evidence internationally that integrated health systems with a strong focus on primary care will produce more efficient outcomes than fragmented systems. Such integration can be difficult given the power of hospitals and the different professional groups in the health system.

Role of the Consumer and Technology

The success of providing patient-centred, integrated and coordinated care is reliant on developing technology and the role of the consumer. We have seen a paradigm shift in how people access health care and the role of social media, social networks and digital communities (see Chapter 16). There has been an upsurge in digital health with consumers progressively taking control of their health information and being involved in managing their own health care. In many countries consumers now have access to their personally controlled **electronic health record (EHR)** and new opportunities exist as a result of wearable apps and interactive systems enabling health service delivery to be managed in their own homes (Labrique et al. 2018). This is vital to achieving the health reform many systems desire, but here in Australia there continue to be major trust issues between consumers and governments on who should have access to this data or how this data should be used. This then results in a fragmentation of the use of personally controlled EHRs, particularly in an Australian health care context, in spite of the evidence that suggests improvements in both patient engagement and health care outcomes (AIHW 2022).

Moving from Volume to Value

Many health care systems around the globe have a dominant fee-for-service model and this incentivises over-provision of services, which contributes nothing to improving health. We are seeing a shift in focus from rewarding activity and volume to models that reward value and effective patient outcomes (Institute of Healthcare Improvement 2019). The work by Piña, Allen and Desai (2021) suggests that if the focus and goals of health systems are to provide high-quality care, and if this is realised, then this will lead to efficiency savings. This suggests that, in Australia, consideration needs to be given to how to incorporate incentives to reward outcomes that focus on value and quality (Hall et al. 2021). This will require a shift in thinking by many health care systems that will need to continue to reduce waste and unnecessary variation, changing health care delivery models using data more effectively to drive the change and engaging with all stakeholders to transform health care systems to providing economically sustainable quality care.

Governance and Stewardship Leadership

Although effective policy is important to system reform, it is cultures and behaviours that shape the system, and as such they will have considerable impact on the development and implementation of health policy (Yeoh et al. 2019). Shifting mindsets and changing culture is a major challenge for system integration, especially in systems like Australia that have privileged silo-based working (Glover & Woods 2020). Reform of this nature will require effective leadership that can navigate the complex system and its different organisations and powerful professions. Bigdeli et al. (2020) emphasise the importance of taking a collective leadership approach, rather than traditional command and control structures; they suggest that the former will 'provide the optimum basis for caring cultures'.

Workforce Challenges

Health workforce recruitment and retention continues to be an issue for many countries, with a global shortage of health workers (Hines et al. 2020), which means the pool of workers is less and migration of workers across countries is impacted. Attracting and retaining health professionals is often more difficult for rural and remote settings compared to well-resourced urban centres. Such staff shortages can lead to challenges for both equity and access of health services, along with impacts on quality of health care. There are a number of studies that have looked at retention strategies and these need to be considered at both national and international levels with policies and legislation being focused on addressing this problem (Hines et al. 2020).

Current and Future Pandemics

The impacts of the COVID-19 pandemic will have profound implications for health systems for years to come. These include the impacts of long COVID on longer term health outcomes, evidence of which is currently limited. The impacts of COVID-19 on mental health and well-being will require a focus on access to appropriate mental health services across education systems, workplaces and health systems (OECD 2021). The impact of the COVID-19 pandemic on non-communicable disease (NCD) related morbidity and mortality will have long-term implications for population health and well-being. Kluge et al. (2020) note that the stress of the COVID-19 pandemic, through restrictions, economic situations and changes to normal health behaviour coupled with the postponement of routine medical appointments and services for those with and at risk of NCDs, could increase the prevalence and incidence of NCDs. Going forward, health systems will need to adapt to support and manage the increased risk for those with underlying chronic conditions and those at increased risk of developing them. The challenge will be to support public health measures that go beyond health services and incorporate the policies focused on the broader social determinants of health.

> **Pause *for* Reflection …**
> * What are the dominant and powerful professions in health care systems? Give reasons for your answers.
> * Who are the dominant stakeholder groups in health care systems? Why?
> * Are there any differences in these groups between the UK, the USA and Australia? If so, what are they and what could be the reasons for this?
> * What are the three biggest challenges, in your view, facing the Australian health care system now and into the future? Why?

SUMMARY

In this chapter we focus on the different systems of health care found worldwide.

- This included a brief description of what we mean by a health system, including the goals, elements and characteristics of international health systems.
- Health systems have similar building blocks but differ in the way they are organised, funded, function and perform based on a number of factors, including a society's views, values and cultures; we have also seen that future policy reforms are often influenced by past choices.
- The chapter explored the performance of systems and compared two very different health system models – that of a predominantly market-based model (US) and a predominantly public-based model (UK).
- Four features distinguish top-performing countries: (1) they provide for universal coverage and remove cost barriers, (2) they invest in primary care systems to ensure that high-value services are equitably available in all communities to all people, (3) they reduce administrative burdens that divert time, efforts and spending from health improvement efforts and (4) they invest in social services, especially for children and working-age adults.

- International lessons for Australia include that, although systems strive for efficiency, policies that reward activity can actually have a negative impact on efficiency, and we are seeing a number of systems moving from a focus on volume to one on value and patient experience.
- International policy directions are shifting to more integrated systems of care that focus on the whole patient experience – this involves breaking down the traditional silos and power structures.
- It is early days in terms of this policy direction; however, early evidence suggests that system integration will require policies that incentivise this type of approach and have access to data that can measure performance and governance. It will also require effective leadership, throughout the system, that can motivate and drive change.
- Finally, Australia has much to learn from other countries while also having much to offer – policy-makers need to look to international evidence and consider how this evidence translates to their own health system setting.

REVIEW QUESTIONS

1. Is it possible to have a health service that is free for all? Give reasons for why or why not in your answer.
2. Discuss whether health care is a *right* or a *commodity*. Should health care be treated like a commodity and traded in the marketplace? Give reasons for your answers.
3. What characteristics would you say the perfect health care system should have? Explain each characteristic.
4. Do you think the population in general needs more education about the health care system? Talk about the reasons why this may be important.
5. Identify the key aspects of the US health care system.
6. Identify the key aspects of the UK health care system.
7. Reflect on how the US and UK systems have changed over the past 20 years. Why have they changed?

REFERENCES

Asian Development Bank and World Trade Organization, 2011. Aid for trade in the Asia–Pacific: its role in trade-driven growth. Report from the Co-Chairs of the Regional Technical Group on Aid for Trade for the Asia–Pacific. https://www.wto.org/english/tratop_e/devel_e/a4t_e/a4t_asia_pacific11_e.pdf.

Australian Institute of Health and Welfare (AIHW), 2022. Australia's health 2022: in brief. Cat. no. AUS 241. Australia's health series number 18. AIHW, Canberra. https://www.aihw.gov.au/reports/australias-health/australias-health-2022-in-brief/summary. (25 July 2022).

Bacchi, C., 2016. Problematizations in health policy: questioning how "problems" are constituted in policies. SAGE Open, Sydney. doi: 10.1177/2158244016653986.

Bigdeli, M., Rouffy, B., Lane, B.D., et al., 2020. Health systems governance: the missing links. BMJ Glob Health 5 (8), e002533.

Braithwaite, T., Winford, B., Bailey, H., et al., 2020. Health system dynamics analysis of eyecare services in Trinidad and Tobago and progress towards Vision 2020 Goals. Health Policy Plan 33 (1), 70–84.

Chapman, A.R., 2016. Assessing the universal health coverage target in the Sustainable Development Goals from a human rights perspective. BMC Int Health Hum Rights 16 (33), 1–9.

Department of Health, 2020. Health Policy Analysis 2020. Evaluation of the Health Care Homes program – interim evaluation report 2020, Volume 1: Summary report. Department of Health, Canberra.

Ghebreyesus, T.A., 2020. Strengthening our resolve for primary health care. Bull World Health Org 98 (11), 726–726A.

Global Access Partners, 2019. Ensuring the sustainability of the Australian health system: Australia's Health 2040 Task Force Report. Global Access Partners, Sydney.

Glover, L., Woods, M., 2020. The Australian health system. In: Tikkanen, R., Osborn, R., Mossialos, E., et al. (Eds), International Profiles of Health Care Systems. Commonwealth Fund, New York, pp. 7–17. https://www.commonwealth-fund.org/international-health-policy-center/countries/australia.

Hall, D.S., Desborough, J., de Toca, L., et al., 2021. "A decade's worth of work in a matter of days": The journey to tele-health for the whole population in Australia. Int J Med Inform 151, 104483.

Hasanovna, B.N., 2019. Models of financing and organization of health care system – international experience. IJMSBR 5 (5), 7–12.

Health Economic Forum, 2020. Healthcare system models and how they work. https://www.weforum.org/agenda/2020/10/covid-19-healthcare-health-service-vaccine-health-insurance-pandemic/.

Hines, S., Wakerman, J., Carey, T.A., et al., 2020. Retention strategies and interventions for health workers in rural and remote areas: a systematic review protocol. JBI Evid Synth 18 (1), 87–96.

Ibeneme, S., Ongom, M., Ukor, N., et al., 2020. Realigning health systems strategies and approaches; what should African countries do to strengthen health systems for the Sustainable Development Goals? Front Public Health 8, 372.

Institute for Healthcare Improvement, 2019. Moving from Volume to Value: IHI National Forum: December 8–11, 2019 in Orlando, FL, USA. https://www.ihi.org/education/Conferences/National-Forum/Pages/track-volume-to-value.aspx.

Islam M.M., 2019. Social Determinants of Health and related inequalities: confusion and implications. Front Public Health 7 (11), 1–4.

Jarvis, T., Scott, F., El-Jardali, F., et al., 2020. Defining and classifying public health systems: a critical interpretive synthesis. Health Res Policy Syst 18 (1), 68.

Kämpfen, F., Wijemunige, N., Evangelista, B., 2018. Aging, non-communicable diseases, and old-age disability in low- and middle-income countries: a challenge for global health. Int J Public Health 63, 1011–1012.

Klinga, C., Hasson H, Andreen, S.M., et al., 2018. Understanding the dynamics of sustainable change: a 20-year case study of integrated health and social care. BMC Health Serv Res 18 (1), 400.

Kluge, H.H.P., Wickramasinghe, K., Rippin, H.L., et al. 2020. Prevention and control of non-communicable diseases in the COVID-19 response. Lancet 30, 395 (10238), 1678–1680.

Kumah, E., Ankomah, S.E., Fusheini, A., et al., 2020. Frameworks for health systems performance assessment: how comprehensive is Ghana's holistic assessment tool? Glob Health Res Policy 9 (5), 10.

Labrique, A., Vasudevan, L., Mehl, G., et al., 2018. Digital health and health systems of the future. Glob Health Science and Practice, 6 (suppl 1), S1–S4.

Mannion, R., Davies, H., 2018. Understanding organisational culture for healthcare quality improvement. BMJ 363, k4907.

Manyazewal, T., 2017. Using the World Health Organization health system building blocks through survey of healthcare professionals to determine the performance of public healthcare facilities. Arch Public Health 75 (50), 1–9.

Metusela, C., Usherwood, T., Lawson, K., et al., 2020. Patient Centred Medical Home (PCMH) transitions in western Sydney, Australia: a qualitative study. BMC Health Serv Res 20 (1), 285.

Organisation for Economic Co-operation and Development (OECD), 2021. OECD Policy responses to Coronavirus (COVID-19), Supporting young people's mental health through the COVID-19 crisis. https://www.oecd.org/coronavirus/policy-responses/supporting-young-peoples-mental-health-through-the-covid-19-crisis-84e143e5/.

Papanicolas, I., Rajan, D., Karanikolos, M., et al., 2022. Health System Performance Assessment: A Framework for Policy Aanalysis. World Health Organization, Geneva.

Piña, I.L., Allen, L.A., Desai, N.R., 2021. Policy and payment challenges in the post pandemic treatment of heart failure: value-based care and telehealth. J Card Fail S1071–9164 (21), 00360.

Sacks, E., Morrow, M., Story, W.T., et al. 2019. Beyond the building blocks: integrating community roles into health systems frameworks to achieve health for all. BMJ Glob Health 3 (Suppl 3), e001384.

Scanlon, D.P., 2021. Redesigning health care: keeping the patient connected and at the center of a system that learns in real time. American Journal of Accountable Care 9 (4), 1.

Schneider, E.C., Shah, A., Doty, M.M., et al., 2021. Mirror, mirror 2021 — reflecting poorly: health care in the US compared to other high-income countries. Commonwealth Fund, New York. https://www.commonwealthfund.org/publications/fund-reports/2021/aug/mirror-mirror-2021-reflecting-poorly.

Shatrov, K., Pessina, C., Huber, K., et al., Improving health care from the bottom up: Factors for the successful implementation of kaizen in acute care hospitals. PLOS ONE, 16 (9),e0257412.

Shaw, J., Gray, C.S., Baker, G.R., et al., 2018. Mechanisms, contexts, and points of contention: operationalizing realist-informed research for complex health interventions. BMC Med Res Methodol 18 (1), 178.

Tikkanen, R., Osborn, R., Mossialos, E., et al., 2020. International profiles of health care systems. Commonwealth Fund, New York.

Tumusiime, P., Karamagi, H., Titi-Ofei, R., et al., 2020. Building health system resilience in the context of primary health care revitalization for attainment of UHC: proceedings from the Fifth Health Sector Directors' Policy and Planning Meeting for the WHO African Region. BMC Proceedings 3 14 (Suppl 19), (16), 1–8.

Valentelyte, G., Keegan, C., Sorensen, J., 2021. Analytical methods to assess the impacts of Activity-Based Funding (ABF): a scoping review. Health Economic Review 11 (1), 17.

Wenham, C., Katz, R., Birungi, C., et al., 2019. Global health security and universal health coverage: from a marriage of convenience to a strategic, effective partnership. BMJ Glob Health 4 (1), e001145.

Witter, S., Palmer, N., Balabanova, D., et al., 2019. Health system strengthening: Reflections on its meaning, assessment, and our state of knowledge. Int J Health Planning and Management 34, e1980–e1989.

World Health Organization (WHO), 2009. Health financing strategy for the Asia Pacific region (2010–2015). World Health Organization Regional Office for the Western Pacific. Manila, Philippines.

World Health Organization (WHO), 2014a. Achieving the health-related Millennium Development Goals in the Western Pacific Region, 2014. World Health Organization Regional Office for the Western Pacific, Manila, Philippines.

World Health Organization (WHO), 2014b. Western Pacific Regional Action Plan for the Prevention and Control of Noncommunicable Diseases (2014–2020). World Health Organization Regional Office for the Western Pacific, Manila, Philippines.

World Health Organization (WHO), 2016. Universal health coverage: moving towards better health: action framework for the Western Pacific Region. World Health Organization Regional Office for the Western Pacific, Manila, Philippines.

World Health Organization (WHO), 2019. Health systems strengthening glossary. https://www.who.int/docs/default-source/documents/health-systems-strengthening-glossary.pdf?sfvrsn=b871d95f_4.

World Health Organization (WHO), 2021. Building health systems resilience for universal health coverage and health security during the COVID-19 pandemic and beyond: WHO position paper. World Health Organization, Geneva.

Yeoh, E.K., Johnston, C., Chau, P.Y.K,. et al., 2019. Governance functions to accelerate progress toward universal health coverage (UHC) in the Asia-Pacific Region. Health System Reform 5 (1), 48–58.

FURTHER READING

Braithwaite, J., Tran, Y., Ellis, L.A., et al., 2020. Inside the black box of comparative national healthcare performance in 35 OECD countries: issues of culture, systems performance, and sustainability. PLOS ONE 15 (9), e0239776.

Jain, B., Cheong, E., Bugeja, L., et al., 2019. International transferability of research evidence in residential long-term care: a comparative analysis of aged care systems in 7 nations. J Am Med Dir Assoc 20 (12), 1558–1565.

Dudley, L., Mamdoo, P., Naidoo, S., et al., 2022. Towards a harmonised framework for developing quality of care indicators for global health: a scoping review of existing conceptual and methodological practices. BMJ Health Care Inform, 29 (1), e100469.

Karamagi, H.C., Titi-Ofei, R., Kipruto, H.K., et al., 2022. On the resilience of health systems: A methodological exploration across countries in the WHO African Region. PLOS ONE 7 (2), e0261904.

Komashie, A., Ward, J., Bashford, T., et al., 2021. Systems approach to health service design, delivery, and improvement: a systematic review and meta-analysis. BMJ open, 11 (1), e037667.

Takkanen, R., Osborn, R., Mossialos, E., et al., 2020. International profiles of health care systems. Commonwealth Fund, New York. https://www.commonwealthfund.org/international-health-policy-center/system-profiles.

ONLINE RESOURCES

Australian Institute of Health and Welfare (AIHW) and the Australian Bureau of Statistics (ABS) – both the AIHW and ABS have a range of resources and publications illustrating the health of the Australian population: https://www.aihw.gov.au and https://www.abs.gov.au.

Organisation for Economic Co-operation and Development (OECD) – the OECD brings together the governments of countries committed to democracy and the market economy from around the world. The OECD analyses the financial sustainability, efficiency and quality of health and long-term care systems in member countries: https://www.oecd.org/health/.

Universal Health Coverage 2030 – UHC2030 provides a multi-stakeholder platform to promote collaborative working at global and country levels on health systems strengthening. The participating stakeholders advocate increased political commitment to UHC and facilitate accountability and knowledge sharing: https://www.uhc2030.org.

World Health Organization (WHO) – the WHO website provides many resources for comparing health care systems in other countries: https://www.who.int/countries/.

5

Public Health in Australia

Helen Keleher

KEY LEARNING OUTCOMES

When you finish this chapter you should be able to:
- understand public health and population health and their aims
- describe the very real anti-science challenges to public health
- consider the consequences of challenges to the science and practices of public health

- describe pathways into public health careers
- describe the public health system in Australia and the responsibilities of different levels of government for public health
- provide an overview of how major public health issues are handled
- consider the politics of public health.

KEY TERMS AND ABBREVIATIONS

acquired immune deficiency syndrome (AIDS)
Council of Academic Public Health Institutions Australia (CAPHIA)
environmental health officer (EHO)
health equity

health gap
high-risk strategy
human immunodeficiency virus (HIV)
intersectoral collaboration
Master of Public Health (MPH)
new public health
old public health

population strategy
prevention paradox
Public Health Association of Australia (PHAA)
social determinants of health (SDH)
targeted public health
universal approaches

INTRODUCTION

Public health is a global field of practice, research and advocacy designed to protect and improve the health of individuals, families, communities and populations (Association of Schools and Programs of Public Health (ASPPH) 2018) (Box 5.1). Using sound evidence, public health finds solutions to the problems that cause illness, disease and death among populations, in efforts that have been remarkably successful. Public health actions have created longer life expectancy and lower death rates from conditions that otherwise might reduce life

expectancy and people's quality of life. Measures such as ensuring clean drinking water, rather than water contaminated by typhoid or gastroenteritis-causing pathogens; vaccinations for polio, measles, diphtheria, tetanus and smallpox; and actions to reduce deaths and trauma from road traffic accidents are now widely accepted as necessary for a healthy population. It is often said that medicine saves one life at a time, but public health saves millions of lives, every day.

But, increasingly over the last few decades, the science of public health has been challenged by anti-science

BOX 5.1 **This is Public Health**

Public Health is Your Health
On a global scale, public health improves the conditions of living that affect the health of all of us. Public health is at the forefront of containing deadly contagious diseases such as Ebola, measles, malaria and HIV/AIDS. Public health seeks to reduce the incidence of preventable diseases, minimise the consequences of catastrophic events, provide the basics of sanitation, safe food and safe water, and promote healthier lifestyles.

You are Only as Healthy as the World You Live in
Your health is determined not only by your own genetics and personal choices, but also by the environment around you. Public health investigates the ecology of health – from social networks and economic circumstances to our environment – and then minimises health risks.

Public Health is Moral and Smart
Public health efforts allow us to save lives – your life, the lives of your family and friends, and the lives of people around the world. If we can save lives, we should. We'll not only make people healthier, but we'll also address soaring health care costs by preventing unnecessary death and disease.

Source: Association of Schools and Program of Public Health (2018). https://www.aspph.org.

groups, targeting, for example, vaccinations for childhood conditions and even challenging the science of climate change and its threats to human health. This has undermined trust in public health measures. During the COVID-19 pandemic, the science of pandemic controls was challenged to such an extent that the anti-science agenda itself became a 'wicked problem' (MacDougall & Pettman 2021). This means that public health practitioners must learn how to manage the world of misinformation, disinformation and fake news (Keleher 2021a) that undermines and disputes public health evidence.

This chapter will introduce you to public health, its underpinning values as well as some of its challenges; discuss pathways into public health careers, and the connections between public health and the social determinants of health. It will also be useful for you to know how public health is organised and delivered in Australia, including the public health responsibilities of Australia's three levels of government.

The classic definition of public health, from Winslow (1920), is that public health is the art and science of preventing disease and injury, prolonging life and promoting health through the organised efforts of society. However, a more contemporary explanation of public health considers:

- the distribution and determinants of patterns of health, sickness and disabilities in communities, and the distribution of health care, health services and other resources
- the impact of the physical and social environment on health, and the prevention and control of disease
- the structure and organisation and function, planning and management of health services and health information systems
- the causes and likely remedies for a reduction of social and economic inequities in health status, especially the inequities between Indigenous and non-Indigenous populations.

It is also worth noting that public health is different to clinical care, and is not the same as public hospitals, as important as they are.

'OLD' AND 'NEW' PUBLIC HEALTH

'**Old public health**' in the 19th and early 20th centuries focused on hygiene, sanitation, control of infectious diseases and the provision of clean water. '**New public health**' developed in the latter part of the 20th century, emphasising knowledge to action on the social determinants of health and the conditions of life where people live, work and play. New public health focuses on deliberate efforts to redress health inequities without forgetting about the foundations provided by old public health measures such as clean water and air, sanitation, vaccinations and population-focused strategies. New public health has become a movement that has learnt from the political and practical experience of past successes and failures in public health, and aims to achieve higher standards of health for populations, particularly those who have the least resources and experience disadvantages of various types (Keleher 2021b).

The drivers for public health are both philosophical and economic. However, both the philosophical and economic drivers for public health were challenged during the first two years of the COVID-19 pandemic, when both the philosophy of protecting people from infections and death, and the economics related to re-ducing people's social interactions in order to contain the virus, were not just challenged but undermined and politicised. The pandemic has fundamentally challenged what have been seen as strong economic drivers under-pinning public health in terms of preventing ill-health and promoting and protecting the public's health, and maintaining a healthy workforce (Baum 2016).

While public health measures taken to limit the spread of the COVID-19 virus have certainly saved lives, simultaneously they had an enormous impact on so many other aspects of health, particularly mental health, and both the public health and health care workforces have been pushed to their limits. The public health workforce has been very stretched to keep up with the scale and breadth of health prevention, protec-tion and promotion work while the health care work-force has struggled to maintain sufficient staff because of the heavy demands due to COVID-19, and the burdens on hospitals.

In Tuohy's terms (Tuohy 1999), public health is maintained by strong networks, which is characteristic of public health delivery systems. No single organisation can effectively deliver a public health service. While public health is primarily a public-sector government activity, delivery of some activities is reliant on sound relationships between governments at all levels, univer-sities and research institutes, as well as with the private sector such as general practice, cancer screening ser-vices, road safety organisations, the alcohol and drug sector, water utilities and so on. All societies need public health, provided in the most efficient and effective ways, and if those networks fail or there are policy failures, there are almost inevitably increased death rates, espe-cially among the more vulnerable, and reduced quality of life for vast numbers of people.

Pathways into Public Health

Public health practitioners come from a wide range of disciplines including medicine, nursing, epidemiology, biostatistics, economics, social sciences, political science, psychology, allied health, environmental health and health promotion. Public health can be studied as a dis-cipline at undergraduate and postgraduate levels.

The peak body for academic schools of public health is the **Council of Academic Public Health Institutions Australia (CAPHIA**; https://www.caphia.com.au). This is an organisation of schools of public health that work together to advance public health education.

The Public Health Workforce

Public health systems rely on the infrastructure of good education and an experienced workforce. The public health workforce is necessarily multidisciplinary, stem-ming from occupational groups that include medicine, epidemiology, biostatistics, social sciences, environmen-tal health, nursing, health promotion, health communi-cation, the various allied health groups, public policy, health service management and health economics (Gebbie et al. 2003). People with these disciplinary back-grounds have often studied public health at postgraduate level and find a wide range of careers in government and non-government sectors and in academia. For example, a social science graduate from a **Master of Public Health (MPH)** course may discover a strong affinity with epide-miology and biostatistics, while a graduate from health promotion may study a Master of Public Policy course and find a career in government, working on policy issues associated with health promotion or health inequalities.

Any single public health issue requires a multidisci-plinary response. Many major public health programs represent 'investments in large-scale, longer term public health programs over 30–50 years that utilise a breadth of strategies and methods to achieve reductions in harm' (Keleher 2017, p. 2). Public health programs seek improved population health outcomes from significant, and often socially entrenched, problems, analysing what is needed to improve health outcomes from those prob-lems from the evidence, and often building the evidence over time. For example, global road safety efforts to reduce deaths from vehicle and bike accidents have required legislative, institutional, policy and program responses that have aimed to 'change the story' behind the problems, which are complex and therefore cannot be solved by simplistic solutions.

Public health efforts are coordinated and evidence based, backed by clear legislative and policy frameworks that inform road safety campaigns. The legislation is complemented by national strategies that provide clear roles and responsibilities across levels of government within agreed national goals, objectives and priorities. However, the acceptance of legislation has been depen-dent on law enforcement backed by concerted public education programs.

To inform public education, researchers in biostatistics and epidemiology interpret the trends in the incidence and prevalence of road deaths and injuries, engineers and police advise on the causes of road traffic accidents, and program managers develop the overall program plans, budgets and the various components of the whole program. The campaign materials have often included graphic footage that involves all of the people associated with film- or documentary-making, while the health communication experts work on shaping the key messages, designing them to influence people's behaviour on roads.

Public health professionals are distinguished by their preparedness to advocate for neglected public health issues and to stand up for what might be politically unpopular solutions to public health problems. This is called public health advocacy, which is a mechanism to influence public policy, legislation and education.

Pause *for* Reflection …
What social conditions and settings have had the greatest impact on your life? How might they reflect public health issues?

POPULATION HEALTH

Population health can be narrowly defined in terms of risks and associated health outcomes, but also more broadly to encompass the multiple determinants of health. The narrow view of population health is that 'population health rests largely on shaping the distribution of risk in a population so that fewer people are exposed to risky situations' (Berkman & Melchior 2006, p. 55). A broader view is that population health is a framework for thinking about why some populations are healthier than others, as well as policy development, research and resource allocation for investment in population health (Keleher 2021a; Young 2004). The aims of population health are twofold: to improve the health of the whole population, and to decrease the inequities in health status between different social groups.

Geoffrey Rose (1981, 1992, 2001), now regarded as a classic thinker and researcher about public and population health, posed a key question for public health: '*Why are some people healthy and others not?*'

To answer that question, Rose said (1992, p. 62):

In order to grasp the principles of public health, one must understand that society is not merely a collection of individuals but is also a collectivity, and the behavior and health of its individual members are profoundly influenced by its collective characteristics and social norms.

Pause *for* Reflection …
How did the handling of the COVID-19 pandemic employ both narrow and broad efforts to protect us from exposure and risk? What measures influenced health outcomes across the population?

Population health is a growing field of practice that encompasses the generation of data, data mining and data analysis, which are the foundation of population health research. As the availability of data grows, there is increasing demand for professionals who see through the lens of populations rather than individuals. Priority population groups are those most impacted by social conditions and are therefore most likely to be exposed to factors that cause significant health conditions (Keleher & MacDougall 2021). Understanding the characteristics of populations who do not enjoy the same levels of health as the general population is the work of population health (Keleher 2015, p. 65).

Both high-risk and population strategies have been developed to influence the distribution of illness across the population. A **high-risk strategy** is one that targets the right patient at high risk of developing a more serious condition, such as pregnant women or overweight men who are smokers. A **population strategy** is one that attempts to control the determinants of incidence, and thus to shift the distribution of exposure across the whole population. This gives rise to the **prevention paradox**, which is that a large number of people at low risk may give rise to more cases than the small number who are at high risk – that is, 'a preventive measure that brings large benefits to the community offers little to each participating individual' (Rose 1992, p. 38). Limiting where people can smoke is one such measure – it is an inconvenience to smokers but protects large numbers of people from second-hand smoke.

Health Equity

Health inequities are caused by avoidable circumstances (such as homelessness) and unfair socio-economic conditions such as insecure low-paid work. **Health equity** means that all people have the same rights to equitable access to services on the basis of need. Public hospitals are an example of that principle.

Health equity rights extend to the principle that people have the resources, capacities and power they need to act upon the circumstances of their lives that determine their health. So if a person has a health condition such as diabetes or HIV/AIDS, they should be able to get the medicines they need to stay well, the health education they need to understand how to stay well, and to feel empowered to manage their health. In Australia, the '**health gap**' describes the inequities between population groups that may happen because of circumstances related to where they live, or their socio-economic status.

Social Determinants of Health

The **social determinants of health (SDH)** are the social conditions in which people live and work, and they represent a significant shift in thinking about how to resolve issues of health inequity and disadvantage (Commission on the Social Determinants of Health 2008). Collectively, the SDH are recognised as the best predictors of health – the causal pathways for both individuals and populations. The evidence that has been systematically collected and analysed demonstrates how pathways through societal, political, environmental and economic determinants translate into illness and disease. The social conditions and settings in which people live not only influence how people behave, but also have a direct impact on the health of individuals, families, communities and populations.

Public health is concerned with the evidence about how to address the determinants of health. The worldviews of the social science disciplines involved in public health are influenced by contemporary social–ecology/ equity debates, and since the early 21st century 'new public health' has increasingly been influenced by the evidence emerging about the social, economic, political and environmental determinants of health (Baum 2016). The new public health is a socio-political movement that argues for the need for social and political action to control disease and improve the health of populations while simultaneously addressing inequities. Its proponents see the need for action on social and economic environments to improve the public's health and to reduce health inequalities where these are avoidable, and especially where they are unjust or unfair (Commission on the Social Determinants of Health

2008). These determinants include quality early childhood education, secure employment, access to health care and public health interventions, social support, gender and culture, and the quality of physical environments including urban design, access to green spaces, clean air and water.

In theory, population health work should take account of the patterns of health determinants, and the policies and interventions that link outcomes with determinants. But in reality only a narrow range of determinants is considered in population health work by governments when they focus on behavioural issues and disregard socio-economic and environmental factors. Good population health requires **intersectoral collaboration** and programs that focus on the needs of those with disadvantaged health status in order to impact on health and social inequities. Typically, both public health and population health strategies are more 'upstream' than medical treatment services, which are classified primarily as 'downstream'. Upstream strategies are focused on social and environmental change and on health-promoting policies and practices.

Universal and Targeted Public Health Approaches

Universal approaches to public health are those available to everyone at no cost or very little cost, such as immunisation, maternal and child health and cancer screening programs. **Targeted public health** approaches are those focused on particular population groups – those at higher risk for contracting a communicable disease, for example.

FUNDING OF PUBLIC HEALTH

Overall, public health receives about 2–2.5% of the total recurrent allocations from Commonwealth and state/territory health budgets. The **Public Health Association of Australia (PHAA)** notes the extent to which the economy and public health are intertwined; or in other words, public health policy *is* economic policy (PHAA 2022) – an association which cannot be ignored.

Given the COVID-19 pandemic, and the rise of other communicable diseases, the PHAA is advocating for a long-term vision in order to build a more sustainable and equitable public health system and making the case in many states for an increase in public health investment from 2% to 5% of the total annual health expenditure by 2030 (PHAA 2021, 2022).

RESPONSIBILITIES FOR PUBLIC AND POPULATION HEALTH

Different levels of government carry diverse and distinct levels of responsibility for the work involved in public health. Australia has three levels of government: the federal government, the governments of the six states and two territories, and local governments in all states and territories, all with their own jurisdictions. All levels of government have responsibilities for public health policy, planning and implementation.

Federal Responsibilities

The main federal bureaucracy with public health responsibilities is the Department of Health. Apart from Medicare (see Chapter 2), the Pharmaceutical Benefits Scheme (see Chapter 7) and aged care (see Chapter 8), the Department of Health is responsible for the funding of the supply of blood products (mainly through the Red Cross), and food safety such as applications for genetic modification of foods and the labelling of products, and specific health promotion programs, such as harm reduction from drugs and the prevention of violence against women, although the states and territories are also funding programs for these priorities.

State and Territory Government Responsibilities

The responsibilities for public and population health activities are directed by public health departments in state/territory governments, each of which is headed by the Chief Health Officer, or Manager of Public Health, who has statutory responsibility to the Minister for Health for the health of the population.

Public health units in government departments are responsible for population-based programs (such as immunisation and vaccination) in disease control and health protection, to ensure that the whole population is protected from preventable communicable (or infectious) diseases which covers communicable diseases such as legionellosis, tuberculosis, HIV/AIDS, SARS and COVID-19, and for managing disease outbreaks (such as *Salmonella* poisoning from contaminated food).

State and territory governments are required by federal law to manage effective epidemiological surveillance systems for the identification of public health issues, for the development and implementation of interventions to protect people's health, and for the monitoring of the outcomes of interventions. State and territory governments are also responsible for the administration of many public health issues, including dangerous drugs and poisons, emergency responses (e.g. floods, fires, bioterrorism), immunisation, maternal and child health, school health and dental health. State governments are also responsible for health promotion such as healthy nutrition, physical activity, mental health promotion, promoting safe environments, sexual and reproductive health, and reducing tobacco-related harm.

Every jurisdiction in Australia has a *Public Health Act* that sets out the requirements for individuals, organisations and governments and their agencies for the control of infectious diseases, the control of a range of risks to public health, and measures that must be taken to promote and protect health. Policy for public health frequently combines diverse but complementary approaches to creating better health, including legislation, fiscal measures, taxation, and organisational and behavioural change. Public health policy influences the actions that can be taken by public health professionals. The strong evidence-based policy platforms for the regulation and management of public health issues ensures that the practices of public health are more effective.

Local Government Responsibilities

Local government is a key player in public health as well as the health and well-being of local populations. For example, local governments are involved in the promotion of healthy environments through local amenities such as footpaths, walkways and bicycle paths linked to active transport strategies, reduction of harm from illicit drugs and alcohol abuse, and early childhood programs. Specific local government public health responsibilities include:

- legislative responsibility for the administration of legislation for food safety, food premises, food production, food selling (*Victorian Government Food Act 1984*)
- the built and social environment, including cultural, community and recreational development
- environmental hazards, including waste disposal and exposure to second-hand smoke
- providing community services
- land use planning, roads, drains and footpaths.

Pause *for* Reflection ...
There has been continued well-funded resistance from industry to undermine and oppose public health

efforts to control tobacco use. In what ways have legislation, taxation, organisational change and behavioural change been effective in tobacco control?

How Are Public Health Issues Handled?

Federal, state, territory and local governments all have public health staff who have responsibility for particular issues such as communicable disease, non-communicable disease, health protection and so on. Frequently, governments work across jurisdictions to develop responses to specific issues. **Environmental health officers (EHOs)** in local government have statutory responsibilities – they are responsible for the development, regulation, enforcement and monitoring of laws and regulations governing public health, building and environmental management of significant incidents.

All levels of government undertake strategic planning for the prevention and management of diseases and conditions that feature highly in the burden of disease data. Strategic planning processes can be quite extensive to work out how governments should approach issues; where responsibilities lie for action; how prevention, health protection and health promotion should be addressed; and how action will be monitored using indicators to track and measure progress. For example, the Department of Health has a National HIV/AIDS Strategy (Department of Health 2018–22), which was first developed in 1989 and has been reviewed and renewed every few years since. It sets out requirements for epidemiology and surveillance so that the incidence and prevalence of new infections are carefully monitored along with the treatment and support for people living with HIV/AIDS (see Case study 5.1).

PUBLIC HEALTH: LIBERTARIAN TO EGALITARIAN

Tensions between narrow and broad approaches to public health continue as individual versus broad approaches are debated by governments, bureaucrats, advocates, academics and practitioners. Just as previous chapters have discussed the role of the public and private sectors in health insurance, public health must be debated on the spectrum from libertarian to egalitarian:

- Libertarian positions represent choice and personal responsibility for health needs.
- Egalitarian positions represent a rights-based universality with equal access for equal need.

CASE STUDY 5.1 HIV/AIDS Prevention

In the field of HIV prevention and control, the rapid and coordinated mobilisation of governments and community has enabled significant activity through community education and awareness-building and behaviour change, both in the most at-risk groups from contracting HIV and in the general community. The response to HIV/AIDS has achieved progress towards its targets in a shorter timeframe compared with other public health issues. It has done so despite raising controversial social questions about sexuality and human rights that had not previously been openly discussed, and despite requiring difficult conversations at the individual and also policy level. How did this happen? Leadership came from the Minister for Health at the time, the Hon Neal Blewett, who advocated for both public policy and social change. Government and civil society organisations then worked closely together to ensure efforts to change attitudes and behaviours were well targeted and involved mobilisation of opinion and action within key groups. This enabled introduction of policies and regulations that may otherwise have become points of resistance. However, while the achievements in this health area are remarkable, there is some concern that Australia is becoming complacent about HIV/AIDS prevention, and winding back strategies rather than embedding them (Keleher 2017).

Sources: Keleher, H. (2017). Review of prevention and public health strategies to inform the primary prevention of family violence and violence against women. Report commissioned to VicHealth by the Department of Premier and Cabinet. VicHealth and Victorian State Government, Melbourne.

Neither health care for individuals nor public health for populations is a typical commodity. It might be, some argue, that the private sector is more efficient, but in Australia the reverse is true in the provision of public health: the public sector is not only more efficient but also carries more of the risks and is able to handle emergencies and the seriously complex issues that the private sector would find unprofitable, such as policy development and disease prevention that relies on complex solutions.

Case study 5.2 discusses public health messaging during the COVID-19 pandemic.

Public health suffers from lack of funding, but additional funding will make a real difference only if there are more concerted intersectoral efforts to tackle the causes of problems such as poverty, low levels of education and

CASE STUDY 5.2 Public Health Messaging During the COVID-19 Pandemic

The COVID-19 pandemic caused high anxiety across the population; as the months went on, public health messaging became more and more important. Messaging was vital to communicate risk, to explain the progress of the virus, to minimise anxiety and to reassure people that governments were doing all they could to manage and control the spread of the virus. But, messaging was not straightforward and advice was regularly changing. As vaccines became available, vaccine hesitancy arose, but while vaccines were vital in controlling the virus, it was not sufficient as a single measure. Masks are a cheap and easy technology but the politics of masks became entrenched and raised debates about the role of governments in the lives of the public and, therefore, government's role in public health.

Case Study Questions
1. Looking back, how do you think masking became politicised?
2. Was the role of government sufficient from a public health perspective?
3. What do you think were the concerns of people who challenged public health during 2020–22 and what have been the consequences?

literacy, and degraded environments, rather than 'soft' targets such as physical activity and obesity. The failure of public health systems is more likely to occur if public health maintains a narrow rather than broad focus, because health is mostly created outside the health sector, so intersectoral activity is essential for public health success.

SUMMARY

In this chapter, the following have been addressed:
- an explanation of the breadth of public and population health
- the importance of public health infrastructure within the public sector
- approaches to public health, including upstream–downstream approaches
- a brief overview of the public health workforce
- an introduction to how public health issues are handled
- the responsibilities of different levels of government for public health
- public health futures and what is required to promote and protect the health of the public.

An accompanying video exploring the themes of this chapter is hosted on Evolve: http://evolve.elsevier.com/AU/Reynolds/understanding/.

REVIEW QUESTIONS

1. What are three key characteristics of the population health approach?
2. What are the implications for policy and programs of a narrow approach to population health that is focused on diseases?
3. Critically reflect on how well Australia's public health efforts are doing in increasing health equity and reducing inequities among the population.
4. Whose business in the health sector is not related to public health?

REFERENCES

Association of Schools and Programs of Public Health, 2018. Homepage. https://www.aspph.org.

Baum, F., 2016. The New Public Health, fourth ed. OUP, Oxford.

Berkman, L.F., Melchior, M., 2006. The shape of things to come. How social policy impacts social integration and family structure to produce population health. In: Siegrist, J., Marmot, M. (Eds), Social Inequalities in Health. OUP, Oxford, pp. 55–72.

Commission on the Social Determinants of Health, 2008. Closing the Gap in a generation: health equity through action on the social determinants of health. World Health Organization, Geneva.

Department of Health, 2018. Eighth National HIV Strategy 2018–2022. DOH, Australian Government, Canberra.

Gebbie, K., Rosenstock, L., Hernandez, L.M., 2003. Who Will Keep the Public Healthy? Educating Public Health Professionals for the 21st Century. National Academies Press, Washington, DC.

Keleher, H., 2015. Population health. In: Keleher, H., MacDougall, C. (Eds), Understanding Health, fourth ed. OUP, Melbourne.

Keleher, H., 2017. Review of prevention and public health strategies to inform the primary prevention of family violence and violence against women. Report commissioned to VicHealth by the Department of Premier and Cabinet. VicHealth and Victorian State Government, Melbourne.

Keleher, H., 2021a. Public health in the post-truth world. In: Keleher, H., MacDougall, C. (Eds), Understanding Health, fifth ed. OUP, Melbourne, Chapter 19.

Keleher, H., 2021b. Population health and prevention. In: Keleher, H., MacDougall, C. (Eds), Understanding Health, fifth ed. OUP, Melbourne, Chapter 4.

Keleher, H., MacDougall, C. (Eds), 2021 Glossary. In: Understanding Health, fifth ed. OUP, Melbourne.

MacDougall C., Pettman T., 2021. Anti-science and public health. In: Understanding Health, fifth ed. OUP, Melbourne, Chapter 18.

Public Health Association of Australia, 2021. Striving towards a healthier Western Australia: 2021 and beyond. https://www.phaa.net.au/documents/item/5085.

Public Health Association of Australia, 2022. Budget submission shows how Commonwealth can generate $17b+ in revenue, and improve public health. https://www.phaa.net.au/news/budget-submission-shows-how-commonwealth-can-generate-17b-in-revenue-and-improve-public-health-phaa.

Rose, G., 1981. Strategy of prevention: lessons from cardiovascular disease. Br Med J 282 (6279), 1847–1851.

Rose, G., 1992. The Strategy for Preventative Medicine. OUP, New York.

Rose, G., 2001. Sick individuals and sick populations. Int J Epidemiol 30 (3), 427–432.

Tuohy, C., 1999. Accidental Logics: The Dynamics of Change in the Health Care Arena in United States, Britain and Canada. OUP, New York.

Victorian State Government, 1984. The Food Act 1984.

Winslow, C., 1920. The untilled fields of public health. Science 51 (1306), 23–33.

World Health Organization (WHO), 2018. Health inequities and their causes. https://www.who.int/news-room/facts-in-pictures/detail/health-inequities-and-their-causes.

Young, T.K., 2004. Population health: concepts and methods. OUP, Oxford.

FURTHER READING

Australian Institute of Health and Welfare (AIHW), 2020. Australia's health data insights 2020. AIHW, Canberra.

Keleher, H., MacDougall, C. Understanding health, fifth ed. OUP, Melbourne.

UCL Institute of Health Equity, 2010. Fair Society, Healthy Lives: the Marmot Review. UCL Institute of Health Equity, London.

Oosthuizen, J., Stoneham, M., Hannelly, T., et al., 2022. Environmental health responses to COVID 19 in Western Australia: lessons for the future. Int J Environ Res Public Health 19, 9393. https://doi.org/10.3390/ ijerph19159393.

ONLINE RESOURCES

Association of Schools and Programs of Public Health – resource-rich site for students of public health, established to assist them to prepare for careers in education, advocacy, research and practice: https://www.aspph.org.

UCL Institute of Health Equity – provides a wealth of resources on the social determinants of health and public health. Available from: https://www.instituteofhealthequity.org.

6

Primary Health Care in Australia

Paresh Dawda and Angelene True

KEY LEARNING OUTCOMES

When you finish this chapter you should be able to:
- define primary health care
- describe the primary health care system in Australia
- explain the importance of primary health care
- identify the multidisciplinary professionals who work in community-based health settings
- describe the current state of primary health care in Australia and the future health reform agenda for primary health care.

KEY TERMS AND ABBREVIATIONS

Aboriginal Community Controlled Health Organisation (ACCHO)

Aged Care Assessment Team (ACAT)

Australian Institute of Health and Welfare (AIHW)

Community Health Program (CHP)

community health service (CHS)

comprehensive needs assessment (CAN)

Department of Veterans' Affairs (DVA)

general practice

general practitioner (GP)

health system

Indigenous Australians' Health Programme (IAHP)

National Aboriginal Community Controlled Health Organisation (NACCHO)

non-communicable diseases (NCD)

Organisation for Economic Co-operation and Development (OECD)

primary care (or primary medical care)

primary care organisation (PCO)

primary health care (PHC)

Primary Health Networks (PHN)

Primary Health Reform Steering Group (PHRSG)

Sustainable Development Goals (SDG)

universal health coverage (UHC)

World Health Organization (WHO)

CASE STUDY 6.1

Joan is a 79-year-old Australian women, married to Mario, who is 82 years old and an Italian migrant to Australia. They live in the western suburbs of Sydney and have three children, one of whom lives in Sydney, another interstate and the third overseas.

Joan had enjoyed relatively good health until her early 70s. She has diabetes, high blood pressure and osteoarthritis of both her hip and knees, which gives her chronic pain and is making walking difficult. This is frustrating as she is the carer for Mario. Mario too has diabetes, high blood pressure and high cholesterol, and has had a stroke and many mini-strokes. He has also had heart issues and has a cardiac pacemaker. In the last two years he has developed dementia, diagnosed after an admission to hospital following a fall.

CASE STUDY 6.1—cont'd

His mobility is poor and he needs assistance with dressing and washing. Joan used to do this for him but with her declining health is finding it more and more difficult. They now have a carer coming to help him every morning. He tends to fall and has had three falls in the last couple of months. Fortunately, he has not injured himself, but Joan had to call the ambulance each time to see him and help him get up as she cannot lift him anymore. They both take multiple medications, the costs of which are increasing, and Joan often wonders whether they need to take all the medications. Mario regularly sees the cardiologist and has to pay an out-of-pocket fee for this. The geriatrician he sees bulk-bills them and their GP usually also bulk-bills them. This is important because Joan is worried about her medical bills. She has to see an orthopaedic surgeon for her osteoarthritis and may need joint replacement surgery for both her hips. The waiting list in the public system is very long and so Joan is considering having these privately so she can

continue to look after Mario. She will need to dip into their retirement savings to be able to afford the surgery.

They have known their GP for 7 years. They both see their GP regularly and have care plans, which the practice nurse helps them to develop. This is helpful because the care plans focus on preventing health issues with regular checks on their feet and eyes, and also blood tests. Mario has been seeing the GP less often, initially because of COVID-19 outbreaks and then because it is so hard for him to leave the home. Sadly, the GP practice no longer conducts home visits. However, Joan was grateful because the practice nurse helped her to obtain an **Aged Care Assessment Team (ACAT)** assessment for Mario. Joan just did not know how to go about doing this or sorting out the carers for him.

As we consider primary health care in Australia, reflect on Joan and Mario and consider Australian primary health care from their perspective.

WHAT IS PRIMARY HEALTH CARE?

The **World Health Organization (WHO)** in its vision for **primary health care (PHC)** called for a unified definition as:

> a whole-of-society approach to health that aims at ensuring the highest possible level of health and well-being and their equitable distribution by focusing on people's needs and as early as possible along the continuum from health promotion and disease prevention to treatment, rehabilitation and palliative care, and as close as feasible to people's everyday environment.
>
> **(World Health Organization and United Nations Children's Fund 2018, p. 2)**

There are differing definitions of primary health care and sometimes the terms 'primary health care' and 'primary care' are erroneously used as synonyms. Common elements in the definition of primary health care include (Muldoon et al. 2006):

- the part of the health system that forms the frontline and where the public usually have their first contact with the health system (i.e. first level care)
- care delivered outside the hospital system and usually does not require a referral
- care is as close as possible to where the person lives or works

- care is across the lifespan from cradle to grave
- care is comprehensive
- care is accessible
- care is coordinated.

Primary care has a narrower scope of definition and often refers to **general practice** or family doctor services delivered to individuals. It is important to recognise and appreciate the differences between the two definitions and to not use them interchangeably because primary health care is a much broader concept and includes a wider range of health care professionals and services.

The term 'primary care' has been used since the 1920s and has formed the cornerstone of many health systems. However, it was in 1978 that the Declaration of Alma-Ata became a major milestone for PHC (World Health Organization (WHO) and UNICEF 1978). This was where the concept of PHC was articulated and documented at the first International Conference on Primary Health Care in 1978, held in the city of Alma-Ata, Kazakhstan. The Declaration of Alma-Ata describes the principles of the social model of health in the following terms:

- Health is a fundamental human right, and the attainment of the highest possible level of health is a most important worldwide social goal whose realisation requires the action of many other social and economic sectors in addition to the health sector.

- The existing gross inequality in the health status of people, particularly between developed and developing countries as well as within countries, is politically, socially, and economically unacceptable and is, therefore, of common concern to all countries.
- The people have a right and duty to participate individually and collectively in the planning and implementation of their health care.
- PHC is essential health care based on practical, scientifically sound and socially acceptable methods and technology made universally accessible to individuals and families in the community through their full participation and at a cost that the community and country can afford to maintain at every stage of their development in the spirit of self-reliance and self-determination. It forms an integral part both of the country's health system, of which it is the central function and main focus, and of the overall social and economic development of the community. It is the first level of contact of individuals, the family and community with the national health system, bringing health care as close as possible to where people live and work, and constitutes the first elements of a continuing health care process (World Health Organization and UNICEF 1978).

In 2018 the Declaration of Astana was made (World Health Organization 2018). This declaration was made by heads of state and government, ministers and representatives of states and governments, participating in the Global Conference on Primary Health Care. It reaffirmed the Declaration of Alma-Ata of 1978 and also the United Nation's 2030 Agenda for Sustainable Development. Seven assertions and commitments were made:

1. The highest attainable standard of health is a fundamental right of every human being.
2. PHC is a cornerstone of a sustainable health system for **universal health coverage (UHC)** and health-related **Sustainable Development Goals (SDG)**. PHC is the most inclusive, effective and efficient approach to enhance people's physical and mental health, as well as social well-being.
3. It is ethically, politically, socially and economically unacceptable that inequity in health and disparities in health outcomes persist. The growing burden of **non-communicable diseases (NCD)** needs to be addressed. Promotive, preventive, curative, rehabilitative services and palliative care must be accessible to all.
4. PHC will be strengthened and take an inclusive and engaging multi-sectorial approach to address economic, social and environmental determinants of health.
5. Health systems will focus on investing in PHC, to meet all people's health needs across the life course through comprehensive preventive, promotive, curative, rehabilitative services and palliative care.
6. Individuals and communities will be empowered so they can develop the knowledge, skills, resources and confidence needed to maintain their health or the health of those for whom they care in collaboration with health providers.
7. Countries and stakeholders will work together in a spirit of partnership and effective development cooperation, sharing knowledge and good practices.

The 2030 Agenda for Sustainable Development was adopted by all the United Nations members as a blueprint for prosperity and peace for people of the whole world and the planet (United Nations 2021). The SDG constitute 17 goals at the heart of the blueprint. The third goal is one that seeks to ensure healthy lives and promote well-being for all at all ages. This third goal itself is made up of 13 targets, each of which has a set of indicators.

Pause *for* Reflection ...

Consider the commitments from the Declaration of Astana from the perspective of Joan and Mario in Case study 6.1 from the beginning of the chapter.

Is the highest attainable standard of health being achieved for Joan and Mario? Are their physical, emotional and social care needs being met? Is their care comprehensive? What else needs to be provided to help them? What sectors, other than health, need to be involved?

WHY IS PHC IMPORTANT?

The Alma-Ata and Astana Declaration provide a commitment to PHC and point to why PHC is important. PHC is one of the most effective and efficient ways for health care systems to achieve positive population health outcomes. Effective primary health care helps achieve better outcomes of care and a more equitable distribution of health across the population, and it does so more efficiently (Starfield et al. 2005). There are six mechanisms it achieves this through:

1. improved access to care including for hard-to-reach or deprived populations

2. care that is at least as effective as that provided by specialist care for a range of common conditions
3. preventive care activities are often led and delivered in primary care
4. early management of health problems
5. a focus on person-centred care rather than condition-specific care
6. the gateway (gatekeeping) role reduces unnecessary or inappropriate care.

THE PRIMARY CARE SYSTEM IN AUSTRALIA

The Australian health system spent $66.9 billion on PHC services in Australia in 2019–20, representing 33% of the total health spend (Australian Institute of Health and Welfare (AIHW), updated 2021a). Fig. 6.1 shows this and places it in the context of other expenditure on health. This diagram also shows that while the Australian

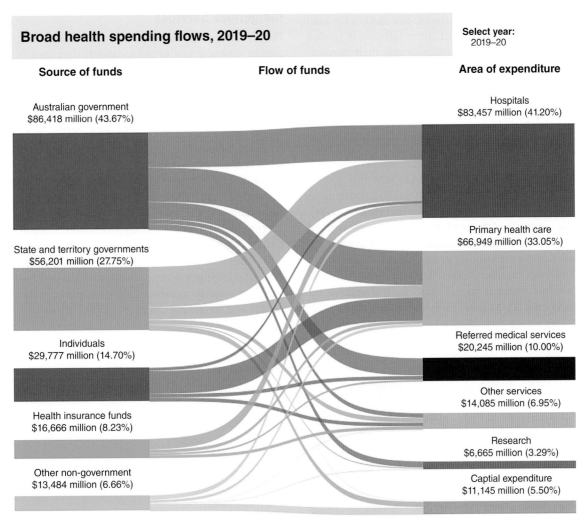

Broad health spending flows, 2019–20

Select year: 2019–20

Source of funds

Flow of funds

Area of expenditure

Australian government
$86,418 million (43.67%)

State and territory governments
$56,201 million (27.75%)

Individuals
$29,777 million (14.70%)

Health insurance funds
$16,666 million (8.23%)

Other non-government
$13,484 million (6.66%)

Hospitals
$83,457 million (41.20%)

Primary health care
$66,949 million (33.05%)

Referred medical services
$20,245 million (10.00%)

Other services
$14,085 million (6.95%)

Research
$6,665 million (3.29%)

Captial expenditure
$11,145 million (5.50%)

Note:
1. This analysis excludes spending on the medical expenses tax rebate.
2. Constant price health spending is in 2019–20 prices.

Figure 6.1 Health Spending Flows. *Source*: Australian Institute of Health and Welfare (AIHW) (2021a). Health expenditure Australia 2019–20, broad flows. AIHW, Canberra. https://www.aihw.gov.au/reports/health-welfare-expenditure/health-expenditure-australia-2019-20/contents/main-visualisations/broad-flows.

federal government is the major contributor to PHC cost it is individuals who are the second largest contributor, followed by state and territory governments. Health insurance and other funding sources make up a small amount of the PHC spend.

PHC is delivered in different settings and includes general practice, community health centres and allied health practices. Primary care professionals include general practitioners, nurses, nurse practitioners, allied health professionals, midwives, pharmacists, dentists and Aboriginal health practitioners. Fig. 6.2 illustrates the breakdown of the PHC spend. You can see for Joan and Mario in Case study 6.1, their GP care is funded from the 'Unreferred medical services', their medications from the 'Benefit paid pharmaceuticals and all other medications' category. The cost of them seeing the podiatrist and optometrist is the 'Other health practitioners' category.

General Practice

General practices are primary care medical services which provide primary care but many may also provide additional elements of PHC. Professionals working in general practices include **general practitioners (GPs)**, practice nurses and nurse practitioners, as well as allied health and sometimes specialists. GPs are the most accessed health professionals in Australia.

The exact number of GP clinics in Australia is unknown but estimates suggest 7185 general practice establishments (IBISWorld 2018 cited in Swerissen et al.

2018), of which over 6500 are accredited (Australian Medical Association 2019). The National General Practice Accreditation Scheme supports the voluntary accreditation of Australian general practices against the Royal Australian College of General Practitioners (RACGP) Standards for general practices (RACGP 2018). Accreditation entitles general practices and general practitioners to additional incentives. There are over 25,000 full-time equivalent GPs in Australia (Australian Medical Association 2019).

Indigenous Services

Health for Aboriginal and/or Torres Strait Islander peoples in Australia is a broader concept than merely the absence of disease and illness (see also Chapter 10). It is a more holistic concept that aligns well to a vision for health and well-being and incorporates physical, emotional, social, cultural and spiritual well-being for individuals and the community.

Fig. 6.3 shows the significant difference in life expectancy between Indigenous and non-Indigenous Australians. Other data highlight additional gaps between the health enjoyed by non-Indigenous Australians and Indigenous Australians. For example, the burden of disease is 2.3 times greater in Indigenous Australians. Most of this burden is because of chronic diseases such as cardiovascular diseases, mental and substance use disorders, cancer, chronic kidney disease, diabetes, vision and hearing loss and selected musculoskeletal, respiratory, neurological and congenital disorders (AIHW 2016).

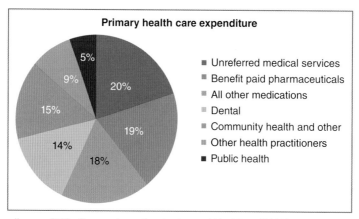

Figure 6.2 Spending on PHC. *Source*: Australian Institute of Health and Welfare (AIHW) (2021b). Health expenditure Australia 2019–20, expenditure table. https://www.aihw.gov.au/reports/health-welfare-expenditure/health-expenditure-australia-2019-20/contents/main-visualisations/expenditure-table.

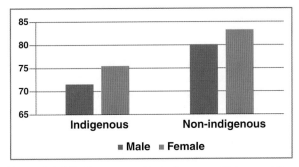

Figure 6.3 Life Expectancy By Indigenous Status and Sex (2015–17). *Source*: Australian Institute of Health and Welfare (AIHW) (2020a). Indigenous life expectancy and deaths. AIHW, Canberra. https://www.aihw.gov.au/reports/australias-health/indigenous-life-expectancy-and-deaths.

Indigenous Australians represent many diverse groups and many cultures. It is therefore critical that health services for Indigenous Australians acknowledge this diversity and are culturally responsive.

Indigenous people may access care from mainstream services. The **Indigenous Australians' Health Programme (IAHP)** specifically aims to improve the health of Indigenous people, improve access to comprehensive culturally responsive PHC and support PHC services to improve the way they operate to better cater for Aboriginal and Torres Strait Islander peoples. The IAHP operates through four themes:

- specific primary health care services such as immunisation or smoking cessation
- improving access to culturally responsive primary health care and facilitating additional services such as coordinating care or supporting outreach services
- targeted health activities, for example, managing chronic conditions or improving the ear and eye health of children
- funding capital works (e.g. upgrading infrastructure).

One of the main beneficiaries of the IAHP program are **Aboriginal Community Controlled Health Organisation(s) (ACCHO)**. They are primary care services that provide culturally responsive holistic and comprehensive care and are operated by the local Aboriginal community. The first ACCHO was formed in 1971 and there are now more than 140 ACCHOs across Australia, represented by a national peak body, the **National Aboriginal Community Controlled Health Organisation (NACCHO)**. In addition to the usual workforce that makes up primary care, Aboriginal and Torres Strait Islander health workers and Aboriginal and Torres Strait Islander health practitioners may also work in primary care (see also Chapter 10).

A new national policy, the National Aboriginal and Torres Strait Islander Health Plan 2021–2031, seeks to realise a vision where Aboriginal and Torres Strait Islander people enjoy long, healthy lives that are centred in culture, with access to services that are prevention-focused, culturally safe and responsive, equitable and free of racism (Department of Health 2021). The plan seeks to achieve this through 12 priority areas across four categories, as follows.

Enablers for Change
- Priority 1: Genuine shared decision-making and partnerships
- Priority 2: Aboriginal and Torres Strait Islander community-controlled comprehensive primary health care
- Priority 3: Workforce

Focusing on Prevention
- Priority 4: Health promotion
- Priority 5: Early intervention
- Priority 6: Social and emotional well-being and trauma-aware, healing-informed approaches
- Priority 7: Healthy environments, sustainability and preparedness

Improving the Health System
- Priority 8: Identify and eliminate racism
- Priority 9: Access to person-centred and family-centred care
- Priority 10: Mental health and suicide prevention

Culturally Informed Evidence Base
- Priority 11: Culturally informed and evidence-based evaluation, research and practice
- Priority 12: Shared access to data and information at a regional level

Private Allied Health and Pharmacy Services

The range of allied health professionals is broad and there is no universally accepted list of disciplines that constitute allied health. Commonly it includes optometrists, physiotherapists, occupational therapists, dietitians, speech pathologists, audiologists and psychologists. This diverse group apply their discipline-specific skills and knowledge to prevent, diagnose and treat health conditions either individually or as part of a multidisciplinary team.

Community Health and Community-Based Services

In the early 1970s the Whitlam Federal Labor Government established the **Community Health Program (CHP)**. This program established a service sector for the delivery of primary health care across Australia through locally managed community health centres that provided 'integrated primary health care'. Based on a social model of health and with a strong focus on equity and participation, the centres comprised multidisciplinary teams that provided medical and nursing services as well as community development and advocacy/social action on social and environmental problems of concern to the community (Baum 2013). Many provided low-cost financial counselling and support referrals to housing services. By 1981, the Fraser Liberal Government had ended its involvement in the CHP and the program effectively ceased to exist.

In 1983, the Hawke Labor Government restored 1975 levels of community support, but in the absence of any overarching policy for primary health care the program was vulnerable. Funding community health had become the responsibility of the states and territories. Victoria and South Australia led the way, continuing to establish community health centres in areas of social and economic deprivation and pioneering new models of service delivery.

The original service profiles of the **community health services (CHS)** were designed to meet the needs of local communities and were established to promote the social model of health. Services included community (or district) nursing, allied health, women's health, drug and alcohol services, child, youth and family services, community mental health and sexual health services. In recent years, drug and alcohol services have largely been moved to specialist services. In Victoria, public dental health services are being integrated into community health services and programs – a trend which is likely to increase as chronic disease and early intervention programs are strengthened across all states and territories. Chronic disease programs increasingly focus on early intervention and education and support for self-management, with an emphasis on effective strategies to facilitate access to early CHS interventions and disease management for people living in disadvantaged circumstances.

Today, across the states and territories, CHSs vary in their governance arrangements, how they employ staff, and the types of programs they fund. Community health services are now funded through a mix of block grants from the Commonwealth and from state and territory funding. Victoria is the only state to have CHSs report directly to boards of management. Staff members of CHSs in Western Australia, Queensland, South Australia and Tasmania are employees of their respective state departments of health, and report directly to district managers. Queensland also funds non-government organisations to provide CHS. The CHSs in Western Australia and New South Wales are part of population health units in state-run, area-based health services.

Most jurisdictions now fund health promotion, community development and capacity-building, although some of this funding may be limited to a focus on prevention and early intervention for chronic disease, such as diabetes. Community development in health has not been well supported, with governments preferring to fund primary care through clinical streaming, and chronic disease programs focused on self-management gaining momentum in all states. Programs funded for disease management strive to maintain a primary health focus by organising work through multidisciplinary teams, working from a social model of health as much as possible, and developing collaborations and partnerships with other service providers and sectors in order to improve health outcomes.

Supporters of community health models continue to advocate for services that address the lack of equity in the distribution and delivery of primary care services, and the need to strengthen primary health care approaches in order to address social inequity. A strong emphasis is placed on multidisciplinary teams and partnerships with, for example, schools, workplaces, migrant services and welfare and social services.

Dedicated women's health services have also been established in each state and territory, supported through Australia's National Policy on Women's Health. Founded solidly on the social model of health, participation and local management, this network of women's health services has a particular focus on the development of information and resources (e.g. on violence against women and on reproductive health), education and training, health promotion and community development.

Dental Services

Dental services do not have any Medicare funding available. They are funded either privately through public dental clinics, through the **Department of Veterans' Affairs (DVA)** (where eligible) or through the Australian Government's Child Dental Benefits Schedule, which provides limited basic dental care for those who meet eligibility criteria (see Chapter 15).

Primary Care Organisations (PCOs)

Primary Health Networks (PHNs), 31 in total across Australia, were developed in 2015 to replace an earlier model of PCOs called Medicare Locals, which ran from 2013 to 2015. These, in turn, were a reform of the Divisions of General Practice, which had operated since 1992 until 2013. Divisions were GP membership organisations to support general practices, but Medicare Locals and now PHNs were given a much broader brief and objectives. The two key objectives of PHNs are (Department of Health 2018):

1. to increase the efficiency and effectiveness of medical services for patients, particularly those at risk of poor health outcomes
2. to improve coordination of care to ensure patients receive the right care in the right place at the right time. PHNs achieve these tasks by:
   - assessing the health needs of their region using a people-centred approach and undertaking a **comprehensive needs assessment (CNA).** Based on this CNA health services may be commissioned to meet the prioritised health needs of the people in their region
   - working closely with providers to build health workforce capacity and ensuring they deliver high-quality care
   - connecting health services for people to encourage better use of health resources and avoid duplication.

An evaluation of PHNs identified a key challenge was to develop levers to encourage Local Hospital Networks (LHNs), state and territory health departments and other agencies to more actively engage in regional planning and support integrated service delivery at the local level (Lane et al. 2018). The evaluation presented its findings and related opportunities for the further development of the PHN program along 11 common themes.

Pause *for* Reflection ...

Consider Joan and Mario's case. If you were a PHN executive, what questions would you want to have answered in a CNA to better understand the needs of older people living with long-term conditions?

THE CURRENT STATE OF PRIMARY HEALTH CARE IN AUSTRALIA

The Australian health care system generally performs well and most health care is associated with good clinical outcomes. A recent report from the Commonwealth Fund showed that Australia's health system overall ranked third from all the OECD countries after Norway and Netherlands. Fig. 6.4 shows that Australia achieved higher health system performance with a relatively lower health care spend compared to other countries.

However, there is significant variation in quality and safety. The health care system faces significant challenges including provision of reliable effective care, coordination of care, workforce pressures, an ageing population and increasing rates of risk factors for chronic conditions such as obesity and lack of physical activity. This is translating into an increasing prevalence of multimorbidity. Furthermore, there is growing concern that for a significant minority of the population, cost is becoming an increasing barrier. For example, in the same report Australia ranked low when the dimensions of access to care and care processes were compared. Access to care includes measures of health care's affordability and timeliness and other studies have demonstrated a significant minority of the population are not accessing health care because of the cost of care (Zurynski et al. 2022). Care processes include measures of preventive care, safe care, coordinated care, and engagement and patient preferences. This included a lack of achieving good communication between the primary care and hospital, emergency department, and home-based care provider or coordination with local social services providers.

Specific research measuring the different nations on timeliness and coordination of health care for older adults suggested delays in accessing primary care (17%), not hearing back from usual care provider (19%) and the majority (54%) reporting difficulty accessing after-hours care (Doty et al. 2021). On a positive note Australia ranked high with respect to telehealth access for people with chronic conditions and care plans, with the majority of older adults with chronic conditions feeling confident that they could control and manage their health conditions.

In evidencing the contribution of primary health care to health outcomes, one problem is the access to limited yet reliable data on Australia's PHC. The limited access makes it difficult to build a comprehensive

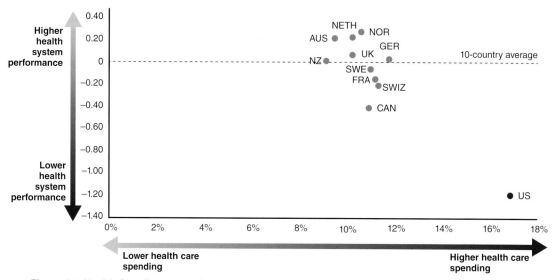

Figure 6.4 Health Care System Performance. *Source*: Schneider, E.C., Shah, A., Doty, M.M., et al. (2021). Mirror, mirror 2021 — reflecting poorly: health care in the US compared to other high-income countries. Commonwealth Fund, New York. https://www.commonwealthfund.org/publications/fund-reports/2021/aug/mirror-mirror-2021-reflecting-poorly.

picture to understand the consumer journey and experience of care. Notwithstanding this, most health care services are delivered in primary health care and PHC accounts for just over one-third of all Australian health care expenditure as shown earlier. The **Australian Institute of Health and Welfare (AIHW)** reports 83% of people over the age of 15 have seen their GP in the previous 12 months and 12% of the population report seeing their GP 12 or more times per year. Moreover, the utilisation of primary health care services has been increasing over time. GP attendances over the decade 2009–19 have increased from 5.3 consultations per person per year to 6.3 consultations per person per year. Indigenous-specific primary health care service attendances have increased by 72%. The range of conditions seen vary and mental health conditions and chronic conditions are increasing. The changing trends in utilisation of health services are illustrated in Fig. 6.5.

Like general practice services, the trend for allied health services shows increasing utilisation with the rate of number of services having increased from 49 to 88 per 100 people in the decade ending 2018–19 (Fig. 6.6). About 15% of the cost of accessing allied health is met by consumers as an out-of-pocket cost.

Just under half of the population over the age of 15 had seen a dentist in the previous 12 months and over a

quarter of the population delayed accessing a dentist because of cost (AIHW 2020c) (see also Chapter 15).

Australian researchers investigated Australian PHC for lessons in relation to UHC for NCD and health equity (Fisher et al. 2020). They identified:
- a predominant biomedical and behavioural approach to health policy
- a focus of policy to strengthen the general practice sector to better manage NCD in order to reduce hospitalisations
- that the Medicare system was broadly favourable to equity of access for general practice but identified concerns in relation to:
  - low level of PHC funding in relation to acute care
  - the emphasis on general practices in the PHC system
  - fee-for-service funding for PHC
  - structural separation of PHC funding between federal and state governments.

Furthermore, there is geographical inequity of health services for rural and regional communities. Consumers report more difficulty in accessing care, with an unequally distributed workforce favouring metro areas. This translated into higher rates of disease burden, potentially preventable hospitalisations and reduced life expectancy (AIHW 2019) (see also Chapter 9).

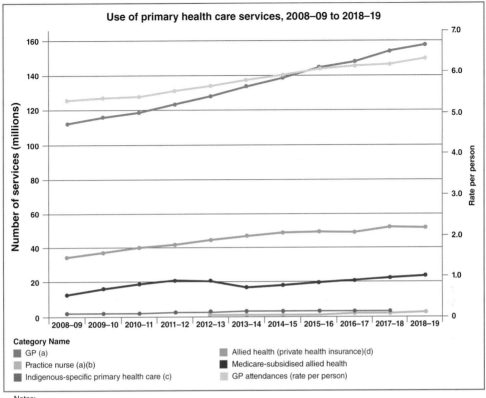

Figure 6.5 Trends in the Utilisation of Primary Health Care Services. *Source*: Australian Institute of Health and Welfare (AIHW) (2020b). Primary health care. AIHW, Canberra. https://www.aihw.gov.au/reports/australias-health/primary-health-care.

The Australian Government Department of Health (2019) recognises several challenges facing the health system:

- an ageing population and increasing demand on health services
- increasing rates of chronic disease
- costs of medical research and innovations
- making the best use of emerging health technologies
- making better use of health data.

Pause *for* Reflection ...

Reflect on the data and commentary on the current state of the Australian PHC system.

What do you consider are the strengths of the current system and what are the opportunities for improvement?

THE REFORM AGENDA AND FUTURE OF PRIMARY HEALTH CARE

Recognising the challenges facing health care and PHC the Australian government has embarked on a National Health Plan aspiring to build the world's best **health system** (Department of Health 2019). The first pillar of this National Health Plan is to strengthen primary care with a goal to make 'primary health care more patient-focused, more accessible, and better able to provide preventive health and management of chronic conditions' (Department of Health 2019).

Included in this 10-year plan is a mental health vision, 10-year Preventive Health Strategy, a 10-year Medical Research Future Fund investment plan and a 10-year Primary Health Care Plan. The formulation of the

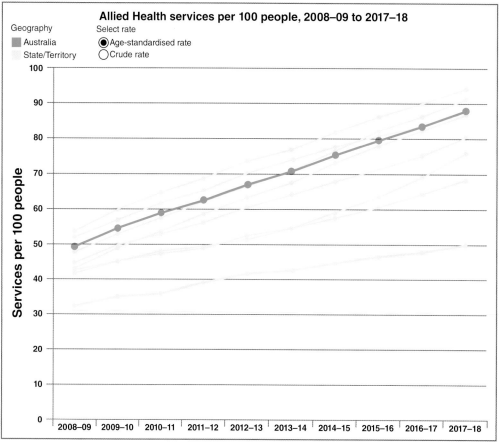

Figure 6.6 Trends in the Utilisation of Allied Health Services. *Source*: Australian Institute of Health and Welfare (AIHW) (2020b). Primary health care. AIHW, Canberra. https://www.aihw.gov.au/reports/australias-health/primary-health-care.

10-year primary care plan was an inclusive process led by the **Primary Health Reform Steering Group (PHRSG)** and a set of recommendations to Government (Primary Health Reform Steering Group 2021) and the federal government's plan entitled Australia's Primary Health Care 10 Year Plan 2022–2032 (Department of Health 2022a). However, there has been a change of government since the publication of this plan and so this chapter will focus on the recommendations of the PHRSG.

The PHRSG took an inclusive approach in formulating its recommendations and incorporated learnings from the COVID-19 health reforms, and the **Organisation for Economic Co-operation and Development** **(OECD)** report, Realising the Potential of Primary Health Care (OECD 2020). The OECD report stated:

- Strong primary health care makes health systems more effective, efficient and equitable.
- Most health systems are still failing to reach the full potential of primary health care.
- New models of care, more economic incentives and broader role for patients are needed.

During the term of the PHRSG the Australian health system was in the first two years of the COVID-19 pandemic. The pandemic had significant impact on the health system including primary health care and general practice. The impact of the COVID-19 pandemic on general practice and care is summarised in a series of snapshot reports:

- a decrease in pathology testing, particularly for older or socially disadvantaged cohorts (Imai et al. 2021a)
- a decrease in face-to-face visits by GPs to residential aged care, particularly in areas with higher prevalence of COVID-19 (Dai et al. 2021)
- the suggestion of delays in managing people with chronic diseases, as evidenced by reduction in measuring HbA1c (a measure of control of diabetes) in people with diabetes (Imai et al. 2021b)
- large decreases in cancer screening (Imai et al. 2021c).

The introduction of Medicare rebates during COVID-19 allowed the system to pivot to alternative virtual modes of care delivery for ongoing care. For PHC, only synchronous telephone consultations and video consultations were funded. Health providers including general practices pivoted to using telehealth and many have continued to incorporate telehealth in their practice. Thirty percent of general practice consultations are by telehealth, 33% of mental health consultations and 2% of allied health consultations (Snoswell et al. 2020). Furthermore, the Department of Health funded 100 GP respiratory clinics around the country to supplement the states' and territories' response to assess, test and treat people with suspected COVID-19. GP clinics and pharmacies around the country were extensively involved in the administration of COVID-19 vaccination with more than 60% of all doses being administered in primary care (Department of Health 2022b).

The PHRSG formulated 20 recommendations. Importantly the first recommendation was to take a one-system view and focus on integrated care. The second recommendation was a single primary health care destination, where people would enrol on a voluntary basis and hence support a shift from episodic care to comprehensive, relationship-based longitudinal care with data systems providing the platform for service delivery and planning insights and accountability. The PHRSG used the quadruple aim (Bodenheimer & Sinsky 2014) as a guiding framework. The quadruple aim is to:

- improve the patient experience of care (including quality of care and satisfaction)
- improve the health of populations
- improve the cost-efficiency of the health system
- improve the work life of health care providers.

Australia can build on the strengths of its PHC system through the reform agenda but this will require an 'equal contribution from all stakeholders and aligned resources to co-create a future delivering value-based health care' (Janamian et al. 2022).

SUMMARY

In summary, primary health care is a broad model of care that incorporates primary care in community-based services that are delivered by a range of practitioners. These services are guided by Australia's health system policy frameworks as well as by service delivery models, characterised by the type of care provided, the settings in which that care is provided, the people providing the care and the specific activities or goals involved or the models' underlying values.

Australian's PHC system is a mature system that performs well when compared with other developed nations. However, we should not be under the illusion that, in a relatively rich country like Australia, there is no need for improved primary health care systems and programs. The need for primary health care in Australia has never been greater than now. System improvements require goals to first increase efficiency and effectiveness of the vast number of health providers across Australia. Second, system goals must also seek to increase access to affordable health services, which is likely to impact on a reduction in health inequalities in Australia as the social divide expands. Thirdly, as technologies emerge and new models of care evolve these need to be tested, adapted and scaled at pace for the benefit of consumers, communities and the health system.

In this chapter, we have explored the concepts of primary health care, primary care and community-based service delivery in the context of the Australian health care system. Key points include:

- the global context for primary health care and its history
- the makeup of Australian PHC
- the challenges facing PHC and the importance of strengthening it to create a sustainable health system
- the role of Primary Health Networks and the potential opportunities presented by future health reform.

REVIEW QUESTIONS

1. What are the differences and synergies between primary care and primary health care? How would you expect these to affect your work as a health care practitioner in the future?
2. For what reasons, and for which groups of people, might Australia need to develop a stronger primary health care service delivery system?
3. What contribution does PHC make to a country's health system and more broadly to that country?
4. What is the connection between public health and PHC in Australia? Consider the COVID-19 pandemic and Australia's response as an example.
5. Any health system should be oriented to providing a person-centred approach to care. What features in the Australian PHC need to be maintained or adapted to create a truly person-centred health system and what new features are needed?

REFERENCES

Australian Government Department of Health, 2019. The Australian health system. https://www.health.gov.au/about-us/the-australian-health-system.

Australian Institute of Health and Welfare (AIHW), 2016. Australian Burden of Disease Study: Impact and causes of illness and death in Aboriginal and Torres Strait Islander people 2011. Australian Burden of Disease Study series no. 6. Cat. no. BOD 7. AIHW, Canberra.

Australian Institute of Health and Welfare (AIHW), 2019. Rural & remote health, Access to health care. AIHW, Canberra. https://www.aihw.gov.au/reports/rural-remote-australians/rural-remote-health/contents/access-to-health-care.

Australian Institute of Health and Welfare (AIHW), 2020a. Indigenous life expectancy and deaths. AIHW, Canberra. https://www.aihw.gov.au/reports/australias-health/indigenous-life-expectancy-and-deaths.

Australian Institute of Health and Welfare (AIHW), 2020b. Primary health care. AIHW, Canberra. https://www.aihw.gov.au/reports/australias-health/primary-health-care.

Australian Institute of Health and Welfare (AIHW), 2020c. Allied health and dental services. AIHW, Canberra. https://www.aihw.gov.au/reports/australias-health/allied-health-and-dental-services.

Australian Institute of Health and Welfare (AIHW), 2021a. Health expenditure Australia 2019–20, broad flows. AIHW, Canberra. https://www.aihw.gov.au/reports/health-welfare-expenditure/health-expenditure-australia-2019-20/contents/main-visualisations/broad-flows.

Australian Institute of Health and Welfare (AIHW), 2021b. Health expenditure Australia 2019–20, expenditure table. https://www.aihw.gov.au/reports/health-welfare-expenditure/health-expenditure-australia-2019-20/contents/main-visualisations/expenditure-table.

Australian Medical Association (AMA), 2019. General practice facts. https://www.ama.com.au/article/general-practice-facts.

Baum, F., 2013. Community health services in Australia. In: Germov, J. (Ed.), Second Opinion: An Introduction to Health Sociology, fifth ed. OUP, Melbourne, pp. 484–502.

Bodenheimer, T., Sinsky, C., 2014. From triple to quadruple aim: care of the patient requires care of the provider. Ann Fam Medicine 12, 573–576. doi:10.1370/afm.1713.

Dai, Z., Franco, G.S., Datta. S., et al., 2021. The impact of the COVID-19 pandemic on general practice consultations in residential aged care facilities. General Practice Snapshot 4. doi:10.25949/71JM-QG60.

Department of Health, 2018. Primary Health Networks (PHNs). http://www.health.gov.au/internet/main/publishing.nsf/Content/PHN-Home.

Department of Health, 2019. Long term national health plan to build the world's best health system. https://www.health.gov.au/sites/default/files/australia-s-long-term-national-health-plan_0.pdf.

Department of Health, 2021. National Aboriginal and Torres Strait Islander Health Plan 2021–2031. https://www.health.gov.au/resources/publications/national-aboriginal-and-torres-strait-islander-health-plan-2021-2031?language=en.

Department of Health, 2022a. Future focused primary health care: Australia's Primary Health Care 10 Year Plan 2022–32. https://www.health.gov.au/sites/default/files/documents/2022/03/australia-s-primary-health-care-10-year-plan-2022-2032-future-focused-primary-health-care-australia-s-primary-health-care-10-year-plan-2022-2032.pdf.

Department of Health, 2022b. COVID-19 vaccination – vaccination data – 31 July 2022. https://www.health.gov.au/resources/publications/covid-19-vaccination-vaccination-data-31-july-2022.

Doty, M., Shah, A., Fields, K., et al., 2021. Comparing nations on timeliness and coordination of health care: findings from the 2021 Commonwealth Fund International Health Policy Survey of Older Adults. Commonwealth Fund, New York.

Fisher, M., Freeman, T., Mackean, T., et al., 2020. Universal Health Coverage for Non-communicable Diseases and Health Equity: Lessons From Australian Primary Healthcare. Int J Health Policy Manag. doi:10.34172/ijhpm.2020.232.

Imai, C., Hardie, R-A., Dai, Z., et al., 2021a. The impact of the COVID-19 pandemic on cancer screening in general practice. General Practice Snapshot 7. doi:10.25949/5Z8Y-2E49.

Imai, C., Hardie, R-A., Thomas, J., et al., 2021b. The impact of the COVID-19 pandemic on general practice-based HbA1c monitoring in type 2 diabetes. General Practice Snapshot 5. doi:10.25949/Q9BE-BJ06.

Imai, C., Thomas, J., Hardie R-A., et al., 2021c. The impact of the COVID-19 pandemic on pathology testing in general practice. General Practice Snapshot 3. doi:10.25949/ZX36-8S49.

Janamian, T., Dawda, P., Jammal, W., 2022. Achieving person-centred primary health care through value co-creation. Med J Aust 216 (10). doi:10.5694/mja2.51538.

Lane, R.I., Russels, G.M., Francis, C., et al., 2018. Evaluation of the Primary Health Networks Program: final report. UNSW, Monash University, EY. https://www.health.gov.au/sites/default/files/documents/2021/06/evaluation-of-the-primary-health-networks-program.pdf.

Muldoon, L.K., Hogg, W.E., Levitt, M., 2006. Primary Care (PC) and Primary Health Care (PHC). Can J Public Health 97 (5), 409–411. doi:10.1007/bf03405354.

Organisation for Economic Co-operation and Development (OECD), 2020. Realising the Potential of Primary Health Care, OECD Health Policy Studies. OECD Publishing, Paris. doi:10.1787/a92adee4-en.

Primary Health Reform Steering Group, 2021. Recommendations on the Australian Government's Primary Health Care 10 Year Plan. Australian Government Department of Healthhttps://consultations.health.gov.au/primary-care-mental-health-division/draft-primary-health-care-10-year-plan/supporting_documents/Primary%20Health%20Reform%20Steering%20Group%20%20Recommendations%20September%202021.pdf.

RACGP, 2018. RACGP – Standards fifth ed. https://www.racgp.org.au/running-a-practice/practice-standards/standards-5th-edition.

Schneider, E.C., Shah, A., Doty, M.M., et al., 2021. Mirror, mirror 2021 — reflecting poorly: health care in the US compared to other high-income countries. Commonwealth Fund, New York. https://www.commonwealthfund.org/publications/fund-reports/2021/aug/mirror-mirror-2021-reflecting-poorly.

Snoswell, C.L., Caffery, L.J., Taylor, M.L., et al,. 2020. Centre for Online Health, The University of Queensland. Telehealth and coronavirus: Medicare Benefits Schedule (MBS) activity in Australia. https://coh.centre.uq.edu.au/telehealth-and-coronavirus-medicare-benefits-schedule-mbs-activity-australia.

Starfield, B., Shi, L., Macinko, J., 2005. Contribution of primary care to health systems and health. Milbank Q 83 (3), 457–502. doi:10.1111/j.1468-0009.2005.00409.x.

Swerissen, H., Duckett, S., Moran, G., 2018. Mapping primary care in Australia. Grattan Institute.

United Nations, 2021. Home. Department of Economic and Social Affairs. https://sdgs.un.org.

World Health Organization (WHO) and UNICEF, 1978. Declaration of Alma-Ata, International Conference on Primary Health Care, Alma-Ata, USSR. WHO, Geneva.

World Health Organization (WHO), 2007. Everybody's Business: Strengthening health systems to improve health outcomes. WHO's Framework for action. WHO, Geneva.

World Health Organization (WHO) and United Nations Children's Fund (UNICEF), 2018. A vision for primary health care in the 21st century: towards universal health coverage and the Sustainable Development Goals. World Health Organization. https://apps.who.int/iris/handle/10665/328065.

World Health Organization (WHO), 2018. Astana Declaration: From Alma-Ata Towards Universal Health Coverage and the Sustainable Development Goals. Astana, Kazakhstan: Global Conference on Primary Health Care. https://www.who.int/docs/default-source/primary-health/declaration/gcphc-declaration.pdf.

Zurynski, Y., Ellis, L. A., Dammery, G., et al., 2022. The Voice of Australian Health Consumers: The 2021 Australian Health Consumer Sentiment Survey. Report prepared for the Consumers Health Forum of Australia, 2022.

FURTHER READING

Guzys, D., Brown, R., Halcomb, E., et al., 2020. Introduction to Community and Primary Health Care, third ed. Cambridge University Press, Melbourne.

Coleman, K., Wagner, E., Schaefer, J., et al., 2016. Redefining Primary Care for the 21st Century. White Paper. Prepared by Abt Associates, in partnership with the MacColl Center for Health Care Innovation and Bailit Health Purchasing. Agency for Healthcare Research and Quality. https://www.ahrq.gov/sites/default/files/wysiwyg/professionals/systems/primary-care/workforce-financing/white_paper.pdf.

ONLINE RESOURCES

AIHW, Primary Health Care: https://www.aihw.gov.au/reports-data/health-welfare-services/primary-health-care/overview.

International Profiles of Health Care Systems, Commonwealth Fund: https://www.commonwealthfund.org/sites/default/files/2020-12/International_Profiles_of_Health_Care_Systems_Dec2020.pdf.

OECD Health Policy Studies Realising the Potential of Primary Health Care, 2020:https://www.google.com.au/books/edition/OECD_Health_Policy_Studies_Realising_the/OwzoDwAAQBAJ?hl=en&gbpv=0.

Primary Health Care. World Health Organization: https://www.who.int/health-topics/primary-health-care#tab=tab_1.

WONCA. The Barbara Starfield Collection: https://www.globalfamilydoctor.com/internationalissues/barbarastarfield.aspx.

7

The Pharmaceutical Benefits Scheme

Lisa Pont

KEY LEARNING OUTCOMES

When you finish this chapter you should be able to:

- explain the purpose of the Pharmaceutical Benefits Scheme (PBS) and its relationship to government health and medicines policy
- describe the key elements of the PBS including types of benefits, the Schedule of Benefits, eligibility requirements, co-payments, the Safety Net scheme, generic substitution, and Closing the Gap
- explain why the cost of the Pharmaceutical Benefits Scheme is high
- describe key reforms to the PBS which have been undertaken to contain cost increases
- identify key challenges to the sustainability of the PBS in the future.

KEY TERMS AND ABBREVIATIONS

authority required benefit

authority required (streamlined) benefit

bioequivalent

Closing the Gap (CTG) PBS co-payment program

concessional beneficiaries

co-payment

Efficient Funding of Chemotherapy

general patients

generic brand

generic substitution

highly specialised drugs (HSD)

incremental cost-effectiveness ratio (ICER)

inpatient

National Medicines Policy (NMP)

originator brand

outpatient

patent

Pharmaceutical Benefits Advisory Committee (PBAC)

Pharmaceutical Benefits Scheme (PBS)

pharmaceutical reform

private prescriptions

quality-adjusted life-year (QALY)

quality use of medicine (QUM)

reciprocal health care agreement (RHCA)

reference pricing

Repatriation Pharmaceutical Benefits Scheme (RPBS)

repeats

restricted benefit

Safety Net scheme

Schedule of Pharmaceutical Benefits

section 100

Therapeutic Goods Administration (TGA)

unrestricted benefits

WHAT IS THE PHARMACEUTICAL BENEFITS SCHEME?

The **Pharmaceutical Benefits Scheme (PBS)** provides the Australian population with access to necessary and lifesaving medicines at an affordable price (Biggs 2003). Under the PBS the Australian Government subsidises the cost of medicines for most medical conditions (Department of Health and Ageing 2022).

The PBS is a key part of the Australian Government's **National Medicines Policy (NMP)**. The aim of the NMP is to meet the medication needs of the Australian population enabling optimal health outcomes across the population as well as for the individual. The NMP takes a comprehensive rationalist approach to health care, with the policy aiming to address the problem of fair and equitable allocation of medicines, as a resource, at a cost which is affordable to the individual as well as to the government (Bacchi 2016).

The NMP has four central objectives:

- *timely access to the medicines that Australians need, at a cost individuals and the community can afford*
- *medicines meeting appropriate standards of quality, safety, and efficacy*
- **quality use of medicines (QUM),** *and*
- *maintenance of a responsible and viable medicines industry.*
        (Department of Health and Ageing 1999, p. 1)

The key elements of the National Medicines Policy addressed by the PBS are:
- ensuring that medicines are affordable for the individual who needs them
- ensuring that medicines are affordable for society since they are subsidised via taxation
- ensuring that the scheme benefits Australian citizens and residents.

With the NMP launched over 20 years ago, ensuring that the policy remains relevant is critical. A review of the NMP commenced in 2021 and is currently in progress (Department of Health and Ageing 2021).

Pause *for* Reflection ...

The COVID-19 pandemic has had a critical impact on health systems worldwide. How has COVID-19 impacted access to and use of medicines in Australia? What changes could be considered as part of a revision of the NMP to ensure that the policy remains relevant in current and future health care contexts?

What Led To Development of the PBS?

While the concept of social responsibility for health and the introduction of schemes to provide health care to the poor had been established in a small number of countries such as France, Britain, Germany and the United States, it wasn't until after the end of the second world war that Australia's journey towards universal access to health care and access to medicines began, stimulated by three pre-conditions: discovery and commercial production of antibiotics; public demand for access to effective treatment for tuberculosis; and political interest in universal health care and access to medicines.

The discovery of penicillin in 1928 saw the advent of the antibiotic era. While chemicals with antibacterial action had been discovered in the late 19th century, it was the discovery of penicillin (Gaynes 2017) and the subsequent commercialisation and mass production of antibiotics such as penicillin and sulphonamides that dramatically changed clinical practice and improved health outcomes. Availability of these medicines meant that previously fatal bacterial infections such as pneumonia, meningitis and dysentery could now be treated.

At the same time, a new antibiotic called streptomycin was discovered. Prior to the discovery of streptomycin, tuberculosis, an infectious disease caused by the *mycobacterium tuberculosis* bacteria, was a major cause of mortality and morbidity for which no effective treatment existed. With the discovery of streptomycin, there was now an effective medicine to reduce the burden of tuberculosis; however, until the introduction of the revised tuberculosis act in 1948 (National Health and Medical Research Council (NHMRC) 2020), access to streptomycin was limited to those able to afford the cost.

Universal access to medicine was already on the Australian political agenda in the early 20th century. The Australian Government introduced the **Repatriation Pharmaceutical Benefits Scheme (RPBS)** in 1919 to provide medicines, free of charge, to ex-service men and women (Biggs 2003). Initial attempts to introduce government policy to allow free-of-charge access to medicines for the Australian population was opposed by the medical association. The concept of a Pharmaceutical Benefits Act was introduced in 1944 and, under this Act, the Australian Government would reimburse pharmacists for the cost of medicines provided to Australian residents. Medicines would be prescribed from a formulary, or list of approved medicines, by a medical doctor and then supplied by the pharmacist at no cost to the individual on receipt of the doctor's prescription (Goddard 2014). Medical uptake of the scheme was low, and by 1949 only 157 of the 7000 doctors practising had prescribed a medicine under the scheme. Despite this the Australian Pharmaceutical Benefits Scheme (PBS) operated under the Pharmaceutical Benefits Act until 1953, when the National Health Act was introduced. The National Health Act strengthened the role of the PBS and saw the establishment of the **Pharmaceutical Benefits Advisory Committee (PBAC)** to recommend which medicines should be included on the national formulary. PBAC continues to take this role, meeting four times a year (Department of Health 2021b). Medicines available via the PBS remained free of charge for Australians until 1960 when a patient co-payment was introduced.

Pause *for* Reflection ...

If the aim of the PBS is to help make prescribed medicines more affordable for Australians, why not cover the costs of all medicines completely? What might be the reason behind the introduction of the patient co-payment?

Who is Eligible for the PBS?

Australian citizens, eligible residents and visitors from countries with which Australia has **reciprocal health care agreements (RHCA)** (United Kingdom, Ireland, New Zealand, Malta, Italy, Sweden, the Netherlands, Finland, Norway, Belgium and Slovenia) are eligible to access subsidised medicines via the PBS (Department of Health and Ageing 2022). Australian veterans and their eligible family members have access to the PBS as well as to the RPBS, which includes additional pharmaceutical items subsidised by the Department of Veterans' Affairs. To access medicines on the PBS, eligible Australians show their Medicare card at the pharmacy when presenting a prescription for a PBS-subsidised medicine. Eligible overseas visitors either show their passport, or a Reciprocal Health Care Agreement card. Australian residents and overseas visitors who are not eligible for the PBS are still able to access medicines, however the Australian Government does not provide any subsidy for these medicines and the individual is required to pay the full cost of the medicine.

Which Medicines are Subsidised via the PBS?

The Australian Government considers two key elements when deciding which medicines to subsidise via the PBS. The medicines need to demonstrate that they provide a therapeutic benefit to the Australian community, and that this health benefit is cost-effective. The balance between therapeutic need and national and individual affordability draws back to Fuch's observation that each society must determine how much health care to provide, and how to distribute it, balancing health care needs with financial resource limitations (Tuohy 1999). In assessing therapeutic need and cost-effectiveness, medicines may be recommended for inclusion in the PBS if they treat or prevent a significant medical condition for which there is not subsidised medicine currently available on the PBS, if the proposed medicine is more effective and/or less harmful than a currently listed medicine or if the proposed medicine is as effective and safe as an existing listed medicine (Department of Health and Ageing 2022). Medicines available via the PBS are listed in the **Schedule of Pharmaceutical Benefits** available at https://www.pbs.gov.au. Medicines listed on the PBS have a fixed price which the government pays for the medicines, a fixed co-payment paid by the patient, a maximum quantity and maximum number of **repeats** that can be supplied each time the medicine is dispensed from the pharmacy.

How do Medicines Get Listed on the PBS?

The **Pharmaceutical Benefits Advisory Committee (PBAC)** is an independent expert committee comprising doctors, health professionals, health economists and consumers who are appointed by the Australian Government. PBAC is responsible for all four stages of policy-making outlined by Bacchi (1999), including setting the agenda regarding the need for the medicines being proposed for the PBS; policy formation such as price negotiation; policy implementation, such as articulation of any therapeutic restrictions associated with a particular medicine; and policy review, including the monitoring and reporting of the PBS operations. The role of PBAC is to recommend new medicines to the Australian Government for inclusion on the PBS. When considering a medicine for inclusion on the PBS, PBAC considers the clinical effectiveness, safety and cost-effectiveness of the proposed medicine compared with existing treatments. In the past, only medicines that were approved for use in Australia by the Australian **Therapeutic Goods Administration (TGA)** could apply to PBAC for listing on the PBS, however in 2011 a parallel pathway was introduced where manufacturers can simultaneously apply to the TGA for marketing approval and to PBAC for PBS listing to reduce delays in the approval processes (Pearce et al. 2012).

How Does the PBS Ensure Affordability of Medicines for Patients?

Patients prescribed PBS medicines pay a capped **co-payment** for each medicine supplied which is listed on the PBS, with the Australian Government covering the remainder of the medicine cost. The PBS co-payment varies depending on socio-economic status. In 2022, the co-payment for **concessional beneficiaries**, that is, patients receiving an Australian pension or other welfare- eligible benefit along with ex-service men and women, was $6.80 and the price per medicine for **general patients** was $42.50 (Department of Health and Ageing 2022). In 2020–21 approximately half of all PBS expenditure was for medicines for concessional beneficiaries (Table 7.1). Where the total cost of the medicine is below the patient co-payment, the patient pays the full medicine cost. Prescribed medicines not included on the PBS are known as **private prescriptions** and the full price of the medicine is paid by the patient without any subsidy from the government. Pricing of private prescriptions is set by market demand.

Pricing of Medicines on the PBS

Part of the PBAC approval process is a recommendation regarding the basis on which the medicine will be priced. When a new medicine is listed on the PBS, if the medicine is considered therapeutically equivalent in terms of safety and efficacy to one or more medicines already listed on the PBS, the listing of the medicine may be recommended based on cost-minimisation and **reference pricing** used. With reference pricing, medicines on the PBS that are considered therapeutically equivalent are linked, and the lowest priced medicine is used as a price benchmark for all other medicines in the same group (Department of Health 2017). If there are no therapeutically equivalent medicines already on the PBS, then the pricing of the listing is considered based on cost-effectiveness, and the manufacturer negotiates with the Australian Government an agreed price that the government is willing to pay for the medicine. Cost-effectiveness pricing considers the **incremental cost-effectiveness ratio (ICER)** in terms of **quality-adjusted life-years (QALYs)** that the medicine offers over existing treatments (Vitry et al. 2015).

Prescribing Medicines on the PBS

There are three main categories of restriction of therapeutic use of the medicines listed on the PBS, with the therapeutic restriction indicated on the listing in the PBS schedule in red. Medicines listed on the PBS which can be prescribed without **unrestricted benefits** are medicines that can be prescribed under the PBS or RPBS without any restrictions on therapeutic use. **Restricted benefit** medicines can only be prescribed for the indication specified in the PBS schedule listing (Table 7.2).

'Authority benefits' are medicines for which the prescriber must obtain authority, or permission, in order to prescribe them for a patient. There are two types of authority benefits listed on the PBS, **authority required benefits** and **authority required (streamlined) benefits**. Authority required benefits require the prescriber to seek approval either electronically, by phone or in writing from the Department of Health and Aged Care (PBS) or Department of Veterans' Affairs (RPBS) prior to prescribing the medicine. During the approval process the prescriber receives an authority approval number which must be included on the prescription. For

TABLE 7.1 PBS Expenditure in 2020–21		
PBS Category	**Expenditure**	**Percentage of Total PBS Expenditure**
Concessional items	$6,884,024,680	50.1%
General items	$2,405,632,262	17.5%
Doctor's bag	$16,685,943	0.1%
Section 100	$4,429,279,015	32.2%
Safety Net Cards	$15,034,724	0.1%
Total	$13,750,656,624	100.0%

Source: Department of Health (2021a). PBS Expenditure and prescriptions report 1 July 2020 to 30 June 2021. https://www.pbs.gov.au/info/statistics/expenditure-prescriptions/pbs-expenditure-and-prescriptions-report-30-june-2021.

TABLE 7.2 Examples of Restricted, Authority Required, and Authority Required Streamlined Benefit Criteria

Type of Benefit and Medicine	Medical Condition	Clinical Criteria
Restricted benefit – alendronate	Established osteoporosis	Patient must have fracture due to minimal trauma, AND Patient must not receive concomitant treatment with any other PBS-subsidised anti-resorptive agent for this condition.
Authority required benefit – voriconazole	Prophylaxis of invasive fungal infections including both yeasts and moulds	Patient must be considered at high risk of developing an invasive fungal infection due to anticipated neutropenia (an absolute neutrophil count less than 500 cells per cubic millimetre) for at least 10 days while receiving chemotherapy for acute myeloid leukaemia or myelodysplastic syndrome; OR Patient must be considered at high risk of developing an invasive fungal infection due to having acute graft versus host disease (GVHD) grade II, III or IV, or, extensive chronic GVHD, while receiving intensive immunosuppressive therapy after allogeneic haematopoietic stem cell transplant; OR Patient must be undergoing allogeneic haematopoietic stem cell transplant using either bone marrow from an unrelated donor or umbilical cord blood (related or unrelated), and, be considered to be at high risk of developing an invasive fungal infection during the neutropenic phase prior to engraftment.
Authority required (streamlined) benefit – glatiramer	Multiple sclerosis treatment phase: continuing treatment	The condition must be diagnosed as clinically definite relapsing-remitting multiple sclerosis, AND Patient must have previously received PBS-subsidised treatment with this drug for this condition, AND Patient must not show continuing progression of disability while on treatment with this drug, AND Patient must have demonstrated compliance with, and an ability to tolerate this therapy.

Source: https://www.pbs.gov.au

authority required (streamlined) benefits, the streamlined approval code is accessed via the PBS schedule. The prescriber is responsible for ensuring that the patient meets the therapeutic criteria associated with the PBS listing and inclusion of the streamlined authority approval code on the prescription by the prescriber confirms that the patient meets the relevant eligibility criteria. Restricted, authority required and authority required (streamlined) benefits are indicated in the PBS schedule.

THE SAFETY NET

The PBS **Safety Net scheme** is designed to protect individuals that need a large number of medicines from burdensome out-of-pocket costs, by ensuring those medicines remain affordable. Under the PBS Safety Net scheme there is a co-payment threshold, and once individuals and their eligible family members have reached the threshold, general beneficiaries receive further PBS medicines that year at the concessional co-payment price, and concessional beneficiaries receive the remainder of PBS medicines for that year for free. The Safety Net co-payment threshold for 2022 differs for general and concessional beneficiaries, and in 2022 was $1542.10 for general beneficiaries and $326.40 for concessional beneficiaries (Australian Government Services Australia 2022).

CLOSING THE GAP

The **Closing the Gap (CTG) PBS co-payment program** was implemented in July 2010 to improve access to PBS medicines for Australia's First Nations peoples. The CTG program allows First Nations Australians living with, or at risk of, chronic disease access to further subsidies in the form of reduced co-payments for PBS medicines. Under CTG, First Nations Australians who would normally pay the general co-payment, instead pay the concessional co-payment and those who would generally pay the concessional co-payment received PBS medicines without any co-payment (Department of Health 2022). In addition to reducing the cost of medicines, the CTG program also includes other measures to increase access to medicines. These measures include permission for Remote Area Aboriginal and Torres Strait Islander Health Services to provide medicines without charge and without the need for the usual PBS prescription form. Since the introduction of the CTG program use of the program has grown from 823,583 items with a value of $6,069,589 in 2010–11, to 7,557,846 items with a value of $55,823,320 in 2020–21 (Department of Health 2022).

MEDICINES WITH SPECIAL ARRANGEMENTS

The **section 100** programs within the PBS provide access to a wide range of highly specialised medicines for the management of chronic conditions under section 100 of the *National Health Act 1953*. The section 100 programs include the **Highly Specialised Drugs (HSD) Program, Efficient Funding of Chemotherapy**, Botulinum Toxin Program, Growth Hormone Program, In Vitro Fertilisation (IVF) Program, Opiate Dependence Treatment Program and the Remote Area Aboriginal Health Services (RAAHS) Program. In 2020–21, section 100 programs accounted for 30.8% of all PBS expenditure with the Highly Specialised Drugs and Efficient Supply of Chemotherapy programs accounting for the majority of government costs associated with supply of medicines under the programs (Table 7.3) (Department of Health 2021a).

The Highly Specialised Drugs (HSD) program facilitates access to specialised medicines used for the treatment of complex conditions that require specialist management or specialist monitoring. Many of the medicines included in the HSD program are considered high-cost medicines and the majority of highly specialised medicines are prescribed and supplied via public hospitals (Harvey & De Boer 2015), however some HSD can also be provided via private hospitals and community pharmacies under the HSD program. The HSD program includes medicines for HIV/AIDS, hepatitis,

TABLE 7.3 Annual Expenditure and Growth for PBS Section 100 Programs 2020–21		
Section 100 Category	**Expenditure**	**Percentage of Total Section 100 Expenditure**
Highly Specialised Drugs	$2,102,049,020	47.5%
Chemotherapy (EFC & Chemotherapy-related)	$1,895,181,306	42.8%
In Vitro Fertilisation	$157,416,057	3.6%
Opiate Dependence Treatment Program	$90,681,291	2.0%
Aboriginal Health Services	$50,012,059	1.1%
Botulinum Toxin Program	$68,154,459	1.5%
Growth Hormone	$34,352,692	0.8%
Closing the Gap (CTG) PBS Co-payment Program	$31,066,492	0.7%
Other	$365,639	0.0
Total	$4,429,279,015	100.0%

Source: Adapted from Department of Health (2021a). PBS Expenditure and prescriptions report 1 July 2020 to 30 June 2021. https://www.pbs.gov.au/info/statistics/expenditure-prescriptions/pbs-expenditure-and-prescriptions-report-30-june-2021.

cancer, severe and chronic arthritic, autoimmune diseases, osteoporosis and organ transplant. In 2019, 9 of the top 10 medicines provided via the PBS/RPBS by cost were provided under the HSD program ('Top 10 drugs 2019–20', 2020).

EFFICIENT FUNDING OF CHEMOTHERAPY

The Efficient Funding of Chemotherapy program provides funding for certain chemotherapy injections and infusions that are administered in public and private hospitals within Australia. The program aims to provide efficient supply and minimise wastage of injectable chemotherapy medicines. Some medicines used to treat chemotherapy side effects, such as medicines to prevent and treat nausea, are also covered by the program. Under the program, in addition to a dispensing fee, pharmacists receive additional preparation, distribution and diluent fees to cover the specialised preparation required for supply of injectable chemotherapy.

MANAGING INCREASING PBS COSTS

Initially, reference pricing was effective at containing PBS costs with the Productivity Commission's reporting in 2000 concluding that reference pricing resulted in the cost of medicines to the government being lower than those in Canada, Sweden, the UK and the USA and similar to prices in France, New Zealand and Spain (Australian Productivity Commission 2001). However, medicine costs in Australia increased over time and, by 2011, the price to the Australian Government for medicines was higher than the prices in many other countries (Duckett et al. 2001).

To address rising PBS costs, major PBS reforms were introduced in 2007 and 2010. These reforms had three elements (Vitry et al. 2015):
1. division of the PBS into two lists or formularies, F1 and F2
2. regular mandatory reduction in price
3. mandatory price disclosure.

Under the reforms all PBS medicines were classified as either F1 or F2. Medicines where only a single brand was available were classified as F1 and those with multiple brands available on the PBS as F2. F1 medicines are re-classified as F2 medicines once an alternative brand, generally a generic brand, is PBS listed.

Generic Substitution

Generic substitution is another strategy which has been introduced to reduce medicine costs associated with the PBS. When a new medicine is first approved for use within Australia by the TGA the pharmaceutical company that has sponsored the TGA approval process receives a 20-year **patent** preventing other companies from developing their own version of the medicine for 20 years. The brand of the first new medicine which holds the 20-year patent is known as the **originator brand**. Once the patent expires, other companies can manufacture and market their own version of the medicine, known as **generic brands**. Generic brands are generally much cheaper than the originator brands since development and approval costs are lower. Since 1994, legislation has allowed pharmacists to substitute a generic brand for the originator brand when they are considered **bioequivalent,** that is equivalent in terms of their absorption into the body (Beecroft 2007), and there may be multiple generics available on the PBS, at the same price, for the one medicine. Generic substitution is one measure that reduces medicine costs on the PBS with the generic brands being significantly cheaper than originator brands, resulting in price reduction over time.

The PBS and Medicines in the Hospital Setting

The PBS was initially developed to provide affordable medicines in the community setting, however, over time access to the PBS has expanded to include provision of medicines in the hospital setting. While some PBS medicines under the Highly Specialised Drugs and Efficient Funding of Chemotherapy programs are supplied from public and private hospital pharmacies, hospital medicines used while a patient is in hospital are funded from state/territory budgets (Australian Healthcare Associates 2017). The introduction from 2001 of **pharmaceutical reform** agreements between the Commonwealth and state governments has allowed some hospital access to PBS medicines beyond that under the HSD and chemotherapy programs. Under the pharmaceutical reform agreements, public hospitals are allowed to prescribe and dispense PBS medicines to **outpatients** and patients being discharged from hospital. The reforms also provided hospitals with access to a range of government-subsidised chemotherapy medicines which could be used for both **inpatients** and outpatients

(Department of Health 2013). Patients receiving PBS-subsidised medicine from a hospital pay the same co-payment as community-based patients. The Australian Government has individual pharmaceutical reform agreements with each state, with Victoria the first state to agree to the reforms in 2001. In 2022, all states and territories with the exception of NSW and ACT have signed pharmaceutical reform agreements allowing access to the PBS for public hospitals (Australian Healthcare Associates 2017).

Pause *for* Reflection …

NSW and ACT are the last states to join the pharmaceutical reforms allowing access to medicines on discharge from public hospitals. What impact would access to the reform agreements provide Australians living in those states?

FUTURE CHALLENGES

One of the key challenges for the PBS is ensuring that medicine remains affordable, not only for the individual but also for Australian society. PBS expenditure is uncapped and therefore increases as demand for medicines and the number of medicines subsidised by the scheme grows (Grove 2016/2022). In 2017–18, over one-third of Australians aged over 65 were taking at least five medicines (Page et al. 2019) and Australians spent $22.3 billion on medicines. Around half of all expenditure on medicines in Australia was funded by the PBS/RPBS with the PBS/RPBS providing 302.6 million prescriptions in 2017–18 at a cost of $11.9 billion, or roughly $485 for every Australian (AIHW 2020). Australians are living longer and relying on medicines to remain healthy, both of which places increasing burden on the PBS.

The type of medicines subsidised by the PBS is also changing. Innovative new medicines such as biological medicines are being used to treat an ever-increasing range of diseases and while this brings health care benefits to the population, the high development and manufacture costs of these medicines is reflected in their high prices. Looking at trends in PBS expenditure, biological medicines account for a large proportion of PBS/RPBS funded medicines by cost, and as new biologicals and new indications for existing biologicals develop, increased impact on the PBS is expected.

With an ageing population, increased reliance on medicines, and changes to the types of medicine being funded on the PBS, additional funding will be needed to ensure that the PBS continues to provide medicines to the Australian population at a cost that both the individual and society can afford. See Case study 7.1.

CASE STUDY 7.1

To see how the PBS provides access to affordable effective medicines for the Australian population, let's consider the COVID-19 pandemic. Robyne contracts COVID-19 after attending a party at a local restaurant. Robyne has been fully vaccinated under the National Immunisation Program under which COVID-19 vaccination is provided free of charge to all Australian citizens and residents.

As Robyne is 81 years old, her doctor would like to prescribe her antiviral medicines which have been shown to reduce the mortality and morbidity associated with COVID-19. While the antiviral medicines have been shown to reduce COVID-19-related death and hospitalisation, they are quite expensive, with a single course costing over $1100 per patient. Such a high price would be unaffordable for Robyne and the majority of Australians, forming a major barrier to accessing such an important and potentially lifesaving medicine.

Antiviral medicines for the management of COVID-19 have been available on the PBS since early 2022. Robyne is a concessional beneficiary as she is a pensioner, so for her the price of her antivirals is $6.80 rather than the market price of $1100. Robyne pays the $6.80 co-payment and the Australian Government pays the difference between her co-payment and the $1100 market price.

Robyne's antiviral medicines are an authority required (streamlined) benefit meaning that before her doctor is able to prescribe them for Robyne they must confirm that she meets the clinical criteria, which in this case includes having a positive result on a test for COVID-19, having mild COVID-19 symptoms and not needing hospitalisation, treatment being initiated within 5 days of having symptoms and being over 70 years of age. These restrictions help to ensure that these expensive medicines are available to those with the greatest clinical need while limiting use to ensure that the cost remains affordable to the Australian Government.

With her antivirals Robyne's COVID remains mild and after 4 days she has recovered and is symptom free. For Robyne, the PBS has provided her access to a medicine that would otherwise be unaffordable to her as an individual, while the restrictions limiting access to antivirals to those with the greatest need ensure that the cost to the Australian Government and Australian society remains affordable.

SUMMARY

The PBS/RPBS is a key part of the Australian National Medicines Policy aiming to provide safe and effective medicines at a cost that is affordable for the individual as well as for Australian society. The Pharmaceutical Benefits Scheme provides access to medicines which have been shown to be effective, safe and cost-effective. Capped patient co-payments ensure that medicines remain affordable for individuals and special programs within the PBS provide access to high-cost drugs and chemotherapy. Additional support is given to individuals and families with high medicines needs and to First Nations Australians to ensure that access to medicines is facilitated for people with high health needs. A variety of measures such as reference pricing and generic substitution have been implemented to contain costs within the PBS, however, an ageing population, increased reliance on medicines and development of new and expensive medicines such as biologicals will increase the pressure on the PBS. Ongoing policy and pharmaceutical reforms will be needed to ensure that medicines remain affordable for all Australians.

REVIEW QUESTIONS

1. What is the aim of the Pharmaceutical Benefits Scheme and how does it relate to the Australian National Medicines Policy?
2. Who is eligible to access the PBS and why might access to the scheme be restricted?
3. How does the Safety Net scheme assist individuals and their families with complex health needs?
4. What is the Closing the Gap scheme and how does it contribute to better health outcomes for First Nations Australians?
5. Describe the process for a new medicine to be added to the PBS. What are the key considerations and who is involved in making them?
6. What strategies have been used to contain or limit PBS expenditure?
7. What are the critical challenges for the PBS to ensure that access to safe, effective and affordable medicines remains for future generations?

REFERENCES

Australian Government Services Australia, 2022. PBS Safety Net thresholds. https://www.servicesaustralia.gov.au/pbs-safety-net-thresholds?context=22016.

Australian Healthcare Associates, 2017. PBS Pharmaceuticals in Hospital Review final report. https://www.pbs.gov.au/reviews/pbs-pharmaceuticals-in-hospitals-review-files/PBS-Pharmaceuticals-in-Hospitals-Review.pdf.

Australian Institute of Health and Welfare (AIHW), 2020. Medicines in the health system. https://www.aihw.gov.au/reports/australias-health/medicines-in-the-health-system.

Australian Productivity Comission, 2001. International pharmaceutical price differences. https://www.pc.gov.au/inquiries/completed/pharmaceutical-prices/report.

Bacchi, C., 2016. Problematizations in health policy: questioning how "problems" are constituted in policies. SAGE Open, Sydney. doi: 10.1177/2158244016653986.

Beecroft, G., 2007. Generic drug policy in Australia: a community pharmacy perspective. Aust New Zealand Health Policy 4, 7. doi:10.1186/1743-8462-4-7.

Biggs, A., 2003. The Pharmaceutical Benefits Scheme an overview. Parlimentary Library. https://www.aph.gov.au/About_Parliament/Parliamentary_Departments/Parliamentary_Library/Publications_Archive/archive/pbs.

Department of Health, 2013. Report to the Minister of Health: Review of funding arrangements for chemotherapy services. https://www1.health.gov.au/internet/main/publishing.nsf/Content/chemotherapy-review/$File/review-of-chemotherapy-funding-arrangements.pdf.

Department of Health, 2017. Fact sheet: Setting an approved ex-manufacturer price for new or extended listings. https://www.pbs.gov.au/info/industry/pricing/pbs-items/fact-sheet-setting-an-approved-ex-manufacturer-price.

Department of Health, 2021a. PBS Expenditure and prescriptions report 1 July 2020 to 30 June 2021. https://www.pbs.gov.au/info/statistics/expenditure-prescriptions/pbs-expenditure-and-prescriptions-report-30-june-2021.

Department of Health, 2021b. Pharmaceutical Benefits Advisory Committee (PBAC) membership. https://www.pbs.gov.au/info/industry/listing/participants/pbac.

Department of Health, 2022. The Closing the Gap (CTG)-PBS Co-payment Program. https://www.pbs.gov.au/info/publication/factsheets/closing-the-gap-pbs-co-payment-measure.

Department of Health and Ageing, 1999. National Medicines Policy. https://www1.health.gov.au/internet/main/publishing.nsf/Content/B2FFBF72029EEAC8CA257BF0001BAF3F/$File/NMP2000.pdf.

Department of Health and Ageing, 2021. National Medicines Policy Review to begin in August 2021. https://www.pbs.gov.au/info/news/2021/06/national-medicines-policy-review-to-begin-in-august-2021.

Department of Health and Ageing, 2022. About the PBS. https://www.pbs.gov.au/info/about-the-pbs.

Duckett, S., Breadon, P., Ginnivan, L., et al., 2001. Australia's bad drug deal: high pharmaceutical prices. Grattan Institute, Melbourne.

Gaynes, R., 2017. The discovery of penicillin—new insights after more than 75 years of clinical use. Emerg Infect Dis 23 (5), 849–853. doi:10.3201/eid2305.161556.

Goddard, M. S., 2014. How the Pharmaceutical Benefits Scheme began. Med J Aust 201 (1 Suppl), S23–25. doi:10.5694/mja14.00124.

Grove, A., 2016 updated 23 February 2022. The Pharmaceutical Benefits Scheme: a quick guide. https://www.aph.gov.au/About_Parliament/Parliamentary_Departments/Parliamentary_Library/pubs/rp/rp1516/Quick_Guides/PBS.

Harvey, R., De Boer, R., 2015. Growth in expenditure on high cost drugs in Australia. https://parlinfo.aph.gov.au/parlInfo/download/library/prspub/3599565/upload_binary/3599565.pdf;fileType=application/pdf.

National Health and Medical Research Council (NHMRC), 2020. History of tuberculosis control in Australia: Case Study. https://www.nhmrc.gov.au/about-us/resources/impact-case-studies.

Page, A.T., Falster, M.O., Litchfield, M., et al., 2019. Polypharmacy among older Australians, 2006–2017: a population-based study. Med J Aust 211 (2), 71–75. doi:10.5694/mja2.50244.

Pearce, A., van Gool, K., Haywood, P., et al., 2012. Delays in access to affordable medicines: putting policy into perspective. Aust Health Rev 36 (4), 412–418. doi:10.1071/AH11110.

Top 10 drugs 2019–20, 2020. Australian Prescriber 43, 209. https://www.nps.org.au/australian-prescriber/articles/top-10-drugs-2019-20.

Tuohy, C.H., 1999. Accidental Logics: The Dynamics of Change in the Health Care Arena in the United States, Britain, and Canada. OUP, New York.

Vitry, A., Thai, L., Roughead, R., 2015. Pharmaceutical pricing policies in Australia. In Z. Barbar (Ed.), Pharmaceutical Prices in the 21st Century. Springer International, Switzerland.

FURTHER READING

Babar, Z. (Ed.), 2015. Pharmaceutical Prices in the 21st Century. Springer International, Switzerland (in particular Chapter 1: Vitry, A., Thai, L., Roughead, E., Pharmaceutical pricing policies in Australia).

Birkett, D.J., 2003. Generics – equal or not? Aust Prescr 26, 857. doi:10.18773/austprescr.2003.063.

Goddard, M., 2014. How the Pharmaceutical Benefits Scheme began. Med J Aust. 201 (1 Suppl.), S23–S25.

Lu, C.Y., Day, R.O., Williams, K.M., 2007. The funding and use of high-cost medicines in Australia: the example of anti-rheumatic biological medicines. Aust NZ Health Policy 4 (1).

NPS Medicinewise, 2021. Biologics, biosimilars and PBS sustainability. Medicinewise News. https://www.nps.org.au/news/biologics-biosimilars-and-pbs-sustainability.

ONLINE RESOURCES

Department of Health – The Pharmaceutical Benefits Scheme: http://www.pbs.gov.au/pbs/home.

8

The Aged Care Sector: Residential and Community Care

Hamish Robertson and David Smith

KEY LEARNING OUTCOMES

When you finish this chapter you should be able to:

- understand the implications of an ageing population for health and social care systems in Australia
- describe recent aged care reforms that have impacted on policy and funding

- critically assess the impact of government policy on aged-care service delivery
- understand community care for older people
- have a critical understanding of the Australian aged-care system.

KEY TERMS AND ABBREVIATIONS

Aged Care Assessment Teams (ACATs)
Commonwealth Home Support Program (CHSP)
population ageing
daily accommodation payment (DAP)

dementia
diversity
formal services
health workforce shortages
Home and Community Care (HACC)
home care package (HCP)

integration of care
life expectancy
not-for-profit
refundable accommodation deposit (RAD)
residential services

INTRODUCTION

This chapter explores the importance, topicality and complexities of ageing and aged care in Australia. In particular, the emergence of population ageing as a global demographic trend, one in which Australia is also enmeshed and which has considerable implications for traditional models of aged care and established funding arrangements. In addition, recent inquiries such as the Royal Commission into Aged Care Quality and Safety (2018–21) have reset the underlying assumptions of that model and provided an impetus for changes that may yet make the Australian aged-care system 'future ready', as population ageing progresses towards its

anticipated peak in 2050. In order that aged care be future-proofed, many other policy and funding adaptations will be necessary as aged care is contextualised with respect to its links to the health and disability care sectors and also, more broadly, to an environmental context which, at the time of writing, indicates major concerns for safe and effective care in the coming decades. The two factors of climate change, including floods and fires in recent years, and the SARS-CoV-2 pandemic, illustrate that assumptions about the stability of the aged-care environment need to be radically altered. As of 2023, we can expect to see a need for major developments across many aspects of aged care if the needs of older Australians are to be met effectively in coming decades.

AUSTRALIAN AGED-CARE CONTEXT

Currently, the Australian aged-care system can be described as complex in design and regulation, as well as being inadequate for the current and emerging level of need. This scenario is driven in part by rising population ageing on the one hand and various systemic limitations on the other. This situation has been compounded by the SARS-CoV-2 pandemic as the majority of deaths from COVID-19 were, and still are, being experienced in residential aged-care facilities (e.g. Aitken et al. 2021; Ibrahim et al. 2021). This points to persistent structural as well as regulatory and strategy problems with the sector as this group is clearly among the most vulnerable in the community. In addition, workforce issues have always been a problem (including **health workforce shortages**, wages and conditions). This connects to Bacchi's (2012) work on how policies can generate rather than resolve specific problems in the health and social care environments. COVID-19, and the responses to COVID-19, has contributed to this destabilising environment in which systemic change is even more relevant than ever.

While there is a complex *historical* context to aged care in Australia (see below), there is also a growing need for reforms and redesign to better accommodate the growing number of older people, their increasingly complex health issues, and the social and associated supports available (or not) to them. This chapter, written in an election year, works on the assumption that more changes are coming and, following the Royal Commission findings, quite probably some significant ones in funding and regulation arrangements at a minimum, but also hopefully in improvements to models of care and more integration across care domains.

Historical Context

The aged-care environment in Australia has a deep historical connection to the British system as a foundational influence not only on how aged care was and is provided but also in terms of the ideological issues at play in aged-care quality, funding and delivery, as well as broader societal representations of 'dependent' older people. More specifically, the British system was for more than 300 years heavily influenced by the Poor Laws and the Workhouse system which dictated societal responses to poverty and housing issues for many of the most vulnerable in society (Boyer & Schmidle 2009). This system was only finally broken up with the advent of universal health care through the National Health Service in the United Kingdom in 1948.

In Australia, similar conditions applied in that religious and charitable institutions were often responsible for the limited care provided to indigent older people in the community (e.g. Draper 2021). The Australian Medical Association, for example, resisted universal public health care until the 1970s when Medicare was introduced. These complicated funding and regulatory relationships between governments (both federal and state/territory), the broader charitable sector and the private sector add to this complexity with, in our opinion, a persistent bias by government towards the charitable and religious provider sector. The effect over the past two decades or so has been to produce both a varied private-sector response (ranging from excellent to very poor) and a growth of religious and quasi-religious corporate entities (e.g. Uniting Care, Anglicare) receiving billions of dollars in tax-payer funded support (e.g. Fine & Davidson 2018).

The situation for older Indigenous people is even more varied and the impact of the Stolen Generations has meant that many ageing Aboriginal people, in particular, did not officially exist due to a lack of birth certificates, Medicare cards and so on (Calabro 2013). In addition, the issues around age-related disease in Aboriginal peoples has tended to focus on mid-life illnesses due to lower **life expectancies** than non-Indigenous people (Wilson et al. 2019). In recent years, a growing evidence base on the impacts of the **dementias** on Aboriginal and Torres Strait Islander peoples has been growing (e.g. Cox et al. 2019; Arkles et al. 2020). This also suggests that 'ageing' and the ageing experience are the result of an often complex mix of biological, social and systemic factors.

Pause *for* Reflection ...

Thinking about how complex the Australian aged-care environment is, what additional complications do you think the COVID-19 pandemic may have added to the mix of factors impacting older people's health and well-being?

POPULATION AGEING IN AUSTRALIA

As noted above, **population ageing** is a global phenomenon but also one with explicit national and sub-national considerations in the Australian context. Globally, Australia is part of a scientific research environment inquiring on ageing, aged care and associated factors such as geriatric medicine and it is currently mid-tier in terms of population ageing across the OECD countries (Organisation for Economic Co-operation and Development (OECD) 2023). At the national level, population ageing was flagged as a key consideration as early as the 1970s by the demographic researcher Jack Caldwell at the Australian National University based on his research into the fertility transition shared across several English-speaking countries (e.g. Caldwell & Ruzkicka 1978).

More recently, the pattern of ageing has become quite distinct, and more obvious, in that between 2000 and 2020 the older segment of the population increased from just over 12% to just over 16% as illustrated in Fig. 8.1. This is not rapid ageing as such, as has been seen in Japan or China for example, but it is progressive and growing. It is also a rising rate which we discuss in more detail later in this chapter. In addition, that compositional effect has major implications for health care and **residential services** because, as you can see, the proportion of people aged 85 and over is rising already and anticipated to rise further in the coming decades. Planning to respond to such demographic trends is important because the quality-of-life factors will be considerable and the systemic needs to provide and support a high-quality aged-care environment – for both those in the community and those in residential care.

Pause *for* Reflection ...

What do you think the implications of progressive population ageing, especially growth in the oldest old segment, are for health and social care? What might facilitate or inhibit the capacity to meet those complex emerging needs?

It is also important to note the gendered nature of older age, especially very old age, and the situational contexts that this produces for older women living in the community and in residential aged care. Women live longer than men on average and are likely to continue to do so, with rising levels of **chronic disease**, disability and dementia (e.g. ABS 2018). Female cohorts aged 55 and over have increased significantly and especially so among the younger cohorts meaning that these women will be the older old in the coming decades (AIHW 2021a).

In addition, the growth in the number of older men is also significant although clearly not as marked by comparison with older women. Nonetheless, this indicates shrinking of the gap between older men and women. What these data do not tell us is what the impacts on

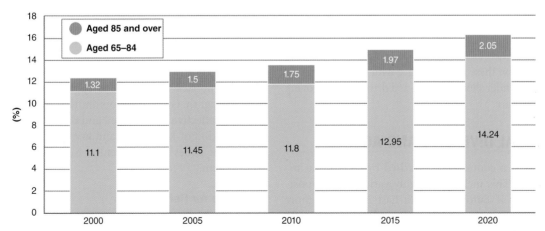

Figure 8.1 Proportion of population aged 65 years and over. *Source*: Australian Bureau of Statistics (ABS) (2020). Twenty years of population change. ABS, Canberra. https://www.abs.gov.au/articles/twenty-years-population-change.

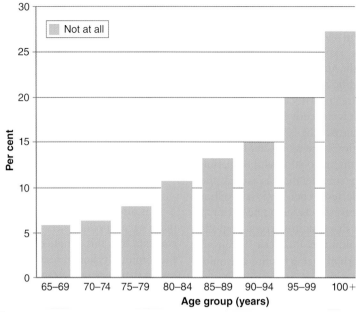

Notes
1. Data exclude 'not stated – both language and proficiency not stated', 'not stated – language stated, proficiency not stated' and 'overseas visitor'.
2. 'Older Australians' refers to people aged 65 and over.

Figure 8.2 English language proficiency for older Australians who spoke another language other than English by age group, 2016. *Source*: AIHW analysis of ABS Census of Population and Housing (2016). Tablebuilder. http://www.aihw.gov.au.

health status will be and associated demands for aged-care services including both residential and community-level supports. However, if current illness patterns are indicative, we can expect a growing number of older people living with multiple chronic diseases including cognitive impairments and associated trajectories towards some form of dementia (see Harrison et al. 2020). This too has implications for the current aged-care funding and service arrangements and suggests a growing need to revise these in accordance with emerging needs. Here too, gender should be seen as a driver for improving models of care.

CULTURAL DIVERSITY AND AGEING

Australia is a country characterised by significant immigration. This includes a highly varied mix of post-World War II European, South-East Asian and more recently African (e.g. Sudanese) settlement (e.g. ABS 2022). While the majority are economic and 'lifestyle' immigrants, there is a significant humanitarian component too. Thus, the complexities of ageing in Australia include Holocaust Survivors with prior trauma (often exacerbated by the ageing process and dementias) through to skilled technology workers from South and East Asia. Obviously, family migration becomes a factor in these scenarios, as does the need for cultural and language skills in the design and delivery of care for ageing population cohorts.

One factor highly relevant to health and aged care is English language capacity as people age. Fig. 8.2 shows how quickly the rate rises across the age cohorts for people who lack (or lose) their capacity to communicate in English. Given that communication is central to safe and effective health, aged and disability care, having this kind of knowledge and knowing how to work with these issues are both central to an effective aged-care system.

> **Pause *for* Reflection ...**
> Given the diversity of the ageing population what sorts of issues might emerge in providing appropriate care to older people in smaller communities or cultural groups?

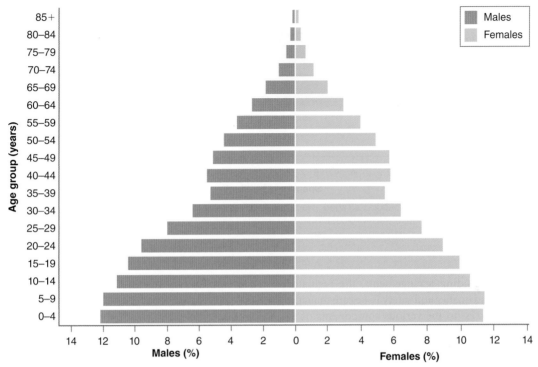

Figure 8.3 Estimated resident Indigenous Australian population by age group and sex, 2016. *Source*: Australian Institute of Health and Welfare (AIHW) (2021b). Older Australians Web Report. AIHW, Canberra. https://www.aihw.gov.au/reports/older-people/older-australia-at-a-glance/contents/diverse-groups-of-older-australians/aboriginal-and-torres-strait-islander-people.

ABORIGINAL AND TORRES STRAIT ISLANDER AGEING

Australia's Aboriginal and Torres Strait Islander population is significantly younger than the non-Indigenous population and growing fast. Indeed, the population pyramid for this group looks like a low- to middle-income country demographically (see Fig. 8.3). The similarities don't end there but for this chapter we note that one of the key issues is that this group does not have equal health inputs and outcomes compared to the rest of the population. Research into Aboriginal and Torres Strait Islander people's ageing often looks at younger age groups in order to have study samples that are large enough to generalise on, because ongoing morbidity and mortality do not readily permit the type of sampling typical in non-Indigenous populations (e.g. Radford et al. 2014).

Over the past decade several studies have worked with Aboriginal and Torres Strait Islander communities to investigate age-related health problems including the dementias, and differences between urban Aboriginal and Torres Strait Islander populations and those living in rural and remote contexts. These include the KICA (Kimberley Indigenous Cognitive Assessment) and KGOWS (Koori Growing Old Well) studies, both of which evidenced dementia rates at least three times those of non-Indigenous Australians (e.g. Racine et al. 2021). A key issue here was the list of co-morbidities, including intergenerational trauma, that characterised these studies (Menzies 2019). These factors all have important implications for the development of improved health outcomes in older Aboriginal and Torres Strait Islander people across Australia.

THE AGED CARE LEGISLATIVE AND FUNDING ENVIRONMENT

A key technique for governmental intervention in the aged-care 'system' is legislation since it is through

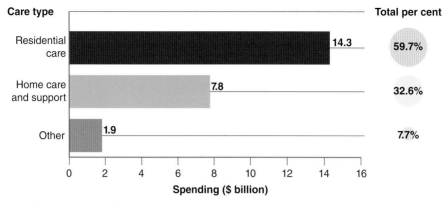

Figure 8.4 Government spending on aged care services by spending type, 2020–21. *Source*: Australian Institute of Health and Welfare (AIHW) (2022). Spending on aged care. AIHW, Canberra. https://www.gen-aged-caredata.gov.au/Topics/Spending-on-aged-care.

legislation that funding arrangements, the regulatory environment, and quality and safety issues are managed. It is also how *access* to the various components of the aged-care system are mediated, including residential aged care and community aged-care supports such as the **Commonwealth Home Support Program (CHSP)**, **refundable accommodation deposits (RADs)** and so on (note that since the 2022 federal election result, many of these factors are being re-negotiated). The legislative environment also impacts on how, for example, the many not-for-profits also engage with and are supported by the aged-care funding system (e.g. Meals on Wheels, CHSPs and **home care packages (HCPs)**).

How aged care is funded depends to a considerable extent on the ideological and philosophical precommitments of governments (e.g. private versus public provision). The resulting funding model(s) and processes are important factors in generating not only the current situation but, potentially, improving future ones. At present, one key outcome appears to be a growth in the regulatory environment. Whether or not this will lead to actual improvements in care, and a reduction in the failures documented by the Royal Commission, is yet to be seen. Certainly, given the nearly 50 years of mixed policy outcomes in this area, the level of change may still not meet what is generally accepted as being necessary. In effect, funding models create their own effects and, when the funding envelope is finite, costs that may still be managed by reducing the quality and quantity of care provided. This has proven to be an ongoing problem across the residential aged-care sector as low wages

and casualisation for direct care providers has driven, and is still driving, a variety of effects such as casual staff chasing better paying shifts and working across multiple facilities. For example, see Bacchi (2016) on how problems are framed and their sometimes inevitable contradictions and, even, perverse outcomes.

Fig 8.4 briefly describes how the formal costs of care are currently allocated by government with just under 60% going to residential aged care in 2020–21, another third (32.6%) to home-based care through the CHSP and HCP schemes, and the remaining 8% (7.75) to the 'other' category. However, even prior to the 2022 election result, the funded home care model was already set for significant change in 2023 going into, more likely, 2024. The change in government will make some of this information date very quickly but funding to the sector will have to grow if only to maintain current level of services for a growing aged population.

The anticipated growth in necessary aged-care funding is supported by the data in Fig. 8.5 showing accelerating growth in funding across the period 2015–16 to 2020–21. While the major categories are residential aged care and home care and support, the category of workforce and service improvement has experienced noticeable growth, especially in the most recent year. The anticipated changes to the CHSP and HPC funding streams, along with developments in the funded supports such as Meals on Wheels, indicate that we may see increased diversification in what is funded and potentially *how* these services are funded. The workforce and service improvement funding suggests that organisational and workforce development are, or

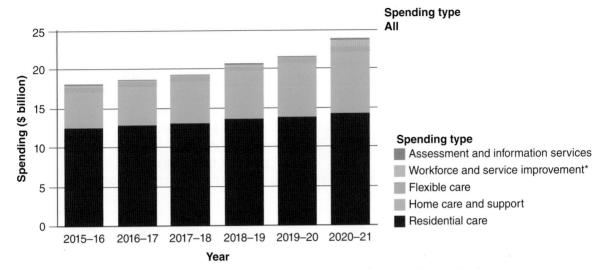

Figure 8.5 Government spending on aged care services by spending type, 2015–16 to 2020–21. *Source*: Report of Government Services 2022: Part F, Section 14 Aged Care Services report.

will increasingly become, a focus for governments as many traditional models of community support have seen limited change in decades. The shift in health and residential aged care to digital technologies, for example, will have flow-on effects for funding, practices and skills that will require further support.

THE ROYAL COMMISSION INTO AGED CARE

Aged care, and more particularly major failures in aged care, have been the focus of inquiries of various kinds for many years in Australia. Indeed, inquiring on the aged-care system is a process that has been going on for decades. However, it is fair to say that the Royal Commission into Aged Care (2018–21) was a unique investment in time, money and effort to establish what currently does and does not work effectively in aged care, and to investigate how the aged-care system might be improved as the population begins to age more rapidly.

Over the decades there have been as many as 40 inquiries into various aspects of the aged-care system and very few of their findings have been incorporated into the government's policy and legislative framework response to aged care. The result is not only what we see currently but also the spectrum of issues identified in detail by the recent Royal Commission in its 148 recommendations (see https://agedcare.royalcommission.gov.au/sites/default/files/2021-03/final-report-recommendations.pdf).

The very first of these recommendations was to replace the existing Aged Care Act (1997) by 2023. At the time of writing, the Australian government had passed the *Aged Care and Other Legislation Amendment (Royal Commission Response) Bill 2022*. The focus of this amendment relates to aged care, health and aged-care pricing, and information sharing in relation to veterans and military rehabilitation and compensation.

RESIDENTIAL AGED CARE AND SUPPORT

The current system is federally funded but responsibilities vary depending on the type of service provided. Prior to 'decentralisation', **Aged Care Assessment Teams (ACATs)** were run through state-managed hospitals. That system has changed significantly over the past decade. Meanwhile, residential aged care was traditionally a mix of government, **not-for-profit** and charitable or religious providers. This scenario changed dramatically to include an expanded private-sector involvement

TABLE 8.1   Aged-Care Provision in Australia

People Receiving Aged-Care Services
(a), (b), (c)

Number of People 2020–2021	NSW	Vic	Qld	WA	SA	Tas	ACT	NT	Aust
Residential care — permanent	79,676	63,249	47,747	21,576	21,424	6,121	3,079	642	243,117
Residential care — respite	25,452	15,566	12,898	3,649	8,053	1,535	602	207	67,775
Home Care Levels 1–2	46,870	35,967	23,027	7,410	8,860	2,877	1,427	465	125,597
Home Care Levels 3–4	34,017	29,090	22,324	12,423	9,658	2,773	1,581	583	110,957
Transition Care	7,638	5,528	4,587	2,512	2,406	614	335	196	23,802
Commonwealth Home Support Program	228,581	224,789	192,120	60,861	79,935	24,678	9,820	4,598	825,383
									1,396,631

Source: Productivity Commission (2022). Report on government services 2022, Part F, Section 14. Released on 25 January 2022. https://www.pc.gov.au/ongoing/report-on-government-services/2022/community-services/aged-care-services.

(Fine & Davidson 2018) and a retreat from or change in operators of aged-care services by many traditional providers. Some, such as Uniting Care and Anglicare, remain major operators but the system is plagued by fiscal sustainability and quality and safety issues, as illustrated by the Royal Commission and others (Sutton et al. 2022). The proposed new Aged Care Act may resolve some of these concerns, but opinions remain mixed at this time on whether tighter regulation will have the desired effect.

The current state and scale of Australian aged-care provision is summarised in Table 8.1. The largest single scheme is the Commonwealth Home Support Program (CHSP) with just over 825,000 recipients (waiting times have been an issue with this scheme). Following that, permanent residential aged care with approximately 243,000 residents is the next largest program. Home care packages (HCPs) range from moderate to high support (levels 1–4) for another 236,000 people's receipt of **formal services**. It may be too obvious to state, but it is important to note, that this only covers formal, funded care provision and that volunteers, families, carers and others constitute another large tranche of the care that is actually delivered in the community, in particular. Thus, both formal and informal care, as they are termed, constitute the larger 'universe' of aged-care service provision across the country and should not be taken as separate elements in the care that older people need and/or receive.

Since their introduction, refundable accommodation deposits (RADs) seem to both hypnotise and blindside governments. It is interesting to note that while the government amends the Means Tested Accommodation Supplement (the amount paid by the government for those residents with insufficient means to pay a RAD or daily accommodation payment (DAP)), the maximum RAD level has not been increased since its inception on 1 July 2014. This means that, with the decreasing Maximum Permissible Interest Rate (MPIR), the Means Tested Accommodation Supplement has increased to a level where it is slightly below the maximum RAD level. Providers can apply to the Pricing Commissioner for permission to set RADs in excess of the Maximum Level ($550,000) but again this is a drawn out bureaucratic and administrative process.

COMMUNITY AGED CARE AND SUPPORTS

Prior to 1985, when the Home and Community Care (HACC) Act was introduced, community care was provided through four separate programs under the following pieces of legislation: the *Home Nursing Subsidy Act 1957*; the *States Grants (Home Care) Act 1969*; the *States Grants (Paramedical Services) Act 1969*; and the *Delivered Meals Subsidy Act 1970* (see Australia Parliament 1994).

The **Home and Community Care (HACC)** program was introduced following a series of reports and inquiries, including the McLeay Report (1982), which illustrated that existing arrangements were insufficient to meet existing community need for both older people and younger people with disabilities. HACC was established under the *Home and Community Care Act 1985* and was a joint Australian Commonwealth (federal) and state/territory government program (Centre for Policy on Ageing 2016).

Then in 2015 the Commonwealth Home Support Program (CHSP) was introduced, which replaced or consolidated several existing programs including: the Commonwealth Home and Community Care (HACC) program; planned respite from the National Respite for Carers Program (NRCP); the Day Therapy Centres (DTC) program; and the Assistance with Care and Housing for the Aged (ACHA) program. As of 2022, these arrangements have been targeted, yet again, for revision in 2023 or possibly pushed out to 2024. This too will be an interesting area to focus on in terms of future policy and funding directions in aged care.

The last key component we need to consider here is the Aged Care Assessment Teams (ACATs) originally designed to assess frail older people's capacity to live in the community with supports (e.g. HCP package levels) or if they need residential care (e.g. Khadka et al. 2019). This program is funded by the Commonwealth but operated out of state/territory health service providers. Currently, anyone can request an ACAT assessment through the MyAgedCare portal operated by the federal government (https://www.myagedcare.gov.au/assessment).

A key issue to consider in all of this complexity is that these arrangements, both historical and contemporary, do not provide the majority of care that is needed or received in the community. Informal care provided by families, carers and communities remains the bulk of actual care and support provided to older people. In a 2015 report for Carers Australia developed by Access Economics Australia, it was estimated that informal carers provided 1.9 billion hours of care with a potential replacement cost of $60.3 billion.

FUTURE TRENDS AND DIRECTIONS

One of the key features of population ageing in Australia is that the rate of ageing is projected to increase in coming years. This includes an increase in the speed at which the population ages and an increase in the older and oldest old (80+) age cohorts, and in the overall numbers of older people. In other words, population ageing will intensify as a societal and demographic process. A key factor will be the changing health status of these much older people including their physical and cognitive health as well as their psychological wellbeing. Given the issues with chronic disease rates mentioned earlier, it will be important to make positive inroads into current rates of chronic diseases in older people including co-morbidities. As with the experience of Aboriginal and Torres Strait Islander older people, social improvements offer potential health improvements. In addition, the realisation of Fries's (1980, 2000) concept of the 'compression of morbidity' offers a socio-medical perspective on how these various factors might work together for improved population health among older people specifically but also across the life cycle of the population more generally.

Central to this, we suggest, will be major improvements in the **integration of care** provision. Presently, especially with activity-based funding arrangements, there is little driving integration from the supply side of the equation. Instead, older people experience a hub and spoke model that requires time and effort to negotiate. Going forwards, the inefficiencies and even perversities this produces will need to be addressed if only to ensure sustainability. Case study 8.1 explores the issues discussed in this chapter.

SUMMARY

Aged care is intrinsically enmeshed in a variety of factors including the objective reality of population ageing but also the various historical, political, economic and cultural factors that frame the status of old age within society, the older person, and the ageing process itself. In addition, the lag effect between the key issues identified by the sector and the quality and timelessness of federal government responses has contributed significantly to the current complexity and inequalities associated with the existing aged-care system. As mentioned above, informal care remains the bulk of *all* care provided to older people in this context but societal changes may affect this situation (e.g. smaller or more geographically distant families, older people living alone).

Two other trends of current significance to aged care are: (1) ongoing issues with workforce supply, quality

CASE STUDY 8.1

Bill is an 84-year-old man living alone in the house he shared with his wife for many years, prior to her death two years ago. She did most of the cooking and house-work and, while his skills have improved, he is also experiencing some cognitive impairment and is more forgetful than previously. He lives alone now and is on a pension with no other means of financial support.

He currently receives a small package of home support services including some cleaning once a week, shopping assistance and dinners delivered by Meals on Wheels volunteers. The volunteers also stay long enough to chat to him about how he is going but beyond this he has limited social contacts and no immediate family nearby.

The meals he receives are actually of good quality and nutritionally balanced (this is not always the case) for a person his age. Due to his declining memory, sometimes he forgets to eat the meals provided and they sit in the fridge, sometimes for days until someone visits and checks. Likewise, no one is entirely sure if he eats break-fast and lunch on a regular basis. Occasionally, when he remembers, he splits the meals in two to stretch them out for reasons of cost.

In addition, his dental health is also in decline, and he has not seen a dentist for some time. Consequently, he is finding it difficult to eat all of his meals even when he remembers that they are there to be eaten. He is beginning to lose weight and even the volunteers are becoming concerned. He has not yet had a fall of any seriousness but they are also aware that this could be a risk to Bill and his risk of an acute hospital admission.

They suspect but are not qualified to say that the combination of poor or inconsistent nutrition and dental health is adding to his cognitive and memory problems. Their suspicion is that Bill needs an ACAT assessment in the near future to see if residential aged care might be the safer option for him. Like many people in his position, Bill is not keen on this option when it is discussed with him as he has lived in his home and neighbourhood for many years and feels safe in these familiar surroundings.

Case Study Questions

What questions or concerns does this case study raise for you about:
- the integration or lack of it for community care services and older people?
- the importance of nutrition and nutritional support in older community-dwelling individuals?
- the service, cost and quality-of-life issues associated with a lack of effective dental care and oversight for many older people in the community and, also, in aged care?
- the capacity of older people to age safely in the community given the lack of service integration or, in many cases, the lack of appropriate services?

and skills; and (2) the COVID-19-induced migration from major urban areas to regional locations over the past two years. The workforce issue has always existed in Australia, especially for regional, rural and remote areas, but population ageing is making the issue of the ageing-health-disability nexus even more profound. The supply of general health and aged-care workforce is and remains problematic, and that of more highly skilled, and scarce, workers such as geriatricians, dementia nurses and the like is more problematic still in many areas (e.g. Howe 2022). While the specific situations may vary in Australia, compared to other countries, there is a bigger picture in terms of how ideological commitments can produce quite similar outcomes across health and social care systems (e.g. Tuohy 1999).

This complex mix of push and pull factors in addition to progressive population ageing means that we can expect further changes. The future of aged care is fundamental to Australian society as an indicator of how we value older people and the resources committed to their care. However, the way that care is expressed in formal systems funded by governments is enmeshed in ideas about economic sustainability, the responsibility of people to 'fund' their retirement (and health care), and associated political and philosophical positions. The key issue will be if such changes improve the aged-care system as it currently stands and if the consequences for older people will be positive. The consequences of failing in this space risk a considerable and growing human cost.

REFERENCES

Australian Bureau of Statistics (ABS), 2018. Disability, ageing and carers, Australia: summary of findings. ABS, Canberra. https://www.abs.gov.au/statistics/health/disability/disability-ageing-and-carers-australia-summary-findings/latest-release#articles.

Australian Bureau of Statistics (ABS), 2020. Twenty years of population change. ABS, Canberra. https://www.abs.gov.au/articles/twenty-years-population-change.

Australian Bureau of Statistics (ABS), 2022. Cultural diversity: Census data on country of birth, year of arrival, ancestry, language, and religion, 2021. Census update. ABS, Canberra. https://www.abs.gov.au/statistics/people/people-and-communities/cultural-diversity-census/2021.

Australian Institute of Health and Welfare (AIHW), 2021a. Aged care. AIHW, Canberra. https://www.aihw.gov.au/reports/australias-welfare/aged-care.

Australian Institute of Health and Welfare (AIHW), 2021b. Older Australians web report: older Australians, older Aboriginal and Torres Strait Islander people. AIHW, Canberra. https://www.aihw.gov.au/reports/older-people/older-australians/contents/about.

Australian Institute of Health and Welfare (AIHW), 2022. Spending on aged care. AIHW, Canberra. https://www.gen-agedcaredata.gov.au/Topics/Spending-on-aged-care.

Aitken, G.E., Holmes, A.L., Ibrahim, J.E., 2021. COVID-19 and residential aged care: priorities for optimising preparation and management of outbreaks. Med J Aust 214 (1), 6–8.

Arkles, R., Jankelson, C., Radford, K., et al., 2020. Family caregiving for older Aboriginal people in urban Australia: disclosing worlds of meaning in the dementia experience. Dementia 19 (2), 397–415.

Australia Parliament, 1994. House of Representatives. Standing Committee on Community Affairs. Home but not alone: a report on the Home and Community Care Program. Australian Government. Canberra. Pub. Service, https://nla.gov.au/nla.obj-2013212571.

Bacchi, C., 2012. Introducing the 'What's the Problem Represented to be?' approach. In: Bletsas, A., Beasley, C. (Eds.), Engaging with Carol Bacchi: Strategic Interventions and Exchanges. University of Adelaide Press, Adelaide, pp. 21–24.

Bacchi, C., 2016. Problematizations in health policy: questioning how "problems" are constituted in policies. SAGE Open, Sydney. doi: 10.1177/2158244016653986.

Boyer, G.R., Schmidle, T.P., 2009. Poverty among the elderly in late Victorian England 1. Econ Hist Rev 62 (2), 249–278.

Calabro, A. (2013). Registering the births of indigenous Australians: has New South Wales got it right? University of New South Wales Law Journal, 36 (3), 809–838.

Caldwell, J.C., Ruzicka, L.T., 1978. The Australian fertility transition: an analysis. JSTOR 4 (1), 81–103.

Centre for Policy on Ageing, 2016. Case study 3: Long-term care in Australia – the Home and Community Care (HACC) /Commonwealth Home Support (CHSP) program, International Case Studies Series. http://www.cpa.org.uk/information/reviews/CPA-International-Case-Study-3-Long-term-care-in-Australia-the-HACC-programme.pdf.

Cox, T., Hoang, H., Goldberg, L.R., et al., 2019. Aboriginal community understandings of dementia and responses to dementia care. Public Health 172, 15–21.

Draper, B., 2021. Older people in hospitals for the insane in New South Wales, Australia, 1849–1905. Hist Psychiatry 32 (4), 436–448.

Fine, M., Davidson, B., 2018. The marketization of care: Global challenges and national responses in Australia. Current Sociology 66 (4), 503–516.

Fries, J.F., 1980. Aging, natural death, and the compression of morbidity. N Engl J Med 303 (3), 130–135.

Fries, J.F., 2000. Compression of morbidity in the elderly. Vaccine 18 (16), 1584–1589.

Harrison, S.L., Lang, C., Whitehead, C., et al., 2020. Trends in prevalence of dementia for people accessing aged-care services in Australia. J Gerontol: Series A, 75 (2), 318–325.

Howe, A., 2022. The 2020 Aged Care Workforce Census and Issues Arising for Residential Care Workforce Planning and Policy. Aust Econ Rev. doi 10.1111/1467-8462.12480.

Ibrahim, J.E., Li, Y., McKee, G., et al., 2021. Characteristics of nursing homes associated with COVID-19 outbreaks and mortality among residents in Victoria, Australia. Australas J Ageing 40 (3), 283–292.

Khadka, J., Lang, C., Ratcliffe, J., et al., 2019. Trends in the utilisation of aged-care services in Australia, 2008–2016. BMC Geriatr 19 (1), 1–9.

Menzies, K., 2019. Forcible separation and assimilation as trauma: The historical and sociopolitical experiences of Australian Aboriginal people. Soc Work Soc 17 (1), 1–8.

Organisation for Economic Co-operation and Development (OECD), 2023. Elderly population (indicator). doi:10.1787/8d805ea1-en.

Racine, L., Johnson, L., Fowler-Kerry, S., 2021. An integrative review of empirical literature on indigenous cognitive impairment and dementia. J Adv Nurs 77 (3), 1155–1171.

Radford, K., Mack, H.A., Robertson, H., et al., 2014. The Koori growing old well study: investigating aging and dementia in urban Aboriginal Australians. Int Psychogeriatr 26 (6), 1033–1043.

Sutton, N., Ma, N., Yang, J.S., et al., 2022. Australia's aged care sector: mid-year report (2021–22). The University of Technology, Sydney.

Tuohy, C.H., 1999. Understanding the dynamics of change in the health care arena. In: Tuohy, C.H. (Ed.), Accidental Logics: The Dynamics of Change in the Health Care Arena in the United States, Britain, and Canada. OUP, New York, pp. 3–34.

Wilson, T., Zhao, Y., Condon, J., 2019. Limited progress in closing the mortality gap for Aboriginal and Torres Strait Islander Australians of the Northern Territory. Aust N Z J Public Health 43 (4), 340–345.

9

Equity and Access: A Spotlight on Rural Health

Bernadette Ward and Pam Harvey

KEY LEARNING OUTCOMES

When you finish this chapter you should be able to:
- explain the concepts of equity and access and how these impact upon health status
- explain the dynamic relationship between health need and health outcomes
- understand the link between equity and the social determinants of health
- discuss the population health profile of people living in rural and urban Australia
- explain the factors that influence health service utilisation

- outline historical understandings of rural health and why this is changing
- understand interventions (e.g. workforce, models of care, funding) aimed at reducing inequitable health outcomes
- explain the underpinning principles and rationale for geographical classification systems
- discuss what might be needed to improve the health status of disadvantaged populations living in rural Australia.

KEY TERMS AND ABBREVIATIONS

Aboriginal Community Controlled Health Organisations (ACCHOs)
acceptability
access
Access Relative to Need (ARN)
Accessibility/Remoteness Index of Australia (ARIA)
affordability
approachability
appropriateness
Australian Institute of Health and Welfare (AIHW)
Australian Standard Geographic Classification – Remoteness Areas (ASGC-RA)

availability and accommodation
Extension for Community Healthcare Outcomes (ECHO)
geographical classification system
horizontal equity
Index of Economic Resources (IER)
Index of Education and Occupation (IEO)
Index of Relative Socio-economic Disadvantage (IRSD)
Index of Relative Socio-economic Advantage and Disadvantage (IRSAD)
Modified Monash Model (MMM)

primary health care (PHC)
Primary Health Network (PHN)
Public Health Information Development Unit (PHIDU)
rural, remote and metropolitan areas (RRMA)
SARS-CoV-2 pandemic
small rural health services (SRHS)
Socio-Economic Indexes for Areas (SEIFA)
United Nations (UN)
utilisation
vertical equity
World Health Organization (WHO)

INTRODUCTION

One of the goals resulting from the **United Nations (UN)** General Assembly 2015 publication on Sustainable Development is to 'ensure healthy lives and promote well-being for all at all ages' (UN 2015). To do this, there must be a focus on health equity and access. Using health services is a much more complex matter than simply having them available. No matter where people live, everyone has different levels of need that are closely linked to the social determinants of health. In this chapter, you will learn about the concepts of equity and access, and how they influence the provision of health services and health outcomes. You will also learn of the challenges of providing equitable health care, and some of the initiatives developed to overcome these, using the health and well-being of rural people as an example.

The majority (72%) of the 26 million people living in Australia live in major cities, while the rest are spread across regional, rural and remote communities within an area of 7.5 million square kilometres (Australian Bureau of Statistics (ABS) 2021a). Generally speaking, the health of people living in rural areas is poorer than those who live in the cities, but it is essential to note not all rural populations have poor health status, and not everyone living in a major city has good health. You might have heard of the 'Blue Zones' project that identified places in the world where the average life expectancy of the population is above the world's average (Buettner & Skemp 2016). Many of these locations are small rural towns. We can learn from these communities, but most importantly, they demonstrate that health is not only about where you live.

Before we investigate rural health, let's begin with the key principles of equity and **access**.

Equity

Health care is a fundamental human right but is influenced by equity issues. Health equity is attained when people are able to reach their full health potential. Inequality and inequity are two quite different concepts but are sometimes used interchangeably, particularly in relation to health care. What is the difference between these two, and how is equity addressed within the delivery of health services?

Health inequality refers to the uneven distribution of health outcomes because of biological differences (e.g. cystic fibrosis, an inherited, genetic condition) or predetermined factors (e.g. age). Equal treatment would mean everyone gets the same treatment even if the result is different because of the biological variations.

With health inequity, the differences in health outcomes can be overcome or avoided altogether (e.g. ensuring the inclusion of people in health care despite ethnic background or gender identity). Equity involves people getting what they need to achieve similar health outcomes for their condition. The concept is represented in Fig. 9.1.

There are different types of equity. When people with similar needs have similar or equivalent care, it is referred to as **horizontal equity**. An example of this would be when two people with respiratory failure in a large emergency department both get admitted to the intensive care unit. In contrast, when people with different levels of need receive different levels of care,

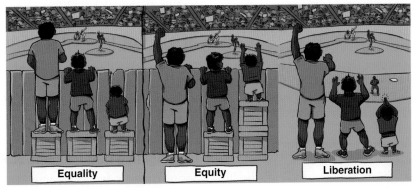

Figure 9.1 Equality and Equity. *Source:* Interaction Institute for Social Change / artist: Angus Maguire. www.interactioninstitute.org and www.madewithangus.com.

it is referred to as **vertical equity.** So, a woman with a low-risk pregnancy receives midwifery team care while another with a high-risk pregnancy receives care that is led by an obstetrician.

The causes of health inequity are closely linked to the social determinants of health. The **SARS-CoV-2 pandemic** has highlighted how health inequities, such as access to stable housing, chronic health conditions and poverty, affect health outcomes. Internationally, people who are most likely to be infected with SARS-CoV-2 virus (e.g. socially excluded vulnerable populations, those in the casual workforce or people unable to 'work from home') are those least able to withstand the associated consequences of Commonwealth and state pandemic-related public health orders (e.g. difficulties quarantining because of living circumstances, loss of income resulting in financial hardship) (Paremoer et al. 2021). Similarly, the limited distribution and administration of COVID-19 vaccines in low-income countries reflects global health inequities (**World Health Organization (WHO)** 2021).

Access

In Australia, we subscribe to having a health care system where there is universal (equitable) access, but what exactly is meant by *access*?

Access to health care is central to health service systems around the world, but as a concept, access is complex. It is defined as the degree of 'fit' between the characteristics of health care services and the ability of the clients to receive them (known as their *potential* access) (Penchansky & Thomas 1981). The act of accessing health care is generally referred to as **utilisation** (also termed *realised* access).

There are five dimensions of access:
- **Approachability:** identifying that a service exists, can be used, and can change a client's health status.
- **Acceptability:** social and cultural factors that influence a client's preference for a service.
- **Availability and accommodation:** the existence and geographical location of a service and appropriately skilled personnel who can potentially be reached by clients.
- **Affordability:** financial and time costs related to using the service.
- **Appropriateness:** the fit between a client's health care needs, the timeliness and care taken to provide the correct treatment and care (Levesque et al. 2013).

As outlined in Fig. 9.2, access is a dynamic interaction between the 'health system' (upper part of the figure) and consumers (lower part of the figure). It is the characteristics of access within the health system that interact with the ability of the client to perceive their own needs, seek health care, reach and pay for the service, and ultimately utilise it.

The dimensions of access are dependent on each other. For example, if you consider the health system, the use of bulk-billing (when a health service provider bills Medicare directly for the rebate fee only) may improve the *affordability* of a service. However, this could inadvertently affect the viability and resultant *availability* of some health services if the Medicare rebate does not cover the true cost of delivering a service. From the client's perspective, increasing *acceptability* (e.g. reconfiguring the gender and cultural mix of staff) for one group in the population may compromise acceptability for another group or reduce service availability (Ward et al. 2015).

The dynamic interplay between *accessibility* and service *utilisation* can also be described as the interaction between the 'supply' and 'demand' for health services. Policy-makers charged with allocating funds and planning (and supplying) services require information to assist their decision-making. This includes understanding the relationship between service utilisation as discussed before, and health care *need*.

There are many definitions of health care need, but policy-makers commonly equate *need* to *health outcomes*, meaning that sometimes services are placed in areas that are not accessed by the population because they don't address their needs. For example, a sole practitioner who is male may be unacceptable to females seeking gynaecological care.

SPOTLIGHT ON RURAL HEALTH

Now that we've discussed the complex interplay of equity, access and other health care concepts, we can use the example of rural health to highlight their importance. Let's begin by exploring what contributes to health status.

Investigating Determinants of Health

Socio-economic factors are important determinants of your potential to live a life of advantage or relative poverty, which in turn affects your well-being. One way of

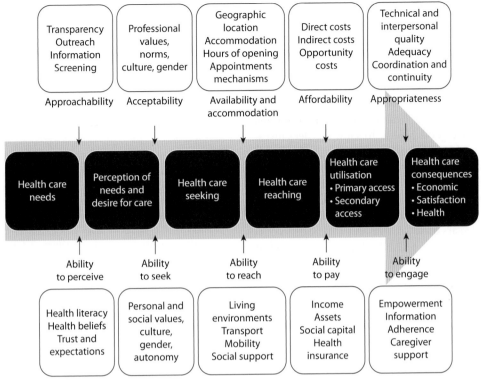

Figure 9.2 A Conceptual Framework of Access to Health Care. *Source:* Levesque, J.F., Harris, M.F., Russell, G. (2013). Patient-centred access to health care: conceptualising access at the interface of health systems and populations. Int J Equity Health, 12, p. 8.

measuring these is the **Socio-Economic Indexes for Areas (SEIFA)**. SEIFA is based on the ABS census data and ranks geographical locations according to relative socio-economic advantage and disadvantage. It includes four indexes:

- Index of Relative Socio-economic Disadvantage (IRSD)
- Index of Relative Socio-economic Advantage and Disadvantage (IRSAD)
- Index of Education and Occupation (IEO)
- Index of Economic Resources (IER) (ABS 2018).

Irrespective of the indicator you examine, the socio-economic profile of those who are most advantaged is not confined to those living in metropolitan areas. Within major cities and non-metropolitan areas, there are populations who are the most advantaged *and* disadvantaged. For example, the socio-economic disadvantage of Indigenous peoples is stark: 48% of this population live in geographical areas in the bottom quintile of disadvantage.

This compares with 18% of non-Indigenous peoples. Similarly, 5% of Indigenous peoples live in areas in the top quintile of advantage areas compared to 22% of non-Indigenous people (ABS 2018). This is consistent with the fact that socio-economic disadvantage accounts for 33–50% of the gap in life expectancy between Indigenous and non-Indigenous people in the Northern Territory (Zhao et al. 2013).

Pause *for* Reflection …

Go to the SIEFA Index interactive maps and type in the postcode or name of any rural town or metropolitan suburb to identify geographically advantaged and disadvantaged areas across the four indexes listed above: https://www.abs.gov.au/ausstats/abs@. nsf/Lookup/by%20Subject/2033.0.55.001~ 2016~Main%20Features~Interactive%20Maps~7.

What does this mean in terms of health inequity (horizontal and vertical)?

Health Status and Behaviours

Overall, Australians living in rural and remote areas generally experience poorer health outcomes than their metropolitan counterparts and there is a plethora of aggregated statistics to support this view (**Australian Institute of Health and Welfare (AIHW)** 2020a). As discussed previously, this does not mean that all rural populations have poor health and all metropolitan populations have 'good' health. To show this, let's investigate some health indicators.

In Australia, life expectancy at birth for females is 84 years and 79.5 years for males, although this differs according to where you live. Life expectancy for males at birth on the Gold Coast, for example, is 81.9 years compared to 79.4 years in Townsville and 73.0 years in outback Northern Territory (ABS 2021b). Irrespective of location, those with the lowest levels of education have a 20–25% reduction in life expectancy (Welsh et al. 2021).

These differences are also apparent in the prevalence of chronic disease. For example, in NSW the estimated prevalence of diabetes (based on 2017–18 data) in Riverwood (a western suburb of Sydney) is 7.3/100 population (age-standardised) compared to 3.4/100 in Colo Vale (107 kilometres from Sydney) (**Public Health Information Development Unit (PHIDU)** 2021). Again, socio-economic disadvantage is associated with higher prevalence of chronic disease (AIHW 2020b). Similarly, health screening behaviour is not consistent across people living in different geographical areas. The age-standardised breast screening participation rate for women aged 50–74 years by **Primary Health Network (PHN)** Area shows the Murrumbidgee PHN participation rate (60.7%) was higher than the national participation rate (54.8%) (PHIDU 2021).

While there are limitations to the use of any data, there are inconsistencies in health statistics across geographical areas, and between metropolitan and rural areas. Geography alone does not explain the differences noted above. Although a relatively higher proportion of Indigenous Australians live in more remote locations compared with non-Indigenous Australians, this does not entirely account for the generally lower health status reported by people living in these remote areas. Also, data does not always reflect the current state of any region. For example, the SARS-CoV-2 pandemic resulted in many people relocating from cities to regional areas (Centre for Population 2020). This may further increase the heterogeneity of the non-metropolitan population and their associated health determinants and status but this is yet to be confirmed.

Pause *for* Reflection …

Go to some of the key health statistics sites to examine the health status and behaviours of Australians across geographical areas:

https://www.aihw.gov.au/reports/cancer-screening/national-cancer-screening-programs-participation/contents/breastscreen-australia; https://phidu.torrens.edu.au/social-health-atlases/maps#social-health-atlases-of-australia-population-health-areas.

What differences can you see if the data is aggregated at the national level compared to looking at smaller geographical areas? What differences can you see within and between metropolitan and rural areas?

Access Relative to Need

By now you will realise that increasing the availability of health services may not result in improved health outcomes, particularly for those with the greatest health needs. Service planning should consider geographical areas' health determinants, status and service data in determining need. One approach would be to utilise a tool such as the sentinel 'Index of Access' that incorporates population size, the number and type of existing health services, the population need for health care (as measured by health care status indicators) and the availability of public transport (McGrail & Humphreys 2009).

The AIHW has done just that. Building on the 'Index of Access', the AIHW developed a geospatial '**Access Relative to Need' (ARN)** index. This index is the only measure that uses GP workforce, census, hospital, and morbidity and mortality data to report on people's access to GPs relative to their predicted need for **primary health care (PHC)** across Australia (AIHW 2014). The ARN index shows health outcomes are enhanced when consumers have improved access to GPs in geographical areas of high health need more than they do when there is improved access to GPs in areas of low health need. This is a very important outcome as it demonstrates the need for PHC services is not only dependent upon where you live – it is also about your health status. The ARN index (see Fig. 9.3) demonstrates that, when you

Indigenous population

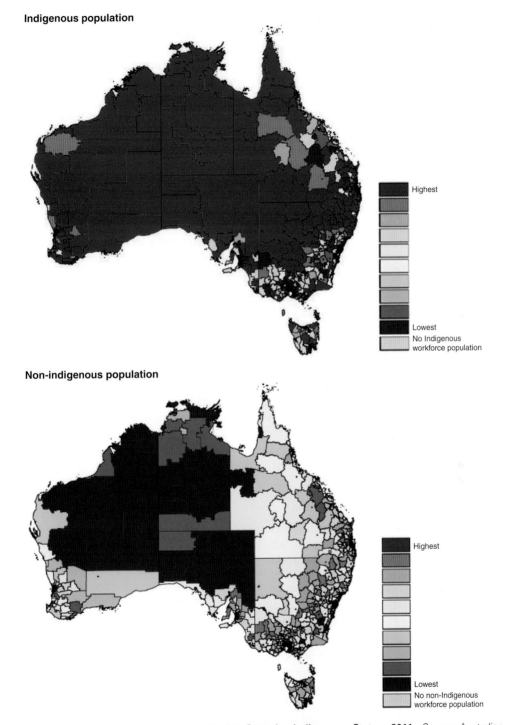

Non-indigenous population

Figure 9.3 Predicted Need for Primary Health Care, by Indigenous Status, 2011. *Source:* Australian Institute of Health and Welfare (AIHW), 2014. Access to primary health care relative to need for Indigenous Australians. AIHW, Canberra. Cat. no. IHW 128. https://www.aihw.gov.au/reports/indigenous-australians/access-to-primary-health-care-relative-to-need/summary.

take health status into account, the predicted need for PHC services in rural and remote areas is very different for Indigenous and non-Indigenous populations. For Indigenous Australians, the need for PHC services is very high throughout these areas, but for non-Indigenous Australians, the need is very low. To address inequitable health outcomes, both *health need* and *socio-demographic factors* (e.g. the ARN index) should be considered when planning PHC services.

> **Pause *for* Reflection …**
> What might explain the discrepancies that are seen comparing the two maps shown in Fig. 9.3? Why, for example, is there an area of highest predicted need next to an area of lowest predicted need in Queensland? What could be influencing the lightly coloured area in western Queensland?

Minimum Health Service Provision

One of the difficulties for policy-makers charged with improving access is equity and therefore systematically determining which health services should be provided for a population. In response, Thomas, Wakerman and Humphreys (2015) identified 'core' primary health care (PHC) services that Australians can expect to access which include mental health and services for children. These were identified using a panel of health service managers, clinicians, academics and consumers, ensuring that representative voices informed the list.

Health Service Utilisation

The social determinants of health are directly correlated with health status but the picture in terms of health service utilisation is not as transparent. Across the world, for example, there are socio-economic inequities in the utilisation of doctors. People who are most disadvantaged are more likely to use primary care doctors while those who are most advantaged are more likely to utilise specialist medical services (Lueckman et al. 2021). Further information is needed to understand how socio-economic and health status impacts the utilisation of different types of health care and their frequency of use.

People's ability to perceive they have needs, and then to seek and receive care, will vary (Fig. 9.2). To add to the complexity, accessibility of services may vary. These factors together can lead to delays in health care utilisation and may result in potentially avoidable hospitalisations.

For example, in 2017–18, hospitalisations for complications of diabetes were markedly higher among people who are socio-economically disadvantaged (who may have poorer health status) and in people from remote areas (where there may be fewer accessible services) (Australian Commission on Safety and Quality in Health Care 2021). Policy-makers charged with improving population health outcomes need to consider both the population and health system characteristics in order to determine resource allocation.

In Australia, most of the policy emphasis on improving access has been on increasing the availability of health professionals. Increased availability of GPs, though, has been associated with increased use of GP services, with less than one-third of the variance explained by population health care need (Mu & Hall 2020). For example, despite the fact that Australia's Indigenous peoples have double the burden of disease and mortality than those of non-Indigenous Australians, their use of GP services is only 1.2 times that of non-Indigenous Australians (AIHW 2020c). More needs to be done to ensure those who most need the service (i.e. disadvantaged with poor health status) are able to access services, remembering that 'access' means an available, acceptable, appropriate, affordable, approachable service. Or, put simply, the right service at the right time.

> **Pause *for* Reflection …**
> Examine patterns of health service utilisation for a range of conditions and potentially avoidable hospitalisations, using the following resources:
> - https://www.heartfoundation.org.au/health-professional-tools/interactive-heart-map-australia
> - https://www.safetyandquality.gov.au/sites/default/files/2021-04/The%20Fourth%20Australian%20Atlas%20of%20Healthcare%20Variation%202021_Full%20publication.pdf
> - https://phidu.torrens.edu.au/current/maps/sha-topics/pph/Total/atlas.html?indicator=i5
>
> Examine also the factors associated with *not* utilising a service:
> - https://www.aihw.gov.au/reports-data/indicators/healthy-community-indicators/national/all-australia/expenditure/health-welfare-expenditure?tab=IND0015|Map&tab=IND0027|Map&tab=IND0030|Map.
>
> If you were charged with improving the 'fit' between the population and the health service (i.e. access), what factors would you consider to be the most important?

INTERVENTIONS TO REDUCE INEQUITABLE HEALTH OUTCOMES

By now, you probably have in your mind a picture of the complexities of providing equitable health care for all Australians. In this section, we'll explore the following four high-level solutions that aim to improve health care for populations across Australia and whether they have been successful: (1) classification of the location of populations, (2) rural workforce initiatives, (3) models of care and (4) funding arrangements (including payment for rural patient travel). While we present them as separate items, they often work together and also depend on those social determinants of health that influence equitable outcomes for people's health and well-being (e.g. employment opportunities, housing).

Systems that Classify the Geographical Location of Populations

Definitions and classifications are important because they assist policy-makers and health service planners to allocate financial and human resources to the health system within and across locations, service models and disciplinary groups. Internationally, though, policy-makers struggle to reach a consensus on the definition of 'rural health', resulting in no consistent definition of this term. Definitions range between geographical, demographical, sociological and cultural perspectives owing to diverse settings and health needs.

In Australia, several **geographical classification systems** have evolved in the attempt to differentiate rural locality and remoteness from urban (metropolitan) areas. Initially, the **RRMA (rural, remote and metropolitan** areas) and **ARIA (Accessibility/Remoteness Index of Australia)** classifications were developed based on population size and road distance to service centres (AIHW 2004). It was soon recognised that more accurate measures were needed. The **ASGC-RA (Australian Standard Geographical Classification—Remoteness Areas)** classification was based on a refinement of enhanced ARIA (Department of Health 2021). It differentiates between levels of accessibility and location as follows: (RA 1) major cities, (RA 2) inner regional, (RA 3) outer regional, (RA 4) remote and (RA 5) very remote. ASGC-RA differentiates between major cities (e.g. capital cities such as Sydney (RA 1)) or outer regional cities (e.g. Darwin (RA 2)). ASGC-RA defines remote areas more tightly than ARIA (AIHW 2004).

The **Modified Monash Model (MMM)** was developed from the ASGC-RA to create a new seven-level geographical classification system that distinguishes different town sizes in inner and outer regional Australia (Table 9.1) in order to overcome distributional inequities, particularly in relation to recruitment and retention incentives for the health workforce (GPs in particular). This system takes six sentinel indicators of rural health workforce recruitment and retention into account: hours worked, work in a public hospital, working after hours, ability to have time off, employment opportunities for a partner and choice of schools available locally (Humphreys et al. 2012).

Although there is no perfect geographical classification system, the MMM addresses some deficiencies of previous systems. Despite it being primarily developed for workforce, the MMM is now the classification system of choice for funding a range of health activities

Table 9.1 Comparison of Modified Monash Model and ASGC-RA Geographical Classification Systems

MMM	Population Size	ASGC-RA	Example Locations
1	All	RA 1	Most capital cities, Newcastle, Geelong, Gold Coast
2	>50,000	RA 2 & 3	Ballarat, Mackay, Toowoomba, Kiama, Albury, Bunbury
3	15,000–50,000	RA 2 & 3	Dubbo, Lismore, Yeppoon, Busselton
4	5000–15,000	RA 2 & 3	Port Augusta, Charters Towers
5	0–5000	RA 2 & 3	Mount Buller, Moruya, Renmark, Condamine
6	0–5000	RA 4	Cape Tribulation, Lightning Ridge, Alice Springs, Mallacoota, Port Hedland
7	0–5000	RA 5	Longreach, Coober Pedy, Thursday Island

Source: Modified from Department of Health and Aged Care (2020). Health Workforce Locator, https://www.health.gov.au/resources/apps-and-tools/health-workforce-locator/health-workforce-locator.

including the National Disability Insurance Scheme (NDIS), aged-care services and workforce incentive and training programs (Department of Health 2020; NDIS 2020; Services Australia 2017).

The use of geographical classifications systems alone for developing appropriate policy can be problematic, as they do not account for socio-demographic indicators such as health status, population density, environmental factors, community resources, availability of communication and transport systems and health literacy (Levesque et al. 2013; McGrail & Humphreys 2009). For example, using the MMM, Macedon in Victoria and Emerald in Queensland are two towns classified as MMM 4 yet Macedon (high advantage ranking) is a forty-five minute drive from Melbourne whereas Emerald (high disadvantage ranking) is a nine hour drive to Brisbane.

Rural Workforce Initiatives

There is inequitable distribution of health workers relative to population need across Australia, within both the suburbs of our cities and the remotest areas of our country. The geographical spread of the health workforce does not reflect the distribution or health need of the population and highlights the reduced access to health practitioners in rural and remote areas. The majority of health professionals are located in MMM 1 (major cities). This might seem reasonable if the number of health practitioners in any geographical location was based on the size of the population but as previously discussed in this chapter, services would be more effective if they were based on health care need.

Health professionals in general report substantial barriers to entering and staying in rural and remote locations including excessive workload and limited opportunities for partners and children (McGrail et al. 2017). It is well documented that medical students from a rural background, who spend placement time in rural areas while linked to a rural medical school, are more likely to return to a rural area to work. A study of medical graduates has found those who spent at least one year studying in rural hospital or PHC settings were more likely to be practising in a rural location nine years post-graduation (Noya et al. 2021). There is growing evidence that other health professions students from rural backgrounds who spend placement time in rural areas are also more likely to return to work in rural areas (Farrugia et al. 2021).

Rural workforce incentive programs are often aimed at medical students and practitioners and have varying degrees of success (McGrail et al. 2018). These funded incentives don't necessarily focus on interdisciplinary practice. For example, accommodation funding is often provided to GPs in small towns but not always to other health professionals who may be on lower salaries.

Models of Health Care in Rural Regions

Due to the extensive geographical distances that separate rural communities, no single health service model can meet the diverse health needs of rural Australians while maintaining economic and operational efficiency. Hence, a variety of service models are needed to ensure equitable health outcomes. Research has shown that a comprehensive PHC approach (see Chapter 6), yields the best health outcomes in situations characterised by limited resources.

Many rural health services have developed innovative service models to meet communities' needs in diverse geographical and cultural settings, evolving to be 'fit for purpose'. Examples include:
- transitioning to integrated and comprehensive PHC services
- **Aboriginal Community Controlled Health Organisations (ACCHOs)**
- outreach services such as the Royal Flying Doctor Service, and other fly-in, fly-out (FIFO) health services
- integrated interprofessional models where allied health, mental health and community health services work across populations
- GP-based and nurse practitioner (NP)-supported hospitals
- expanded and extended use of telehealth services.

Improving access in rural and remote Australia has generally focused on health system characteristics. This has included adapted models of care and workforce initiatives, such as fly-in, fly-out women's health practitioners, which have improved the availability and acceptability of services that are available to women both in Australia and overseas (for example, www.birdsofparadise.clinic). In some locations, practitioners such as nurse practitioners or paramedics have extended scopes of practice that enable them to provide clinical services that another discipline would usually provide (Laurant et al. 2018). Health care workers such as Allied Health Assistants can do some of the routine work of other

CASE STUDY 9.1 The Virtual Rural Generalist Service (VRGS)

Like many rural areas of Australia, Western NSW experiences many challenges recruiting and retaining health care workers to an area already feeling the effects of an ageing rural workforce and decreased numbers of general practice registrars (Playford et al. 2020). The Western New South Wales Local Health District (WNSWLHD) worked with local communities to build on existing health care innovations such as the Remote Medical Consultation Service (RMCS) to create a tele/video health service that provides consultation for emergency departments, acute inpatient wards, ward rounds and aged care when in-situ doctors are not available (NSW Agency for Clinical Innovation 2021).

This innovation involves a team of virtual rural generalist medical practitioners who cover health care across the day. Shifts are structured to meet the anticipated demands of places such as emergency departments. Patients cared for in this structure have usually undergone triage by a nurse, and are non-critical. Health care staff elicit normal transfer procedures if patients need to be seen by other services. The service aims to provide in-person care as well as virtual consultations if possible.

Recently, the VRGS has utilised Australian-trained rural generalist medical practitioners residing in other countries (Marer 2022). This has enabled continuity of service to areas needing GPs who have advanced practice skills.

Case Study Questions

1. What elements of co-design have produced this model of health care? (Which local people and services helped to form this model?)
2. What circumstances may make medical practitioners unavailable to this health service? (Think beyond workforce shortages.)
3. What particular training may health care workers in this model need? (Consider the geographical location of this area, its population and its potential needs.)
4. How do other health care workers support patients in their community when medical practitioners are in short supply? (What skills do other health professions need in rural areas?)

---

allied health professionals, while some worker shortage issues are stop-gapped by employing professionals altogether (an exercise physiologist, for example, instead of a physiotherapist). The approaches and underlying evidence of success are influenced by several health professional and patient factors (Karimi-Shahanjarini et al. 2019).

Digital technology has also meant increased support for health professionals in rural, remote and poorly serviced locations. The **ECHO (Extension for Community Healthcare Outcomes**, see https://hsc.unm.edu/echo/) model of telemonitoring is now widely used by many health professionals and provides specialist knowledge (e.g. alcohol and other drugs, mental health, paediatrics) and support to health professionals across Australia. This means more people can receive high-quality care without having to travel. See also Case study 9.1.

people, the Bendigo and District Aboriginal Co-operative (BDAC) recognised that a vaccination program would have more impact if 'led, managed and administered' by their own Aboriginal and Torres Strait Islander health practitioners. Within six months, the vaccination rate for patients of BDAC had increased to 70% of the eligible Indigenous population, a figure well above the average Victorian Indigenous population at the time (45%) (Naren et al. 2021).

The BDAC vaccination initiative is a great example of an innovative workforce model with acceptable, appropriate and available care that responded to identified need. It resulted in higher levels of utilisation (high vaccination rates) that achieved better outcomes than other existing programs.

How could other health service programs use the success of the BDAC program to provide more equitable health care?

Pause *for* Reflection …

The response to public health concerns regarding the SARS-CoV-2 pandemic has led to many initiatives to increase vaccination rates, with varying success. One of the more productive changes in Victorian legislation was to allow Aboriginal and Torres Strait Islander health practitioners to administer COVID-19 vaccinations under the Public Health Emergency Order. To improve vaccination status of local Indigenous

Health Service Funding

Inequitable access to good-quality health services in rural and remote areas highlights the need for more equitable resourcing mechanisms for those with the greatest health needs. As well as funding for health practitioners and services, it also needs to consider costs to the patient. Every state, for example, has its own patient travel and accommodation allowance scheme for people who have to travel long distances to see health care professionals. The allowance, however, rarely covers the full cost of these visits (National Rural Health Alliance (NRHA) 2019).

Funding of rural and remote services is typically based on geographical classification systems, population–health service provider ratios and/or estimates of population need. Funding models for **small rural health services (SRHS)** differ from the activity-based funding (known also as case-mixed funding) model for larger hospitals where funding is linked to diagnosis and treatment. Because of the difficulties SRHS would have with economies of scale based on activity, SRHS receive block-funding, which allows the health service to channel funds into resources most appropriate for their population.

The reduced availability of doctors means that many rural health services have been unable to access additional Medicare funding because the doctors are not present to generate fees. Programs such as the Medical Specialist Outreach Assistance Program and the Medical Outreach Indigenous Chronic Disease Program use salaried or Medicare-billing doctors in an effort to address these inequities but, to date, funding policies have failed to adequately take the burden of disease into account for rural and remote health service delivery. There is evidence that the funding of ACCHO services addresses some social determinants of health by providing economic benefits to local communities (Pearson et al. 2020), and there is some evidence that digital applications may be able to address the maldistribution of medical services in rural areas (O'Sullivan et al. 2022).

There is substantial evidence that PHC is a cost-effective approach to health care in rural and remote areas (Zhao et al. 2014).

WHERE TO FROM HERE?

Addressing the relatively poor health status of rural populations is a national priority in many countries and, in Australia, the health of rural communities is frequently highlighted in the media. The reality of equity in health care, however, is that most of what would assist people with their health and well-being lies outside the health system (Zhao et al. 2013). Maybe what we need to focus on is not health care itself, but reducing socio-economic disadvantage. What if everyone had safe and secure housing, good nutrition and well-balanced social support? What if people had financial security, regular public transport and better educational opportunities? Investment in these areas may well decrease health care need, which could result in (positive) decreases in health care utilisation.

From reading about these initiatives, you can see the complexities involved in gaining equity in rural health care. Complexity, however, is not necessarily a bad thing, but it does require decision-making that responds to broad concepts situated in heterogenous locations. 'Rural health' is not one problem requiring one solution. It needs dynamic interplay of all factors discussed in this chapter combined with innovation of the most expansive kind, some of which is happening right now.

How will *you* contribute to health care innovation?

SUMMARY

- Equity is not the same as equality.
- The concept of access is multidimensional and invariably involves trade-offs linked to measures of equity.
- Aggregated data suggests some residents of rural Australia have poorer health status than their metropolitan counterparts, but this is not always the case.

- Innovative solutions are needed to address workforce maldistribution and develop models of care that meet the health care needs of disadvantaged populations.
- Health status is closely linked to the social determinants of health so some 'answers' to improving health outcomes may lie outside the health system.

▌ REVIEW QUESTIONS

1. What can policy-makers do to address the underlying inequities in health outcomes?
2. Think about some health services you know. Based on your understanding of the dimensions of access, how accessible are those services? Does your answer apply to all population groups or is access better for some than others?
3. What are some of the limitations of geographical classification systems?
4. How can workforce incentives be equitably distributed to recruit and retain health professionals?
5. How can we use telehealth effectively to provide health care for people with high levels of need?

REFERENCES

Australian Bureau of Statistics (ABS), 2018. Census of Population and Housing 2016: Socio-Economic Indexes for Areas (SEIFA), 2033.0.55.001. Australian Government, Canberra. https://www.abs.gov.au/ausstats/abs@.nsf/Lookup/by%20Subject/2033.0.55.001~2016~Media%20Release~Census%20shows%20our%20most%20advantaged%20&%20disadvantaged%20areas%20(Media%20Release)~25.

Australian Bureau of Statistics (ABS), 2021a. Population clock. ABS, Canberra. https://www.abs.gov.au/statistics/people/population.

Australian Bureau of Statistics (ABS), 2021b. Life tables. ABS, Canberra. https://www.abs.gov.au/statistics/people/population/life-tables/latest-release#:~:text=and%20technological%20advances-~States%20and%20territories,for%20Australian%20males%20and%20females.

Australian Commission on Safety and Quality in Health Care (ACSQHC), 2021. The Fourth Australian Atlas of Healthcare Variation. ACSQHC, Canberra. https://www.safetyandquality.gov.au/sites/default/files/2021-04/The%20Fourth%20Australian%20Atlas%20of%20Healthcare%20Variation%202021_Full%20publication.pdf.

Australian Institute of Health and Welfare (AIHW), 2004. Rural, regional and remote health: a guide to remoteness classifications. Cat. no. PHE 53. AIHW, Canberra.

Australian Institute of Health and Welfare (AIHW), 2014. Access to primary health care relative to need for Indigenous Australians. AIHW, Canberra. Cat. no. IHW 128. https://www.aihw.gov.au/reports/indigenous-australians/access-to-primary-health-care-relative-to-need/summary.

Australian Institute of Health and Welfare (AIHW), 2020a. Australia's health 2020 data insights. Australia's health series no. 17. Cat. no. AUS 231. AIHW, Canberra. https://www.aihw.gov.au/reports/australias-health/australias-health-2020-data-insights/contents/table-of-contents.

Australian Institute of Health and Welfare (AIHW), 2020b. Diabetes. Cat. no. CVD 82. AIHW, Canberra. https://www.aihw.gov.au/reports/diabetes/diabetes.

Australian Institute of Health and Welfare (AIHW), 2020c. Aboriginal and Torres Strait Islander Health Performance Framework 2020 summary report. Cat. no. IHPF 2. AIHW, Canberra. https://www.indigenoushpf.gov.au/getattachment/65fbaaf3-100c-4df5-941c-a8455922693c/2020-summary-ihpf-2.pdf.

Buettner, D., Skemp, S., 2016. Blue zones: lessons from the world's longest lived. Am J Lifestyle Med 10, 318–321. doi:10.1177/1559827616637066.

Centre for Population, 2020. Migration between cities and regions: a quick guide to COVID-19 impacts. Canberra, Australian Government. https://population.gov.au/sites/population.gov.au/files/2021-09/the-impacts-of-covid-on-migration-between-cities-and-regions.pdf.

Department of Health, 2020. Workforce Incentive Program. Australian Government, Canberra. https://www.health.gov.au/initiatives-and-programs/workforce-incentive-program?utm_source=health.gov.au&utm_medium=callout-auto-custom&utm_campaign=digital_transformation.

Department of Health and Aged Care, 2021. Australian statistical geographical classification – remoteness area. https://www.health.gov.au/topics/rural-health-workforce/classifications/asgc-ra.

Farrugia, L., Smith, T., Depczynski, J., 2021. Factors influencing medical radiation science graduates' early career principal place of practice: a retrospective cohort study. J Med Radiat Sci 1–9. doi:10.1002/jmrs.559.

Humphreys, J., McGrail, M., Joyce, C., et al., 2012. Who should receive recruitment and retention incentives? Improved targeting of rural doctors using medical workforce data. Aust J Rural Health 20, 3–10. doi:10.1111/j.1440-1584.2011.01252.x.

Karimi-Shahanjarini, A., Shakibazadeh, E., Rashidian, A., et al., 2019. Barriers and facilitators to the implementation of doctor-nurse substitution strategies in primary care: a qualitative evidence synthesis. Cochrane Database Sys Rev 4, Art. No.: CD010412. doi:10.1002/14651858.CD010412.pub2.

Laurant, M., van der Beizen, M., Wijers, N., et al., 2018. (2018). Nurses as substitutes for doctors in primary care.

Cochrane Database Sys Rev 16 (7), 7. doi:10.1002/14651858.CD001271.pub3.

Levesque, J.F., Harris, M.F., Russell, G., 2013. Patient-centred access to health care: conceptualising access at the interface of health systems and populations. Int J Equity Health 12 (18), 1475–9276. doi.org/10.1186/1475-9276-12-18.

Lueckmann, S.L., Hoebel, J., Roick, J., et al., 2021. Socioeconomic inequalities in primary-care and specialist physician visits: a systematic review. Int J Equity Health 20, 58 (2021). doi.org/10.1186/s12939-020-01375-1.

Marer, L., 2022. 'He said, I'm in Canada': the doctor will see you now – but not from Australia. The Guardian, 17 January. https://www.theguardian.com/australia-news/2022/jan/17/he-said-im-in-canada-the-doctor-will-see-you-now-but-not-from-australia.

McGrail, M.R., Humphreys, J.S., 2009. The index of rural access: an innovative integrated approach for measuring primary care access. BMC Health Serv Res 9 (124), 1472–6963. doi.org/10.1186/1472-6963-9-124.

McGrail, M.R., Russell, D.J., O'Sullivan, B.G., 2017. Family effects on the rurality of GP's work location: a longitudinal panel study. Hum Resour Health 15, 75. doi:10.1186/s12960-017-0250-z.

McGrail, M.R., O'Sullivan, B.G., Russell, D.J., 2018. Rural training pathways: the return rate of doctors to work in the same region as their basic medical training. Hum Resour Health 16, 56. doi:10.1186/s12960-018-0323-7.

Mu, C., Hall, J., 2020. What explains the regional variation in the use of general practitioners in Australia? BMC Health Serv Res 19;20 (1), 325. doi:10.1186/s12913-020-05137-1.

Naren T., Burzacott J., West C., et al., 2021. Role of Aboriginal Health Practitioners in administering and increasing COVID-19 vaccination rates in a Victorian Aboriginal Community Controlled Health Organisation. Rural Remote Health 2021; 21: 7043. doi.org/10.22605/RRH7043.

National Disability Insurance Scheme (NDIS), 2020. NDIS price guide update. NDIS, Canberra. https://www.ndis.gov.au/news/5503-ndis-price-guide-update.

National Rural Health Alliance (NRHA), 2019. Patient assisted travel schemes. NRHA, Canberra. https://www.ruralhealth.org.au/sites/default/files/publications/nrha-pats-fact-sheet-2019.pdf.

Noya, F., Carr, S., Freeman, K., et al., 2021. Strategies to facilitate improved recruitment, development, and retention of the rural and remote medical workforce: a scoping review. Int J Health Policy Manag. doi:10.34172/ijhpm.2021.160.

NSW Agency for Clinical Innovation, 2021. Virtual care: virtual rural generalist service – Western NSW Local Health District. ACI, Sydney. https://aci.health.nsw.gov.au/__data/assets/pdf_file/0005/662234/ACI-virtual-rural-generalist-service.pdf.

O'Sullivan, B., Couch, D., Naik, I., 2022. Using mobile phone apps to deliver rural general practitioner services: critical review using the walkthrough method. JMIR Form Res 25;6 (1), e30387. doi:10.2196/30387.

Paremoer, L., Nandi, S., Serag, H., et al., 2021. Covid-19 pandemic and the social determinants of health. BMJ 372: n129. doi:10.1136/bmj.n129.

Pearson, O., Schwartzkopff, K., Dawson, A., et al., 2020. Aboriginal community controlled health organisations address health equity through action on the social determinants of health of Aboriginal and Torres Strait Islander peoples in Australia. BMC Public Health 20, 1859. doi.org/10.1186/s12889-020-09943-4.

Penchansky, R., Thomas, J.W., 1981. The concept of access: definition and relationship to consumer satisfaction. Med Care 19 (2), 127–140. doi:10.1097/00005650-198102000-00001.

Playford, D., May AM, J.A., Ngo, H., et al., 2020. Decline in new medical graduates registered as general practitioners. Med J Aust 212, 421–422. doi:10.5694/mja2.50563.

Public Health Information Development Unit (PHIDU), 2021. Social Health Atlas of Australia: Population Health Areas. Torrens University Australia. https://phidu.torrens.edu.au/current/maps/sha-aust/pha-single-map/aust/atlas.html.

Services Australia, 2017. Aged Care Viability Supplement for care providers. Australian Government, Canberra. https://www.servicesaustralia.gov.au/aged-care-viability-supplement-for-care-providers#a5.

Thomas, S.L., Wakerman, J., Humphreys, J.S., 2015. Ensuring equity of access to primary health care in rural and remote Australia – what core services should be locally available? Int J Equity Health 14 (1), 111. doi.org/10.1186/s12939-015-0228-1.

UN General Assembly, 2015. Transforming our world : the 2030 Agenda for Sustainable Development, 21 October 2015, A/RES/70/1. https://www.refworld.org/docid/57b6e3e44.html.

Ward, B., Humphreys, J., McGrail, M., et al., 2015. Which dimensions of access are most important when rural residents decide to visit a general practitioner for non-emergency care? Aust Health Rev 39 (2), 121–126. doi.org/10.1071/AH14030.

Welsh, J., Bishop, K., Booth, H., et al., 2021. Inequalities in life expectancy in Australia according to education level: a whole-of-population record linkage study. Int J Equity Health 20, 178. doi.org/10.1186/s12939-021-01513-3.

World Health Organization (WHO), 2021. It's time to build a fairer, healthier world for everyone, everywhere. WHO, Geneva. https://cdn.who.int/media/docs/default-source/world-health-day-2021/health-equity-and-its-determinants.pdf?sfvrsn=6c36f0a5_1&download=true.

Zhao, Y., Wright, J., Begg, S., et al., 2013. Decomposing Indigenous life expectancy gap by risk factors: a life table

analysis. Popul Health Metrics 11, 1. doi:10.1186/
1478-7954-11-1.

Zhao, Y., Thomas, S., Guthridge, S., et al., 2014. Better health outcomes at lower costs: the benefits of primary care utilisation
for chronic disease management in remote Indigenous communities in Australia's Northern Territory. BMC Health Serv
Res 14 (1), 463.

FURTHER READING

Beks H., Walsh S., Alston L., et al., 2022. Approaches used to
describe, measure, and analyze place of practice in dentistry, medical, nursing, and allied health rural graduate
workforce research in Australia: a systematic scoping
review. Int J Environ Res Public Health 19 (3).

Bradford, N., Caffery, L., Smith, A., 2016. Telehealth services
in rural and remote Australia: a systematic review of
models of care and factors influencing success and
sustainability. Rural Remote Health 16, 3808. https://
www.rrh.org.au/journal/article/3808.

Department of Health and Aged Care, 2022. Australia's
primary health care 10 year plan 2022–2032. Commonwealth of Australia, Canberra. https://www.health.gov.au/
resources/publications/australias-primary-health-care-
10-year-plan-2022-2032.

Duckett, S., Stobat, A., Lin, L. March 2022. Not so universal:
How to reduce out-of-pocket healthcare payments.
Grattan Institute, Melbourne. https://grattan.edu.au/wp-
content/uploads/2022/03/Not-so-universal-how-to-
reduce-out-of-pocket-healthcare-payments-Grattan-
Report.pdf.

McGrail, M.R., Russell, D.J., O'Sullivan, B.G., et al., 2018.
Demonstrating a new approach to planning and monitoring rural medical training distribution to meet population need in North West Queensland. BMC Health Serv
Res. 2018 Dec 22;18(1):993. doi:10.1186/s12913-018-
3788-0.

ONLINE RESOURCES

Doctor What? Doctor Where? Stories of Rural Medicine in
Victoria – podcast from Monash University: https://
podcasts.apple.com/gb/podcast/doctor-what-doctor-
where-stories-of-rural-medicine/id1482993048.

Health Direct – Rural Health Services: https://www.healthdi-
rect.gov.au/rural-health-services-in-australia.

National Aboriginal Community Controlled Health Organisation (NACCHO): https://www.naccho.org.au/.

National Rural Health Alliance: https://www.ruralhealth.org.au.

Telehealth Victoria Community of Practice: https://telehealth-
victoria.org.au/.

10

Indigenous Health Systems and Services

Colleen Hayes and Kerry Taylor[a]

KEY LEARNING OUTCOMES

When you finish this chapter you should be able to:
- identify the key elements of Indigenous health systems and services in Australia, including both traditional and contemporary models
- understand the factors that make Indigenous-controlled health systems and services still relevant and necessary
- identify specific features of an Indigenous health service
- critique current funding and policy priorities for Indigenous health services
- examine responses of health services and Government to the SARS-CoV-2 pandemic among First Nations Peoples
- reflect on what practitioners and organisations can do to sustain and collaborate successfully with Indigenous health systems and services.

KEY TERMS AND ABBREVIATIONS

Aboriginal Community Controlled Health Services (ACCHS)
Australian Human Rights Commission (AHRC)
Close the Gap
Closing the Gap
Colonisation
community control
cultural competence

cultural safety
First Nations Peoples
Indigenous
knowledges
mainstream
National Aboriginal Community Controlled Health Organisation (NACCHO)

Ngaanyatjarra, Pitjantjatjara and Yankunytjatjara (NPY)
Ngaanyatjarra, Pitjantjatjara, Yankunytjatjara Women's Council (NPYWC)
primary health care (PHC)
self-determination
social determinants of health (SDH)
traditional

INTRODUCTION

Indigenous[1] health systems and services have been in place for thousands of years prior to the arrival of Western health care. However, **colonisation** has undeniably had detrimental effects on both these systems and the health and well-being of **First Nations People**. To date, **mainstream** health services have been ineffective in dealing with the ongoing impact of our colonising history and reducing the disparity in health status that now exists between Indigenous and non-Indigenous Australians.

In this chapter we will look at the contemporary contexts of Indigenous health but begin with an overview of the pre-existing and continuing systems and services that First Nations People relied on prior to and

[a]Revised and updated from John Reid, Kerry Taylor and Colleen Hayes, 2016.

[1]'Indigenous' is used advisedly throughout this chapter. Although commonly seen in policy and literature to imply First Nations People or Aboriginal and Torres Strait Islander people, not all communities and individuals will identify with this terminology.

since colonisation. We will discuss the interface between what is labelled '**traditional**' and '**non-Indigenous or mainstream**' systems and consider the key elements of Indigenous health services today. We will also examine the role of governments and Indigenous health services and systems in dealing with the SARS-CoV-2 pandemic and consider what health professionals can do to support First Nations People's rights to culturally safe and accessible health care.

THE OLDEST HEALTH CARE SYSTEMS AND SERVICES IN THE WORLD

Evidence suggests that prior to colonisation Indigenous people enjoyed a level of health once envied by the British (Gammage 2011), and that existing health systems were robust (Barnabe 2021). Indigenous health care drew upon **knowledges** and skills developed over thousands of years. Within a relatively short period of contact with non-Indigenous people, however, health and well-being deteriorated owing to introduced diseases, decimation of populations through conflict, dispossession and dislocation and profound and rapid changes in lifestyle that continue to have impacts today (see Fig. 10.1). The experience of colonisation around the world has often resulted in similarly poorer health outcomes for Indigenous peoples (Barnabe 2021; Taylor & Guerin 2019).

For additional information on the current health state of Indigenous Australians, see Australian Indigenous HealthInfoNet (2021), listed in the Online Resources.

Indigenous health focuses on physical, psychological and social well-being. The statistics for First Nations People fail to show the resilience and systems that are health promoting and preventative. Far from rejecting Western health care, many First Nations People access it for dealing with introduced illnesses but also undertake their own health and healing practices, which can include working with **traditional** healers and medicines.

Colonisation resulted in considerable losses in knowledge and health practices, but traditional Indigenous systems and services remain in use throughout Australia today. Although the extent is difficult to quantify, there is a growing recognition of the value and benefits of traditional approaches (Oliver 2013). Even in areas where these practices may have diminished, communities are undergoing cultural revival and reclamation of Indigenous medicinal plants and holistic practices. Terms such as 'traditional' can suggest something of a past era, but it should be recognised that Indigenous health care systems and services are ongoing and adaptive and can offer users an holistic and culturally safe experience.

In Central, South and Western Australia, for example, traditional healers are currently employed within some **Aboriginal Community Controlled Health Services (ACCHS)**. Where they are not formally employed, many traditional healers retain ongoing relationships with patients within mainstream health services. Aboriginal Liaison Officers (ALOs) and/or family members can help hospital patients to access the services of traditional healers when requested. Although this call out might be by phone today, the principles underlying their practice remain consistent and tied to the unique and diverse worldviews of Indigenous peoples.

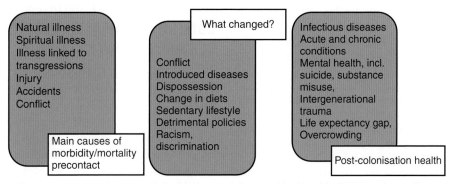

Figure 10.1 Links between Colonisation and Current Health of Indigenous Australians

One organisation that employs traditional healers is the **Ngaanyatjarra, Pitjantjatjara, Yankunytjatjara Women's Council (NPYWC)**[2]. According to the NPYWC:

> **Ngangkari** are Anangu[3] traditional healers, who have received special tools and training from their grandparents. Anangu have a culturally based view of causation and recovery from physical and mental illness and attribute many illnesses and emotional states to harmful elements in the Anangu spiritual world.
>
> *(Ngaanyatjarra, Pitjantjatjara, Yankunytjatjara Women's Council Ngangkari Program 2019).*

Ngangkari believe that collaboration and mutual respect between Western health services and Ngangkari lead to the best outcomes for their communities. Both have valuable skills and knowledge, and both are needed to address the significant problems people face today (NPYWC Ngangkari Program 2019). The aims of the Ngangkari (traditional healers) Project of the Ngaanyatjarra, Pitjantjatjara, Yankunytjatjara (NPY) Women's Council are presented in Box 10.1.

For more information about the work of Ngangkari today, we recommend the award-winning publication *Traditional Healers of Central Australia: Ngangkari*, by NPYWC (see Further Reading section) and the DVD 'Ngangkari', available through Ronin Films (see Online Resources).

The Akeyulerre Healing Centre in Mparntwe/Alice Springs, also offers bush medicines and access to traditional healing and healers (Oliver 2013). A review of literature by Oliver (2013) identified traditional healers and practices as being more apparent in remote areas, but not exclusively. Anecdotal evidence suggests that First Nations People in urban areas may also utilise traditional practices. What is known is that First Nations People have had a longstanding knowledge of medicinal plants across the continent. (For further information, see Low's book *Bush Medicine: A Pharmacopoeia of Natural Remedies*, listed in Further Reading.)

---

[2]**Ngaanyatjarra, Pitjantjatjara and Yankunytjatjara (NPY)** are the major language groups of people whose lands cover the tri-state regions of the top of South Australia, Western Australia and the Northern Territory.

[3]Ngangkari is the NPY word for traditional healer; Anangu is the NPY term for people and has come to imply Aboriginal people.

BOX 10.1   The Ngangkari Program

The Ngangkari (traditional healers) Project of the Ngaanyatjarra, Pitjantjatjara, Yankunytjatjara (NPY) Women's Council aims to:

- provide Anangu and Yarnangu (people) from the NPY region in central Australia with ngangkari traditional healing to promote the work and skills of ngangkari, as a means of ensuring that their work is highly valued and respected within the broader mainstream mental health and public health system
- educate health and mental health workers about the role and work of ngangkari
- provide direction for the development of culturally appropriate mental health services in the region.

The effectiveness of their work in Indigenous mental health was acknowledged in 2009 with a prestigious award from the Royal Australian and New Zealand College of Psychiatrists, and also with the Dr Margaret Tobin Award for excellence in mental health service delivery.

(Reproduced with permission from Ngaanyatjarra, Pitjantjatjara, Yankunytjatjara Women's Council Ngangkari Program 2019.)

Rather than asking people to choose between one practice over another, optimum health outcomes may be achieved by facilitating collaborative responses, as in Case study 10.1.

Pause *for* Reflection …

Readers of this text will usually be undergoing or have undergone education in a Western model of health care. What role would you see for yourself in Colleen's case study as a health professional? How would you find out how best to support this family to ensure they experienced culturally safe care?

WHY DO WE HAVE INDIGENOUS-CONTROLLED HEALTH SYSTEMS AND SERVICES TODAY?

Access to mainstream health care for First Nations People was and still is hampered by systemic and individual barriers. Racism, discrimination, mistrust, miscommunication and a lack of **cultural awareness** meant that even when people had access, this did not always translate into positive health care experiences. Remoteness hampered access for some. Services were simply unavailable or required extensive separation from families

CASE STUDY 10.1 Best of Both Worlds

As an Aboriginal person, my definition of health was and still is about traditional healing and the beliefs and values that come with that; but today for me, I can't go one without the other. Western health care is also needed to deal with the things that my cultural healing practices did not have to deal with before colonisation. As an example, from my own experience of caring for a very sick child, I wanted to try to draw on every option available to him. I did not close one door to the other. I did not think any less of the treatments – both were a priority and of value. When my son was only little, I found him one day, feverish, hot, and unsettled ... the usual things we would do for a hot child did not seem to help as he became sicker throughout the day. I had taken him to the Aboriginal Congress (in Alice Springs) but this was a new illness for me to understand ... so we went to hospital for treatment where they told me he had meningitis.

While we were waiting with him, my mother, who was also a trained health worker in Western health care, said, 'You have to go and pick up that old man ... grandfather.' My grandfather was a healer and I had stopped thinking about what other treatment my son might need because I was only thinking about what the hospital could do for him. My grandfather knew that his grandson was sick before I even told him ... his own healer's messages had already told him and he was waiting for me to pick him up from out bush. When he came to hospital we had prepared the room, telling the nurses what he was going to

do, and asked them to respect us, be quiet and stand back. Even though I felt it was a Western sickness, I still needed my grandfather's healing hands to make sure that my son would get fully better.

He strengthened him by rubbing his hands over his body, and especially his head to help him fight the sickness. This happened around 6 p.m. and by 9 p.m. he was sitting up in bed playing.

While we have trust and value Western medicine for dealing with certain health problems, it would not have been enough for our son to recover. For us, we needed to have access to the depth of knowledge, skills and healing practices that would heal not only his body but his whole being. I felt so much better knowing that my grandfather was coming to do this. And he not only healed my son, but he strengthened my son who has grown into a very healthy and strong young man today. Some people might say this is about faith and the power of belief. How is that any different to Western health practice? People believe antibiotics work and they would say they have a lot of scientific evidence to prove this. Well, Aboriginal people believe in their practices that have thousands of years of evidence as proof as well. The two systems don't have to compete. They can work together for the best outcome for the patient and that is the most important thing.

(Colleen Hayes, personal communication, revised 2022)

and communities to use them. A lack of transport and finances also affected people's uptake of mainstream services. Overall, however, the major gap for Indigenous Australians was the absence of a comprehensive primary health care service. Whereas most Australians today enjoy the benefits of a First World health care system, Indigenous Australians are still experiencing health outcomes that are more commonly associated with Third World conditions. This disparity suggests that something was and is wrong with the system.

The first of the contemporary Aboriginal Community Controlled Health Services (ACCHSs) was established in Redfern, Sydney in 1971 'by community activists in response to ongoing discrimination against Aboriginal people within mainstream health services; to address the poor health and premature deaths of Aboriginal people; and to provide a culturally appropriate system of health care' (Aboriginal Medical Service 2022a).

Primary health care (PHC) emerged internationally as the approach with the greatest potential to address disparities in health for vulnerable and marginalised populations including Indigenous Australians (see Chapter 6 for more information on primary health care). As both a model of service and a philosophy, PHC aligned well with Indigenous concepts of holistic health, which is about maintaining harmony between body, mind and spirit. The establishment of the ACCHSs was a political movement based on the premise of the principle of **self-determination** – proving to the mainstream community that First Nations People could organise and raise funds to set up health care centres and systems that could cater for the culturally diverse needs of their communities.

Redfern Aboriginal Medical Service (AMS), the Central Australian Aboriginal Congress (CAAC) in Mparntwe/Alice Springs and others that followed also represented the political voice of the Aboriginal community, who were fighting for human rights in health, education and employment: important factors in enhancing a person's social capital and maintaining their subjective and communal well-being. The early ACCHSs were a staunch statement about the importance of self-determination (see Box 10.2). Although this occurred some fifty plus years ago, ACCHSs today are still fighting for the same things.

Most ACCHSs have good information on their web pages about their histories, services and systems of care. A common theme in the histories of ACCHSs has been the persistence of a few individuals in striving to improve health outcomes for their communities. It would be worth checking your local region for information relevant to your interests. We have provided some web addresses in the Online Resources.

BOX 10.2   Perspectives from Some of the Pioneering ACCHSs

Redfern Aboriginal Medical Service, Sydney, New South Wales

The Aboriginal Medical Service (AMS) pioneered the concept of Aboriginal community-controlled health care services as the only successful way of improving the health of Aboriginal communities.

Our experience in Redfern has proved that Aboriginal people are capable of solving their own problems: if we are given control of the resources and facilities and allowed to do it our way.

(Aboriginal Medical Service 2022b)

Central Australian Aboriginal Congress (CAAC), Alice Springs, Northern Territory

[The CAAC's] first service was a 'Tent Program', providing shelter to Aboriginal people in town. As time went by, other Aboriginal organisations grew up to take care of issues like housing, education, and land. But health remained a great concern for Aboriginal people, and in 1975, Congress started a Medical Service in a house in Hartley Street. A doctor was employed, and transport and welfare services set up.

(Central Australian Aboriginal Congress 2022)

Pika Wiya Health Service, Port Augusta, South Australia

The Pika Wiya Health Service Aboriginal Corporation provides services to Aboriginal and Torres Strait Islanders of Port Augusta and Davenport, with outreach services to the Northern Flinders Ranges community: Copley, Leigh Creek, Nepabunna and communities isolated in this area as well as Roxby Downs, Andamooka and surrounding areas ... Pika (meaning 'sickness') Wiya (meaning 'no') is derived from the Pitjantjatjara language, which is one of the many Aboriginal languages spoken in the area covered by the health service. The Pika Wiya Health Service Aboriginal Corporation was established by the determination of three local Aboriginal women.

Early in the 1970s, a group of Aboriginal women met in Port Augusta. One of them was a nurse. At the meeting they were told that a sick man was lying in the sand hills just out of town. The women went out and gave what assistance they could and called an ambulance. As a result of the sharing of this and other stories, the women decided that Port Augusta needed a medical service for Aboriginal people. But at the time, neither state nor federal government were interested in providing money, so the women wrote to the World Council of Churches in Geneva, Switzerland and outlined their plight. The World Council of Churches gave them a grant and with this money the Aboriginal Medical Service, Port Augusta was formed.

The Aboriginal Medical Service in Redfern, although struggling themselves, loaned them a doctor, who came over regularly. There were no funds for accommodation, so the doctor had to sleep on the floor of the clinic, and bandages had to be washed and re-used. The Aboriginal Medical Service evolved into the Pika Wiya Health Service Inc. in 1984.

Since then, Pika Wiya has gone through a number of transformations. The Service has grown and has evolved into one of the largest leading Aboriginal Medical Services in South Australia.

(Deadly Vibe 2022)

Kambu Health, Southeast Queensland

Kambu Health was founded by a group of local residents – Ken Dalton, Cecil Fisher, Roberta Thompson, Faye Carr, Bill Robinson, and Doreen Thompson – to address the growing health needs of the local Aboriginal and Torres Strait Islander community. Originally there was a meeting called by the people of the community to get a housing co-operative to be incorporated with Southern Suburbs Football Team. The health service was run from a room in the home of Doreen Thompson. It provided culturally appropriate health care by doctors who travelled up from Aboriginal and Islander Community Health Service Brisbane for one day a week.

BOX 10.2   Perspectives from Some of the Pioneering ACCHSs—cont'd

In 1975–6, a house was purchased by the housing co-op, and the medical staff moved into one of the rooms there. It was from there the doctor and [nursing] sister would go to Wacol Hostel and conduct an outside clinic ... The growth of the co-op and the medical centre was such that there was soon a need to expand, so a new medical centre was built beside the old nursing house at 27 Roderick Street, Ipswich. The staff now consisted of a doctor, nursing sister, bookkeeper, CEO, and medical receptionist.

In 1988 the medical centre became incorporated in its own right and was named the Aboriginal and Islander Community Health Service Ipswich. By

1994 the staff had increased again to a CEO, finance officer, doctor, two health workers, a trainee health worker, a driver, nutrition field officer, trainee receptionist and trainee admin assistant, all managed by a community-elected Board of Directors.

Today, Kambu Aboriginal and Torres Strait Islander Corporation for Health employs over 60 staff (not including visiting specialists) and provides comprehensive medical and specialist services to Ipswich and the surrounding areas. Clinics are now located in Ipswich, Goodna, and Laidley.

(Kambu Aboriginal and Torres Strait Islander Corporation for Health 2022)

ACCHSs differ from one another in their structure, policy implementation, service focus and workforces, reflecting the diversity of Indigenous Australia. What works in one area may not always work in another. The **National Aboriginal Community Controlled Health Organisation (NACCHO)** is Australia's peak national representative body for Indigenous health, representing 144 ACCHSs (NACCHO 2022).

ACCHSs differ from mainstream services in that they are initiated by the community and located within First Nations communities and, importantly, have governance structures that ensure **community control**. Being incorporated provides a legal accountability. Workforces are majority First Nations People and non-Indigenous staff receive cultural awareness training. Fig. 10.2 illustrates the common principles underpinning all ACCHSs.

The links between colonisation and the complex state of Indigenous health today are both explicit and implicit. The consequences of dislocation, dispossession and radical changes in living conditions over several generations has had a profound physiological and psychological effect on Indigenous peoples, showing up in many diverse and complex ways: heart disease, high blood pressure and other forms of chronic disease, mental health issues, including suicide, alcohol abuse, elevated levels of smoking and family violence.

Look at the increased incidence of diabetes as an illustrative example. The diet of Indigenous people prior to colonisation was believed to be well balanced and nutritionally sound. It required considerable physical energy to obtain food. With the loss of lands came a loss of access to traditional diets. Instead, successive governments and other groups provided Indigenous Australians with inferior and potentially harmful food through the periods of missions and reserves and even in lieu of wages in some employment settings such as the cattle industries. The staples of these diets were most often flour, sugar, tea, low-quality fatty meat, and tobacco. Ecologically and environmentally safe shelter was replaced by inappropriate housing that led to overcrowding, and high rates of infectious illness. The pathways to chronic diseases were established. It will take considerable collaboration and a willingness to work differently to turn around this trajectory.

Pause *for* Reflection ...

Fig. 10.1 examines just some of the overt links between colonisation and health today.

What other examples of contemporary health issues can you identify that disproportionately affect First Nations People today?

For pre-colonisation illnesses and, to some extent, injuries and accidents, protocols and practices to minimise risks existed. With changes brought on by colonisation, the risks and exposure to health are amplified. Not recognising and responding to the role of colonisation in health today perpetuates a deficit approach to individuals and specific populations that overlooks underlying structural and systemic causes.

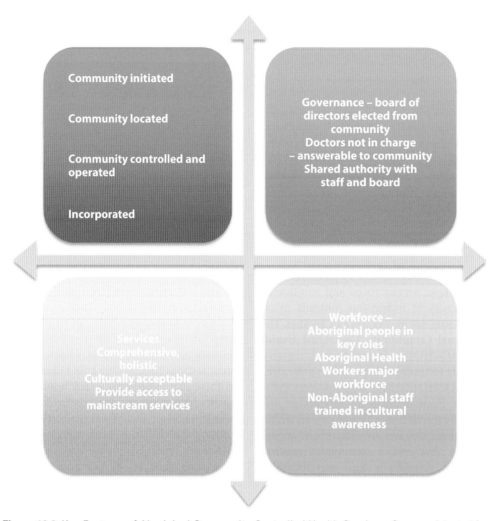

Figure 10.2 Key Features of Aboriginal Community-Controlled Health Services. *Sources*: Adapted from http://www.ntgpe.org/workingwell/working_well1_1.htm; Miller & Speare (in Willis et al. 2012).

Funding for ACCHSs

Funding insecurity is possibly the greatest threat to the successful achievement of the original goals of ACCHSs. ACCHSs commonly had to develop with relatively little financial support in their early days. While health care services are often taken for granted for most Australians, Indigenous Australians have had to fight to secure funding and, even now, to maintain adequate funding.

Despite strong evidence for the effectiveness and value of ACCHSs, there is an ongoing need to fight for their place in Australian health care (Baba et al. 2014; Rollins 2014). Successive governments have found it difficult to separate their responsibility for funding from trying to assert control.

Pause *for* Reflection …

Bacchi's approach to critically analysing public policy suggests that 'what one proposes to do about something reveals what one thinks is problematic (needs to change)' (2012, p. 21). First Nations People have been 'problematised' in public policy since colonisation commenced as the ones who need to change. What changes might the government make instead to facilitate better health and social outcomes for First Nations People?

CASE STUDY 10.2   An Example of the Principles That Define ACCHSs: The Purple House (Western Desert Dialysis) – Alice Springs

The Purple House is the name of a health care service that has arisen from the tenacity and persistence of a small group of people for whom today's impressive renal and holistic services have come too late. Purple House is the operational base for a network of services that seeks to provide an ongoing connection to family and country for those people affected by renal failure. The organisation's full name, Western Desert Nganampa Walytja Palyantjaku Tjutaku, means 'making all our families well'.

With the knowledge that what they were setting out to achieve would not benefit them directly, the group's thoughts were for the future and their countrymen and women who would experience the almost inevitable trajectory towards renal failure, which is at epidemic proportions throughout many First Nations populations. The Purple House story is well worth hearing. When Pintupi people from the Western Desert found themselves faced with the need to leave their homes to access renal services, the genesis for this unique and innovative health service emerged. After being repeatedly told by governments that dialysis services in remote homelands was unviable, this group took matters into their own hands by using the growing regard for contemporary Indigenous art. They sold two major works at auction raising over a million dollars.

For Pintupi, receiving dialysis treatment meant little if the person's spirit was sick. Health is more than physical well-being and this holistic view of health is reflected in the service's core values of compassion, caring for family and connection to country. A major goal of the Purple House and the satellite centres now established is to ensure this ongoing connection for people.

Far from living on the machines, away from family and culture, the original Purple House is a vibrant environment for patients, where the CEO, along with any other staff member, can be found making cups of tea for families, who are working in the yard preparing bush medicines or cooking kangaroo in a fire pit. As the model demonstrated its success and sustainability, other remote populations sought to partner with Western Desert Dialysis and there are now mobile and permanent dialysis services in some eighteen remote communities.

Reflecting on the key elements outlined in Fig.10.2: Purple House was initiated by the community it serves and is governed by local people, to meet a need that they identified. The service provides employment and training opportunities for Indigenous staff and non-Indigenous employees are committed to the cultural values of the organisation. For more information, see Western Desert Nganampa Walytja Palyantjaku Tjutaku Corporation (2018).

The benefits of ACCHSs are more than health-related. They are political, cultural, economic, educational and more. Case study 10.2 is a powerful example of resilience and self-determination to address the lack of culturally safe care for renal patients.

Indigenous Australia is culturally diverse, and the models of health systems and services are by necessity reflective of this diversity (Baba et al. 2014). What works in one region may not work in another. As you might have noticed with each of the examples of ACCHSs in Box 10.2, the common impetus for development was a lack of access or acceptable services. ACCHSs filled a service delivery gap; all commenced as initiatives of the local communities that they serve and are controlled by them.

While a gap in health outcomes between Indigenous and non-Indigenous Australians exists, the need for such services remains. This of course does not mean that mainstream services cannot do much to improve the effectiveness and experience of health care they provide to Indigenous Australians. Increased employment of Indigenous people across all sectors of mainstream health services, better cultural safety education, policy and accountability, and greater partnering with Indigenous organisations will all go a long way to improving outcomes for Indigenous clients.

The Role of ACCHSs in Dealing with the COVID-19 (SARS-CoV-2) Pandemic

Despite a recognised need for a tailored response to the SARS-CoV-2 pandemic, ACCHSs were left underfunded and under-resourced to deal with the expected high morbidity and mortality rates within Indigenous populations (McCalm et al. 2021). The Gurriny Yealamucka Health Service is one example of how locally led solutions managed to keep people safe in the community of Yarrabah, North Queensland. Research by McCalm et al. (2021) identified the service's capacity to pivot in response to the pandemic and resource shortfalls, to find solutions locally which also highlighted the need for dedicated funding and resources to manage such events going forward. Lowitja Institute 2021 highlights other successful responses to protecting First Nations People in their 2021 Close the Gap Report. 'Aboriginal and Torres Strait Islander leaders moved rapidly to safeguard communities when the COVID-19 [SARS-CoV-2] pandemic took hold. Their actions were decisive and designed with each local community in mind and avoided a potential catastrophe. Some of our homelands, once threatened with closure by governments in the past, became some of the safest places in Australia' (Lowitja Institute 2021, p. 3).

WHERE TO FROM HERE?

The **social determinants of health** (**SDH**) demonstrate that health is determined by the social circumstances of individuals and groups, such as education, housing and employment. Over the last decade, the disparities between Indigenous and non-Indigenous Australians have highlighted more than ever the need for Indigenous control over and participation in health services. Two campaigns aimed at addressing inequalities in outcomes have been rolled out since 2008 – **Close the Gap** and **Closing the Gap**.

Close the Gap is a public awareness campaign focused on closing the health gap. It is run by numerous **non-government organisations** (**NGOs**), Indigenous health bodies and human rights organisations, including the **Australian Human Rights Commission** (**AHRC**). The Lowitja Institute (2022) Close the Gap Report provides an update on progress and shares some of the individual and community-level success stories in Indigenous-led health policy, service delivery and human rights sectors.

Closing the Gap has been the government's program with six key targets:

- *To close the life-expectancy gap within a generation*
- *To halve the gap in mortality rates for Indigenous children under five within a decade*
- *To ensure access to early childhood education for all Indigenous four-year-olds in remote communities within five years*
- *To halve the gap in reading, writing and numeracy achievements for children within a decade*
- *To halve the gap in Indigenous Year 12 achievement by 2020*
- *To halve the gap in employment outcomes between Indigenous and non-Indigenous Australians within a decade.*

(Davidson 2014)

Unfortunately, in 2018 the report card for Closing the Gap did not score well in the majority target areas, but in 2020, the Lowitja Institute reported that:

> *our leaders finally sat with government, negotiated and co-signed the New National Agreement on Closing the Gap as partners. The investment for health equity is relatively small but must be relative to a burden of disease 2.3 times that of other Australians. As repeated often, a country as 'great' and wealthy as Australia is capable of delivering health equity for and with its First Nations Peoples – just three per cent of the population.*

(Lowitja Institute 2021, p. 2)

In 2022 the key themes of the Closing the Gap Report were: Aboriginal and Torres Strait Islander-led Transformation; Gender Justice: equality and equity; and Allyship (Lowitja Institute 2022) in recognition of the need to move away from deficit approaches to holistic, culturally safe, community-led initiatives.

Far from being less necessary since their inception in the 1970s, ACCHSs remain essential to reduce disparities in health outcomes. Sustainability for ACCHSs will require strategic partnerships with mainstream services to achieve the best outcomes for Indigenous consumers (Lloyd & Wise 2011). Working together and/or allyship however, 'should not be approached as simply 'improving' or 'helping' others; ... allyship implies respectful relationship building and addressing power imbalances' (Barnabe 2021, p. 4). We know that, irrespective of financial support, Indigenous Australians will rightfully continue to hold their own health beliefs and conduct their own health care practices at the individual and community levels. However, there are health care challenges today that have been beyond successive governments' resources to manage. It will only be through sustained and collaborative efforts that improvements in the health of Indigenous Australians will be made.

Racism remains a major barrier to health for Indigenous Australians. While some improvements have resulted from the uptake of key philosophical frameworks such as **cultural safety** and **cultural competence** within mainstream services, more needs to be done by government. Inadequate funding and resources, along with efforts to control the autonomy of organisations, may be hampering the original goals of putting Indigenous health into Indigenous hands. Indigenous health services and systems have proven their worth in ensuring better outcomes for Indigenous Australians. Both traditional and contemporary models of Indigenous health services remain relevant and active today. Working together with mainstream services offers the greatest potential for improving the health and well-being of Indigenous Australians today.

SUMMARY

Indigenous health systems and services existed well before the introduction of Western medical services and remain relevant and necessary across Australia today.

Aboriginal-controlled services arose from the paradigm of self-determination for Aboriginal people and a failure of mainstream services to adequately provide for Indigenous people. There are fundamental differences in the way Indigenous services are structured that reflect Indigenous ways of thinking, feeling and valuing.

Some positive examples of Indigenous health care systems and services are found in the case studies.

Changes to funding and governance may be impacting on the original aims of Aboriginal-controlled health services. Positive and respectful partnerships are necessary.

REVIEW QUESTIONS

1. From your reading of this chapter and reviewing information on their web site, what are the key features that make the Purple House an example of an ACCHS?
2. There is a tension between mainstream health systems and Indigenous health systems. What are the advantages and disadvantages of Australia having multiple health systems, e.g. Indigenous, private, complementary?
3. How can traditional health care systems and services play a role improving outcomes for First Nations People in contemporary Australia?
4. What are some of the current challenges to the sustainability of ACCHSs today?
5. How can mainstream services improve the experience of health care for Indigenous Australians?

REFERENCES

Aboriginal Medical Service, 2022a. Our history. https://amsredfern.org.au/.

Aboriginal Medical Service, 2022b. redfernoralhistory.org/Organisations/AboriginalMedicalService/tabid/208/Default.aspx.

Baba, J., Brolan, C., Hill, P., 2014. Aboriginal medical services cure more than illness: a qualitative study of how Indigenous services address the health impacts of discrimination in Brisbane communities. Int J Equity Health 13, 56. http://www.equityhealthj.com/content/13/1/56.

Bacchi, C., 2012. Introducing the 'What's the Problem Represented to be?' approach. In: Bletsas, A., Beasley, C. (Eds.), Engaging with Carol Bacchi: Strategic Interventions and Exchanges. University of Adelaide Press, Adelaide, pp. 21–24.

Barnabe C., 2021. Towards attainment of Indigenous health through empowerment: resetting health systems, services, and provider approaches. BMJ Glob 6, e004052. doi:10.1136/ bmjgh-2020-004052.

Central Australian Aboriginal Congress (CAAC), 2022. Past, present, future, Alice Springs, CAAC. http://www.caac.org.au/about-congress/past-present-future.

Davidson, H., 2014. Close the Gap and Closing the Gap – what's the difference? The Guardian. https://www.the-guardian.com/world/blog/2014/feb/12/close-the-gap-and-closing-the-gap-whats-the-difference. 12 Feb.

Deadly Vibe, 2022. Pika Wiya means 'no sickness'. Deadly Vibe Group. https://www.deadlyvibe.com.au/2013/08/pika-wiya-means-no-sickness-2.

Gammage, B., 2011. The Biggest Estate on Earth: How Aborigines Made Australia. Allen & Unwin, Sydney.

Kambu Aboriginal and Torres Strait Islander Corporation for Health, 2022. Ipswich and West Moreton Areas. https://kambuhealth.com.au/ipswich-and-west-moreton-areas.php.

Lloyd, J., Wise, M., 2011. Improving Aboriginal health: how might the health sector do things differently? Aust Rev Public Affairs 2.

Lowitja Institute, 2021. Close the Gap: Leadership and legacy through crises: keeping our mob safe, Close the Gap

Report 2021. The Close the Gap Campaign Steering Committee, Melbourne.

Lowitja Institute, 2022. Close the Gap: Transforming power: voices for generational change, Close the Gap Report 2022. The Close the Gap Campaign Steering Committee, Melbourne.

McCalman, J., Longbottom, M., Fagan, S., et al., 2021. Leading with local solutions to keep Yarrabah safe: a grounded theory study of an Aboriginal community-controlled health organisation's response to COVID-19. BMC Health Serv Res 21, 732. doi:10.1186/s12913-021-06761-1.

Miller, A., Speare, R., 2012. Health care for Indigenous Australians. In: Willis, E., Reynolds, L., Keleher, H. (Eds.), Understanding the Australian Health Care System, second ed. Elsevier, Australia.

National Aboriginal Community Controlled Health Organisation (NACCHO), 2022. Government announces new funding model for ACCHS. https://www.naccho.org.au/wp-content/uploads/Government-announces-new-funding-model-for-ACCHS.pdf.

National Aboriginal Community Controlled Health Organisation (NACCHO), 2022. About us. https://www.naccho.org.au/about/.

Ngaanyatjarra, Pitjantjatjara, Yankunytjatjara Women's Council, 2019. 2017–2018 annual report: Ngangkari Program. http://www.npywc.org.au/wp-content/uploads/NPWC-AR-2017-18.pdf.

Oliver, S. 2013 The role of traditional medicine practice in primary health care within Aboriginal Australia: a review of the literature. J Ethnobiol Ethnomed 9, 46. http://www.ethnobiomed.com/content/9/1/46.

Rollins, A., 2014. End funding uncertainty in Aboriginal controlled health care. Med J Aust 26 (7), 11. https://ama.com.au/ausmed/end-funding-uncertainty-aboriginal-controlled-health-care-ama.

Taylor, K., Guerin, P., 2019. Health Care and Indigenous Australians: Cultural Safety in Practice, third ed. Palgrave MacMillan, Melbourne.

Western Desert Nganampa Walytja Palyantjaku Tjutaku Corporation, 2018. Purple House. https://www.purple-house.org.au.

FURTHER READING

Funding of ACCHSs – Aboriginal Community Controlled Health Service funding: report to the sector 2011. https://www.lowitja.org.au/sites/default/files/docs/Overburden_Funding-Report-to-ACCHS-2011.pdf.

Hayman, N., Armstrong, R., 2014. Health services for Aboriginal and Torres Strait Islander people: handle with care. Med J Aust 200 (11), 613.

Low, T., 1990. Bush Medicine: A Pharmacopoeia of Natural Remedies. Angus & Robertson, Sydney.

Ngaanyatjarra, Pitjantjatjara, Yankunytjatjara Women's Council, 2013. Traditional Healers of Central Australia; Ngangkari, by the Ngaanyatjarra, Pitjantjatjara, Yankunytjatjara.

Reilly, L., Adams, M., Rees, S., 2021. The intensifying threat of COVID-19 among First Nations People of Australia: making up for lost time. AMA Health Forum 2 (12), e214356. doi:10.1001/jamahealthforum.2021.4356.

ONLINE RESOURCES

For a history of the various ACCHSs or AMSs the following websites are useful.

Central Australian Aboriginal Congress: https://www.caac.org.au.

Information about traditional healers – watch the film Ngangkari (National Indigenous Documentary Fund Series 5), Dir. Erica Glynn: https://www.roninfilms.com.au/feature/778.html.

Kambu Health in Southeast Queensland: http://kambuhealth.com.au/our-history.php.

Ngaanyatjarra, Pitjantjatjara, Yankunytjatjara Women's Council: https://www.npywc.org.au/.

Northern Territory General Practice Education online resources: https://www.ntgpe.org/workingwell/working_well1_1.htm.

Australian Indigenous HealthInfoNet (2021). Overview of Aboriginal and Torres Strait Islander health status 2020: https://healthinfonet.ecu.edu.au/learn/health-facts/overview-aboriginal-torres-strait-islander-health-status/

Redfern AMS: http://redfernoralhistory.org/Organisations/AboriginalMedicalService/tabid/208/Default.aspx.

The Indigenous Health and Cultural Competency (IH&CC) education resources for emergency department staff: https://acem.org.au/Content-Sources/Advancing-Emergency-Medicine/Cultural-competency/Indigenous-Health-and-Cultural-Competency-Resource/Indigenous-Health-and-Cultural-Competency.

Ngaanyatjarra, Pitjantjatjara, Yankunytjatjara Women's Council: http://www.npywc.org.au/shop/.

11

Mental Health and Recovery-Oriented Mental Health Services

Fiona Orr

KEY LEARNING OUTCOMES

When you finish this chapter you should be able to:
- identify the prevalence of mental disorder in the Australian population
- identify the major changes in the delivery of mental health services, including the role of the consumer movement
- outline the components of recovery-oriented mental health practice and services
- differentiate the key mental health professional workforce – consumer peer, carer peer and clinical
- describe the components of the Australian mental health care system.

KEY TERMS AND ABBREVIATIONS

biopsychosocial model
Community Mental Health Services (CMHS)
consumer[1]
deinstitutionalisation
emergency departments (EDs)
general practitioners (GPs)
lived experience

mental disorder
Mental Health Coordinating Council (MHCC)
National Mental Health Commission (NMHC)
National Disability Insurance Scheme (NDIS)
peer worker

personal recovery
social determinants of health (SDH)
stigma
World Health Organization (WHO)

INTRODUCTION

This chapter presents an introduction to mental health and well-being and the prevalence of mental disorders in the Australian population. It explores an overview of Australian mental health services and the major mental health reforms that shaped them, including the role of the mental health **consumer** rights movement, the *National Mental Health Strategy*, and a recovery-oriented model of mental health practice.

MENTAL HEALTH AND WELL-BEING

The **World Health Organization (WHO)** (2021) refers to mental health as 'a state of well-being in which the individual realizes his or her own abilities, can cope with the normal stresses of life, can work productively and fruitfully, and is able to make a contribution to his or her community' (p. 1).

[1]Various terms have been adopted by people with lived experiences of mental disorder and using mental health services. These include psychiatric survivors, ex-patients, consumers, lived experience consumers, experts by experience and service users. While no single term is adequate to represent the experiences of everyone, the term 'consumer' will be used in this chapter to refer to people with lived experiences of mental distress and disorder and of using mental health services.

The **social determinants of health (SDH)** also affect mental health, and include financial means, living conditions, working environment, long-term health conditions, access to health care, the quality of social relationships and supports, experience of violence and abuse, and geographic and climatic conditions (WHO 2021). Employment, physical activity, strong social relationships and networks, adequate diet, alcohol reduction and green space can act as protective factors (Rickwood & Thomas 2019, p. 22). The promotion of mental health is important in the prevention of mental distress and disorder.

A **mental disorder** refers to 'a clinically diagnosable disorder that significantly interferes with a person's cognitive, emotional or social abilities. Examples include anxiety disorders, depression, bipolar disorder, eating disorders, and schizophrenia' (Council of Australian Governments (COAG) 2017, p. 67). Worldwide there are about 284 million people affected by anxiety, 264 million affected by depression, 45 million who have bipolar disorder and 20 million people who have schizophrenia (Abate et al. 2018; WHO 2022). While there are several explanations for the genesis of mental disorders, the **biopsychosocial model** views mental disorder as the complex interactions between biological, psychological and social factors (Papadimitriou 2017). Holistic and person-centred approaches to mental health recovery are vital.

Prevalence of Mental Disorders in Australia

What is the state of Australians' mental health? For many people who experience a mental disorder, it occurs before the age of 25 years (Productivity Commission 2020), a time when young adults are undertaking work and studies, living independently and forming relationships. The *National Study of Mental Health and Wellbeing* provides some insight into the prevalence of mental disorders in Australia (Australian Bureau of Statistics (ABS) 2022). Between 2020 and 2021, over 43% of Australians aged 16–85 years reported experiencing a mental disorder at some time in their life. More than one in five people had symptoms of a mental disorder in the previous 12 months, with the most frequently experienced disorders being anxiety (16.8%), affective (mood disorders) (7.5%) and substance use (3.3%). Women were more likely than men to have an anxiety or affective disorder, while men were more likely than women to have a substance use disorder. Overall, more women than men, and younger rather than older adults, experience a mental disorder (ABS 2022).

The prevalence of psychotic disorders in the Australian population, such as schizophrenia, bipolar disorder and brief psychosis, was estimated at 4.5 per 1000 population. The prevalence for men was higher than for women in every age group (Morgan et al. 2011).

Aboriginal and Torres Strait Islander People

Aboriginal and Torres Strait Islander people have higher rates of mental distress and disorders compared to non-Aboriginal and Torres Strait Islander people. When compared with non-Indigenous Australians, psychological distress was 2.3 times the rate for Aboriginal and Torres Strait Islanders, particularly for people living in non-remote areas, with 24% of Aboriginal and Torres Strait Islander people experiencing a mental disorder or behavioural condition (ABS 2019). Racism has been associated with poor mental health outcomes in Aboriginal and Torres Strait Islander people, with some evidence linking it to the development of anxiety and depression (Kairuz et al. 2021).

> **Pause *for* Reflection …**
> Why might more women than men be diagnosed with a mental disorder? Think about the social, cultural, biological and psychological factors that could contribute to these prevalence rates.
> Why might men more often than women experience substance use disorders?
> How might the social determinants of health explain the higher rates of mental distress and disorders in Aboriginal and Torres Strait Islander people?

SUICIDALITY AND SUICIDE

This section of the chapter discusses suicide. Anyone can be affected by suicide, including health professionals. If the following causes you distress, the suicide and mental health support services in Table 11.1 could assist you.

Suicide can be confronting to discuss, and professional practice can involve interactions with health care consumers who are suicidal. Prevention of suicide is possible, so it is important for health professionals to capably discuss suicidality with health care consumers and those who support them.

Intentional self-harm is deliberately causing physical harm to oneself, with or without the intent to die; therefore, it includes suicide attempts and non-suicidal

Table 11.1   Suicide and Mental Health Support Services

Service	Telephone	Website
Lifeline	13 11 14	lifeline.org.au
Suicide Call Back Service	1300 659 467	suicidecallbackservice.org.au
Beyond Blue	1300 22 46 36	beyondblue.org.au
MensLine Australia	1300 78 99 78	mensline.org.au
Q life (LGBTIQ+)	1800 184 527	qlife.org.au
Kids Helpline	1800 55 1800	kidshelpline.com.au

self-harm (Australian Institute of Health and Welfare (AIHW) 2022a). Suicide is the act of deliberately ending one's life, and suicidality refers to thoughts about suicide, making plans for suicide, and suicide attempts (AIHW 2022a). The **Mental Health Coordinating Council (MHCC)** (2018) advises the use of the following non-stigmatising language when speaking about suicide: 'died by suicide' or 'ended their life'. When talking about attempted suicide, they advise this wording: 'an attempt to end their own life'.

Suicide is a complex phenomenon, and several psychological and socio-economic factors are associated with an increased risk for suicide; however, the presence of risk factors in any individual does not predict the future occurrence of suicide. The factors associated with a higher risk for suicide include a personal history of intentional self-harm, being male, being widowed, divorced or separated, living in a lone household, being unemployed and having a lower income (AIHW 2022a).

Prevalence of Intentional Self-Harm and Suicide

Since 2008, the rate of hospitalisation for intentional self-harm has risen, with the rate for Indigenous Australians being three times that of non-Indigenous Australians (AIHW 2022a). Between 2019 and 2020 females made up almost two-thirds of people hospitalised for intentional self-harm, with the highest rate of hospitalisations in those 15–19 years of age (AIHW 2022a). Over ten years, the suicide rate in Australia increased by 13% to 12.1 per 100,000 population, with 3139 deaths by suicide in 2020 (AIHW 2022a). Latest figures suggest that while there has been increased mental distress due to the SARS-CoV-2 pandemic, the pandemic has not been associated with a rise in suspected deaths by suicide (AIHW 2022b).

Across all age groups, the number of suicides by males was higher than for females, occurring at a ratio of approximately 3:1, and rates for Indigenous people are more than twice as high as for non-Indigenous people. Suicide is the leading cause of death among all people aged 15–44, however, males 85 years and older have the highest age-specific rate of suicide at 32.9 per 100,000, and the Northern Territory had the highest rate of all states and territories (AIHW 2022a).

Costs of Mental Disorder and Suicide

The Productivity Commission (2022, p. 9) estimated that mental disorder costs the Australian economy within the range of $200–220 billion per year, including costs of health and other services, lost productivity and economic participation and informal care by families. While the social and emotional costs are less able to be quantified, they can adversely affect individuals and those who support them, and include reduced health and well-being, distress, stigma and discrimination, social isolation, reduced participation in communities and premature death (Productivity Commission 2020, p. 151).

Suicide of any individual is a tragedy and has far-reaching effects for family, friends and the wider community, and the importance of accessible mental health and suicide prevention programs and timely support services for people who have attempted suicide cannot be overstated. It is estimated that adequate follow-up after a suicide attempt, and specific support services for Aboriginal and Torres Strait Islanders provided by Indigenous-led organisations, could reduce the number of people presenting to **emergency departments (EDs)** for a suicide attempt by 20% and decrease deaths due to suicide by 1%; that is, 35 people each year who would not die by suicide (Productivity Commission 2020, p. 22).

Pause *for* Reflection ...

How does an understanding of the psychological, social and economic risk factors for suicide contribute to its prevention and the development of effective supports and interventions?

Why do health professionals need to be aware of the prevalence of intentional self-harm and suicide?

STIGMA AND DISCRIMINATION

People living with a mental disorder can experience **stigma** and discrimination, social isolation and violation of their human rights (WHO 2021). Despite mental health reforms and campaigns to address stigma and discrimination, it continues today. Stigma is 'a negative opinion or judgment that excludes, rejects, shames or devalues a person or group of people' (COAG 2017, p. 70) that can lead to public discrimination, internalisation and self-stigma, and non-engagement with mental health services (Carrara et al. 2019; Corrigan et al. 2014; Thornicroft et al. 2007). While programs to address stigma have increased awareness and knowledge of anxiety and depression, the public's understanding of schizophrenia and bipolar disorder are limited and attitudes toward people diagnosed with these conditions are more negative (COAG 2017). But stigma is not confined to the public; stigma by health professionals also occurs and is related in part to beliefs about negative treatment and recovery outcomes (Carrara et al. 2019; Charles 2013; Economou et al. 2019). Acknowledging and actively addressing our own stigmatising attitudes and behaviours and their impact on individuals' recovery and well-being is the responsibility of all health professionals. The **National Mental Health Commission (NMHC)** (2022b) is currently developing a National Stigma and Discrimination Reduction Strategy to reduce structural and public stigma across a range of sectors, including health, social services, legal, and education and training.

DEINSTITUTIONALISATION AND COMMUNITY MENTAL HEALTH

Until the second half of the 20th century, mental health services in Australia were predominantly provided in large psychiatric hospitals or institutions. Originally referred to as asylums in the 19th century, they were often situated on large, secluded grounds, custodial in nature, and funded by governments, with the first institution operating from 1838 (Coleborne & MacKinnon 2006; Lewis & Garton 2017). The 20th century witnessed changing views, with the emerging idea of mental illness as opposed to insanity, a range of new therapies – talking therapies, therapeutic communities and psychotropic medications – and changes to legislation governing the care and control of people in psychiatric hospitals (Lewis & Garton 2017). While there were improvements in some therapeutic practices, criticisms of psychiatric services included overcrowding, abuses of human rights, injuries and death (Lewis & Garton 2017).

By the 1960s with the beginning of community psychiatry, psychiatric services in institutions were reduced. Referred to as **deinstitutionalisation**, the focus of care gradually shifted from hospitals to the community (Smith & Gridley 2006). While the early 1970s saw a rise in community mental health services, many recently discharged people were unsupported in the community (Dunlop & Pols 2022; Lewis & Garton 2017). During the 1980s, the principle of the 'least restrictive care' facilitated community mental health treatment and the establishment of community mental health centres, some with extended hours of service (Smith & Gridley 2006). In the early 1990s, the Burdekin inquiry into human rights and people with a mental illness was a damning account, identifying them as some of the most vulnerable and disadvantaged people (Human Rights and Equal Opportunity Commission (HREOC) 1993). Consequently, the last decade of the 20th century witnessed further deinstitutionalisation and the closure of many psychiatric institutions across the country (Coleborne & MacKinnon 2006).

Pause *for* Reflection ...

Why do you think the public might hold negative views and attitudes about people diagnosed with schizophrenia, bipolar and other psychotic disorders? Consider the role that popular culture plays in informing those views.

MENTAL HEALTH CONSUMER MOVEMENT: 'NOTHING ABOUT US WITHOUT US'

Historically, people diagnosed with a mental disorder had few opportunities to influence decisions about the treatment they received, or the services provided. The gross violations of the human rights of people in psychiatric hospitals, and their subsequent discharge to unsupported communities, led to the rise of the mental health consumer movement, born from the 'ground up', by those who had direct experiences of psychiatric treatment and abuse (Dunlop & Pols 2022). In Australia, the 1980s saw the burgeoning of the mental health consumer movement, a rights-based movement informed in part by the health consumer rights movement, that viewed consumers as having rights to adequate services and choices about the services they used. Further, the term 'consumer' was considered non-stigmatising as it was not linked to a diagnosis, and it implied active participation in medical and other treatments (Dunlop & Pols 2022). The rights statement 'Nothing about us without us' that evolved from the disability rights movement in reaction to the oppression of people living with disabilities, recognition of their human rights and their knowledge of what was best for them (Charlton 1998), was adopted by mental health consumers. Today, central to decision-making about the development of mental health policy and mental health services is the inclusion of the people affected by those decisions: consumers (COAG 2017).

The development of organisations to assist people discharged from psychiatric hospitals focused on what people needed to recover, well before it was incorporated in mental health policy. Initially comprising health professionals and community members, they developed alliances with consumers to influence decision-making about mental health policy and services (Dunlop & Pols 2022; Smith & Gridley 2006). These partnerships contributed to the de-stigmatisation of people living with mental disorders, facilitated consumer advocacy and created the opportunity to affect change in the mental health system (Dunlop & Pols 2022). Many consumer advocates have leadership roles within mental health organisations and government departments, including Mary O'Hagan who was appointed as the first Executive Director of Lived Experience in the Victorian health department (Victoria Health 2021). The mental health consumer movement demonstrated that recovering from mental disorder and leading a meaningful life were achievable.

MENTAL HEALTH REFORM

National Mental Health Strategy (1992)

The *Mental Health Strategy* was established by the Australian Government to guide the development and delivery of mental health services by each of the state and territory governments (Australian Health Ministers 1992). It comprises the *National Mental Health Policy, National Mental Health Plan* (National Plan), the *Mental Health Statement of Rights and Responsibilities*, and the *National Standards for Mental Health Services*. Each of the National Plans are for a period of five years (COAG 2017).

The first *National Mental Health Policy* (1992) and the *First National Plan* (1993–98) provided the impetus for the transfer of mental health services from psychiatric institutions to the community sector, protected consumers' rights and integrated mental health services within general health services (Whiteford 1993). The reforms of the first three National Plans (1993–2008) were not without criticism, including inadequate funding of services, limited consumer advocacy and little focus on prevention of mental disorder (Rosen 2006; Whiteford et al. 2002). The current *National Mental Health Policy* was released in 2009 (Department of Health and Ageing 2009), and the National Mental Health Commission was established in 2012 (NMHC 2022a). Key to the work of the NMHC is the notion of a 'Contributing Life', which views an individual's recovery as living as fulfilling and complete a life as possible. The NMHC independently monitors and evaluates the implementation of the National Plan (NMHC 2022a).

The *Fifth National Mental Health and Suicide Prevention Plan* promotes consumer and carer participation at all levels of service design, delivery and evaluation: 'nothing about us, without us' (COAG 2017, p. 4). It focuses on services for people who experience complex mental disorders, a national approach to the prevention of suicide, particularly Aboriginal and Torres Strait Islander suicide prevention, and reduction of stigma and discrimination (COAG 2017).

Productivity Commission Inquiry 2020

The Productivity Commission, an independent research and advisory body to the federal government, recently undertook a whole-of-system and whole-of-life inquiry into mental health and social and economic participation. The cost benefits of reforming the mental health system and the subsequent improved quality of life and social participation equated to $18 billion annually, with a further benefit of $1.3 billion related to increased economic participation (Productivity Commission 2020, p. 2). The reforms prioritised five areas: prevention and early intervention for mental health issues and suicide risk; a person-centred mental health system adaptable to changing consumer needs; access to community support services beyond the health care system; participation in education and employment; and integration of services adopting a whole-of-governments approach: federal, state and territory. Moreover, the Inquiry proposed that the NMHC lead the development of the *National Mental Health Strategy* and the next *National Mental Health Plan* (Productivity Commission 2020).

RECOVERY-ORIENTED MENTAL HEALTH SERVICES

The most recent paradigm shift in Australian mental health practice and service delivery was the implementation of a recovery-oriented model (Australian Health Ministers' Advisory Council (AHMAC) 2013). Underpinning this model is the notion of personal recovery.

Personal Recovery

Historically, mental health services have focused on clinical recovery, a term that refers to the reduction or remission of the symptoms of a mental disorder. **Personal recovery** is not restricted to symptom remission (Roosenschoon et al. 2019; Van Eck et al. 2018), and personal recovery occurs in people who have ongoing symptoms (Van Eck et al. 2018).

The concept of personal recovery originated from the consumer movement. A leader in the international mental health consumer movement, psychologist Pat Deegan described her recovery from schizophrenia as the **lived experiences** of finding a new sense of self and purpose in life despite and beyond any disabling effects of the disorder (Deegan 1988). She highlights that personal recovery – what individuals do to recover, rather than what health professionals and systems do – infers personal responsibility and control. Personal recovery is captured in the following often-quoted definition, based on consumers' lived experiences:

> *A deeply personal, unique process of changing one's attitudes, values, feelings, goals, skills and/or roles. It is a way of living a satisfying, hopeful, and contributing life even with limitations caused by the illness. Recovery involves the development of new meaning and purpose in one's life as one grows beyond the catastrophic effects of mental illness.*
>
> *(Anthony 1993, n.p.)*

A National Framework for Recovery-Oriented Practice and Services

In Australia, the *National Framework for Recovery-oriented Mental Health Services* guides recovery-oriented mental health practice in the public, private and non-government health sectors (AHMAC 2013). Uppermost are consumers' human rights of autonomy and self-determination, an environment of hope and optimism, and a person-centred, collaborative approach that is supportive of personal definitions of recovery and personal responsibility for decision-making (AHMAC 2013).

Recovery-Oriented Practice

Health professionals cannot recover individuals, but they can facilitate an environment in which recovering occurs. Supporting the mental health workforce to develop the requisite knowledge and skills, however, is essential (Meadows et al. 2019; NMHC 2022c).

Importantly, the language of recovery-oriented practitioners should convey hope and optimism (AHMA 2013). Using non-stigmatising language, such as referring to the person rather than the diagnosed mental disorder, focusing on strengths rather than deficits and conveying an expectation of recovering are necessary (Mental Health Coordinating Council (MHCC) 2018).

Many consumers have experienced trauma in their lives, and recovery-oriented practice must also be trauma-informed. Trauma-informed practices and services are cognisant of the pervasiveness of trauma in our society (Kezelman & Stavropoulos 2019). Doing no harm, asking what has happened to the person rather than what is 'wrong' with them, and working with, rather than doing to, the person are trauma-informed practices that all health professionals can adopt (Blue Knot Foundation 2021, p. 1).

Lived Experience Workforce

Instrumental to recovery-oriented services are the lived experience workforce, including the consumer peer workforce, or peer workers, and the carers of people living with a mental disorder – the carer peer workforce. **Peer workers** 'are employed to openly identify and use their lived experience of mental illness and recovery' in their support of consumers of mental health services (MHCC 2018, p. 11). Peer workers are a unique discipline employed in public mental health services and community-managed mental health organisations (Scanlan et al. 2020). The supportive role of peer workers, and reductions in ED presentations and mental health inpatient admissions, attest to their value (Byrne et al. 2021; Productivity Commission 2020).

Pause *for* Reflection ...
The recovery movement has changed the mental health landscape in Australia. How does a biomedical approach differ from a recovery-oriented approach to mental health practice and service provision?

MENTAL HEALTH SERVICE SYSTEM

The funding and regulating of mental health services is provided by the federal, state and territory governments (APH 2019). Responsibilities of the federal government include Medicare-subsidised mental health care provided by **general practitioners (GPs)**, allied health professionals and psychiatrists, prescription medications under the Pharmaceutical Benefits Scheme and primary care from Primary Health Networks (APH 2019). The state and territory governments have responsibilities for specialised mental health in public hospitals with a mental health unit and standalone psychiatric hospitals, community mental health services and residential services (AIHW 2022b; APH 2019). They also have responsibilities for non-specialised health services in EDs of public hospitals and supported accommodation (AIHW 2022b). During 2019 and 2020, $11 billion was spent on mental health related services or 7.6% of total government health expenditure (AIHW 2022b).

Also jointly funded by the federal and state and territory governments, the **National Disability Insurance Scheme (NDIS)** supports the recovery of people living with a mental disorder who have psychosocial disabilities (NDIS 2021). The NDIS reflects a move to a market model of disability support, via individual funding packages to purchase necessary support, which can be empowering for many but not all due to various personal and program barriers (Wilson et al. 2022).

Medicare-Subsidised Services

Mental health care is integrated in general health services. Psychologists provide most services, followed by GPs, psychiatrists and other allied health professionals (AIHW 2022b). Recommendations to increase the consumer peer workforce in primary health care is warranted (Lawn et al. 2021). Better Access is a Medicare Benefits Schedule initiative available for people diagnosed with a mental disorder to receive support from health professionals, including telehealth services (Department of Health 2022).

Specialised Mental Health Facilities

Specialised mental health care is provided in a variety of health services. The majority are community mental health services (1321), followed by government and non-government residential mental health services (181), public hospitals (161) – predominantly mental health units of general hospitals – and private hospitals (68) (AIHW 2022b). Nurses comprise 50% of staff, followed by allied health professionals (20%), and medical officers, psychiatrists, and psychiatry registrars and trainees. Almost half of all specialised mental health organisations employ consumer peer workers and about a third employ carer peer workers (AIHW 2022b).

Community mental health services **(CMHs)** are government-funded, operate in the community, and include mental health centres and hospital-based ambulatory care services, such as outpatient clinics (AIHW 2022b). The majority of people using the services have ongoing conditions and contact with health professionals of 5–15 minutes duration (AIHW 2022b).

CMHs are provided by multidisciplinary teams, offering a range of therapeutic interventions, including assessment, crisis intervention, and pharmacological, or specialist, such as early psychosis, and assertive community treatment (Williams & Smith 2019). Assertive case management with psychosocial interventions is considered superior for recovery (Lau et al. 2017). Current debate about CMHs focuses on continuity of care across inpatient and community settings and increasing the opportunities for co-designed services (Williams & Smith 2019).

Residential care services are provided by government and non-government services. The majority of people using services are 18–24 years of age and have an ongoing mental health condition. Over half of the residents used a service for two weeks or less, and 30% for 2–4 weeks (AIHW 2022b).

Pause *for* Reflection ...

What role do community mental health services play in the early intervention for people with mental health issues? Given that most community mental health contacts are of 5–15 minutes in duration, what therapeutic interventions are most likely provided? Do you think this is adequate for a recovery-oriented approach? Why or why not?

EMERGENCY DEPARTMENTS

Young adults experiencing mental distress frequently present to emergency departments (EDs) of hospitals (AIHW 2022b); however, people experiencing a mental health crisis have reported extended waiting times and care that was traumatising and unwelcoming (Allison et al. 2021; Judkins et al. 2019). Services provided in a lower stimulus setting, utilising multidisciplinary teams, inclusive of peer workers (Judkins et al. 2019), are developing throughout New South Wales. Known as Safe Havens, they are co-designed, confidential, safe, alternative services to EDs for people experiencing mental distress or suicidality, and are staffed by peer workers (NSW Health 2022; South Eastern Sydney Local Health District (SESLHD) 2022).

Another initiative is the Mental Health Acute Assessment Team, a collaboration between paramedics and mental health clinicians (Faddy et al. 2017; Queensland Cabinet & Ministerial Directory 2021). The teams assess people experiencing mental crisis and determine the most appropriate care setting, including remaining at home, rather than the automatic transfer to an ED. This initiative demonstrated a reduction in ED transfers for people without physical health concerns and increased transfers to specialist mental health services in the community (Faddy et al. 2017). Another initiative in New South Wales, the Mental Health Intervention Team, is a collaboration between NSW Health and Police NSW. It aims to facilitate access to appropriate mental health services for people who are experiencing a mental health crisis and to increase advocacy for mental health issues. This initiative demonstrated reduced community stigma related to mental distress (Police NSW n.d.).

Criticisms of specialised mental health services in Australia include resourcing issues, a reliance on ED use and inadequate community services to support people after discharge from hospital services (Allison et al. 2021; Judkins et al. 2019; Perera 2020). The provision of co-designed and adequately resourced specialist mental health and suicide support services, staffed with peer workers, is a vital component of a recovery-oriented mental health care system.

Case study 11.1 presents a young man who experiences a mental health crisis and demonstrates the use of a range of mental health services to support his recovery.

CASE STUDY 11.1 Recovery-Oriented Mental Health Services

Lachlan is a 24-year-old man who lives with his partner and a flatmate in a shared house in a large city. He recently completed a three-year TAFE qualification in electrotechnology, and he is employed as an electrician. He enjoys running, working out at the gym and socialising with his friends.

Lachlan experienced a brief episode of psychosis five years ago. At the time, he used cannabis daily, experienced some paranoid beliefs, was unable to sleep and stopped eating. He was hospitalised for three days in a mental health unit and prescribed antipsychotic medication.

After discharge from hospital, some of his friends reacted negatively and stopped contacting him. He continued taking the medication and was supported by a Community Mental Health Crisis (CMHC) team and then his GP. He stopped using cannabis regularly and gradually ceased the antipsychotic medication with his GP's support.

Three months ago, Lachlan lost his job due to a downturn in work related to the COVID-19 pandemic. He was unable to find work as an electrician, but he obtained casual employment in hospitality. A month ago, after repeated conflict, his partner ended their relationship, and he was left with the total cost of the rent for his room. His parents were supportive and assisted him financially.

Since that time, Lachlan feels anxious about his job and relationship loss. He has difficulty falling asleep and can't stop thinking about what has happened. He can't concentrate at work, and some of his colleagues have expressed a view that 'he has problems and should be let go'. He is smoking cannabis daily to cope with anxiety, and he has lost interest in socialising with his friends. His flatmate has been critical of his changed behaviour, stating that he 'should see a shrink, and take some pills'.

Lachlan told his parents that he was worried about having another psychotic episode and stated that, 'he felt nervous and sick all the time and wanted to sleep and never wake up'. His parents were concerned, and he agreed to go with them to a Safe Haven at a nearby public hospital.

CASE STUDY 11.1 Recovery-Oriented Mental Health Services—cont'd

At the Safe Haven, Lachlan was greeted warmly by peer workers, one of whom was his age and had lived experiences of suicidality and using support services. The peer worker encouraged him to talk about his previous experiences of recovering and what he wanted to happen, now. While he said he didn't want to end his life, he stated the anxiety and fear were overwhelming and he wanted that to end, and that he'd found the CMHC and his GP supportive.

With the peer worker's assistance, Lachlan telephoned the CMHC who met him later that evening. Lachlan discussed his anxiety with the team and stated that he did not want to go to hospital. The CMHC offered Lachlan twice-daily visits to support him at home over the next week, which he accepted. They also discussed the possibility of using the Better Access program.

Over the next few months, Lachlan continued to receive support from the Safe Haven, the CMHC and online mental health support groups. He and his GP developed a mental health treatment plan, which included referral to a psychologist for cognitive therapy. He agreed to the short-term use of medication for anxiety and to improve his

sleep, and he has decreased his cannabis use. His parents have continued to support him while recovering, as have his close friends, and he is starting to think about working as a licensed electrician again.

Case Study Questions

1. What precipitating factors might have contributed to Lachlan's mental health crisis, and what are his strengths and some possible protective factors? Consider psychological, physical and social factors.
2. How might peer workers who are of a similar age to Lachlan assist him?
3. Why are peer workers essential for Safe Havens and other mental health and suicide support services?
4. What evidence is there of public stigma towards Lachlan?
5. How is 'Nothing about us without us' demonstrated in the case study?
6. Using examples from the case study, outline how a personal recovery-oriented approach to mental health care is demonstrated.

SUMMARY

This chapter has presented an overview of mental health, well-being and mental disorder and the development of the Australian mental health service delivery. It addressed the following key points:

- The social determinants of health affect mental health, and therefore overall health and well-being.
- The high-prevalence mental disorders in Australia include anxiety, affective and substance use disorders. The rates of these disorders are higher in Aboriginal and Torres Strait Islander people as compared to non-Aboriginal and Torres Strait Islander people.
- Professional practice can involve interactions with health care consumers who are suicidal. Prevention of suicide is possible, so it is important for health professionals to capably discuss suicidality with consumers and the people who support them.
- Mental health services in Australia were provided in psychiatric institutions until the mid-20th century. Pharmacological and psychosocial treatments, a concern for the human rights of people in psychiatric institutions and the rise of the mental health consumer movement resulted in the closure of many

psychiatric hospitals and the development of community mental health services.

- Deinstitutionalisation and closure of psychiatric hospitals did not translate to adequate funding of community mental health services, resulting in inadequate support for many people discharged and reliance on families as informal carers.
- The *National Mental Health Strategy*, initiated in 1992, reformed Australian mental health care, by transferring services from institutions to mainstream health services and the community sector, and including consumers in the development and evaluation of mental health policy and services.
- The fifth *National Mental Health Plan* focuses on addressing the needs of people who experience complex mental disorders and the development of a national approach to the prevention of suicide. The establishment of the National Mental Health Commission ensures an independent evaluation of the implementation of the National Plan.
- The paradigm shift to a recovery-oriented approach has changed the focus of Australian mental health practice and service delivery. Led by the consumer

movement, the rise of personal, rather than clinical only, understandings of recovery, and the development of the lived experience/peer mental health workforce, have contributed to the expectation of living a fulfilling life and increased social and economic participation for consumers.

- Today, mental health care is predominantly provided by health professionals and peer workers in primary health care, and in specialised mental health services, such as community mental health centres, mental health units in general hospitals, and in residential settings.
- Co-designed co-delivered services are vital for a recovery-oriented mental health and suicide support system.

REVIEW QUESTIONS

1. Most people diagnosed with a mental disorder and using mental health services are younger than 25 years of age. How do the social determinants of mental health contribute to the development of mental distress and disorder in younger adults?
2. Identify two examples of each of the following types of stigma towards people living with a mental illness: personal, public/social and professional stigma.
3. How have changes to the mental health system, over the past sixty years, contributed to person-centred, recovery-oriented mental health practice and services?
4. The consumer movement has been influential in the development of mental health policy and services in Australia. How could consumers influence the practice of health professionals? Consider their influence in education, training and research.
5. What is meant by co-design and co-delivery of mental health services? What are the enablers and barriers to co-designed and co-delivered services?

REFERENCES

Abate, K., Abebe, Z., Abil, O.Z., et al., 2018. Global, regional, and national incidence, prevalence, and years lived with disability for 354 diseases and injuries for 195 countries and territories, 1990–2017: a systematic analysis for the Global Burden of Disease Study 2017. Lancet 392, 1789–1858. doi:10.1016/S0140-6736 (18)32279-7.

Allison, S., Bastiampillai, T., Looi, J.C., et al., 2021. Emergency department–focused mental health policies for people with severe mental illness. Aust N Z J Psychiatry 55 (6), 533–535. doi:10.1177/0004867420976849.

Anthony, W., 1993. Recovery from mental illness: the guiding vision of the mental health system in the 1990s. Psychiatr Rehabil J 16 (4), 11–23. doi.org/10.1037/h0095655.

Australian Bureau of Statistics (ABS), 2022. National study of mental health and wellbeing, 2020–21. ABS, Canberra. https://www.abs.gov.au/statistics/health/mental-health/national-study-mental-health-and-wellbeing/latest-release.

Australian Bureau of Statistics (ABS), 2019. National Aboriginal and Torres Strait Islander health survey. Cat. no. 4715.0. ABS, Caberra. https://www.abs.gov.au/statistics/people/aboriginal-and-torres-strait-islander-peoples/national-aboriginal-and-torres-strait-islander-health-survey/latest-release.

Australian Health Ministers, 1992. National mental health strategy. AGPS, Canberra.

Australian Health Ministers' Advisory Council (AHMAC), 2013. A national framework for recovery-oriented mental health services: Guide for practitioners and providers. Commonwealth of Australia, Canberra. https://www.health.gov.au/sites/default/files/documents/2021/04/a-national-framework-for-recovery-oriented-mental-health-services-guide-for-practitioners-and-providers.pdf.

Australian Institute of Health and Welfare (AIHW), 2022a. Suicide and self-harm monitoring. AIHW, Canberra. https://www.aihw.gov.au/suicide-self-harm-monitoring/data.

Australian Institute of Health and Welfare (AIHW), 2022b. Mental health services in Australia. https://www.aihw.gov.au/reports/mental-health-services/mental-health-services-in-australia/report-contents/summary-of-mental-health-services-in-australia.

Australian Parliament House, 2019. Mental health in Australia: a quick guide. https://www.aph.gov.au/About_Parliament/Parliamentary_Departments/Parliamentary_Library/pubs/rp/rp1819/Quick_Guides/MentalHealth.

Blue Knot Foundation, 2021. Becoming trauma-informed services. https://professionals.blueknot.org.au/wp-content/

uploads/2021/09/45_BK_FS_PRF_BecomingTraumaInformed_Services_July21.pdf.

Byrne, L., Wang, L., Roennfeldt, H., et al., 2021. National lived experience workforce guidelines. National Mental Health Commission. https://www.mentalhealthcommission.gov.au/getmedia/a33cce2a-e7fa-4f90-964d-85dbf1514b6b/NMHC_Lived-Experience-Workforce-Development-Guidelines.

Carrara, B.S., Ventura, C.A., Bobbili, S.J., et al., 2019. Stigma in health professionals towards people with mental illness: An integrative review. Arch Psychiatr Nurs, 33 (4), 311–318. doi:10.1016/j.apnu.2019.01.006.

Charles, J.L., 2013. Mental health provider-based stigma: Understanding the experience of clients and families. Soc Work Ment Health 11 (4), 360–375. doi:10.1080/15332985.2013.775998.

Charlton, J.I., 1998. Nothing About Us Without Us: Disability Oppression and Empowerment. University of California Press, Berkeley.

Coleborne, C., MacKinnon, D., 2006. Psychiatry and its institutions in Australia and New Zealand: An overview. Int Rev Psychiatry, 18 (4), 371–380. doi:10.1080/09540260600813248.

Council of Australian Governments (COAG), 2017. Fifth national mental health and suicide prevention plan. COAG, Canberra. https://www.mentalhealthcommission.gov.au/getmedia/0209d27b-1873-4245-b6e5-49e770084b81/Fifth-National-Mental-Health-and-Suicide-Prevention-Plan.pdf.

Corrigan, P.W., Druss, B.G., Perlick, D.A., 2014. The impact of mental illness stigma on seeking and participating in mental health care. Psychol Sci Public Interest 15 (2), 37–70. doi:10.1177/1529100614531398.

Deegan, P., 1988. Recovery: The lived experience of rehabilitation. Psychiatr Rehabil J 11 (4), 11–19. doi:10.1037/h0099565.

Department of Health, 2022. Better access initiative. https://www.health.gov.au/initiatives-and-programs/better-access-initiative.

Department of Health and Ageing, 2009. National mental health policy 2008. Commonwealth of Australia, Canberra. https://www.health.gov.au/sites/default/files/documents/2020/11/national-mental-health-policy-2008.pdf.

Dunlop, R., Pols, H., 2022. Deinstitutionalisation and mental health activism in Australia: emerging voices of individuals with lived experience of severe mental distress, 1975–1985. Hist Aust 19 (1), 92–114. doi:10.1080/14490854.2022.2028559.

Economou, M., Peppou, L.E., Kontoangelos, K., et al., 2019. Mental health professionals' attitudes to severe mental illness and its correlates in psychiatric hospitals of Attica: The role of workers' empathy. Community Ment Health J 56 (4), 614–625. doi:10.1007/s10597-019-00521-6.

Faddy, S.C., McLaughlin, K.J., Cox, P.T., et al., 2017. The mental health acute assessment team: A collaborative approach to treating mental health patients in the community. Australas Psychiatry 25 (3), 262–265. doi:10.1177/1039856216689655.

Human Rights and Equal Opportunity Commission (HREOC), 1993. Human rights and mental illness: report of the national inquiry into the human rights of people with mental illness. AGPS, Canberra.

Judkins, S., Fatovich, D., Ballenden, N., et al., 2019. Mental health patients in emergency departments are suffering: the national failure and shame of the current system. A report on the Australasian College for Emergency Medicine's Mental Health in the Emergency Department Summit. Australas Psychiatry 27 (6), 615–617. doi:10.1177/1039856219852282.

Kairuz, C.L., Bennett-Brook, K., Coombes, J., et al., 2021. Impact of racism and discrimination on physical and mental health among Aboriginal and Torres Strait Islander peoples living in Australia: A systematic scoping review. BMC Public Health 21 (1), 1302. doi:10.1186/s12889-021-11363-x.

Kezelman, C.A., Stavropoulos, P., 2019. Practice guidelines for clinical treatment of complex trauma. Blue Knot Foundation.

Lau, M., Bennett, S., Crompton, D., et al., 2017. A capability framework to develop leadership for evidence-informed therapies in publicly-funded mental health services. Int J Public Leadership, 13 (3), 151–165. doi:10.1108/IJPL-08-2016-0030.

Lawn, S., Kaine, C., Stevenson, J., et al., 2021. Australian mental health consumers' experiences of service engagement and disengagement: A descriptive study. Int J Environ Res Public Health 18 (19), 10464. doi:10.3390/ijerph181910464.

Lewis, M., Garton, S., 2017. Mental health in Australia, 1788–2015: A history of responses to cultural and social challenges. In: Minas, H., Lewis, M. (Eds), Mental Health in Asia and the Pacific. International and Cultural Psychology. Springer, Boston, pp. 289–313. doi:10.1007/978-1-4899-7999-5_19.

Meadows, G., Brophy, L., Shawyer, F., et al., 2019. REFOCUS-PULSAR recovery-oriented practice training in specialist mental health care: a stepped-wedge cluster randomised controlled trial. Lancet Psychiatry 6 (2), 103–114. doi:10.1016/S2215-0366 (18)30429-2.

Mental Health Coordinating Council (MHCC), 2018. Recovery Oriented Language Guide, second ed. Mental Health Coordinating Council, Rozelle. https://mhcc.org.au/wp-content/uploads/2019/08/Recovery-Oriented-Language-Guide_2019ed_v1_20190809-Web.pdf.

Morgan, V.A., Waterreus, A., Jablensky, A., et al., 2011. People living with psychotic illness 2010: Report of the second Australian national survey. Department of Health, Canberra.

National Disability Insurance Scheme (NDIS), 2021. Psychosocial disability recovery-oriented framework. https://www.ndis.gov.au/understanding/how-ndis-works/mental-health-and-ndis#new-psychosocial-recovery-oriented-framework.

National Mental Health Commission (NMHC), 2022a. Home page. https://www.mentalhealthcommission.gov.au/.

National Mental Health Commission (NMHC), 2022b. National stigma and discrimination strategy. https://haveyoursay.mentalhealthcommission.gov.au/hub-page/national-stigma-and-discrimination-reduction-strategy

National Mental Health Commission (NMHC), 2022c. Monitoring mental health and suicide prevention reform: National Report 2021. NMHC, Sydney. https://www.mentalhealthcommission.gov.au/getmedia/095abc13-4f0a-4244-a648-f2eb9e18f938/National-Report-2021.pdf.

National Mental Health Commission (NMHC), 2017. The National Mental Health Commission's consumer and carer engagement: a practical guide. https://www.mentalhealthcommission.gov.au/getmedia/afef7eba-866f-4775-a386-57645bfb3453/NMHC-Consumer-and-Carer-engagement-a-practical-guide.

New South Wales (NSW) Health, 2022. Safe haven. https://www.health.nsw.gov.au/towardszerosuicides/Pages/safe-haven.aspx.

Police NSW (n.d.), Mental health background. NSW Government. https://www.police.nsw.gov.au/safety_and_prevention/your_community/mental_health/mental_health/background.

Papadimitriou, G., 2017. The "Biopsychosocial Model": 40 years of application in Psychiatry. Psychiatriki 28 (2), 107–110. doi:10.22365/jpsych.2017.282.107.

Perera, I., 2020. The relationship between hospital and community psychiatry: Complements, not substitutes? Psychiatr Serv 71 (9), 964–966. doi:10.1176/appi.ps.201900086.

Productivity Commission, 2020. Mental health report, vol.1 & 2 (95). Commonwealth of Australia, Canberra. https://www.pc.gov.au/inquiries/completed/mental-health/report/mental-health-volume1.pdf; and https://www.pc.gov.au/inquiries/completed/mental-health/report/mental-health-volume2.pdf.

Queensland Cabinet and Ministerial Directory, 2021. Enhanced frontline care for patients experiencing mental health crisis. Queensland Government. https://statements.qld.gov.au/statements/91932.

Roosenschoon, B., Kamperman, A., Deen, M., et al., 2019. Determinants of clinical, functional and personal recovery for people with schizophrenia and other severe mental illnesses: A cross-sectional analysis. PLOS ONE 14 (9), e0222378. doi:10.1371/journal.pone.0222378.

Rosen, A., 2006. Australia's national mental health strategy in historical perspective: Beyond the frontier. International Psychiatry, 3 (4), pp. 19–21. https://www.ncbi.nlm.nih.gov/pmc/articles/PMC6734702/pdf/IP-3-19a.pdf.

Rickwood, D.J., Thomas, K.A., 2019. Mental wellbeing interventions: an Evidence Check rapid review brokered by the Sax Institute for VicHealth. https://www.saxinstitute.org.au/wp-content/uploads/20.10_Evidence-Check_Mental-Wellbeing-Interventions.pdf.

Scanlan, J., Still, M., Radican, J., et al., 2020. Workplace experiences of mental health consumer peer workers in New South Wales, Australia: a survey study exploring job satisfaction, burnout and turnover intention. BMC Psychiatry 20 (1), pp. 270–270. doi:10.1186/s12888-020-02688-9.

Smith, M., Gridley, H., 2006. Living with mental illness in Australia: Changes in policy and practice affecting mental health service consumers. Aust Psychol 41 (2), 130–139. doi:10.1080/00050060600559622.

South Eastern Local Health District (SESLHD), 2022. What is safe haven. https://www.seslhd.health.nsw.gov.au/what-safehaven.

Thornicroft, G., Rose, D., Kassam, A., et al., 2007. Stigma: Ignorance, prejudice or discrimination? Br J Psychiatry 190 (3), 192–193. doi:10.1192/bjp.bp.106.025791.

van Eck, R., Burger, T.J., Vellinga, A., et al., 2018. The relationship between clinical and personal recovery in patients with schizophrenia spectrum disorders: A systematic review and meta-analysis. Schizophr Bull 44 (3), 631–642. doi:10.1093/schbul/sbx088.

Victoria Health, 2021. https://www.health.vic.gov.au/news/mary-ohagan-appointed-to-key-lived-experience-leadership-reform-role.

Whiteford, H., Buckingham, B., Manderscheid, R., 2002. Australia's National Mental Health Strategy. Br J Psychiatry 180 (3), 210–215. doi:10.1192/bjp.180.3.210.

Whiteford, H., 1993. Australia's National Mental Health Policy. Hosp Community Psychiatry 44 (10), 963–966. doi:10.1176/ps.44.10.963.

Williams, T., Smith, G.P., 2019. Laying new foundations for 21st century community mental health services: An Australian perspective. Int J Ment Health Nurs 28 (4), 1008–1014. doi:10.1111/inm.12590.

Wilson, E., Campain, R., Pollock, S., et al., 2022. Exploring the personal, programmatic and market barriers to choice in the NDIS for people with psychosocial disability. Aust J Soc Issues 57 (1), 164–184. doi:10.1002/ajs4.154.

World Health Organization (WHO), 2022. Mental disorders. https://www.who.int/news-room/fact-sheets/detail/mental-disorders.

World Health Organization (WHO), 2021. Comprehensive mental health action plan 2013–2030. WHO, Geneva. Licence: CC BY-NC-SA 3.0 IGO.

FURTHER READING

Farhall, J., Edan, V., Roper, C., et al., 2020. Mental Health and Collaborative Community Practice: An Australian Perspective, fourth ed. Oxford University Press, Melbourne.

Hungerford, C., Hodgson, D., Bostwick, R., et al., 2018. Mental Health Care: An Introduction For Health Professionals, third ed. John Wiley & Sons, Brisbane.

National Mental Health Commission, 2020. Monitoring mental health and suicide prevention reform: National report 2020. https://www.mentalhealthcommission.gov.au/monitoring-and-reporting/national-reports/2020-national-report/2020-national-report.

ONLINE RESOURCES

Australian Bureau of Statistics: https://www.abs.gov.au/.

Australian Government Department of Health and Aged Care: https://www.health.gov.au/.

Australian Institute of Health and Welfare: http://www.aihw.gov.au.

Being – Mental Health Consumers: https://being.org.au/.

Beyond Blue: https://www.beyondblue.org.au/.

Black Dog Institute: https://www.blackdoginstitute.org.au/.

Flourish Australia: https://www.flourishaustralia.org.au/.

Headspace Australia: https://www.headspace.org.au/.

Lifeline: https://www.lifeline.org.au/.

Mental Health Australia: https://mhaustralia.org/.

Mental Health Carers Australia: https://www.mentalhealthcarersaustralia.org.au/.

Mind Australia: https://www.mindaustralia.org.au/.

Mental Health Coordinating Council: https://mhcc.org.au/.

National Mental Health Commission: https://www.mentalhealthcommission.gov.au/.

National Mental Health Consumer and Carer Forum: https://nmhccf.org.au/.

One Door Mental Health: https://www.onedoor.org.au/.

SANE Australia: https://www.sane.org/.

Suicide Prevention Australia: https://www.suicideprevention-aust.org/.

World Health Organization – Mental Health: https://www.who.int/health-topics/mental-health#tab=tab_2.

12

People Living with Disability: Navigating Support and Health Systems

Caroline Ellison[a]

KEY LEARNING OUTCOMES

When you finish this chapter you should be able to:

- identify some key factors and barriers impacting on health and development of a quality life for a diverse range of Australians living with disability
- understand the importance of a holistic approach and challenges faced in providing overall health care for people living with disability
- describe the concepts of **self-management** and **individualised funding models**, and quality and safeguarding, including the **National Disability Insurance Scheme (NDIS)**, and their interface with the Australian health system
- briefly outline roles undertaken by disability professionals in Australian health care and human services systems
- outline some areas in which **developmental educators (DEs)** and other disability professionals engage with the Australian disability support and health systems in assisting individuals living with disability to achieve quality of life.

KEY TERMS AND ABBREVIATIONS

ableist
activities of daily living (ADLs)
block-funded
developmental educators (DEs)
Developmental Educators
    Australia Incorporated (DEAI)
disability
general practitioner (GP)
human rights model

impairment
individualised funding
medical model
National Disability Insurance
    Agency (NDIA)
National Disability Insurance
    Scheme (NDIS)
National Health Priority Areas
    (NHPAs)

person-centred approach
restrictive practices
safeguarding
self-determination
social model
Technical and Further Education
    (TAFE)
transdisciplinary

INTRODUCTION

Approximately 4.4 million Australians live with **disability** (Australian Bureau of Statistics (ABS) 2019), and globally this number is more than a billion, according to the World Health Organization (WHO) (2021). While most individuals living with disability in Australia are not sick, a higher proportion will experience or self-report complex general health issues (Australian Institute of Health and Welfare (AIHW) 2022a; Carey et al. 2017; Fortune et al. 2020; Keramat et al. 2021). Fortune et al. (2020)

---

[a]We acknowledge the contribution by Kerrie Lante to the chapter in the 3rd edition of this book.

report that individuals with long-term disability require supports to engage in **activities of daily living (ADLs)** or to interact with and navigate disability support and health systems. Disability, while a social construct (Jóhannsdóttir et al. 2022), is described as a limitation, restriction or **impairment** lasting, or likely to last, for at least six months and impacting on everyday activities. There are many various impairments that result in living with disabilities, often resulting from accidents, illness or genetic disorders. Impairment may affect a person's mobility, communication or learning. Being a social construct and given society's responses to impairments and resulting disability, employability, income, social connectedness and participation in education can be impacted.

People living with disability are at greater risk of experiencing mental health difficulties (Chapter 11) and having negative physical outcomes associated with ageing sooner than the general population (AIHW 2022b), and are often less able to engage with support systems to achieve positive outcomes (AIHW 2022b; Keane 1996; WHO 2021). The Australian Institute of Health and Welfare (AIHW 2022b) reports that adults living with disability are six times as likely as those without disability to assess their health as 'poor' or 'fair'. They note that people living with significant impairments were more likely to have acquired a long-term health condition related to the **National Health Priority Areas (NHPAs)** at a younger age than people without disability. For example, according to ABS National Health Survey data, people living with disability aged 15–64 years had higher rates of long-term health conditions such as diabetes and arthropathies (Fortune et al. 2021).

This has implications for disability support and health professionals in understanding how an individual's impairment can interplay with and impact on their health, community participation, independence and need for disability support. For example, the Survey of Disability, Ageing and Carers reported that for those living with disability, the most common mental and behavioural disorders were intellectual and development disorders (6.5%) (ABS 2019). Many experiencing these disorders frequently experience communication difficulties and psychiatric disability (ABS 2020), are misunderstood or are misinterpreted by service providers in health and disability support service systems. Research has established that adults living with intellectual disability are more susceptible to sedentary lifestyle diseases owing to low levels of physical activity (Dairo et al. 2016; Hsieh et al. 2017; Tyrer et al.

2019). Emerson (2005) found that 25–34-year-old adults living with intellectual disability have an activity level equivalent to that of a 75-year-old. With such high levels of sedentary behaviour, an increasing demand is placed on health systems (Lante et al. 2014).

Case study 12.1 helps illustrate how an individual's impairment can interplay with and impact on their health and the need for effective communication in the health care setting. The questions following the case study ask you to consider how changes from the allied health professionals and the support worker could impact on Nancy's health care management.

The Productivity Commission (2011) report on disability care and support identified problems with the current disability policy (Bacchi 2016; Horsell 2020) and acknowledged an inadequate, fragmented support system for individuals living with disability in Australia. In response to these concerns, in 2013 the Commission's proposed **National Disability Insurance Scheme (NDIS)** was launched by the Australian Government, giving groups of people living with disability access to individualised packages of resources to support daily living and living a life of their choice.

The *National Disability Insurance Scheme (NDIS) Act* (Cth 2013), based on the United Nations *Convention on the Rights of Persons with Disabilities* which was ratified by the Australian Government in 2008, was first proposed in the Productivity Commission (2011) report. The *NDIS Act* (2013 Cth *s4*) has 17 general principles guiding action; principle one states that 'People with disability have the same right as other members of Australian society to realise their potential for physical, social, emotional and intellectual development' (p. 6). Other principles outline their right to participate in economic and social life in line with their ability to receive support across their life-span, to be supported to exercise choice in the pursuit of their goals, to be respected, to have dignity and to ensure control over their own life is maximised. Despite this, accessing timely and effective health care for people living with disability is often restricted, owing to physical and organisational (i.e. health care staff attitudes) barriers (Victorian Health Promotion Foundation (VicHealth) 2012). International systematic literature reviews concur with these findings and add that barriers around accessing health care stems from factors such as a lack of formal training for health care around understanding disability, lack of communication and advocacy skills between

CASE STUDY 12.1

Nancy, a 25-year-old female living with intellectual disability and mental health needs, presents to a rheumatologist at the local hospital. The rheumatologist notices Nancy's file indicates that four years ago she presented to hospital with her mother who was listed as her carer. No diagnosis was made; however, potential lupus was recorded. Today Nancy has a support worker, Lucy, accompanying her. During the consultation the rheumatologist asks questions including 'What are your symptoms?' and 'When did they start?' Nancy replies, 'My body aches' and then continues to ask what is wrong and why this is happening. To assist, Lucy asks Nancy 'Did your body ache before or after Christmas?' to which the reply is 'Before, it was just before we went away.' From this information Lucy could inform the rheumatologist that this had started two weeks ago, adding that she had heard Nancy complain of body aches on and off over the past year. Lucy then asked Nancy, waiting for a response, between each question, if she could tell the rheumatologist 'What part of your body aches?', 'Can you walk around when your body aches?' and 'When your body aches do you get tired?'

A blood test and 24-hour urine test were ordered. Nancy had to wait some time at pathology for the blood test and became extremely anxious. Lucy reassured Nancy while waiting and tried to explain the process. Nancy was called to have the blood test and said she wanted Lucy to accompany her. The nurse would not allow this, indicating 'It's against the rules, I'll get in trouble from my boss.' Following the test Nancy appeared with some containers and said 'We can go now.' Lucy asked what the containers were for and was told 'For the other test, the nurse told me what to do.' Upon discussion when Lucy dropped Nancy back home it was obvious that Nancy did not understand why or how she had to do the 24-hour urine test. As Lucy was not present when this was explained to Nancy, she could not explain this to Nancy herself. Nancy did not complete the test, but indicated to everyone that she had and that she took the sample back to the hospital the next day. The rheumatologist presumed that something went wrong at pathology's end.

After further tests and upon the return visit to the rheumatologist, Nancy was informed that she had connective tissue disorder and was prescribed medication. Nancy replied 'Okay' and carried on the conversation. She was given a piece of paper and told 'This is about a similar disorder but most of it applies to you, if you want to know more you can Google it.' She was also told that it was important that if she ever had a temperature she must go straight to hospital.

Case Study Questions
1. Given the above, do you believe Nancy understands her condition? What, if any, follow-up steps do you believe are needed and why?
2. What could the (a) rheumatologist, (b) nurse and (c) Lucy have done differently to help Nancy to successfully complete the urine test and understand her newly diagnosed condition?
3. What further information could have been provided to Nancy around the medication she was prescribed? Is Nancy likely to take the medication? Why/why not? What could occur between health and disability professionals to assist Nancy to take and manage her medication? What might the interactions be between the National Disability Insurance Scheme and the health system?

---

individuals living with disability and health care providers, and often complex transport, finance and other access barriers (Ervin et al. 2014; Williamson et al. 2017).

The NDIS is based on a Medicare-type model and is currently funded by directing funds from consolidated revenue. Full roll-out of the NDIS has been achieved in all states with ongoing reviews and evaluations to ensure that the scheme meets its aims and objectives. Cost estimates have increased to $22 billion annually (Productivity Commission 2017).

Four guiding principles govern the NDIS:
- actuarial estimate of long-term costs – to ensure financial sustainability
- long-term view of funding requirements – unlike previous models the NDIS takes a lifelong view of an individual's need for support
- investment in research, innovation and outcome analysis – to facilitate capacity-building
- investment in community participation and building social capital – to further access to and use of mainstream services and increased social and economic participation by people living with disability (**National Disability Insurance Agency (NDIA)** 2014).

The introduction of the NDIS and subsequent funding changes between the Commonwealth and state governments built on existing individualised Australian funding models, particularly in Victoria and Western Australia. However, since the initial pilot sites and completion of the national roll-out, tensions exist between the NDIA and service providers, with concerns around rejection of items to be included in plans as requested by individuals and families, as well as high compliance costs linked to audits and other processes which are not funded, and have made long-term sustainability uncertain for smaller organisations. This is likely to impact on long-term choice and control for individuals, who may find they have a limited number of options to support them. This is particularly an issue in rural and regional communities (Loadsman & Donelly 2021). This continues to undermine the concept of choice and control, and opportunities for a good and ordinary life for people living with disability.

Individualised funding is conceptually and philosophically about maximising independence, choice and control over supports and services, and allowing a person living with disability to have a valued role within their community (Carey et al. 2017; Government of Western Australia 2013). At the forefront of this notion is the individual being at the centre of and involved in decisions affecting their life. However, there is a pricing structure for health, therapeutic and daily living supports provided, and the NDIS worked with service providers to transition from previous block grant funding models to compliance with the new scheme. In addition, new models around the use of **restrictive practices** and increasing **safeguarding** for people living with disability have seen significant changes in services and accountability.

The NDIS already has powerful implications for how disability, health and therapeutic professionals provide services to people living with disability. Developing a collaborative interprofessional model within the health sector focusing on the **medical model**, the **social model** and the **human rights model** of disability (focus on removal of environmental and attitudinal barriers and access to the same human rights as other citizens) (Mallett & Runswick-Cole 2014) needs to be at the forefront of service development in these sectors (Bonyhady 2014). For example, in an article discussing the benefits of reliable, regular, persistent and assertive support, the following case study of Peter, who lives with psychosocial support needs, highlights the importance of his understanding about his diabetes and mental health needs. This was achieved through a holistic support plan that included Peter, his parents, a home visiting nursing support service, a local **general practitioner (GP)** and disability supports. It highlights the need for supports that do not restrict a person but overcome barriers and create opportunities via health and disability staff working collaboratively for **self-determination** (Springgay & Sutton 2014).

Pause *for* Reflection …

Access the Summer 2014 issue of *new paradigm*, the *Australian Journal on Psychosocial Rehabilitation*, at: https://www.yumpu.com/en/document/read/49305098/vicserv-new-paradigm-summer-2014-website.

Go to the article on p. 16 – 'Psychosocial disability: the urgent need for reform in assessment and care' by Springgay & Sutton (2014).

Read the full case study of Peter on p. 19. It is under the heading 'Benefits of reliable, regular, and persistent and assertive support'.

Now consider the following:

- What is the importance of the role for each person in Peter's support plan?
- What were the identified barriers for Peter and how were these identified? Reflect on the outcome for Peter and his family if these barriers were not identified.
- Once an ideal placement is found for Peter, what adjustments need to be made to his support plan, who should initiate this, who should be involved and what steps will need to take place for this to occur?
- What would the potential health outcomes have been for Peter if a collaborative, interprofessional approach had not been not taken?

The NDIS website also has a range of videos, testimonials and other resources that can assist you to understand the role of the NDIS. The worker orientation module is a free online learning opportunity that is necessary for those working or volunteering in disability services. If you complete the module, remember to save and keep your certificate: https://www.ndiscommission.gov.au/workers/training-course.

CONCEPTS OF DISABILITY, HEALTH AND SUPPORT

As stated by Kavanagh (2020), the concept of health can be a difficult construct for some people living with disability to define. In research conducted by Ellison et al.

(2011), participants living with disability most often described health as being free from negative impacts of illness or disease. In addition, participants' comments reflected the perception that having health was linked to being mobile, able to engage in activities of daily living to their satisfaction, having activities to keep busy, and having the opportunity and ability to form and maintain relationships.

Unchanged since 1948, the World Health Organization (WHO 2020) definition of health is 'a state of complete physical, mental and social well-being and not merely the absence of disease and infirmity'. On this basis, no person who identifies as living with disability could attain the status of having health. This raises numerous questions including:

1. Is this an ableist perspective?
2. What are the implications of this for people living with disability and their interactions with Australia's disability support and health system?
3. What are the issues for health professionals educated around this definition and their potential view of the capacity for individuals living with disability to live a quality life and be actively involved in health-related decisions?

In a paper discussing 'Why people are so messed up about dis/ability', Goodley (2014, pp. 117–136) states that we live in an **ableist** culture that provokes responses to individuals living with disability that can be described as fascination, anxiety, projection and devaluation. These are also often the responses of the health and support system professionals. Therefore, there is a need for support professionals to understand a person's differing perception of health, especially when communicating with them. What has been problematic is health professionals who view individuals living with disability as not having the capacity for positive health and participation in decision-making around their health, within the context of their disability (Bacchi 2016; Douglas et al. 2015; Stuifbergen et al. 1990). The challenge for professionals is to ensure information is provided so that the person living with disability understands and comprehends so as to make informed choices and actions. Information needs to be provided in alternative formats to what currently exists.

Pause *for* Reflection ...
Considering the balance between duty of care and an individual's right to make decisions, how can you

professionally ensure people living with disability are involved in decision-making around their health care? In addressing this question, consider people living with various needs, including their cultural background, cognitive impairments, communication difficulties and intellectual disabilities.

What supports and services are needed to facilitate capacity-building for decision-making in individuals living with disability, and understanding of the need to build capacity in health and support providers? Do these supports and services exist?

The NDIS is not the panacea to overcome all challenges and there is a risk it could be seen as a vehicle for resource 'handballing' or 'buck-passing'. The 2013 *NDIS Act* is clear that people living with disability can be supported by the NDIS in a coordinated manner to access generic and mainstream supports available outside of the NDIS. The purpose of the NDIS is not to replace or provide services that are available to the rest of society and for the cost of such services to be transferred to the NDIS. For example, state governments are still obliged to provide accessible and affordable public transport and not defer transport to the responsibility of the NDIS. During COVID-19, and any pandemic, individuals living with disability have the same rights to health service as others in society. There is concern in the disability community that individuals may be denied access to acute health services if the system became strained (Courtenay & Perera 2020; Turk & Mitra 2021). How do we ensure that decision-making and rights are upheld for people living with disability in this situation?

Skills and Knowledge Linked to Collaborative Health and Disability Supports

Like the rest of our community, people living with disability are not a homogeneous group. People may have lifelong conditions with which they are born, their disability may be invisible or visible, the effects of their disability may be constant or episodic, and levels of care and support required may range from occasional to 24 hours per day. However, there is specific knowledge about living with the interaction between impairment, disability and health that can be useful for support professionals to consider. The *NDIS Act* indicates a strong need for individuals to be at the centre of decision-making around planning for support, and the scheme is seeking outcomes that reflect this. So, disability, therapy and health professionals need to work collaboratively with each other, the individual and their family and supports.

Professionals working with people living with disability, their families and supports to achieve the individual's expressed goals and choices need to listen and discuss with the individual and those who support the person:

1. health care issues which may impact on support, management and education of the person
2. the effect of impairments on some bodily systems and how this impacts on daily living and community participation for the person
3. specific personal care, communication issues and the link to a person-centred approach to managing health implications of some impairments and syndromes on the person
4. specific health care issues relevant to some people living with disability, which can include the use of medication, epilepsy, incontinence, impact of ageing and increased risk of psychological and mental health issues
5. lifestyle issues, which may affect or be affected by the person's physical and emotional well-being, including nutrition, housing and accommodation, relationships, sexuality, grief and loss and vulnerability to abusive relationships
6. the interaction between the disability and health professionals' duty of care and a person's freedom to choose and the right to 'dignity of risk'
7. provision of opportunities for capacity-building and experience around decision-making that allows for experience, learning, skill development and growth in the ability to make decisions.

To ensure these discussions can occur in a way that is accessible and understandable to all, allied health professionals, disability professionals and **developmental educators (DEs)** need to work collaboratively to ensure the person living with disability can make informed decisions.

Pause *for* Reflection ...

1. Search for health education material and general information on informed consent and consider how you can (a) provide accessible and understandable information to people living with intellectual disability and (b) ensure they have the capacity to give informed consent for a routine medical procedure.
2. What does current research on the COVID-19 pandemic identify as the main issues surrounding access to information about vaccines, antivirals and other medical supports and consent for people living with disability?
3. Currently, there are government-mandated COVID-19 vaccinations for staff who work with persons living with a disability. Is this mandate the same for the person living with disability, and what are **their** rights around consent?

DISABILITY PROFESSIONALS IN AUSTRALIA

Disability professionals constitute a relatively new stream in Australia and in most states and territories there is developing recognition that they comprise an allied health profession. One of the first associations to lobby for a discrete group of disability professionals, **Developmental Educators Australia Incorporated (DEAI)** was established in South Australia where DEs were recognised in the allied health professional stream in 2012, alongside and equivalent to speech pathologists, psychologists, occupational therapists and other allied health disciplines. The DEAI is pursuing national recognition and registration with Allied Health Professions Australia (AHPA).

DEs are part of the human service system, educated to understand the myriad functions and roles of health and support professionals in the lives of people living with disability (Bottroff et al. 2000). DEs and other disability professionals use this understanding to enhance the health, self-determination and control of people living with disability and their supports through promoting a **person-centred approach** to support and advocacy and assisting individuals to navigate access to relevant support and health services (Bottroff et al. 2000). Person-centred approaches put the individual at the centre of decision-making processes and create opportunities to inform and empower individuals to be actively involved in the management of their health (Nankervis 2006).

The roles of disability professionals are complex, with a need for varied but specific skills and knowledge. DEs are multi-skilled professionals who can work within a **transdisciplinary** and interprofessional framework with other professionals, such as speech pathologists, occupational therapists, physiotherapists, psychologists and social workers. Rather than *replace* these professions, the DE *facilitates* a holistic, coherent response to supports for people living with disability, primarily in their local community as opposed to a particular 'centre-based' response.

Prior to the mid 1990s, relatively untrained personnel were often in the position of providing core services and support to people living with disability. This often led to suboptimal outcomes and a lack of opportunity for self-determination and control over their lives for individuals and their families. This is being highlighted in the outcomes of the current Royal Commission into Violence, Abuse, Neglect and Exploitation of People with Disability (Royal Commission) (Kayess & Sands 2020). Encouragingly, government policy continues to advocate that people working in the sector have at least Certificate III level training in disability and related areas. Increasingly, this has resulted in vocational graduates moving onto university-training and increasing the number of available professionals providing planning, support coordination and direct support services to ensure the individual and their family are in control of supports. The Royal Commission Public Hearing 10 Report (Royal Commission 2022) presents a number of recommendations about the training and capacity-building of health workers around providing services to people living with cognitive impairment in particular. Recommendation 1 states that the Australian Medical Council and Medical Deans Australia and New Zealand should develop and co-design a cognitive disability health capability framework and embed the capabilities in education and training programs for health practitioners across all training stages (Royal Commission 2022). DEs continue to be in high demand and often pursue further qualifications in areas such as social work, counselling, special education, occupational therapy, speech pathology, rehabilitation counselling, community development and/or management to meet the needs of engaging in such diverse environments.

Pause *for* Reflection …

Much of the work done by DEs and other disability professionals may appear similar to that of other allied health professionals such as speech pathologists, psychologists, physiotherapists and occupational therapists. Can you foresee any potential difficulties emerging due to these professional similarities? How might these issues be resolved? What role does transdisciplinary health and human services play in supporting successful holistic care? Is workforce diversity important? How do we ensure that there are opportunities and roles for Aboriginal and Torres Strait Islanders to build skills and capacity as Developmental Educators, Behaviour Support Practitioners, Early Interventionists and other specialist disability supports?

The Changing Face of the Disability Profession

The work of disability professionals may range from one-to-one services and localised group supports to policy development and involvement in disability campaigns. Regarding interactions between community-based allied health and disability professionals, there is a need for disability professionals to be employed in primary health care, positive behaviour support to ensure a reduction in restrictive practices and safeguarding, not just within disability support systems that deal with education, employment, social connection, community participation and daily living. The acute health care system has a clear need for community disability professionals to be involved in clinical care pathways to assist individuals living with disability who are re-entering the community from acute or community-based health care settings.

The disability profession has to date been publicly funded at no cost to service consumers or their families. However, there are increasing private disability support services with costs generally covered by the individual living with disability or his/her family if not covered by the NDIS. The broader availability of individualised funding under the NDIS has not necessarily increased opportunities for individual services and practices to emerge and the shift has required workers to undertake training and develop 'new skills to support choice and control, to be more customer-orientated and, to move from task-focused to person-centred care' (Moskos & Isherwood 2019, p. 34). There is also an opportunity under the NDIS for individuals and families to choose who provides support and assists in the achievement of goals and development of a chosen life and lifestyle (Bigby 2014). This can include support from service providers who may not have specific disability training and skills but are valued by the individual and/or their family. Although this may seem a move away from quality, it is not necessarily so. The NDIS is about ensuring that people living with disability have maximum choice and control over their lives and is likely to see the need for building capacity of such supports.

Increasingly, disability professionals in Australia are working in their own private practice. The NDIS provides increased opportunities for DEs and disability professionals to establish private practices because individuals living with disability and their families are no longer restricted to trying to access supports from already '**block-funded**' state services and having the case manager, coordinator or support worker allocated. The NDIS provides resources to the individual and/or their family so they can purchase the services and supports of their choice. Disability professionals can also be found working as consultants in a broad range of non-disability-specific settings including research, education, family support and sexuality and with other disadvantaged individuals such as those from refugee backgrounds. Their work is often varied and can include advocacy, individual counselling, group education, public presentations and the production of written materials such as audits, resources, articles and reports, and individual lifestyle, positive behaviour support and skills development programs. Areas of employment for disability professionals include:

- disability-specific non-government organisations
- generic human service non-government organisations
- government and health departments
- educational institutions, such as universities and **Technical and Further Education (TAFE)** campuses, where DEs are involved in professional training and research
- local government.

Responsibility for Disability Health Care – Specialised or Generic Services, Segregated or Community?

There is ongoing debate as to whether people living with disability should have specialised segregated health care services or whether they should access mainstream generic community-based services. The 2013 *NDIS Act* and current government policy is a move away from specialised disability services towards people living with disability and their supports to access mainstream services and resources via an individualised package. There have been changes to the NDIS whereby some health supports and costs related to functionality and living with impairment and disability are now supported by

the NDIS. Details can be found on the NDIS website: https://www.ndis.gov.au/understanding/supports-funded-ndis/disability-related-health-supports/disability-related-health-supports-health-sector.

Pause *for* Reflection …

Should people living with disability access disability-specific health services or generic health services?

What added pressure does accessing generic health services put on allied health professionals? How may they need to adjust their practice to accommodate people living with disability accessing their services?

Decisions about health and lifestyle are impacted upon by economic, social and systems issues combining to affect the well-being of people living with disability. Healthy foods, medications, therapies and support to be active are difficult to afford on a disability support pension. Although risk factors for a range of health conditions are higher than in typical community members, individuals living with disability are often not targeted in primary health campaigns on healthy lifestyle (Keane 1996). In addition, individuals living with disability often receive support from a myriad of allied health professionals all with discipline-specific jargon and strategies, who are not always aware of strategies, equipment or advice being suggested by another and how this advice can contradict or compete for limited time and fiscal resources. This, along with the dominant paradigms apparent in the Australian health system around curing illness and the promotion of lifestyle changes with emphasis on the individual being responsible for their own health, can be challenging to individuals living with disability who have limited economic and social resources. Also to be considered is the impact on the health of carers and significant others supporting individuals living with disability. As both health and disability support resources become stretched, the negative impacts on the health of the non-paid supports in an individual's life are emerging rapidly (AIHW 2022b).

Disability professionals have much to contribute to the provision of quality health services. Concepts such as consumer self-determination, person-centred approaches and consumer contribution to planning have been part of disability research and practice for over 25 years. A further shift from multidisciplinary approaches to better-developed collaboration, interprofessional practice and a transdisciplinary approach is needed. In a transdisciplinary approach, allied health professionals move beyond traditional disciplinary boundaries to share skills and knowledge with individuals, caregivers and other team members as facilitators of services, acting as consultants providing indirect services rather than just delivering therapies (O'Reilly et al. 2017). This approach has proven effective and it supports the philosophy of person-centred approaches to services. However, the principles and practice of interprofessional and transdisciplinary approaches need to continue to spread through disability support and health care systems.

The NDIS Quality and Safeguards Commission is an independent agency established to improve the quality and safety of NDIS supports and services and it will have implications for practice for all health and disability supports. The Commission aims to regulate the NDIS market, provide national consistency, promote safety and quality services, resolve problems and identify areas for improvement. It brings together, under a nationally consistent approach that applies across Australian regulations, education opportunities, safeguarding functions and regulatory powers around the use of restrictive practices which can include medication, behaviour support strategies, restricting movement and locking doors. Details of the codes of conduct, policies, legislation and rules can be found at https://www.ndiscommission.gov.au/about/legislation-rules-policies. It is critical that all health and human services professionals are aware of and are familiar with these rules and regulations.

SUMMARY

In this chapter, we have outlined key information about supporting people living with disability to navigate disability support in the context of the Australian health care system.

The complexities around people living with disability accessing health care and their daily support needs have been briefly described. In a health and human service environment with limited funding and resources, competition for resources among interest groups representing both the dominant medically oriented clinical services and the broader public health groups continues to be an issue of the health system. The complexities of the relationship between disability and the health care system, especially considering the changing environment with the NDIS, will necessitate the consideration of how disability and health care services manage the care of people living with disability (Department of the Prime Minister and Cabinet 2014).

The roles of disability professionals have been defined within the health care system. These roles are diverse and are undertaken in various settings in the health care system from clinical treatment of patients to primary health care and health promotion advocacy work.

The status of the disability profession in Australia has been described, and although the disability profession is still under-recognised it has growing influence within allied health and human service sectors.

REVIEW QUESTIONS

1. What is the NDIS and why is it significant for the health care of people living with disability?
2. Identify health and human services organisations in your local area that employ professionals with an understanding of disability.
3. List the diversity of roles that are undertaken, or could be undertaken, by DEs and disability professionals in those organisations.
4. Outline what structural changes would need to be introduced into Medicare to allow DEs and other disability professionals to work with GPs and other allied health professionals in providing multidisciplinary primary care. Has the COVID-19 pandemic strengthened the rationale for this?
5. Describe your approach to working under the 2013 *NDIS Act* in supporting a person living with disability around an emergency, short-term or long-term chronic health care situation. What do you need to understand in order to approach this in a person-centred way? Who and/or what information and resources might assist? What do you understand your responsibilities are around restrictive practices and obligations under the NDIS Quality and Safeguarding Commission legislation and rules?

REFERENCES

Australian Bureau of Statistics (ABS), 2019. Disability, ageing and carers, Australia: summary of findings. ABS, Canberra. https://www.abs.gov.au/statistics/health/disability/disability-ageing-and-carers-australia-summary-findings/latest-release#:~:text=In%202018%20there%20were%204.4,years%20and%20over%20had%20disability.

Australian Bureau of Statistics (ABS), 2020. Psychosocial disability. ABS, Canberra. https://www.abs.gov.au/articles/psychosocial-disability.

Australian Institute of Health and Welfare (AIHW), 2022a. Health of people with disability. AIHW, Canberra. https://www.aihw.gov.au/reports/australias-health/health-of-people-with-disability#General%20health.

Australian Institute of Health and Welfare (AIHW), 2022b. People with disability in Australia. AIHW, Canberra. https://www.aihw.gov.au/reports/disability/people-with-disability-in-australia/contents/health/health-risk-factors-and-behaviours.

Bacchi, C., 2016. Problematizations in health policy: questioning how "problems" are constituted in policies. SAGE Open 6 (2). doi:/10.1177/2158244016653986.

Bigby, C., 2014. The NDIS – a quantum leap towards realising social rights for people with intellectual disability. In: Rice, S., Day, A. (Eds), Social Work in the Shadow of the Law. Federation Press, Sydney, pp. 305–321.

Bonyhady, B., 2014. Tides of change: the NDIS and its journey to transform disability support. New Paradigm. Psychiatric Disability Services of Victoria, Melbourne, pp. 7–9. https://dro.deakin.edu.au/eserv/DU:30061988/wilson-consumerchoices-2014.pdf#page=8.

Bottroff, V., Grantley, J., Brown, R.I., 2000. Tertiary education for professionals in the field of disability studies: roads of progress and crossroads. Int J Practical Approaches to Disability 24 (1), 18–24.

Carey, G., Malbon, E., Reeders, D., et al., 2017. Redressing or entrenching social and health inequities through policy implementation? Examining personalised budgets through the Australian National Disability Insurance Scheme. Int J Equity Health 16 (1), 192. doi:/10.1186/s12939-017-0682-z.

Courtenay, K., Perera, B., 2020. COVID-19 and people with intellectual disability: impacts of a pandemic. Ir J Psychol Med 37 (3), 231–236. doi:/10.1017/ipm.2020.45.

Dairo, Y.M., Collett, J., Dawes, H., 2016. Physical activity levels in adults with intellectual disabilities: a systematic review. Prev Med Rep 4, 209–219. doi:10.1016/j.pmedr.2016.06.008.

Department of the Prime Minister and Cabinet, 2014. Reform of the Federation White Paper, roles and responsibilities in health. Issue paper 3, December. Australian Government, Canberra. https://ahha.asn.au/sites/default/files/docs/policy-issue/rotf_issues_paper_3_-_roles_and_responsibilities_in_health.pdf.

Douglas, J., Bigby, C., Knox, L., et al., 2015. Factors that underpin the delivery of effective decision-making support for people with cognitive disability. Res Pract Intellect 2 (1), 37–44. doi:/10.1080/23297018.2015.1036769.

Ellison, C.J., White, A.L., Chapman, L., 2011. Avoiding institutional outcomes for older adults living with disability: the use of community-based aged-care supports. J Intellect Dev Disabil 36 (3), 175–183. doi:/10.3109/13668250.2011.597377.

Emerson, E., 2005. Underweight, obesity and exercise among adults with intellectual disabilities in supported accommodation in Northern England. J Intellect Disabil Res 49 (2), 134–143. doi:/10.1111/j.1365-2788.2004.00617.x.

Ervin, D.A., Hennen, B., Merrick, J., et al., 2014. Healthcare for persons with intellectual and developmental disability in the community. Front Public Health 2, 83. doi:/10.3389/fpubh.2014.00083.

Fortune, N., Badland, H., Clifton, S., et al., 2020. The Disability and Wellbeing Monitoring Framework: data, data gaps, and policy implications. Aust N Z J Public Health 44 (3), 227–232. doi:/10.1111/1753-6405.12983.

Fortune, N., Madden, R.H., Clifton, S., 2021. Health and access to health services for people with disability in Australia: data and data gaps. Int J Environ Res Public Health 18 (21), 11705. doi:/10.3390/ijerph182111705.

Goodley, D., 2014. Dis/ability studies: theorising disablism and ableism. Routledge, New York.

Government of Western Australia, 2013. Disability Services Commission: individualised funding policy. http://www.disability.wa.gov.au/Global/Publications/Reform/Procurement%20reform/Individualised%20Funding%20Policy.pdf.

Horsell, C., 2020. Problematising disability: a critical policy analysis of the Australian National Disability Insurance Scheme. Aust Soc Work 76 (1), 1–13. doi:/10.1080/0312407X.2020.1784969.

Hsieh, K., Hilgenkamp, T.I.M., Murthy, S., et al., 2017. Low levels of physical activity and sedentary behavior in adults with intellectual disabilities. Int J Environ Res Public Health 14 (12), 1503. doi:/10.3390/ijerph14121503.

Jóhannsdóttir, Á., Egilson, S.Þ., Haraldsdóttir, F., 2022. Implications of internalised ableism for the health and wellbeing of disabled young people. Sociol Health Illn 44 (2), 360–376. doi:/10.1111/1467-9566.13425.

Kavanagh, A., 2020. Disability and public health research in Australia. Aust N Z J Public Health 44 (4), 262–264. doi:/10.1111/1753-6405.13003.

Kayess, R., Sands, T., 2020. Convention on the Rights of Persons with Disabilities: shining a light on social transformation (research report). UNSW Social Policy Research

Centre, Sydney. https://disability.royalcommission.gov.au/system/files/2020-09/Research%20Report%20-%20Convention%20on%20the%20Rights%20of%20Persons%20with%20Disabilities%20Shining%20a%20light%20on%20Social%20Transformation.pdf.

Keane, S., 1996. Health medication and consent to intervention. In: Annison, J., Jenkinson, W., Sparrow, W., et al. (Eds), Disability: A Guide for Health Professionals. Nelson, Melbourne, pp. 307–335.

Keramat, S.A., Alam, K., Sathi, N.J., et al., 2021. Self-reported disability and its association with obesity and physical activity in Australian adults: results from a longitudinal study. SSM – Population Health 14, 100765. doi:/10.1016/j.ssmph.2021.100765.

Lante, K, Stancliffe, R.J., Bauman, A., et al., 2014. Embedding sustainable physical activities into the everyday lives of adults with intellectual disabilities: a randomized controlled trial. BMC Public Health 14 (1), p. 1038. doi:10.1186/1471-2458-14-1038.

Loadsman, J.J., Donelly, M., 2021. Exploring the wellbeing of Australian families engaging with the National Disability Insurance Scheme in rural and regional areas. Disabil Soc 36 (9), 1449–1468. doi:/10.1080/09687599.2020.1804327.

Mallett, R., Runswick-Cole, K., 2014. Approaching Disability: Critical Issues and Perspectives. Routledge, New York.

Moskos, M., Isherwood, L., 2019. Individualised funding and its implications for the skills and competencies required by disability support workers in Australia. Labour & Industry 29 (1), 34–51. doi:/10.1080/10301763.2018.1534523.

Nankervis, K., 2006. Planning for support. In: Dempsey, I., Nankervis, K. (Eds), Community Disability Services: An Evidence-Based Approach to Practice. UNSW Press, Sydney, pp. 110–144.

National Disability Insurance Agency, 2014. Annual report 2013–14. National Disability Insurance Agency, Canberra. https://www.ndis.gov.au/about-us/publications/annual-report/annual-report-2013-14.

National Disability Insurance Scheme Act 2013 (Cth), http://www.comlaw.gov.au/Details/C2013A00020.

O'Reilly, P., Lee, S.H., O'Sullivan, M., et al., 2017. Assessing the facilitators and barriers of interdisciplinary team working in primary care using normalisation process theory: an integrative review. PLOS ONE 12 (5), p. e0177026. doi:/10.1371/journal.pone.0177026.

Productivity Commission, 2011. Disability care and support (Productivity Commission inquiry report no. 54). Productivity Commission, Canberra. https://www.pc.gov.au/inquiries/completed/disability-support/report.

Productivity Commission, 2017. National Disability Insurance (NDIS) costs: study report. Productivity Commission, Canberra. https://www.pc.gov.au/inquiries/completed/ndis-costs#report.

Royal Commission into Violence, Abuse, Neglect and Exploitation of People with Disability (Royal Commission), 2022. Public Hearing Report: Public Hearing 10 – Education and training of health professionals in relation to people with cognitive disability. Royal Commission, Canberra. https://disability.royalcommission.gov.au/system/files/2022-03/Report%20-%20Public%20hearing%2010%20-%20Education%20and%20training%20of%20health%20professionals%20in%20relation%20to%20people%20with%20cognitive%20disability.pdf.

Springgay, M., Sutton, P., 2014. Psychosocial disability: the urgent need for reform in assessment and care. New Paradigm. Psychiatric Disability Services of Victoria, Melbourne, pp. 16–19. https://www.yumpu.com/en/document/read/49305098/vicserv-new-paradigm-summer-2014-website.

Stuifbergen, A.K., Becker, H.A., Ingalsbe, K., et al., 1990. Perception of health among adults with disabilities. Health Values 14 (2), pp. 18–26.

Turk, M.A., Mitra, M., 2021. COVID-19 and people with disability: social and economic impacts. Disabil Health J 14 (4), 101184. doi:/10.1016/j.dhjo.2021.101184.

Tyrer, F., Dunkley, A.J., Singh, J., et al., 2019. Multimorbidity and lifestyle factors among adults with intellectual disabilities: a cross-sectional analysis of a UK cohort. J Intellect Disabil Res 63 (3), 255–265. doi:/10.1111/jir.12571.

Victorian Health Promotion Foundation (VicHealth), 2012. Disability and health inequalities in Australia research summary: addressing the social and economic determinants of mental and physical health (publication no. P-053-HI). VicHealth, Vic. https://www.vichealth.vic.gov.au/-/media/ResourceCentre/PublicationsandResources/Health-Inequalities/VH_Disability-Summary_web.pdf?la=en&hash=3347870D3B7ADF0227C5B7B831E02A2ED27AE31E.

Williamson, H.J., Contreras, G.M., Rodriguez, E.S., et al., 2017. Health care access for adults with intellectual and developmental disabilities: a scoping review. OTJR 37 (4), 227–236. doi:/10.1177/1539449217714148.

World Health Organization (WHO), 2020. Basic documents – forty-ninth edition. Preamble to the Constitution of the World Health Organization (WHO). WHO, Geneva. https://apps.who.int/gb/bd/pdf_files/BD_49th-en.pdf#page=1.

World Health Organization (WHO), 2021. Disability and health. WHO, Geneva. https://www.who.int/en/news-room/fact-sheets/detail/disability-and-health.

FURTHER READING

Australian Government, 2018. National Disability Insurance Scheme (Quality Indicators) Guidelines 2018. Australian Government, Canberra. https://www.legislation.gov.au/Details/F2018N00041.

Bigby, C., 2003. Ageing With a Lifelong Disability. A Guide to Practice, Program and Policy Issues for Human Services Professionals. Jessica Kingsley, London.

Brown, I., Percy, M., 2007. A Comprehensive Guide to Intellectual and Developmental Disabilities. Paul H. Brookes, Baltimore, MD.

Browning, M., Bigby, C., Douglas, J., 2014. Supported decision making: understanding how its conceptual link to legal capacity is influencing the development of practice. Res Pract Intellect 1 (1), 34–45.

Crozier, M., Muenchberger, H., Colley, J., et al., 2013. The disability self-direction movement: considering the benefits and challenges for an Australian response. Aust J Soc Issues 48 (4), 455–472.

O'Brien, E., Rosenbloom, L. (Eds), 2009. Developmental Disability and Ageing. Mac Keith Press, Cambridge.

Queensland Health, 2017. Guide to informed decision-making in health care, second ed. State of Queensland. http://www.health.qld.gov.au/consent/documents/ic-guide.pdf.

ONLINE RESOURCES

Developmental Educators Australia Incorporated (DEAI) – provides information on DEs and promoting the profession to the general public: http://www.deai.com.au.

Department of Social Services – has produced a series of short videos explaining the National Disability Advocacy Program. These videos can be viewed at: https://www.youtube.com/playlist?list=PLrjsEoziQmWSJbkTp28wys7MWLBvBcVXH.

NDIS – provides updated information on the NDIS and its roll-out, inclusive of set prices for supports; information is available for people currently involved in the scheme, other people living with disability, family and carers, providers and the community: http://www.ndis.gov.au/.

National Disability Services (NDS) – provides information, representation and policy advice; promotes and advances services which support people with all forms of disability to participate in all domains of life: http://www.nds.org.au.

People with Disability: provides useful information and links around disability and human rights, the social model, advocacy, legislation and disability-specific organisations: http://www.pwd.org.au.

Reports on services provided under the National Disability Agreement: information about people who used disability support services and the agencies and outlets that provided services. Key trends in service provision are examined: http://www.aihw.gov.au/publication-detail/?id=60129547855.

13

Australian Workers' Compensation Systems

Alex Collie and Tyler Lane

KEY LEARNING OUTCOMES

When you finish this chapter you should be able to:

- describe the Australian system of compensation for work-related injury and illness
- understand the interaction between Australia's workers' compensation systems and the health care system

- describe the positive and negative impacts that involvement in compensation processes can have on health and well-being
- understand the impact that work and the employment relationship have on recovery and return to work following work-related injury and illness.

KEY TERMS AND ABBREVIATIONS

benefits

biomedical model

biopsychosocial model

cause-based systems

claim

claims management organisation

claims manager

disability-based systems

iatrogenic

independent medical assessments
 (IMAs)

occupational rehabilitation

presumptive rules

regulator

return to work (RTW)

social contract

social determinants of health
 (SDH)

work disability

work disability duration

INTRODUCTION TO WORK AND HEALTH

Work injury and illness are substantial and costly public health issues. In 2013–14, there were nearly one-quarter of a million work-related injury claims for absence from work that were accepted by the nation's workers' compensation jurisdictions (Collie et al. 2016). The direct and indirect costs of work-related injury and illness for 2012–13 were estimated to be in excess of (AU)$60 billion (Safe Work Australia (SWA) 2016).

Workers' compensation systems are the primary means by which Australian governments have chosen to address the recovery and **occupational rehabilitation** of injured and ill workers. Although Australia has a complex federated system of workers' compensation

systems, they share some common underlying principles and approaches. There is substantial interaction between workers' compensation and public and private health care systems.

Employment and safe work are determinants of health (Marmot 2005; Waddell & Burton 2006). Timely **return to work (RTW)** after injury or illness can promote recovery (Rueda et al. 2012). Despite this, disability due to work injury remains a significant economic and health burden both in Australia and internationally. Prevention of **work disability**, promotion of RTW and effective management of workplace injury are central mandates of Australia's workers' compensation systems.

MODELS OF WORK DISABILITY AND RETURN TO WORK

Initial approaches towards work disability adopted the **biomedical model**, which approached injury and recovery from an entirely physiological perspective: operating on the assumption that treatment of the injury or illness will enable a worker to return to work. However, as evidence accumulated that work disability was psychologically and socially influenced, this model was recognised by many as incomplete. The most current model is therefore the **biopsychosocial model**, which takes a more holistic perspective, recognising the numerous forces that influence how work disability manifests, recovery and return to work (Knauf & Schultz 2016).

The Loisel/Sherbrooke model of work disability prevention is an example of a biopsychosocial model and one of the most comprehensive, placing the injured worker at its centre within four separate systems that influence the extent and duration of work disability: the workplace, health care, legislation/workers' compensation, and the injured workers' physical, psychological and social resources (Loisel et al. 2005).

AUSTRALIAN WORKERS' COMPENSATION SYSTEMS

Australia has a complex and fragmented system of workers' compensation (Case study 13.1). In total there are 11 main workers' compensation systems in operation across Australia (Table 13.1). Each of the eight Australian states and territories have developed their own workers' compensation systems, and there are also three Commonwealth systems. Each system has adopted policy settings and practices to maximise RTW and the recovery of those injured, while also ensuring their ongoing financial sustainability. These systems operate under an 'insurance model', with premiums collected from employers based on the risk of work injury occurring at any given employer/workplace. Some higher risk industries attract higher premiums (e.g. forestry, mining), whereas lower risk industries generally attract lower premiums (e.g. community and public sectors). The systems rely on substantial investments to cover the current and future costs of compensation (i.e. the outstanding liabilities) with the objective of achieving full funding (for their investments and assets to be sufficient to pay for all future costs of the compensation system). The systems thus operate within relatively tight financial constraints.

Each of the main systems is established under state, territory or Commonwealth legislation. All are **cause-based systems**, meaning an injury or illness is only compensated if it can be attributed to work. This is in contrast to **disability-based systems**, where compensation is provided to people with work disability regardless of cause (Lippel & Lötters 2013). The Australian Disability Support Pension (DSP)

CASE STUDY 13.1   Introduction of Workers' Compensation in Australia

Workers' compensation legislation preceded many of the national health care reforms by decades. The first formal workers' compensation system to be enacted was in South Australia in 1900, followed by Western Australia (1902), Queensland (1905) and Tasmania (1910). These statutes were based on similar approaches in the UK and New Zealand. These early compensation systems prescribed the amounts of compensation that employers had to pay if an employee suffered 'personal injury by accident arising out of and in the course of' their employment. They did not remove the right of employees to sue their employers (as modern workers' compensation legislation does except under specific circumstances), although an employee could not both recover damages from a court and receive workers' compensation. The introduction of these systems reflects an underlying, and at that time unstated, proposition that work and working circumstances are an important social determinant of health. The legislation was specifically designed to ensure that, in the event of a worker being harmed in the course of work, the employer should provide compensation. Since the late 20th century it has been increasingly recognised that work, and being in work, is positively associated with health status. The **social determinants of health (SDH)** remind us that work and employment facilitate improved health in many ways, for instance by providing supportive social networks and income to pay for life's necessities, health care and other needs. Modern workers' compensation systems seek to minimise the dislocation from the workplace (period of time off work) and maximise the health status of the injured person. This is both to ensure that the optimal health state is achieved and to reduce the costs of health care provision to injured workers.

TABLE 13.1   Workers' Compensation Regulators in Australia, Coverage of Employed Workforce and Number of Serious Claims with 1 Week or More Incapacity (2017–18)

Jurisdiction	Authority / regulator	Employees covered by workers' compensation	Claims ≥1 week incapacity
New South Wales	State Insurance Regulatory Authority (SIRA)	3,611,821	34,859
Victoria	WorkSafe Victoria	2,967,417	21,716
Queensland	Office of Industrial Relations	2,279,303	26,702
Western Australia	WorkCover WA	1,230,161	11,183
South Australia	ReturnToWork SA	768,214	5904
Tasmania	WorkCover Tasmania	227,064	2629
Northern Territory	NT WorkSafe	141,380	957
Australian Capital Territory	WorkSafe ACT	147,400 (private sector approx.)	1728
Commonwealth	Comcare / Seacare / Department of Veterans Affairs	405,230	1568

Source: Data drawn from the Australian workers' compensation statistics published by Safe Work Australia (SWA 2020).

operated by the Commonwealth Government is an example of a disability-based income support benefit, as it is paid to people with reduced work capacity regardless of whether work was a contributing factor (Collie et al. 2022a). Despite all of Australia's workers' compensation systems adopting cause-based models, there is substantial variability between the systems with respect to their structure, coverage, benefits provided, claims management practices and, in some cases, interactions with health care and legal and financial systems. The limits of each system are defined by legislation. These financial and legal structures within workers' compensation systems mean that, as well as having important public health objectives, Australia's workers' compensation systems can equally be considered from a financial or a legal systems perspective.

Workers' compensation is a good example of a **social contract**. Before the implementation of workers' compensation arrangements, an injured worker's only means of receiving compensation was to sue their employer for negligence at common law. With the onset of workers' compensation, injured workers have forgone the right to sue their employers in return for the provision of health care, wage replacement and other benefits provided by the compensation systems.

In addition to workers' compensation, Australia maintains a variety of other systems of income support for people with health conditions that affect their ability to work. These include life insurance, motor vehicle accident compensation and social security. The most recent estimates demonstrate that more than 750,000 Australians of working age with health-related work disability will receive income support from one of these systems annually, and the total direct cost of income replacement alone is estimated at $37.2 billion (Collie et al. 2019). Workers' compensation represents a substantial component of this overall 'systems of systems'.

System Structure and Operation

Each workers' compensation system is regulated by a government authority. The **regulator** is responsible for ensuring that the system operates within the boundaries of the relevant legislation, and ultimately for achieving the objectives of the workers' compensation legislation. Employers and workers are often considered the 'clients' of workers' compensation systems, as they are the parties involved in, and responsible for, the RTW and rehabilitation process. Management of compensation **claims** is a core function of the systems, but is achieved in different ways in different jurisdictions. Some systems have 'in-house' claims management functions whereby the regulatory authority also conducts the claims management, whereas other systems outsource the claims management function to private insurers or other claims management providers. The operation of claims management can change dramatically from time to time. For example, in 2018 the state of New South Wales moved from a model where five private insurers provided claims management, to a model where a single organisation was responsible for managing all new claims. A subsequent independent review of this new model identified that it contributed to a worsening of return-to-work outcomes in the state (Dore 2019).

Australian workers' compensation systems share many common features. They generally provide coverage for employees of working age within the relevant jurisdiction. Many common work-related physical conditions are eligible for compensation, including acute traumatic injuries and chronic or gradual-onset conditions (e.g. chronic lower-back pain). Musculoskeletal conditions are the most common condition dealt with in Australian workers' compensation systems. Some diseases are also compensable, and each jurisdiction maintains a list of occupational diseases for which workers' compensation may be paid. Most jurisdictions also accept 'psychological injury' or mental health claims, mainly due to workplace stress. However, there are substantial variations between jurisdictions in this area, and the process for demonstrating eligibility for a stress or psychological injury claim is qualitatively different (and usually more difficult to meet) than those for more apparent physical injuries. A summary of the regulators in each Australian jurisdiction, the number of employees covered, and number of 'serious' workers' compensation claims (exceeding 1 week of work incapacity) is provided in Table 13.1.

Benefits or Payments

Benefits are provided to eligible workers with a work-related injury or illness, regardless of fault. Benefits or payments provided by workers' compensation systems typically include health care expenses (medical and hospital costs, fees of allied health practitioners) and income replacement payments to injured workers for the period of time they are away from work. In many cases, systems will also pay the costs associated with occupational or vocational rehabilitation and retraining. Some injured workers with a permanent injury or disability may also be eligible to receive lump-sum payments.

Health care and other medical expenses are typically provided on the basis that they are 'reasonable and necessary' as determined by the **claims management organisation**. In many systems, income replacement payments are capped at a percentage of the worker's pre-injury earnings or a maximum value based on state wage rates (e.g. twice state weekly average earnings in Victoria). Some jurisdictions have time limits on the duration for which benefits will be provided (e.g. 130 weeks in Victoria), whereas others have no such time limit (e.g. Comcare). In nearly all circumstances, compensation systems employ step-downs, which reduce the rate of compensation after a certain amount of time. One of the stated aims is to encourage faster return to work, though a recent study found little evidence that step-downs have any meaningful effect (Lane et al. 2020).

Changes to benefit levels or to the maximum allowable duration of benefits are relatively common. For example, a maximum benefit time limit of five years was introduced in the New South Wales workers' compensation scheme in 2012, whereas the South Australian workers' compensation system restricted benefits to a maximum of two years in 2014.

Pause *for* Reflection ...

The Australian Government provides an annual overview of the performance of the nation's work health and safety and workers' compensation systems. This includes analysis of injury rates, work disability duration and costs of compensation in the major workers' compensation jurisdictions. The annual *Comparative performance monitoring* report is available at the Safe Work Australia website (https://www.safework-australia.gov.au/).

Compare the return-to-work rates between different jurisdictions. Examine the differences in outcomes.

Process

All jurisdictions place substantial emphasis on returning to work as a primary goal of rehabilitation. Most require employers to develop RTW plans for injured workers, and require injured workers to meet certain obligations such as participation in RTW planning and attending assessments, and to make reasonable efforts to return to work.

The process of making a workers' compensation claim is largely consistent between jurisdictions. Workers who have incurred an injury at work and are intending to make a workers' compensation claim must provide their employer, and in some cases their insurer, with information about their injury. This information is captured on a 'claim form', which was historically paper based but is increasingly able to be captured online, and must usually be accompanied by a medical certificate from a general practitioner (GP) or other qualified medical practitioner. The employer must then notify the claims management organisation of the claim within a specified time, and that organisation usually has a period of time to determine whether the claim is eligible for workers' compensation benefits under the legislation, and to accept or deny the claim.

If the claim is accepted, the injured person becomes eligible for benefits; however, these are usually provided on an as-needs basis, with the claims management organisation having policies and work practices in place to determine the need for certain benefits.

In many cases, an RTW plan is developed that involves the employer, the worker and the claims management organisation, and usually health care professionals. The requirements for RTW planning vary somewhat between jurisdictions, and different approaches may be taken depending on the severity of the worker's injury and/or the duration for which they have been away from work (**work disability duration**). A recent study found that the use of RTW plans varies significantly between states and territories, and that not having an RTW plan was associated with a longer period of time off work (Gray et al. 2019). RTW plans usually include a list of actions to be taken to enable a return to work, and the person responsible for each action. They may include:

- suitable duties being offered, including alternative duties or changes in duties
- health care and rehabilitation requirements during the period away from work and while returning to work
- modifications to the working environment, including hours of work, changes to work tasks and changes to the physical work environment
- timeframes for returning to work, often including a graduated re-entry to the workplace
- an approach to monitoring and evaluating progress.

In most jurisdictions, employers have legal obligations with respect to the return to work. These include obligations to:

- consult with the worker and other involved parties, such as medical or rehabilitation practitioners

- develop or be involved in the development of an RTW plan
- provide suitable duties for injured workers who have some work capacity.

INTERACTION WITH THE HEALTH CARE SYSTEM

Workers' compensation systems purchase health care services on behalf of their clients (injured workers and employers) from the public and private health care systems. They do so within certain policy settings and using processes and procedures intended to ensure that workers receive appropriate treatment and rehabilitation in a cost-effective manner. With the exception of acute/critical care, the claims management organisation makes the decisions regarding funding of health care for injured workers with accepted workers' compensation claims. Health care professionals are considered to have an important role in the rehabilitation and RTW process, as an advisor to the worker, the claims manager and the employer regarding reasonable and necessary treatment. The claims management function is the primary interface between the workers' compensation and health care systems.

Until very recently, there have been virtually no peer-reviewed studies of the nature, quality or impact of health care provision in Australian workers' compensation schemes. Development and analysis of new data resources by academic researchers has shed new light into health care service use by injured workers. For example, a series of studies in workers with low back pain has used system-level health care payment data to describe the prevalence of diagnostic spinal imaging (Di Donato et al. 2022a), and has demonstrated statistical associations between high-dose or long duration of opioid use with prolonged periods of time away from work (Di Donato et al. 2022b). Another study examined use of physiotherapy services before and after lumbar spinal surgery and identified significant variation in utilisation and costs (Zadro et al. 2021). There is also emerging evidence that health service utilisation varies between workers' compensation jurisdictions. For example, a recent study of general practice (GP) care observed a higher utilisation of GP services among injured workers in Victoria, South Australia and Western Australia compared with Queensland, and attributed this to differences in policy between jurisdictions

(Collie et al. 2022b). Specifically, the authors proposed that administrative requirements for GPs to provide work capacity certificates in Victoria, South Australia and Western Australia (but not in Queensland) may be contributing to increased service use. Despite these recent advances, knowledge of health care utilisation among injured workers in Australian workers' compensation schemes remains sparse.

Claims Management

Claims management (also known as injury management or case management) is a critical component in all workers' compensation systems. **Claims managers** have a decision-making role regarding payments for treatment, income replacement and the provision of health care and other services to the injured person. There is now substantial evidence that certain approaches to claims management can have positive impacts on recovery (e.g. Arnetz et al. 2003; Orchard et al. 2021) and that other approaches can substantially impede recovery or lead to exacerbation of mental health concerns in some injured people (Collie et al. 2019; Kilgour et al. 2015a; Lippel 2007). Effective and efficient claims management is also considered critical to maintaining the financial viability of workers' compensation systems, and ensuring a positive experience for injured persons and employers engaging with the system. There is relatively little research evidence regarding the features of an effective claims management approach. However, it is commonly accepted in the sector that a holistic approach that engages the multiple parties involved in worker rehabilitation is desirable, with a focus on engaging health care providers, employers and the injured person in developing common treatment and occupational goals. This is supported by systematic review evidence of the effectiveness of multimodal RTW interventions (Cullen et al. 2018).

Claims management within workers' compensation systems is distinct from case management in related systems such as health and disability services. Claims managers act for, or on behalf of, the compensation authority or insurer, and have a dual objective of facilitating the recovery of the injured person while minimising the costs of rehabilitation for the insurer. They do not represent the injured person in their interactions with health care and social policy agencies.

A recent Australian qualitative study identified that claims managers experienced their role as highly stressful, with multiple competing priorities from within their own organisations and from external parties (Newnam et al. 2014). These findings are consistent with reports of a high level of staff turnover in claims management organisations (up to 29% per annum) (Dore 2019) and challenges in embedding good practice and appropriate training and education for those at the 'front line'.

There are many different approaches to claims management within the workers' compensation sector in Australia. At a macro level, some jurisdictions outsource claims management services to private sector insurers; others provide claims management services directly. At a more micro level, there is substantial variation between jurisdictions and between claims management organisations with respect to critical issues such as identification of complex cases (or claims 'triage'), education and training of claims managers, segmentation of cases according to complexity or client needs, and use of independent medical examiners to aid decision-making (Kosny et al. 2013).

Treatment Versus Assessment

Workers' compensation systems utilise health care services for two distinct purposes: treatment and assessment. The primary role of health care practitioners in the workers' compensation systems is to provide diagnostic, treatment and rehabilitation services to injured workers. Combined, Australia's workers' compensation systems spend more than $2 billion annually on payments for health care services. The most common services are provided by medical practitioners, including GPs and physical therapists. Other major categories include psychology, occupational therapy and rehabilitation counsellors.

Many Australian workers' compensation systems provide guidance to health care providers about their expectations regarding what constitutes reasonable treatment. These include policies outlining what services the workers' compensation system will (and at times will not) pay. Emerging from Victoria, but now in place in many jurisdictions, there is also the Clinical Framework for the Delivery of Health Services (Transport Accident Commission and WorkSafe Victoria 2012). This framework outlines a set of five guiding principles for the delivery of health services in workers' compensation and motor vehicle accident compensation systems. The principles have the support of peak health care practitioner groups, and focus on measuring the progress of treatment to determine effectiveness, adopting a biopsychosocial approach to treatment, focusing on empowering the injured person to manage their injury and their recovery, developing and implementing treatment goals focused on optimising function, participation in activities and return to work, and using an evidence-based approach to treatment.

A secondary, but important, role for health care providers in workers' compensation systems is in the assessment of injured workers. Medical and allied health care practitioners may also perform the role of an independent medical assessor. These assessments are used by the claims management organisation as a means of reviewing an injured worker's injury status and progress throughout the claims process. Such assessment may be conducted to establish the work-relatedness of the injury, to identify treatment needs, to establish a worker's functional capacity for RTW purposes, or as a means of determining the degree of impairment once maximum medical progress has been achieved (Busse et al. 2014). These assessments can serve to reinforce the adversarial nature of the workers' compensation system, as assessments can be requested by both claims management organisations and lawyers (Busse et al. 2014) – at times with the purpose of disputing the other party's assessment. In other work disability benefit systems, such as the UK disability pension system, these assessments have been linked with adverse mental health outcomes for benefit recipients including an increase in suicide (Barr et al. 2016).

The reliability of these assessments in fairly determining the existence of a health condition or the degree of impairment has been questioned. Typically, assessments are completed in one consultation and in most cases have no therapeutic purpose (Lax 2004). It has been reported that the vulnerability of the injured worker can be accentuated during assessment, and that the requirement to demonstrate illness symptoms to assessors may fuel the **iatrogenic** nature of the process (Tsushima et al. 1996). Numerous studies demonstrate that injured workers can find these **independent medical assessments (IMAs)** stressful, and that they can exacerbate underlying mental health conditions or lead to their onset (Grant et al. 2014; Kilgour et al. 2015a). IMAs also tend to downgrade condition severity and are less likely to attribute it to employment relative to other medical assessments (Lax 2004).

Factors Affecting Health Care Provider Engagement in Workers' Compensation

There is a body of evidence demonstrating that engagement in workers' compensation systems can affect the interaction between health care providers and their patients (injured workers) (Kilgour et al. 2015a). Although involvement in workers' compensation has the benefit of providing low-income workers with access to health care services that may otherwise be unaffordable, a number of negative consequences have been reported.

A systematic review found some injured workers experience bias by health care providers against workers' compensation clients, in some cases through declining to provide services. This was attributed to the providers' frustration with compensation system administrative demands, and delays with approvals and payment (Kilgour et al. 2015b).

Some conditions are less visible than others, including mental health and some musculoskeletal conditions such as back pain, which can contribute to detrimental interactions. In such cases, determining whether a condition is work-related – and thus eligible for compensation – is difficult. Without obvious physical manifestations, it is harder for injured workers to establish they have been injured, much less that work was the cause. In arguing their case, injured workers must establish that they are unwell, which can contribute to the self-perception of being injured and impede future progress. Such workers are often long-term clients who show little improvement. They can be clinically challenging and may require lengthy consultations to address multiple health concerns, and can represent a significant administrative load for a busy health care provider, which may prevent them from seeing less-demanding clients.

System processes mean that claims managers can contest the health care provider's recommendations for treatment or medications. This can lead to frustration among health care providers, who may view this as disregard of their professional training and expertise.

In Canadian workers' compensation jurisdictions, similar impacts of claims management practices on health care providers have been observed (Kosny et al. 2011) and reported as resulting in a breakdown of trust between health care providers and the compensation system. This can have 'flow-on' effects to the injured people treated by those providers. These findings have been supported by studies of Australian GPs operating within the Victorian workers' compensation system (Brijnath et al. 2014).

SYSTEM IMPACT ON WORKER HEALTH AND WELL-BEING

Somewhat counterintuitively, those who receive compensation for injury or disease have poorer injury recovery and RTW than those with matched injuries who do not receive compensation (Harris et al. 2005). Although most injured workers recover and return to work promptly, there is a minority with complex injuries whose claims are prolonged (Waddell & Burton 2006). Some research has proposed that injured workers may purposefully delay recovery owing to financial considerations and other secondary gains (Zelle et al. 2005); yet other research has suggested that the compensation process itself can exacerbate underlying health conditions or be an independent cause of disability (Kilgour et al. 2015b). Longer term claimants who have delayed recovery with injuries that are not readily seen nor easily diagnosed are more likely to experience stigma and disbelief, attend multiple IMAs and subsequently develop adversarial relationships with claims management organisations and health care providers (Kilgour et al. 2015a, 2015b).

A number of Australian studies shed light on the mechanism by which this system-generated disability occurs. A systematic review of injured workers' experiences in workers' compensation systems has identified that case management practices can negatively influence the psychosocial function and mental health outcomes of injured workers. This review of 14 published qualitative studies identified that, in some instances, claims management practices contribute to a cyclical and pathogenic interaction between the compensation system and the injured person that can reduce access to health care, diminish social engagement and restrict the injured person's ability to participate in productive work (Kilgour et al. 2015b).

A long-term cohort study involving a group of seriously injured workers across three Australian states (Victoria, New South Wales and South Australia) identified that stressful claims experiences were highly prevalent, and that there were strong associations between stressful experiences during the claims process and poorer long-term mental and physical health and quality of life (Grant et al. 2014). Of note, this study identified a small number of specific claims management practices that those injured found particularly stressful.

Workers' compensation policies and practices are associated with differences in work disability, including claim processing times, longer retroactive periods (number of days since injury before a worker is eligible to claim), fee schedules (maximum reimbursement amount that a provider can claim), benefit generosity, choice in health care provider (Collie et al. 2019; Gray et al. 2019b; Lane et al. 2018a; Lane et al. 2019; Shraim et al. 2015).

However, it is often difficult to determine whether the association between system settings and injured worker outcomes is due to an influence on injured worker recovery or changes in who gets into the compensation system (Lane 2021). For instance, New South Wales workers' compensation reform in 2012 restricted access to the system, which substantially reduced the number of new claims while also increasing average duration of time off work (Collie et al. 2020). The cause could be less severely injured workers becoming unable to meet the new, more restrictive compensability threshold, thereby increasing average severity and disability duration of claimants getting into the system without directly affecting their outcomes. Alternatively, the new restrictions may exacerbate iatrogenic effects. Neither explanation is mutually exclusive. These questions become important when trying to determine how systems can be designed to improve injured worker outcomes.

THE EMPLOYMENT RELATIONSHIP – AN IMPORTANT SOCIAL DETERMINANT OF HEALTH IN INJURED WORKERS

There are a number of accepted conceptual models of work disability that attempt to explain the biological, psychological and social factors that affect recovery from work injury. These include the biopsychosocial model of lower-back pain and disability, the WHO International Classification of Function, Disability and Health (WHO-ICF), the Institute of Medicine/National Research Council model of musculoskeletal disorders in the workplace and the Loisel/Sherbrooke model of work disability prevention (Costa-Black et al. 2013). These models share some common features including an emphasis on the importance of social factors in work injury recovery and the prevention of ongoing disability.

The working environment and the injured worker's relationship with the employer are recognised as important social factors that influence recovery and RTW. Employer influence on injured worker outcomes starts as early as the moment of injury. Supervisors who respond to worker injury with sympathy, concern or support improve the likelihood of RTW (Jetha et al. 2018). High levels of social and supervisor support in the workplace have been associated with a reduction in work disability among those injured, whereas problems with colleagues and social isolation at work are associated with an increase in work disability (Shaw et al. 2013). In all of Australia's states and territories, employers are obliged to assist injured workers through the RTW process through interventions such as developing an RTW plan and providing an RTW coordinator, both of which can improve the likelihood of RTW (Gray et al. 2019a; Lane et al. 2018b). Some of our recent work on this provides an interesting window on how workplace interventions could be targeted based on injured worker prognosis: the functional intervention (RTW plan) improved RTW outcomes in only shorter duration claims, whereas the psychosocial intervention (low-stress interactions with an RTW coordinator) improved them only in longer duration claims (Lane et al. 2018b). This aligns with existing research on the changing needs of injured workers over the course of the duration of a claim; injury factors such as severity are more important earlier, whereas psychosocial factors become increasingly important to RTW as the claim persists (Krause et al. 2001).

Within the working environment, there is a complex set of factors that can operate to either enhance or decrease a given individual's recovery or level of function. For example, job demands such as being involved in heavy physical work, being employed in a 'blue-collar' occupation and self-reported levels of high job stress and short job tenure (<2 years) have been reported as increasing the level of work disability (Shaw et al. 2013). The organisation of work and workplace support factors can also affect recovery.

The importance of workplace factors in recovery has led many RTW and work disability prevention intervention studies to focus on modifying workplace factors in efforts to improve RTW outcomes for injured workers. A recent systematic review concluded that workplace-based interventions had better evidence for effectiveness if they were multi-domain (i.e. accompanied by concurrent health- or communication-focused components) (Cullen et al. 2018).

This finding demonstrates that multiple factors, including the workplace, need to be addressed concurrently to improve RTW outcomes and reduce work disability in those injured at work.

WORKERS' COMPENSATION DURING THE SARS-COV-2 PANDEMIC

The workplace has been a focus during the SARS-CoV-2 pandemic, following observations of increased transmission or high rates of infection among some occupational groups and in some industrial settings. For example, health care workers have been identified as a group particularly vulnerable to COVID-19 infection (Gómez-Ochoa et al. 2021), while jobs involving direct exposure to the public and occupational settings that limit ability to enforce preventive measures such as physical distancing are also higher risk for serious COVID-19 infection (Nakamura et al. 2021).

In response, some workers' compensation schemes have introduced **presumptive rules** to support access to the benefits and services provided by workers compensation schemes among COVID-affected workers. Presumptive rules are policy that make it easier for workers to make a claim for compensation in the event they contract an illness or disease. They effectively remove the burden of proof on the worker to demonstrate that their injury or disease occurred in the course of employment, by introducing a presumption that certain diseases (in this case COVID-19) are linked with certain occupations or industrial settings. In the United States, many states have introduced presumptive rules in their workers' compensation systems (Dworsky & Saunders-Medina 2022).

In Australia, two states introduced presumptive rules for COVID-19. In Western Australia the *Workers' Compensation and Injury Management Amendment (COVID-19 Response) Act 2020* came into effect on 20 October 2020 and established a presumption of work-related injury for COVID-19 contracted by health care workers. In New South Wales a broader presumption was introduced, providing automatic workers' compensation rights for workers who contract COVID-19 in industries including health care, education, retail, transport, emergency services, construction, disability and aged care, dining and entertainment.

To date there have been very few analyses of workers compensation claims due to COVID-19 in Australia. Early data provided by Safe Work Australia for the 2020 year shows that there were 1222 claims lodged across Australia, of which 974 (79.7%) were accepted at the time of publication (Safe Work Australia 2021). The vast majority were from the states with the largest outbreaks in 2020 – Victoria and New South Wales. While most (75%) were for workers who had contracted COVID-19 at work, 19% were for the mental health consequences of the SARS-CoV-2 pandemic. The health care industry was the source of over 60% of all claims in that year.

SUMMARY

- Work is good for health, and return to work can facilitate recovery after injury or illness. Prevention of work disability, promotion of RTW and effective management of workplace injury are central mandates of Australia's workers' compensation systems.
- Australia has a complex network of workers' compensation systems that provide health care and income replacement coverage for injured Australian workers.
- Benefits (payments for services) are provided to eligible workers and employers with a work-related injury or illness regardless of fault, and may include health care expenses, income replacement payments, costs of vocational rehabilitation and retraining, and in some cases lump-sum payments for workers with a permanent injury.
- All Australian workers' compensation jurisdictions now place substantial emphasis on returning to work as a primary goal of rehabilitation. Most jurisdictions encourage development of RTW plans for injured workers that identify the roles and responsibilities of employers, workers and health care providers in the RTW process.

- Claims management (also known as injury management or case management) is a critical component in all workers' compensation systems. Claims managers have a decision-making role regarding payments for treatment, income replacement and provision of health care and other services to the injured person.
- Workers' compensation systems utilise health care services for two distinct purposes. The primary role of health care practitioners is to provide diagnostic, treatment and rehabilitation services to injured workers. However, health care practitioners may also be requested to undertake independent medical assessments to assess workers' eligibility for system benefits or their work capacity.
- There is a body of evidence demonstrating that engagement in workers' compensation processes can affect the interaction between health care providers and their patients (injured workers), and that this can in some cases lead to slower recovery and RTW for the injured person.
- The working environment and the injured worker's relationship with their employer are important social factors that influence recovery and RTW.

REVIEW QUESTIONS

1. How many workers' compensation systems are in operation in Australia?
2. What roles might health care providers be asked to undertake in workers' compensation systems?
3. Engagement in work and employment are important social determinants of health. How would being off work affect the health of an injured worker?

4. Workers' compensation system processes and procedures can have a major impact on health outcomes for injured workers in Australia. Can you identify the mechanisms by which these impacts might arise?

5. Considering Tuohy's economics of health care delivery, how does workers' compensation serve the 'agency' role between injured workers and health care providers?

REFERENCES

Arnetz, B.B., Sjogren, B., Rydehn, B., et al., 2003. Early workplace intervention for employees with musculoskeletal-related absenteeism: a prospective controlled intervention study. J Occup Environ Med 45 (5), 499–506.

Barr, B., Taylor-Robinson, D., Stuckler, D., et al., 2016. 'First, do no harm': are disability assessments associated with adverse trends in mental health? A longitudinal ecological study. J Epidemiology Community Health 70 (4), 339–45. doi:10.1136/jech-2015-206209.

Brijnath, B., Mazza, D.S., Kosny, A., et al., 2014. Mental health claims management and return to work: qualitative insights from Melbourne, Australia J Occup Rehabil 24 (4), 766–776. doi:10.1007/s10926-014-9506-9.

Busse, J., Braun-Meyer, S., Ebrahim, S., et al., 2014. A 45-year-old-woman referred for an independent medical evaluation by her insurer. Can Med Assoc J 186 (16), E627–E630.

Collie, A., Sheehan, L., Lane, T.J., et al., 2019. Injured worker experiences of insurance claim processes and return to work: a national, cross-sectional study. BMC Public Health 19 (1), 927. doi:10.1186/s12889-019-7251-x.

Collie, A., Lane, T.J., Hassani-Mahmooei, B., et al., 2016. Does time off work after injury vary by jurisdiction? A comparative study of eight Australian workers' compensation systems. BMJ Open. 6 (5), e010910. doi:10.1136/bmjopen-2015-010910.

Collie, A., Di Donato, M., Iles, R, 2019. Work disability in Australia: an overview of prevalence, expenditure, support systems and services. J Occup Rehabil 29 (3), 526–539. doi: 10.1007/s10926-018-9816-4.

Collie, A., Sheehan, L., Lane, T.J., 2022a. Changes in access to Australian disability support benefits during a period of social welfare reform. J Soc Policy 51 (1), 132–154. doi:10.1017/S0047279420000732.

Collie, A., Sheehan, L., Di Donato, M., 2022b. Variation in general practice services provided to Australian workers with low back pain: a cross-jurisdictional comparative study. J Occup Rehabil 32 (2), 203–214. doi: 10.1007/s10926-021-10013-8.

Collie, A., Beck, D., Gray, S., et al., 2020. Impact of legislative reform on benefit access and disability duration in workers' compensation: an interrupted time series study. Occup Environ Med 77 (1 (January 2020): 32–39. doi:10.1136/oemed-2019-106063.

Costa-Black, K.M., Feuerstein, M., Loisel, P., 2013. Work disability models: past and present. In: Loisel, P., Anema, J.R. (Eds.), Handbook of Work Disability Prevention and Management. Springer, New York.

Cullen, K.L, Irvin, E., Collie, A., et al., 2018. Effectiveness of workplace interventions in return-to-work for musculoskeletal, pain-related and mental health conditions: an update of the evidence and messages for practitioners. J Occup Rehabil 28 (1), 1–15. doi:10.1007/s10926-016-9690-x.

Di Donato, M., Iles, R., Buchbinder, R., et al., 2022a. Prevalence, predictors and wage replacement duration associated with diagnostic imaging in Australian workers with accepted claims for low back pain: a retrospective cohort study. J Occup Rehabil 32 (1), 55–63. doi:10.1007/s10926-021-09981-8.

Di Donato, M., Xia, T., Iles, R., et al., 2022b. Patterns of opioid dispensing and associated wage replacement duration in workers with accepted claims for low back pain: a retrospective cohort study. Pain 163 (8), e942–e952. doi:10.1097/j.pain.0000000000002539.

Dore, J., 2019. Independent reviewer report on the Nominal Insurer of the NSW workers compensation scheme. For the State Insurance Regulatory Authority of New South Wales. https://www.sira.nsw.gov.au/__data/assets/pdf_file/0005/584798/Independent-Reviewer-Report-into-the-Nominal-Insurer.pdf.

Dworsky, M., Saunders-Medina, B., 2022. COVID-19 and workers' compensation: Considerations for policy makers. RAND Corporation.

Grant, G., O'Donnell, M., Spittal, M., et al., 2014. Relationship between stressfulness of claiming for injury compensation and long-term recovery. A prospective cohort study. JAMA Psychiatry 71 (4), 446–453.

Gray, S., Sheehan, L.R., Lane, T.J., et al., 2019. Concerns about claiming, postclaim support, and return to work planning: the workplace's impact on return to work. J Occup Environ Med 61, (4), e139–e145. doi:10.1097/JOM.0000000000001549.

Gómez-Ochoa, S.J., Franco, O.H., Rojas, L.J., 2021. COVID-19 in health-care workers: a living systematic review and meta-analysis of prevalence, risk factors, clinical characteristics, and outcomes. Am J Epidemiol 190 (1), 161–175. doi:10.1093/aje/kwaa191.

Gray, S.E., Sheehan, L.R., Lane, T.J., et al., 2019a. Concerns about claiming, post-claim support, and return to work planning. J Occup Environ Med 61, e139–e145.

Gray, S., Lane, T.J., Sheehan, L., et al., 2019b. Association between workers' compensation claim processing times and work disability duration: analysis of population level claims data. Health Policy 123 (10), 982–91. doi:10.1016/j.healthpol.2019.06.010.

Harris, I., Mulford, J., Soloman, M., et al., 2005. Association between compensation status and outcome after surgery – a meta analysis. J Am Med Assoc 293 (13), 1644–1652.

Jetha, A., LaMontagne, A.D., Lilley, R., et al., 2018. Workplace social system and sustained return-to-work: a study of supervisor and co-worker supportiveness and injury reaction. J Occup Rehabil 28, 486–494.

Kilgour, E., Kosny, A., McKenzie, D., et al., 2015a. Healing or harming? Healthcare providers interactions with injured workers and insurers in workers' compensation systems. J Occup Rehabil 25 (1), 220–239. doi:10.1007/s10926-014-9521-x.

Kilgour, E., Kosny, A., McKenzie, D., et al., 2015b. Interactions between injured workers and insurers in workers' compensation systems: a systematic review of qualitative research literature. J Occup Rehabil 25 (1), 160–181. doi:10.1007/s10926-014-9513-x.

Knauf, M.T., Schultz, I.Z., 2016. Current conceptual models of return to work. In: Schultz, I.Z., Gatchel, R.J. (Eds.), Handbook of Return to Work. Springer US, Boston, pp. 27–51.

Kosny, A., MacEachen, E., Feerier, S., et al., 2011. The role of health care providers in long term and complicated workers' compensation claims. J Occup Rehabil 21 (4), 582–590.

Kosny, A., Allen, A., Collie, A., 2013. Understanding independent medical assessments – a multi-jurisdictional analysis. Institute for Safety, Compensation and Recovery Research, Melbourne.

Krause, N., Dasinger, L.K., Deegan, L.J., et al., 2001. Psychosocial job factors and return-to-work after compensated low back injury: a disability phase-specific analysis. Am J Ind Med 40, 374–392.

Lane, T.J., Gray, S., Hassani-Mahmooei, B., et al., 2018a. Effectiveness of employer financial incentives in reducing time to report worker injury: an interrupted time series study of two Australian workers' compensation jurisdictions. BMC Public Health 18 (1), 100. doi:10.1186/s12889-017-4998-9.

Lane, T.J., Lilley, R., Hogg-Johnson, S., et al., 2018b. A prospective cohort study of the impact of return-to-work coordinators in getting injured workers back on the job. J Occup Rehabil 28, 298–306.

Lane, T.J., Gray S.E., Sheehan, L., 2019: Increased benefit generosity and the impact on workers' compensation claiming behavior: an interrupted time series study in Victoria, Australia. J Occup Environ Med 61 (3), e82–90. doi:10.1097/JOM.0000000000001531.

Lane, T.J., Sheehan, L.R., Gray, S.E., et al., 2020. Step-downs reduce workers compensation payments to encourage return to work. Are they effective? Occup Environ Med 77, 470–77. doi:10.1136/oemed-2019-106325.

Lane, T.J., 2021. Collider bias in administrative workers' compensation claims data: a challenge for cross-jurisdictional research. J Occup Rehabil, 2021, 1–9. doi:10.1007/s10926-021-09988-1.

Lax, M., 2004. Independent of what? The independent medical examination business. New Soluti 14 (3), 219–251.

Lippel, K., 2007. Workers describe the effect of the workers' compensation process on their health: a Québec study. Int J Law Psychiatry 30, 427–443.

Lippel K, Lötters F., 2013. Public insurance systems: a comparison of cause-based and disability-based income support systems. In: Loisel, P., Anema, J.R., Handbook of Work Disability. Springer, New York, pp. 183–202. doi:10.1007/978-1-4614-6214-9_12.

Loisel, P., Buchbinder, R., Hazard, R., et al., 2005. Prevention of work disability due to musculoskeletal disorders: the challenge of implementing evidence. J Occup Rehabil 15 (4), 507–24. doi:10.1007/s10926-005-8031-2.

Marmot, M., 2005. Social determinants of health inequalities. Lancet 365, 1099–1104.

Nakamura, T., Mori, H., Saunders, T., et al., 2022. Impact of workplace on the risk of severe COVID-19. Front Public Health 5 (9), 731239. doi:10.3389/fpubh.2021.731239.

Newnam, S., Collie, A., Vogel, A.P., et al., 2014. The impacts of injury at the individual, community and societal levels: a systematic meta-review. Public Health 128 (7), 587–618. doi:10.1016/j.puhe.2014.04.004.

Orchard, C., Carnide, N., Smith, P., 2021. The association between case manager interactions and serious mental illness following a physical workplace injury or illness: a cross-sectional analysis of workers' compensation claimants in Ontario. J Occup Rehabil 31 (4), 895–902. doi:10.1007/s10926-021-09974-7.

Rueda, S., Chambers, L., Wilson, M., et al., 2012. Association of returning to work with better health in working age adults: a systematic review. Am J Public Health 102, 541–556.

Safe Work Australia (SWA), 2016. The cost of work-related injury and illness for Australian employers, workers and the community: 2012–13. SWA, Canberra. https://www.safeworkaustralia.gov.au/system/files/documents/1702/cost-of-work-related-injury-and-disease-2012-13.docx.pdf.

Safe Work Australia (SWA), 2020. Comparison of workers' compensation arrangements in Australia and New Zealand. Safe Work Australia, Canberra. https://www.safeworkaustralia.gov.au/system/files/documents/2001/comparison-report-2019.pdf.

Safe Work Australia (SWA), 2021. COVID-19 related workers' compensation claims. Canberra: Safe Work Australia. https://www.safeworkaustralia.gov.au/sites/default/files/2021-10/COVID-19%20related%20workers%27%20compensation%20claims%20-%201%20January%20to%2031%20December%202020.pdf.

Shaw, W.S., Kristman, V.L., Vezina, N., 2013. Workplace issues. In: Loisel, P., Anema, J.R. (Eds.), Handbook of Work Disability Prevention and Management. Springer, New York, pp. 163–183.

Shraim, M., Cifuentes, M., Willetts, J.L., et al., 2015. Length of disability and medical costs in low back pain: do state workers' compensation policies make a difference? J Occup Environ Med 57 (12), 1275–1283. doi:10.1097/JOM.0000000000000593.

Transport Accident Commission and WorkSafe Victoria, 2012. Clinical framework for the delivery of health services, Victorian WorkCover Authority and TAC, Melbourne. https://www.worksafe.vic.gov.au/resources/clinical-framework-delivery-health-services.

Tsushima, W., Foote, R., Merrill, T., et al., 1996. How independent are psychological examinations? A workers' compensation dilemma. Prof Psychol Res Pr 27 (6), 626–628.

Waddell, G., Burton, A., 2006. Is Work Good for Your Health and Well-being? The Stationery Office, London.

Zadro, J.R., Lewin, A.M., Kharel, P., 2021. Physiotherapy utilisation and costs before lumbar spine surgery: a retrospective analysis of workers compensation claims in Australia. BMC Musculoskeletal Disorders 22 (1), 248. doi:10.1186/s12891-021-04129-4.

Zelle, B., Panzica, M., Vogt, M.T., et al., 2005. Influence of workers' compensation eligibility on functional recovery 10 to 28 years after polytrauma. Am J Surg 190, 30–36.

FURTHER READING

Loisel, P., Anema, J., 2013. Handbook of Work Disability Prevention and Management. Springer, New York.

Safe Work Australia (SWA), 2013. Comparative performance monitoring report 15th edition: comparison of work health and safety and workers compensation in Australia and New Zealand. SWA, Canberra. http://www.safeworkaustralia.gov.au/sites/SWA/about/Publications/Documents/810/CPM-15.pdf.

Safe Work Australia (SWA), 2014. Comparison of workers' compensation arrangements in Australia and New Zealand. SWA, Canberra. http://www.safeworkaustralia.gov.au/sites/SWA/about/Publications/Documents/875/comparison-wc-aug-2014.pdf.

ONLINE RESOURCES

Heads of Workers' Compensation Authorities: https://www.hwca.asn.au/.

Healthy Working Lives Research Group: https://www.monash.edu/medicine/sphpm/units/healthy-working-lives-research-group.

Personal Injury Education Foundation: https://www.pief.com.au/.

Safe Work Australia: https://www.safeworkaustralia.gov.au/.

14

The Complementary and Alternative Health Care System in Australia

Julia Twohig

KEY LEARNING OUTCOMES

When you finish this chapter you should be able to:

- describe complementary and alternative medicine (CAM) practices, their evidence base and their place in the Australian health system
- explain the holistic nature of CAM and the commonly used modalities
- discuss the increasing growth of and demand for CAM

- outline the current regulatory requirements and questions about statutory registration
- explain the change to natural therapies in the private health insurance reforms
- comment on the current complaint before the Commonwealth Ombudsman.

KEY TERMS AND ABBREVIATIONS

allopathy
Australian Health Practitioner Regulation Agency (Ahpra)
Australian Qualifications Framework (AQF)
Commonwealth Ombudsman
complementary and alternative medicine (CAM)

continuing professional development (CPD)
evidence-based medicine (EBM)
general practitioners (GPs)
holistic
modalities
National Health and Medical Research Council (NHMRC)

National Institute of Complementary Medicine (NICM)
primary contact practices
private health insurance (PHI)
randomised controlled trial (RCT)

INTRODUCTION

In Australia, **complementary and alternative medicine** (CAM) refers to a range of popular but diverse health care practices and products that exist parallel with, but are not regarded as part of, the mainstream biomedical system (McCabe 2005). However, this definition is rather wanting because it defines what CAM is not, rather than what it is (Coulter & Willis 2004). It is impossible to apply a single definition that covers all aspects of CAM. The variety of healing approaches that fall under the umbrella of CAM did not develop by force or persuasion but rather evolved out of a need and demand by people disillusioned with Western medical approaches.

Even the name CAM is controversial, and it could be argued that CAM is not always complementary to Western medicine and that for some people CAM is, in fact, an alternative (O'Brien 2004).

Common Features of All CAM Practices

Although many differences exist in their approaches to treatment, the **modalities** that comprise CAM do share some common features:

- CAM takes a **holistic** view of the individual.
- CAM places emphasis on individualising the treatment.
- Most CAM approaches encourage a partnership approach to the consultation and management of the case.
- Many of the CAM clinical approaches have an underlying belief that people heal themselves, given the right support and stimulus (Weir 2005).

What Sets CAM Apart from Conventional Medicine?

Most CAM practices have at their heart a concept of force or energy that is variously described as a *life force, vital force, vital energy, entelechy or élan vital:* this is a concept that has existed from the earliest days but was first referred to as *vitalism* in the early 19th century. In Traditional Chinese Medicine this concept is referred to as *ch'i* or *qi*, in Ayurvedic or traditional Indian medicine it is known as *prana*, and in homeopathy it is referred to as the *vital force* or *life force*.

Conventional Western medicine does not include such a concept, instead embracing what is increasingly referred to as biomedicine. Although biomedicine has made enormous strides in treating disease, taken to extremes, biomedicine can become a part of the scientific model, where only the parts can explain the whole. It is the opposite of a holistic approach and can result in 'a never-ending search for causes within increasingly smaller parts' (Tesio 2010, p. 108). This approach is very beneficial when a 'part' can be repaired but is somewhat lacking when it comes to complex issues such as chronic disease, mental health and problems of ageing and palliative care.

Pause *for* Reflection ...

A particularly pertinent example of the deficiencies inherent in the Western biomedical model of medicine is the recent conclusion of cancer researchers that the majority of cancers are just 'bad luck' or, rather, random mutations in DNA replication of normal stem cells (Tomasetti & Vogelstein 2015, p. 78). Although it seems perfectly logical that many disease processes are not understood, it is rather surprising that this lack of understanding would be put down to 'bad luck'. If it is acceptable in the world of science to equate not knowing with luck, then it might be reasonable for CAM practitioners to claim that cancer is a complex derangement of *ch'i* or *prana* or the life force.

We might pose the following questions: Is a medical system that develops and operates without a concept of life energy very one-sided? If this imbalance exists, does it result in a health system that is in the complete embrace of technology and pharmacology, encouraging a distancing from the individual and the human being who is sick (Dragos 2010)? Apart from anything else, could it be seen as an approach to health care that is wasteful of resources, very expensive to operate and often unrewarding for both patient and practitioner?

HISTORY OF CAM IN AUSTRALIA

Many of the more established CAM practices have existed in Australia, in some form, since European settlement. Chinese medicine arrived with colonial Chinese immigrants, and homeopathy with those migrating from Europe. These practices were often carried out by lay practitioners or by medical doctors who were also homeopaths. Homeopathic hospitals were established in Melbourne in 1882 and in Sydney in 1901 (Armstrong 2019).

The introduction of antibiotics, the rapid expansion of pharmaceutical treatments and greatly improved public health programs are widely credited with contributing to the decline of CAM, especially after World War II (Gray 2005). Since European settlement, CAM practitioners have often been marginalised by those in the dominant Western biomedical mainstream; despite this, many practices have survived and even prospered, due in large part to the dedication and commitment of the practitioners and the demand of the followers.

Those Who Seek CAM

The increasing use of CAM by Australians mirrors the pattern of use in other Western industrialised countries. In a 2004 South Australian study, CAM was used by 52.2% of the study population, across a range of ages; the highest use was by well-educated, affluent women between the ages of 25 and 34 years, with the majority using CAM for maintenance of general health (MacLennan et al. 2006).

In similar previous research, 57% of CAM users revealed that they did not tell their doctor that they were receiving CAM (MacLennan et al. 2002).

A subset of patients who use CAM are those diagnosed with cancer. Individuals with cancer seek two benefits of CAM: to treat the disease and to treat the side-effects of some conventional treatments, including chemotherapy and radiation therapy. They also tend to seek out CAM when mainstream medicine has no treatments left to offer. The latter is a difficult situation for both patient and practitioner, as the disease is usually very advanced and the patient is also struggling with the debilitating side-effects of the medical treatment they have received.

In the first longitudinal study of its kind, a comparison was made between cancer patients under homeopathic care and a similar group under conventional care (Rostock et al. 2011). The researchers found a significant and stable improvement in quality of life, including spiritual, mental and physical well-being in the homeopathic care group, compared with the conventional care group. The improvement was clinically relevant and statistically significant (Rostock et al. 2011).

Trends in the Rise of Consumer Confidence in CAM

Biomedicine, or allopathic medicine, did not emerge until the late 19th century. As **allopathy** became the dominant system of medicine, the other approaches declined until a resurgence in their popularity occurred in the 1960s (Gray 2005). The reasons why CAM is increasingly in demand are not fully understood nor fully researched, but what is apparent is that the rise in demand for CAM is a social phenomenon (Coulter & Willis 2004).

The impact of globalisation along with rapid social changes that accompany it are regarded as part of the postmodern era in which we live. These changes have also seen a loss of faith in science, technology and medicine to provide all the solutions for living (Coulter & Willis 2007).

After World War II (1939–45), the introduction of antibiotics and immunisations resulted in a dramatic decline in infectious diseases. This decline has resulted in a drop in mortality, with the population in Western countries living longer. This in turn has shifted the pattern of disease from infections to chronic conditions. Chronic illnesses often have no quick-fix solutions and mainstream medicine, with its emphasis on biomedical solutions, may be able to alleviate some of the symptoms but not provide a cure. This has led some researchers to suggest that more emphasis needs to be placed on primary prevention strategies such as exercise (Booth et al. 2000). Living with a chronic disease often motivates patients to turn to CAM.

It has been confirmed that patients seek CAM because of an intuitive feeling that it could offer them a more appropriate medical model for their illness. Patients may therefore not be seeking proof of the efficacy of particular treatments, but instead meaning and context for their illness, thus allowing them the freedom to benefit from therapeutic consultations within their chosen milieu (Case study 14.1). 'Why should we [doctors] impose our medical model on patients? Their use of

---

CASE STUDY 14.1

A 23-year-old woman presented with lingering symptoms after contracting COVID-19, the disease caused by the virus SARS-CoV-2 in mid-2021.

History
The woman had been living and working in the USA when she contracted the Delta variant of COVID-19. Her two flat-mates also contracted the virus. She had been double vaccinated. Despite testing negative for the virus on three occasions, some of her initial symptoms persisted. She had received no medical treatment. As she was too unwell to work she made the decision to return to her family in Australia. This woman had no known health problems before contracting the virus.

Physical Symptoms
- Breathlessness on the slightest exertion
- Desire for fresh, cool air to assist breathing yet at the same time feeling cold
- No appetite, nausea and decreased taste and smell
- Disturbed sleep, restlessness, fatigue and weakness
- A strange 'blueish' discolouration of the palms of her hands and the soles of her feet

Mental Symptoms
- Fear of still being contagious
- Fear of never being well again
- Fear of never being able to return to work
- Frightening dreams of being enveloped by a black mist

Continued

CASE STUDY 14.1—cont'd

Treatment

There is abundant research describing the virus and the importance of diet and nutritional supplementation for supporting the immune system (Skrajnowska et al. 2021). The therapeutic benefits of nutraceuticals for treating respiratory complications is well documented (Tahir et al. 2020).

A complete blood examination showed a low level of vitamin D. Adequate levels of this fat-soluble vitamin, usually boosted by the exposure of the skin to sunlight, have been shown to enhance immune protection against SARS-CoV-2 virus (McCartney & Byrne 2020). Studies have also shown that vitamin C has a role in limiting severe symptoms of COVID-19 (Hemilä & Chalker 2020).

The mineral zinc is often lacking when an individual has no sense of smell or taste. Zinc also has antioxidant and anti-inflammatory effects on the respiratory epithelium. A complete blood examination also revealed a raised C-reactive protein level, a marker of inflammation in the body.

The practitioner recommended supplementation of additional vitamin D, together with limited safe exposure to sunlight, vitamin C and zinc.

The woman's symptoms also indicated she might benefit from the homeopathic medicine Carbo vegetablis in a Q/1 potency and taken as directed. Carbon is a fundamental element of life, and in homeopathy, carbon remedies are often indicated when an individual has a deep level of insecurity about their future survival. They also present with the contradictory symptoms of feeling very cold yet needing fresh, cold air to relieve their air hunger. Dreams of being engulfed by a black mist are interesting to the homeopath, as the medicine is sourced from charcoal, which is made from burnt wood.

Follow-Up Consultations

A telehealth phone consultation was held two weeks after the initial face-to-face consultation.

For the first time in many months, the patient described a lessening of her symptoms, especially her breathlessness. In fact, all of her symptoms were marginally improved. She was advised to continue the treatment.

Two weeks later, the patient was seen in the clinic, and she was at last beginning to have confidence that she was going to get well. The discolouration of her palms and soles had at last resolved. She was now able to go for a short walk each day which did not leave her feeling exhausted. Her appetite was returning, as was her taste and smell. Treatment was continued, and one month later, the patient had returned to part-time work. A follow-up blood test revealed improved vitamin D levels and the reduction of her C-reactive protein levels. The young woman still had to manage her recovery by attention to diet and lifestyle but was encouraged that she would eventually recover her health.

CAM may be their process of empowerment, which in turn allows them to contain and manage their chronic illness' (Lewith 2000, p. 102).

Research Funding – How Serious is It?

Given the high use of CAM in the Australian community the National Institute of Complementary Medicine (NICM) was established in 2007 and hosted by the University of Western Sydney at its Campbelltown campus. 'The National Institute of Complementary Medicine (NICM) was established to provide leadership and support for strategically directed research into complementary medicine and translation of evidence into clinical practice and relevant policy to benefit the health of all Australians' (NICM 2015). Initial seed funding for the establishment of the NICM included $4 million from the Australian Government and $0.6 million from the government of New South Wales (NICM 2015). This support for CAM from the Australian Government began to bring it in to line with international trends. The investment in Australian research looked positive for CAM until the Commonwealth Government stopped funding the operations of the NICM in 2010. The institute is still hosted by the University of Western Sydney, but has had to drastically reduce its staff and operations and rely on substantial donations from the private sector, including CAM manufacturers (NICM 2015).

The NICM is responsible for two significant reports, *Cost effectiveness of complementary medicines* (2010) and *National research priorities in complementary medicine in Australia* (2013). The first report found that Australia could potentially save millions in health care costs without compromising patient outcomes if complementary medicine was more widely used. With more and more Australian consumers seeking out CAM, they would be entitled to ask why support for this institute has been withdrawn. The second report points out that Australians are among the highest users of CAM in the world, with two out of three people using some form of CAM. Despite expenditure of over $3.5 million each year, however, the research investment dollar for CAM is one of the lowest in the world. 'The report focuses on target areas that have a higher burden of disease, that accord with the Australian Government's National Health Priority Areas, and that have a greater probability of success' (NICM 2013, p. v). Rather than simply removing subsidies, perhaps a more positive outcome of the Review of Natural Therapies could have included increasing the funding of research in those areas (Wardle 2016a).

Integrative Medicine – Does It Exist in Australia?

Moves to strengthen the integration of complementary medicine have occurred from within the medical profession. One such example is the formation of the Australasian Integrative Medicine Association (AIMA), which is an independent, not-for-profit group of medical practitioners whose mission statement is 'to lead and facilitate the development of integrative medical care as being core to the health and well-being of individuals and society as a whole' (AIMA 2011). Yet, it is curious to see shifts in attitude toward integrative medicine with the recent move by the Medical Board of Australia (MBA) to begin a consultation process about their intention to restrict medical practitioners from using CAM. This resulted in more than 13,000 submissions in opposition to this proposal and the move was quickly abandoned (Medical Board Ahpra, 2021).

WHY ARE CAM PRACTITIONERS AN UNDER-UTILISED RESOURCE?

Australia's health 2018 is an extensive document developed by the Australian Institute of Health and Welfare (AIHW 2018) on behalf of the Australian Government. One of the questions this document aims to answer is 'Who does what in the health system?' – and yet this detailed account of the health of the nation does not make any mention of CAM, its statutorily *unregulated* practitioners, the services they offer, or the people who pay for these health services. Another example of this lack of inclusion is found in the Gratton Institute report *Access all areas: new solutions for GP shortages in rural Australia* (Duckett et al. 2013), which makes no mention of the rich resource of CAM health practitioners who are well equipped to

make a contribution to a health system that is over-taxed and often understaffed.

Government reports rarely focus on the actual CAM workforce. Because there is no national government register of CAM practitioners, other than for chiropractors, osteopaths and practitioners of Chinese medicine, accurate numbers are difficult to establish, but figures from 2007 suggest that they are in the vicinity of 31,000 (Grace 2012). The increasing demand for CAM services is in complete contrast to the often-negative attitudes displayed towards them by some medical practitioners, other health professionals and even government policy-makers. For example, figures from the Australian Bureau of Statistics (ABS) tell us that the number of people visiting a complementary health professional increased by 51% in the 10 years to 2005. Almost 750,000 people had visited this type of practitioner in a 2-week period, and the number of people working as complementary health professionals nearly doubled from 4800 to 8600 in the 10 years to 2006 (ABS 2008b).

How CAM is Marginalised

Ignoring the CAM workforce in government policies has been common practice until now, although **general practitioners (GPs)** can currently refer patients for a limited number of consultations with chiropractors and osteopaths. These patients are then entitled to claim a government rebate, under the Medicare Benefits Schedule, for a portion of these costs. This is the first time for many years that any CAM service has been included in government funding, even though to access it requires the oversight of a medical practitioner (see Chapter 7). The Australian Government is also committed to a National E-Health Strategy (Australian Health Ministers' Conference 2008). This strategy is intended to streamline the movement of information, facilitate referrals and improve access to care. This system has been devised without the inclusion of CAM practitioners, thus further marginalising them from the Australian health care system (Grace 2012).

CAM practitioners are excluded from national registration despite the benefits of regulation being the method of assuring best-practice and consistent minimum education standards for practitioners, and enabling a legal system rigorous enough to afford protection to the consumer of CAM. Currently, *all CAM practitioners are regulated by systems of self-regulation*, operated by professional associations.

EDUCATION AND TRAINING IN CAM

Towards the close of the 20th century, many CAM professional associations participated in the development of a vocational Health Training Package (Community Services and Health Industry Skills Council 2013), which ensured government endorsement and three nationally recognised components for CAM:

- national competency standards
- a national system of assessment
- national qualifications.

Significant Changes in CAM Education

In 2014, as a result of a review of the Health Training Package, some CAM modalities believed that the knowledge and skills required for primary practice would be more accurately placed in the higher-education sector, and moved to increase the minimum practice standard to an undergraduate (**Australian Qualifications Framework (AQF)** Level 7) Bachelor's degree (Steel & McEwen 2014). From 2018, homeopathy, naturopathy, nutritional medicine and Western herbal medicine moved to the higher education sector, and now require an undergraduate Bachelor's degree as the minimum entry level for practice.

Government-endorsed qualifications still exist for a variety of CAM modalities, however, ranging from Certificate IV (AQF Level 4) to Advanced Diploma (AQF Level 6) and including the following modalities:

- aromatherapy, Ayurvedic medicine, kinesiology, remedial massage, reflexology, shiatsu, Traditional Chinese Medicine, remedial massage.

Pause *for* Reflection …

CAM practitioners are almost entirely involved in clinical care, the work of listening to and supporting people in their goal to wellness. Many of these health practitioners are extremely well educated, graduating with Bachelor's degrees and higher qualifications.

Could these practitioners help to address the targets of such bodies as the National Health Workforce Taskforce, including increasing the numbers of health workers and reforming the health workforce (Australia's Health Workforce Online 2006), or is the ghostly absence of CAM workers in the Australian health workforce yet another example of the 'silences' illuminating their marginalisation (Bacchi 2012a, p. 21)?

TABLE 14.1	Principles of Primary Contact Practice CAMS
Homeopathy	Based on the principle 'let like cure like', homeopathy stimulates the body's ability to fight infection, the susceptibility to disease and treats both acute and chronic disease
Naturopathy	Emphasises prevention, treatment and restoration of the body's natural balance with the use of a variety of natural, holistic approaches
Nutritional medicine	Nutrition is the central focus as a therapeutic tool to achieve and maintain good health
Western herbal medicine	Consultation and preparation of herbal remedies based on an individual's specific treatment needs
Indigenous medicine	A broad range of traditional approaches, such as the use of bush medicines, incorporated into healing practices

Table 14.1 is a brief description of those CAMs that are **primary contact practices**: practices that accept patients directly, or without referral from another practitioner.

Problematising Private Health Insurance Rebates

'Examining alternative therapy claims' was identified by the **National Health and Medical Research Council (NHMRC)** (NHMRC 2010) in their 2010–12 Strategic Plan as a major health issue that needed investigation. The resulting investigation, entitled 'The review of the Australian Government rebate on private health insurance for natural therapies' (Baggoley 2015) set out to examine the evidence of clinical efficacy, cost-effectiveness, safety and quality of natural therapies. The review, chaired by the former Commonwealth Chief Medical Officer, found 'there is no clear evidence demonstrating the efficacy of the listed natural therapies' and resulted in 16 natural therapies losing 'the definition of private health insurance general treatment' and as a consequence from 1st April 2019 they no longer receive the **private health insurance (PHI)** rebate. The natural therapies affected were Alexander technique, aromatherapy, Bowen therapy, Buteyko, Feldenkrais, herbalism, homeopathy, iridology, kinesiology, naturopathy,

Pilates, reflexology, Rolfing, shiatsu, tai chi and yoga (Australian Government 2018).

It should be noted that nutritional medicine and Ayurvedic medicine were not included in the review of natural therapies – nutrition because it was considered out of scope of the review and seen to be covered by dietitians already registered with the **Australian Health Practitioner Regulation Agency (Ahpra),** and Ayurveda because the necessary cooperation from the Indian Ministry did not occur (Baggoley 2015).

A limitation of the investigations into natural therapies was the single research design employed, which was a systematic review – in fact, a review of reviews (Bradbury 2017).

The Private Health Insurance Policy in Australia

Access to natural therapies is not available through Australia's universal health care scheme, Medicare. Private health insurance (PHI) has been available for natural therapies if consumers were prepared to pay the out-of-pocket costs of insurance and this gave them partial reimbursement for consultations (see Chapter 3 for more information on PHI). The PHI rebate covered a portion of the cost of a natural therapy consultation, allowing more people to afford to take out ancillary or 'extras' cover. It is estimated that PHI pays out around $90 million each year on natural therapies, the rebate covering one-third of this (Wardle 2016b). In the June quarter of 2018, benefits paid to natural therapies comprised 4.1% of the total ancillary benefits paid out. It is difficult to see how the withdrawal of natural therapies benefits will have a significant financial impact on PHI premiums (Australian Prudential Regulation Authority 2018). What we may see is a withdrawal from PHI by individuals who took out health insurance solely to support their use of natural therapies. Their potential withdrawal could result in an increase in premiums. The other possibility is that the removal of the partial rebate for natural therapies may create an increased demand on public health services and on general practice, systems which are already under great stress (Leach & Steel 2018).

The Decision to Remove Private Health Insurance Rebates for Natural Therapies is a Change in Government Policy

In many ways the change in policy defies logic when CAM is increasingly in demand by a large proportion of the Australian population. Perhaps, as Tuohy suggests,

not every policy change is entirely a 'rational choice', but it requires the passage of time to expose the broader political factions which seized the opportunity to carry out what seems to have been a concerted attack on the CAM professions (Tuohy 1999). It is also something of an irony that this change, initially introduced by the Labor Government, was enacted by a coalition government whose mantra has always been to support individual choice in health care services (Elliot 2006).

The Health Minister at the time suggested the removal of the subsidy for natural therapies was necessary because the CAM professions are unregulated. The problem with this argument is that enforceable professional standards can be achieved only through statutory regulation with the Australian Health Practitioner Regulation Agency and yet every government, both state and federal and the current Council of Australian Governments, has so far refused all attempts at such regulation (Leach & Steel 2018).

Removal of Natural Therapies from Private Health Insurance and the Consequences

In order for a CAM practitioner to be allocated a provider number by a private health insurer they must meet strict requirements. They must belong to an accredited professional association or national register. All are required to have an adequate level of education, to work in an ethical way by adhering to their profession's standards of practice, to keep up to date with compulsory **continuing professional development (CPD)** requirements, to have adequate professional indemnity insurance and to have a current senior first aid certificate. Unless individuals met all of these requirements they were not eligible for a provider number.

Questioning the Review Process

In 2010, a draft position paper from the NHMRC was leaked to the media (NHMRC 2010). It described homeopathy as *unethical* and *inefficacious*. In response to the wave of criticism and charges of bias and lack of scientific process the NHMRC initiated a formal investigation into homeopathy. Their conclusions found very little in favour of homeopathy (NHMRC 2013b).

The review resulted in the generation of many negative reports about homeopathy (Davidson 2014) and has been used to inform anti-homeopathy policies internationally (European Academies Science Advisory Council 2017). This has influenced Australian and international educators to withdraw their courses in homeopathy (4Homeopathy Group 2018).

In direct contradiction to the Australian NHMRC finding, a press statement from the Swiss Government, in August 2017, confirms that complementary medical services including homeopathy will be compensated by the Swiss Government's compulsory health care insurance in line with all other medical specialties (Federal Council 2017).

The difference between the positive Swiss findings (Bornhoft & Matthiesen 2012) and the negative findings of the Australian Homeopathic Review are in stark contrast. They have met with universal derision by the CAM community. This has resulted in an extensive public campaign by practitioners and consumers of natural medicine to draw attention to the flawed methods and therefore flawed findings of the review and to the potential loss of access to complementary medicines and services that may result (see https://www.yourhealthyourchoice.com.au).

Researchers have found serious procedural and scientific anomalies in the review (Homeopathy Research Institute 2017). In 2016 three of the leading natural medicine professional associations submitted a complaint to the **Commonwealth Ombudsman** challenging the findings of the NHMRC (Complementary Medical Association (CMA) 2016). A response to the complaint has yet to be delivered.

Points Raised in the Complaint to the Commonwealth Ombudsman

- The NHMRC conducted two reviews of homeopathy but only released the first review, which presented positive evidence for the efficacy of homeopathy, in 2019 (Kelso 2019).
- Until 2019 the NHMRC refused all freedom of information (FOI) requests to view the first review.
- The NHMRC outsourced the second review and changed the review protocols without notice, setting an unprecedented minimum number of participants to 150 and an unusually high-quality standard, requiring 5 out of 5 on the 'Jadad' or equivalent quality rating scale.
- The above exclusion criteria resulted in only 5 trials of the 1863 studies presented being considered. The NHMRC decided that none of the 5 was effective.
- Agreeing on a research protocol which details the exact methods used to assess and interpret data is a well-accepted safeguard to protect against scientific bias.
- The NHMRC failed to disclose conflicts of interest of those involved in the review, and included members of the anti-homeopathy group Friends of Science in Medicine.
- The NHMRC failed to consult a single homeopathic expert or researcher.
- The NHMRC reviewed only studies conducted in native English, ignoring excellent research from countries such as Brazil, Italy, Portugal and Spain.

If the process and protocols that the NHMRC used to investigate homeopathy prove to be flawed, then their conclusions that it 'fails to demonstrate that homoeopathy is an effective treatment for any of the reported clinical condition in humans' (NHMRC 2015) must be questioned. If the review stands up to the scrutiny of the Ombudsman, does this imply that the increasing number of patients seeking homeopathic treatment are entirely gullible and unable to make a judgement about efficacy of the treatment?

The Questionable Problem of Evidence for CAM

'Evidence-based medicine is the conscientious, explicit and judicious use of current best evidence in making decisions about the care of individual patients' (Sackett et al. 1996, p. 71). This sounds imminently sensible, for who would not want the best treatment for patients, but practising **evidence-based medicine (EBM)** requires a high degree of clinical expertise; a practitioner must be able to research, retrieve, interpret and then choose from various research findings what will be applied in busy clinical situations. This may prove difficult for any health practitioner, whether mainstream or from CAM. One of the disadvantages of EBM for CAM is that it is much more difficult to apply the research requirements to practice, which in turn diminishes wider acceptability in the clinical community. **Randomised controlled trials (RCTs)** remain the first choice for research into clinical practice medicine, and are often conducted to meet the requirements for the registration of new treatments and drugs despite a plethora of information revealing that RCTs are often flawed and even corrupted by the vested interests of the pharmaceutical industry (Gøtzsche 2013). Chapter 7 explores the process for registering new drugs.

The questionable way that the NHMRC conducted reviews into CAM is a timely example of how evidence is gathering and can be used in creating a position for, or in this case against, certain types of practice. Even the most elegantly designed trials with smart protocols for blinding and including a minimum number of participants only ever measure a narrow set of symptoms and effects.

What seems glaringly absent from reviews of CAM is the fact that any production of sound scientific evidence must also be embedded in the social context and quality of life effects, yet all investigations have actively excluded all reviews of qualitative evidence (Barry 2006).

The NHMRC, the national research institution for Australia, demonstrated a clear resistance to CAM not only by the unscientific way it conducted its reviews, but also by underfunding meaningful research and by not supporting CAM to develop appropriate research models (Clark-Grill 2007).

Problematising this approach to CAM raises some key political questions, such as whether biomedicine perceives the rise in demand for CAM as a threat to its long-standing dominance (Barry 2006). CAM organisations have advocated and challenged the findings of the review into their professions, and in doing so have shone a light on the politics of these marginalised, perhaps soon-to-be-invisible, professions making the wide-ranging, ongoing negative effects on both practitioners and consumers visible (Bacchi 2012a).

The question remains whether this is either ethically or philosophically acceptable. Patients' increasingly positive experiences of CAM are too important to be dismissed and do 'deserve a truly scientific exploration of non-biomedical conceptualisations of health and illness' (Clark-Grill 2007, p. 21), and because 'regimes of truth' (Foucault 1977, p. 23) such as the evidence-based movement currently enjoy a privileged status, scholars have not only a scientific duty, but also an ethical obligation to deconstruct these regimes of power (Holmes et al. 2006).

SUMMARY

This chapter:

- introduces the commonly used CAMs and gives a brief history of CAM in Australia, confirming the reality that many CAMs have been in existence for hundreds of years, and that mainstream biomedicine is, actually, a more recent development
- suggests that people who seek out CAM therapies are generally well educated and economically well-off and seeking to improve their general well-being, or are very sick with cancer or some other chronic disease and are looking for treatment options when mainstream medicine may have little to offer
- outlines the benefits and disadvantages of government statutory regulation by registration for CAMs, and considers other models of regulation
- outlines how CAM is funded and the difficulties of conducting high-quality research without sufficient funding
- highlights the need to design research models that are suited to the multifaceted nature of CAM treatment.

An accompanying video exploring the themes of this chapter is hosted on Evolve: http://evolve.elsevier.com/AU/Reynolds/understanding/.

REVIEW QUESTIONS

1. How is the problem of the PHI rebate represented?
2. One of the aims of the removal of the rebate was to reduce the premiums for private health insurance (Australian Government 2018), but has this occurred?
3. How has the perception of the problem been disseminated and how has it been resisted?
4. Will removing the natural therapies health rebate encourage practitioners to drop their professional memberships and to become lone, unregulated practitioners?
5. If Australia is a democracy, why are CAM therapies not available through the universal health scheme, Medicare?
6. Are patients' preferences and their right to choose being disregarded?
7. Which interest groups might oppose these changes to CAM, and which might support them? (Bacchi 2000, 2012a, 2012b; Tuohy 1999).
8. Does this change in government policy fly in the face of international trends and directives for CAM? Both the WHO Traditional Medicine Strategy 2014–2023 (WHO 2013) and the Beijing Declaration (WHO 2008) gave clear directions to their member nations, including Australia, that they should be doing all they could to improve patient access to natural medicine services and to support the integration of natural medicine into the health care system.

REFERENCES

4Homeopathy Group, 2018. Homeopathy course suspended on basis of European document citing second Australian Report. https://releasethefirstreport.com/lille-faculty-medicine-suspends-homeopathy-diploma.

Armstrong, B., 2019. History of homoeopathy in Australia, Melbourne. http://www.historyofhomeopathy.com.au/articles/item/185-homoeopathy-australian-colonies-early-knowledge.html.

Australasian Integrative Medicine Association (AIMA), 2011. About AIMA. https://www.aima.net.au/about/.

Australian Bureau of Statistics (ABS), 2008. Australian social trends, 2008 (media release). Cat. no. 4102.0. ABS, Canberra. https://www.abs.gov.au/AUSSTATS/abs@.nsf/Lookup/4102.0Main+Features12008.

Australian Government, 2018. Private health insurance reforms: changing coverage for some natural therapies. Australian Government, Canberra.

Australian Health Ministers' Conference (AHMC), 2008. National e-health strategy summary. AHMC, Sydney. https://www.ehealth.gov.au/Internet/ehealth/publishing.nsf/content/home.

Australian Institute of Health and Welfare (AIHW), 2018. Australia's health 2018. Cat. no. AUS 221. AIHW, Canberra. https://www.aihw.gov.au/reports/australias-health/australias-health-2018/contents/table-of-contents.

Australian Prudential Regulation Authority (APRA), 2018. Private health insurance statistical trends, PHI Publications, Sydney. https://www.apra.gov.au/publications/private-health-insurance-statistical-trends.

Australia's Health Workforce Online, 2006. National Health Workforce Taskforce. https://www.ahwo.gov.au/nhwt.asp.

Bacchi, C., 2000. Policy as discourse: what does it mean? Where does it get us? Discourse 21 (1), 45–57.

Bacchi, C., 2012a. Why study problematizations? Making politics visible. Open J Polit Sci 2 (1), 1–8.

Bacchi, C., 2012b. Introducing the 'What's the problem represented to be?' approach. In: Baggoley, C., 2015. Review of the Australian government rebate on natural therapies for private health insurance. Australian Government, Canberra. http://www.health.gov.au/internet/main/publishing.nsf/Content/4899F1657E19A6F4CA2583A50020140D/$File/Natural%20Therapies%20Overview%20Report%20Final%20with%20copyright%2011%20March.pdf.

Barry, C.A., 2006. The role of evidence in alternative medicine: contrasting biomedical and anthropological approaches. Soc Sci Med 62 (11), 2646–2657.

Bletsas, A., Beasley, C. (Eds.), Engaging With Carol Bacchi: Strategic Interventions & Exchanges. University of Adelaide Press, Adelaide.

Booth, F.W., Gordon, S.E., Carlson, C.J., et al., 2000. Waging war on modern chronic diseases: primary prevention through exercise biology. J Appl Physiol 88 (2), 774–787.

Bornhoft, G., Matthiesen, P., 2012. Homeopathy in Healthcare: Effectiveness, Appropriateness, Safety, Costs. Springer, Herdecke.

Bradbury, J., Grace, S., Avila, C., 2017. N-of-1 trials: building the evidence for natural medicine, one patient at a time. J Aust Tradit Med Soc 23 (1), 14–15.

Clark-Grill, M., 2007. Questionable gate-keeping: scientific evidence for complementary and alternative medicines (CAM): response to Malcolm Parker. J Bioeth Inq 4 (1), 21–28.

Community Services and Health Industry Skills Council, 2013. Health training package HLT07. https://training.gov.au/Training/Details/HLT07.

Complementary Medical Association (CMA), 2016. CMA, AHA, ATMS executive summary: Complaint to the Commonwealth Ombudsman regarding the National Health and Medical Research Council (NHMRC) assessment of homeopathy, 2010–2015. https://www.hri-research.org/wp-content/uploads/2017/04/Executive-Summary-to-Ombudsman-Complaint-re-NHMRC-Homeopathy-Review-FINAL.pdf.

Coulter, I.W., Willis, E., 2004. The rise and rise of complementary and alternative medicine: a sociological perspective. Med J Aust 180 (11), 587–589.

Coulter, I., Willis, E., 2007. Explaining the growth of complementary and alternative medicine. Health Sociol Rev 16, 214–225.

Davidson, H., 2014. 'Homeopathy is bunk': study says. The Guardian – Australian Edition, 9 April. https://www.theguardian.com/world/2014/apr/08/homeopathy-is-bunk-study-says.

Dragos, P., 2010. The Copernican Revolution in Homeopathy: The New Way of Dealing With Life Energy. Books on Demand GmbH, Norderstedt.

Duckett, S., Breadon, P., Ginnivan, L. 2013. Access all areas: new solutions for GP shortages in rural Australia. Grattan Institute, Melbourne.

Elliot, A., 2006. 'The best friend Medicare ever had'? Policy narratives and changes in Coalition health policy. Health Sociol Rev 15, 132–143.

European Academies Science Advisory Council, 2017. Homeopathic products and practices: assessing the evidence and ensuring consistency in regulating medical claims in the EU. EASAC, Halle.

Federal Council, 2017. Complementary medicine: regulations of new remuneration. https://www.admin.ch/gov/de/start/dokumentation/medienmitteilungen/bundesrat.msg-id-67050.html.

Foucault, M., 1977. Discipline and Punish: The Birth of the Prison. Vintage Books, New York.

Gøtzsche, P.C., 2013. Deadly Medicine and Organised Crime: How Big Pharma Has Corrupted Healthcare. Radcliffe, London.

Grace, S., 2012. CAM practitioners in the Australian health workforce: an underutilized resource. BMC Complement. Altern Med 12, 205.

Gray, D.E., 2005. Health Sociology: An Australian Perspective. Pearson Education, French's Forest, NSW.

Hemilä, A., Chalker, E., 2020. Vitamin C may reduce the duration of mechanical ventilation in critically ill patients: a meta-regression analysis. J Intensive Care 8 (15).

Holmes, D., Murray, S.J., Perron, A., et al., 2006. Deconstructing the evidence-based discourse in health sciences: truth, power and fascism. Int J Evid Based Healthc. 4 (3), 180–186.

Homeopathy Research Institute (HRI), 2017. World-renowned government research department misled scientists and the public over homeopathy. HRI, London. https://www.hri-research.org/wp-content/uploads/2017/04/20170405_HRI-NHMRC-PRESS-RELEASE-Full-Analysis.pdf.

Kelso, A., 2019. CEO Statement – Release of an annotated version of the 2012 draft report 'The Effectiveness of Homeopathy: an overview review of secondary evidence', Australian Government, Canberra.

Leach, M.J., Steel, A., 2018. The potential downstream effects of proposed changes in Australian private health insurance policy: the case for naturopathy. Adv Integr Med 5 (2), 48–51.

Lewith, G., 2000. Complementary and alternative medicine: an educational, attitudinal, and research challenge. Med J Aust 172, 102–103.

MacLennan, A., Wilson, D., Taylor, A., 2002. The escalating cost and prevalence of alternative medicine. Prev Med 35, 166–173.

MacLennan, A., Myers, S., Taylor, W., 2006. The continuing use of complementary and alternative medicine in South Australia: costs and beliefs in 2004. Med J Aust 184 (1), 27.

McCabe, P., 2005. Complementary and alternative medicine in Australia: a contemporary overview. Complement. Ther Clin Pract 11, 28–31.

McCartney, D.M., Byrne, D.G., 2020. Optimisation of Vitamin D status for enhanced immune-protection against Covid-19. Irish Med J 113 (58).

Medical Board Ahpra, 2021. Board responds to consultation on complementary medicine. https://www.medicalboard.gov.au/News/2021-02-16-Complementary-medicines-consultation.aspx.

National Health and Medical Research Council (NHMRC), 2010. Draft NHMRC public statement on homeopathy. NHMRC, Canberra.

National Health and Medical Research Council (NHMRC), 2013. Effectiveness of homeopathy for clinical conditions: evaluation of the evidence. Overview report prepared for the NHMRC Homeopathy Working Committee by Optum. NHMRC, Canberra. https://www.nhmrc.gov.au/_files_nhmrc/file/your_health/complementary_medicines/nhmrc_homeopathy_overview_report_october_2013_140407.pdf.

National Health and Medical Research Council (NHMRC), 2015. NHMRC statement: statement on homeopathy. NHMRC, Canberra. https://www.nhmrc.gov.au/about-us/publications/homeopathy#block-views-block-file-attachments-content-block-1.

National Institute of Complementary Medicine (NICM), 2010. Cost effectiveness of complementary medicines. Report prepared by Access Economics for the NICM, Penrith, NICM. https://www.westernsydney.edu.au/__data/assets/pdf_file/0006/537657/Cost_effectiveness_of_CM_2010.pdf.

National Institute of Complementary Medicine (NICM), 2013. Research priorities for complementary medicine in Australia, Penrith, NICM. https://www.nicm.edu.au/__data/assets/pdf_file/0009/537840/Research_Priorities_for_CM.pdf.

National Institute of Complementary Medicine (NICM), 2015. About us, Penrith, NICM. https://www.nicm.edu.au/about_us/about_NICM.

O'Brien, K., 2004. Complementary and alternative medicine: the move into mainstream health care. Clin Exp Optom 87 (2), 110.

Rostock, M., Naumann, J., Guethlin, C., et al., 2011. Classical homeopathy in the treatment of cancer patients – a prospective observational study of two independent cohorts. BMC Cancer 11 (19), 1–8.

Sackett, D., Rosenberg, W., Gray, J., et al., 1996. Evidence based medicine: what it is and what it isn't. BMJ 312, 71–72.

Skrajnowska, D., Brumer, M., Kankowska, S., et al., 2021. Covid 19: diet composition and health. Nutrients 13 (9).

Steel, A., McEwen, B., 2014. The need for higher degrees by research for complementary medicine practitioners. Aust J Herbal Med 26 (4), 136–140.

Tahir, A.H., Javen, M.M., Hussain, Z., 2020. Nutraceuticals and herbal extracts: a ray of hope for COVID-19 and related infections (Review). Int J Funct Nutr 1 (6).

Tesio, L., 2010. The good-hearted and the clever: clinical medicine at the bottom of the barrel of science. J Med Person 8 (3), 103–111.

Tomasetti, C., Vogelstein, B., 2015. Variation in cancer risk among tissues can be explained by the number of stem cell divisions. Science 347, 6217.

Tuohy, C., 1999. Accidental Logics: The Dynamics of Change in the Health Care Arena in the United States, Britain and Canada. OUP, Cary, NC.

Wardle, J., 2016a. More integrative research is needed: but where will it come from? Adv Integr Med 3 (1), 1–2.

Wardle, J., 2016b. The Australian government review of natural therapies for private health insurance rebates: what does it say and what does it mean? Adv Integr Med 3 (1), 3–10.

Weir, M., 2005. Alternative Medicine: A New Regulatory Model. Australian Scholarly, Melbourne.

World Health Organization (WHO), 2008. Beijing declaration. WHO Congress on Traditional Medicine, 7–9 November 2008, Beijing, China. WHO, Geneva. http://www.who.int/traditional-complementary-integrative-medicine/about/beijing-congress/en/index4.html.

World Health Organization (WHO), 2013. WHO Traditional Medicine Strategy 2014–2023. WHO, Geneva.

FURTHER READING

Baer, H., 2009. Complementary Medicine in Australia and New Zealand: Its Popularization, Legitimation, and Dilemmas. Verdant House, Australia.

Deans, M., 2004. The Trials of Homeopathy: Origins, Structure and Development. KVC–Verlag, Essen, Germany.

Kaptchuk, T., 2000. The Web That Has No Weaver: Understanding Chinese Medicine. St Martin's Press, New York.

Kennedy, I., 1981. The Unmasking of Medicine. Allen & Unwin, London.

Kotsirilos, V., Vitetta, L., Sali, A., 2011. A Guide to Evidence-Based Integrative and Complementary Medicine. Churchill Livingstone, Sydney.

Ninivaggi, F., 2001. An Elementary Textbook of Ayurveda Medicine With a Six Thousand Year Old Tradition. International Universities Psychosocial Press, Madison, CT.

Phelps, K., Hassed, C., 2010. The Integrative Approach. Churchill Livingstone, Sydney.

Pizzorno, J., Murray, M., 2005. Textbook of Natural Medicine, third ed. Churchill Livingstone, New York.

Schnaubelt, K., 1998. Advanced Aromatherapy: The Science of Essential Oil Therapy. Healing Arts Press, Rochester, Vermont.

Wood, M., 2004. The Practice of Traditional Western Herbalism: Basic Doctrine, Energetics and Classification. North Atlantic Books, Berkeley, CA.

ONLINE RESOURCES

Alliance of International Aromatherapists: https://www.alliance-aromatherapists.org/.

Australian Chiropractors Association – the peak body for chiropractic in Australia: https://www.chiro.org.au/.

Australian Homoeopathic Association – the national professional homeopathic association in Australia: https://www.homeopathyoz.org/.

Australian Natural Therapists Association (ANTA) – natural therapists' professional association covering multiple modalities: https://www.australiannaturaltherapistsassociation.com.au/.

Australian Naturopathic Practitioners Association: https://anpa.asn.au/.

Australian Register of Homoeopaths (AROH) – including their Code of Professional Conduct and Standards of Practice Regulations: https://www.aroh.com.au.

Australian Register of Naturopaths and Herbalists (ARONAH) – national register: https://www.aronah.org.

Australian Traditional Medicine Society (ATMS) – professional association covering multiple modalities: https://www.atms.com.au.

Ayurvedic medicine information and contacts: www.allayurveda.com.

Chinese medicine information: www.chinesemedicineboard.gov.au.

Commonwealth Ombudsman – a government agency which assists members of the public with disputes: https://www.ombudsman.gov.au/.

National Health and Medical Research Council (NHMRC) and research integrity: www.nhmrchomeopathy.com.

Naturopaths and Herbalists Association of Australia: https://nhaa.org.au/.

Osteopathy Australia: https://www.osteopathy.org.au/.

Release the First Report: https://releasethefirstreport.com/.

Therapeutic Goods Administration – contains the TGA regulations governing natural medicines: https://www.tga.gov.au/complementary-medicines-overview.

Your Health Your Choice: https://www.yourhealthyourchoice.com.au/.

15

Oral Health and Dental Services

Julie Satur

KEY LEARNING OUTCOMES

When you finish this chapter you should be able to:
- describe oral health in the context of overall health
- briefly describe the features of the oral health care system and how it intersects with other aspects of the health system
- describe the oral health and dental workforce and the range of activities they undertake, distinguishing between the different practitioners who work in oral health
- describe the educational pathways to these professions
- discuss the professional forces that have led to the current models of supply of dentistry and oral health practitioners
- identify the issues this raises for future service delivery.

KEY TERMS AND ABBREVIATIONS

Cleft Lip and Palate (CLP) Scheme
dental decay / dental caries
dentate
dental hygienist (DH)
dental prosthetists

dental therapist (DT)
dentist
edentulous
general practitioners (GPs)
oral health therapist (OHT)
oral health therapy practitioners

periodontal disease
public dental services
school dental services
Vocational Education and Training (VET)

INTRODUCTION

Dental disease is one of the most prevalent and costly diseases in our community. Oral health is fundamental to overall health, and supports people's ability to eat, sleep and socialise. In Australia, oral health is a significant marker of social inequality. Poor oral health erodes self-esteem and impacts on quality of life; it both affects people's ability to fully participate in society and is an outcome of low socio-economic status. Further, there is increasing evidence of its impact on general health, with links evident between chronic oral infections and stroke, premature births and low birthweight, heart and lung diseases and diabetes. Poor oral health is one of the chronic disease areas that our health service system does not deal with well, at least for those reliant on public-sector dental services. The private dental sector is world class and offers high-quality care to those who can afford it, and indeed around 85% of Australia's dental services are provided through private-sector dentistry. But, for around half of our population who are not able to participate in market-delivered services and instead rely on public-sector services, access to care is poor (Australian Institute of Health and Welfare (AIHW) 2022; Council of Australian Governments (COAG) Health Council 2015; National Advisory Council on Dental Health 2012; Productivity Commission 2017, 2022).

This chapter will demonstrate the necessity of dealing with the problem of unmet need for care among low-income people and those at high risk of oral disease, and at its interface with chronic disease and ageing. It will also discuss some ideas about how to increase the supply of services to those who currently have poor, or no, access to care and reduce demand through much more preventively oriented oral health care and better use of the existing workforce.

SNAPSHOT OF POPULATION ORAL HEALTH AND DISEASE

Oral diseases, including **dental decay/dental caries** and **periodontal disease** (of gum and supporting tissues), are among the most prevalent diseases in Australia and rank as the second most costly diseases to treat (COAG Health Council 2015). Dental trauma, developmental disorders such as cleft lip and palate, and oral cancers also contribute to the (AU)\$9.5 billion spent on oral disease and disorders each year (AIHW 2022). Although disease rates among school children have declined significantly since the 1970s, they are again increasing; in 2018, 34.3% of 5–6-year-olds, 46.2% of 9–10-year-olds and 38.2% of 14-year-olds had tooth decay, and children in low-income families had around 50% more decay-affected teeth than those in the most advantaged families (AIHW 2022).

Dental decay is a disease of cumulative effects, and among adults continues to follow patterns of social inequality. Among all Australians over the age of 18 there are differences in disease experience: on average, low-income adults (those eligible for public dental care) have 15.7 teeth affected by decay, with those on higher incomes having 9.3 teeth affected; for all those over the age of 75, decay has affected 24.4 teeth on average. However, when looking at untreated decay the gap is wider: around 40% of low-income people have untreated decay compared with only around 17% of high-income people (AIHW 2022; Chrisopoulos et al. 2016).

People living in rural and remote areas in 2017–18 had higher levels of untreated decay (32.6%), as did those without dental insurance (38.6%). In 2019–20, only 57% of children aged under 5 years had a dental visit in the previous year, while 87% of 5–14-year-olds and 48% of adults (people aged over 15 years) had visited a dental practitioner for either a check-up or a problem. Among people aged over 15 years, one in five people (20%) reported having a toothache in the past year, with lower-income people being twice as likely to both experience toothache and undergo an extraction as treatment. Alongside this, there were close to 67,000 hospitalisations for dental conditions that could potentially have been prevented with earlier treatment in 2019–20 (AIHW 2022).

Among people over 15 years of age with teeth, 35% reported feeling uncomfortable about their dental appearance, and 33% of those aged 35–54 years had moderate to severe periodontal disease, affecting the soft tissues and bone supporting the teeth which can also result in the loss of teeth. For those aged 55–75 years, these figures were 33.8% and 51% respectively, with 21% of those over 75 years of age edentulous (having no natural teeth). Edentulism is, however, decreasing over time – an outcome that will increase demand for dental services as our population ages with their natural teeth requiring more prevention, treatment and maintenance (AIHW 2022; COAG Health Council 2015).

The consequences of poor access to oral health care increases in significance and impact on general health in the elderly (Case study 15.1). Oral cancer, for example, is the eleventh most common cancer and, often as a consequence of late diagnoses (3329 diagnoses and 622 deaths in 2017), can result in higher mortality than many other cancers (AIHW 2021; AIHW 2022). In 2018, only 61% of **dentate** (those with teeth) individuals and 16% of **edentulous** (those without teeth) individuals over 60 years of age had visited a dentist in the past 12 months. These issues are exacerbated among nursing home residents whose access to care is complicated by immobility, dependence, multiple and chronic medical conditions and medications, and poor oral hygiene (COAG Health Council 2015; Productivity Commission 2018). This situation will worsen as our population ages and people increasingly retain their teeth.

Socio-economic circumstances are clearly related to risk status for dental disease, with the highest levels of disease prevalence occurring in those least able to access care. People from low-income families, refugees, people in rural areas, Aboriginal and Torres Strait Islander people, the elderly, the home-bound and those with disabilities and those with mental health problems all demonstrate higher levels of dental disease and greater difficulty in accessing dental care (AIHW 2022; COAG Health Council 2015). A 2018 Productivity Commission review of Australia's oral health and dental visiting patterns describe two

CASE STUDY 15.1   Oral Health in the Setting of Residential Aged Care

A bed-bound, immobile, high-care patient is not eating, and her health is deteriorating. The nursing-home staff finally determine that toothache is the problem but cannot get the patient to a dentist. The mobile public dental service is booked out and waiting lists are 2 years long. The busy local dentist is fully booked for several months, but finally attends and extracts a tooth for the patient. The staff of the nursing home realise that several of their patients are in need of dental care, and become aware that poor oral health can contribute to poor nutrition, inhalation pneumonia and other quality-of-life compromises for their residents. The local dentist does not have the time or resources to meet the needs of this group of residents. Investigations by the Director of Nursing reveal that there is a funded program operating in South Australia, the Better Oral Health in Residential Care (BOHRC) program (South Australian Department of Health 2014), which covers oral health checks when new residents are admitted and uses the residential aged-care hairdressing salon for dental checks. A study undertaken in Victoria by Hopcraft et al. (2008, 2011) found that dental hygienists can examine, diagnose and provide simple oral health care to the same standard as a dentist for dependent older people in residential aged-care settings, and can reliably identify and refer conditions beyond their scope to dentists and specialists. This study resulted in a change in dental practice regulation in 2000, to allow hygienists and oral health therapists to work in this way. Unfortunately, this model of service still relies on private funding.

Case Study Questions

1. What are the barriers to oral health for these residents?
2. Who is responsible for their oral health?
3. Which dental practitioners could provide care?
4. What sort of models of care would work in this setting?

worlds of dental care. The 39% of adults who inhabit one world have favourable dental visiting patterns (regular check-ups with the same practice and access to timely care) and better oral health. The second world constitutes the majority – some 61% – who have unfavourable (29%) or intermittent (32%) patterns of dental visiting (less than yearly and problem related) and poorer oral health. These people have more untreated oral disease, and their delayed treatment leads to people in pain seeking emergency rather than general care. Further, this second group, who undergo more tooth extractions, also receive fewer preventive services (COAG Health Council 2015; Productivity Commission 2018).

In summary, there are three key aspects to the community's needs for dental care. First, there is the issue of the high levels of disease prevalence across the whole community that require greater attention to oral health promotion and preventive care. Second, there is the issue of unmet need for services that is largely concentrated in lower-income groups and others least able to access services. Third, there are the cohort patterns associated with fluoridation and increasing retention of teeth among an ageing population, which results in a greater need for lower-technology services among the young to middle-aged and an increasing need for higher-technology services among middle-aged and older adults. Our existing system, while providing excellent care for some, is not meeting the needs of all and is not reducing oral disease levels (COAG Health Council 2015; Duckett et al. 2019; Productivity Commission 2018).

THE PROBLEM OF SERVICE DELIVERY SYSTEM POLICY

Dental care sits at the interface between a market model and the welfare state, in that it is excluded from Medicare but is increasingly recognised as being integral to general health and therefore due for broader health policy consideration. The Rudd and Gillard Labor Governments moved to enable this consideration by generating proposals to begin the process of finding more universal approaches to providing services with public funding. The (now-ceased) Chronic Dental Disease Program initiated by the Howard Liberal Government in 2007 was the first of these initiatives, followed in 2012 by the Child Dental Benefits Scheme, which represented something of a revolution in public dental funding, 'looking a lot like the much talked about Denticare' (Dooland 2014, p. 20).

In the 1990s, Lewis and Satur both evaluated the policy environment against Alford's (1975) model of structural interests (dominant interests – professional monopolists, challenging interests – corporate rationalists, and repressed interests – equal health advocates), arguing that the exclusion of dental care from universal health insurance models had preserved the professional hierarchies and power of the market model (for further explanation of these ideas, please see Chapter 1). Dentists (in private practice) had a monopoly over the market thus the freedom to set prices, dominate regulatory systems and protect their sovereignty through professional dominance. This model has served those who can afford to participate in the market well, but excluded many, mostly those with the highest needs for care such as those unable to access (pay for) private dental care (lower income/SES, Indigenous, dependent elderly, new migrants, those with mental or physical health challenges, etc.) (Lewis 2000; Satur 2002).

The National Health Strategy of the early 1990s recognised the high levels of dental disease and included dental care in the reform agenda, driving the consideration of oral health as a social welfare issue and offering opportunities to make proposals that cut across the division of market and welfare models (Dooland 1992). In 1995, for the first time since the development of universal school dental services in the 1970s, the Commonwealth government invested funding in a public dental program (Parliament of Australia 2008), providing services for adults using both public and private clinics. Sadly, this program was de-funded in the first Liberal Government Budget of 1996 (Lewis 2000) presenting a problem for public dental providers who now had visible demand for care from a previously undefined and underserved population group. The de-funding of this scheme set an agenda that drew on the emergence of 'new public management' to drive new models of care, with several states expanding access to adult care using co-payment mechanisms.

The emergence of the National Competition Policy and managerialism challenged and shifted the landscape to redefine the problem as one of powerful interest groups limiting the ability to develop more innovative service models and workforces. This national agenda enabled a change process that diluted the absolute power of the dentist professional monopolists, allowing dental corporate rationalists and equal health advocates to align and challenge the policy monopoly of the dentists (Bacchi 2016; Lewis 2000; National Advisory Committee on Oral Health 2004; Satur 2002; Spencer 2004). In the 2000s, the application of the National Competition Policy and later the development of the National Regulation and Accreditation Scheme and Health Workforce Australia furthered this agenda, resulting in proposals to include dental care in Medicare and enabling challenges to traditional workforce professional hierarchies (see Chapter 1) (National Advisory Committee on Oral Health 2004; National Advisory Council on Dental Health 2012; Parliament of Australia 2013). Ultimately, the problem with the various interest groups and the current health policy approach is that a majority (85%+) of dental care is provided through a market-based private business model that benefits business owners but fails to provide for those who are unable to participate in the market. This model of health care delivery has been replaced by Medicare for all other aspects of health care, but the mouth has been excluded and those who benefit from this market-based delivery continue to work to protect their interests (Duckett et al. 2019).

Dental Services: Funding and Services Overview

Under Section 51 xxiii(a) of the Australian Constitution, the Commonwealth government has the power to legislate for 'the provision of pharmaceutical, sickness and hospital benefits, medical and dental services'; however, the state and territory governments have traditionally been responsible for delivering public oral health services (Commonwealth of Australia 2020). In 2019–20, total expenditure on dental services in Australia was $9.6 billion, representing 5.8% of total health expenditure – a proportion that has not altered much since 2004. Around three-quarters of the expenditure on dental services is borne by individual consumers, compared with just 12% of the expenditure on other health services; this is displayed in Fig. 15.1 (AIHW 2020a; COAG Health Council 2015). Ironically the funding provided to rebate private health insurance for dental services for those who can afford care is roughly equivalent to the direct funding for public dental services (Figure 15.1).

Private-Sector Services

In Australia, the vast majority of services (85%) are delivered through private dental practices under self-funded (or self-insured) arrangements. The private sector offers care on a fee-for-service basis to all children and adults, including emergency, general and specialist care, with access to technology and evidence-based practice that is equivalent to the best international standards. Fees are set on a competitive market basis, and specialist

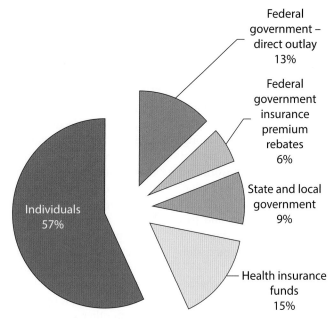

Figure 15.1 Dental Service Expenditure as Percentage by Source. *Source*: Adapted from Australian Institute of Health and Welfare (2021). Health Expenditure Australia 2019–20. AIHW, Canberra.

services do not require referral but often involve one. In 2017–18, about half (51.6%) of Australians had some level of private health insurance that included dental benefits; 76% of these policies contributed to dental services but did not entirely cover their cost (AIHW 2022a). Some health insurance funds own practices and provide care directly to their members, and the Commonwealth government also rebates private health insurance fees through taxation mechanisms.

Public-Sector Services

After the state funded dental hospitals, school dental services have been the longest-running **public dental services** in Australia and New Zealand. Australian **school dental services** have, since their expansion under the Whitlam Government in the 1970s, offered dental care to all primary school children and eligible adolescents, through fixed and mobile dental clinics. Now funded largely by state and territory governments, this service has continued since that time, although eligibility and service delivery models vary from state to state. For example, New South Wales and the Australian Capital Territory (ACT) provide services predominantly through community-based clinics with some outreach

mobile clinics. Western Australia, Queensland and South Australia have dedicated school dental program clinics (both fixed and mobile), and the Northern Territory uses a mixed model consisting of community-based services and school dental clinics with outreach to remote communities (COAG Health Council 2015). Victoria, which had moved their services into community health clinics in the 1990s, has recently implemented a new 'Smile Squad' program which provides mobile dental services in state primary schools delivered by community health services (State Government of Victoria 2019).

Eligibility also varies, from primary and secondary school children in some states to all children and young people aged 0–18 years regardless of school enrolment. Dental care is free (government funded) for all eligible children and adolescents in most states and territories, with ACT and South Australia charging a co-payment for those without concession cards (National Advisory Council on Dental Health 2012). Children are seen as a priority population in the public dental services with no significant waiting periods, but if they require inpatient hospital care then waiting periods can be long (COAG Health Council 2015).

In 2014, following on from the recommendations of the National Advisory Council on Dental Health (NACDH), the Commonwealth government commenced the Child Dental Benefits Schedule, which provides a capped $1000 worth of dental care over a 2-year period to each child eligible for Family Tax Benefit A (around 80% of children). Under the scheme, children between 2 and 17 years old receive basic dental services such as examinations, X-rays, cleaning, fissure sealing, fillings, root canals and extractions. Benefits are not available for orthodontic or cosmetic dental work and cannot be paid for any services provided in a hospital. Services can be provided through private practices and public practices using a fixed scale of items and fees which are rebated through Medicare (Department of Health 2017; Dooland 2014; Productivity Commission 2022).

Public dental services for adults have been characterised over many years by inadequacy; around 36% of Australians are eligible for public dental care; however, current funding for public oral health services allows only around 10% of means-tested adults who are eligible for dental care (those with concession cards and other benefits) to receive care in any one year (AIHW 2018; National Advisory Council on Dental Health 2012; Productivity Commission 2018). For low-income Australians, the impact of dental disease is magnified because they are unable to afford private care and instead choose public-sector care, which usually means being placed on a waiting list. The long wait for care worsens their dental conditions, resulting in problems that could have been fixed relatively easily becoming more complex and costly: prevention becomes a filling, a filling becomes an extraction; local infections become systemic; a problem becomes pain (Case study 15.2). Despite the investment in a range of programs (see Table 15.1), the 'safety net' is inadequate; this results in some services being overwhelmed by 'emergency' visits for pain and infections, and in the need for prioritising care for particularly vulnerable people (e.g. Aboriginal and Torres Strait Islander people, pregnant women, those with mental health problems and disabilities, those who are homeless, and refugees and asylum seekers). Others simply miss out because they are not eligible for care in the public sector and cannot afford care in the private sector.

Delays in being able to access preventive or urgent dental care shifts, compounds and creates other problems for non-dental health services. A downstream effect is that people often seek relief of pain and infections through other services, such as public and private hospitals, hospital outpatient clinics and **general practitioners (GPs)**. In 2019–20, around 67,000 Australians were hospitalised for acute preventable dental conditions (up from 63,000 in 2012–13), the second highest cause of potentially preventable hospitalisations after urinary tract infections. Young children have the highest rates of hospitalisations; in 2019–20, some 7212 children aged 0–4 years and 13,899 aged 5–9 years were admitted to hospital for dental conditions. This rate was greater for Indigenous Australians (4.4 per 1000 people) and those living in remote communities (4.2 per 1000 people)

CASE STUDY 15.2   Oral Health for a Low-Income/Working-Poor Family

Gerrard is a father of four and works as a cleaner; he earns too much to qualify for a Health Care Card or public dental care, but not enough to be able to afford regular dental care. His children see the school dental service, but there is simply not enough money left at the end of the week to afford health insurance or for private dental care for himself or his wife. He has had a hole in his tooth for some time, which has started to ache, but he has been too scared to go to a dentist because he knows there are several teeth needing treatment and fears the embarrassment of being unable to pay. He puts up with toothache until it becomes overwhelming, and finally goes to see his general practitioner and is given antibiotics (bulk-billed to Medicare). This resolves the problem temporarily, but it recurs and a swelling around his neck starts to make it hard to breathe. Gerrard, unable to breathe properly or sleep, finally goes to a hospital emergency department with an infection that is compromising his airway. He requires tracheotomy to maintain his airway and extraction of the tooth under general anaesthesia. Gerrard loses 3 days' work and another tooth.

Case Study Questions
1. What are the costs to Gerrard, the health system and his family?
2. How do you think this affects Gerrard's quality of life?
3. Can you think of better ways to deal with Gerrard's situation? How could this be funded?

TABLE 15.1 Summary of Commonwealth-Funded Dental Programs

Period	Program	Scope
	Veterans' Affairs programs	Members of Australian Defence Force, Army Reserve and eligible veterans
	Aboriginal Community Controlled Dental Services	Dental services provided through some Aboriginal Community Controlled Health Services
	Cleft Lip and Palate (CLP) Scheme	For children 0–18 years of age diagnosed with CLP
	Oral health services for prisoners and asylum seekers in community detention	People in detention facilities and community detention have access to free oral health care but may face long waiting times
1999–	Private Health Insurance Rebate	30%–40% rebate provided to people with private health insurance which includes dental services ($606 million in 2012–13)
2004–07	Enhanced Primary Care Program	People with specific chronic disease impacting on or impacted by their oral health
2007–12	Medicare Chronic Disease Dental Scheme	People with GP-managed chronic disease whose oral health is impacting, or is likely to impact, on their overall health
2008–13	Medicare Teen Dental Program	Children aged 12–17 years receiving Family Tax Benefit A and other income support payments – examination and preventive services only
2013–15	Voluntary Dental Graduate Year Program	Provision of practice experience, professional development and mentoring to new graduate dentists in under-served areas
2014–15	Oral Health Therapist (OHT) Graduate Year Program	Provision of practice experience, professional development and mentoring to new graduate OHTs in under-served areas
2013–14	Dental relocation and infrastructure program	To encourage and support dentists to relocate to regional and remote areas (workforce redistribution)
2012/13– 2021/22	Stronger Futures in the Northern Territory and National Partnership Agreement oral health implementation	Oral health services program for Aboriginal and Torres Strait Islander children under 16 years of age, with a focus on remote communities
2013–21	National Partnership Agreement – treating more public dental patients	Reduction of public dental waiting lists – tied grants allocated to state and territory public dental programs
2014–	Child Dental Benefits Schedule	Basic dental care for children aged 12–17 years receiving Family Tax Benefit A and other income support payments
2016–	Dental Training Expanding Rural Placements (DTERP)	Supports high-quality rural dental student training to address gaps in the rural and remote health workforce

Sources: Adapted from AGDH (2019); Chrisopoulos et al. (2016); COAG Health Council (2015); Department of Health (2017); Duckett et al. (2019); National Advisory Council on Dental Health (2012).

compared to urban populations (2.5 per 1000 people) (AIHW 2020b, 2022; COAG Health Council 2015; Productivity Commission 2018). This downstream problem represents a significant cost-shift arising out of poor access to care, and a considerable cost to the health system and the economy through days lost at work and school.

Pause *for* Reflection ...

Should the government include dental care in Medicare? Why do you think it is not included at present?

Access to dental care has also been impacted by the COVID-19 pandemic. This has affected patients and dental practitioners in terms of the number and type of services provided and the way in which services were delivered. Early in the pandemic, the Australian Health Protection Principal Committee (AHPPC) and National Cabinet recommended restrictions on performing dental treatments that generated aerosols, and that all routine examinations and treatments should be deferred. These restrictions were implemented and eased at various times over the course of the pandemic, which considerably impacted the delivery of dental services between March 2020 and October 2021. It also saw many dental practitioners and their staff work reduced hours or be laid off. This resulted in the provision of emergency care only during those periods and around 1 in 8 (12%) people aged over 15 years delaying or missing at least one dental visit in 12 months due to COVID-19. This impact appears to be greater on those from lower socio-economic families and those with higher disease experience. The flow-on effect of delayed care is increased demand and this has placed pressure on public funding, waiting list times and the availability of care across the sector, which will be long lasting (AIHW 2022; Hopcraft & Farmer 2021; Nguyen et al. 2021).

The challenges for practitioners in continuing to provide care during this time also saw the development of teledentistry, which was used to screen and triage patient care, provide preventive care and advice and extend the capacity of remote diagnostic services. The professional, education and regulatory environments responded rapidly to enable and ensure the delivery of quality services through this mechanism, with this innovation being one of the positive changes to emerge from COVID-19 (Australian Dental Association (ADA) 2021; Dental Board of Australia (DBA) 2020; Holden et al. 2021; Poirier et al. 2022).

Current Workforce or Practitioner Groups and Roles

The dental and oral health workforce comprises registered dental practitioners (dentists, specialist dentists, dental therapists, hygienists and oral health therapists, and dental prosthetists) alongside dental assistants and dental technicians who are not registered (see Table 15.2). Prior to 2004, there was a projected shortage in the workforce which has resulted in considerable increases

TABLE 15.2	Dental and Oral Health Practitioner Role Descriptions	
Role		**Description**
Dentist	✓	Dentists practise all parts of dentistry, including assessment, diagnosis, treatment, management and preventive services for patients of all ages.
Dental therapist	✓	Dental therapists provide oral health assessment, diagnosis, treatment, management and preventive services for children, adolescents and young adults (and, with additional education, for all adults) within a preventive philosophy. They provide fillings and tooth removal, additional oral care, and oral health education and promotion for individuals and communities. Dental therapists are autonomous practitioners who work in collaborative and referral relationships with dentists.
Dental hygienist	✓	Dental hygienists provide oral health assessment, diagnosis, treatment, management and education for the prevention of oral disease to promote oral health for people of all ages. They provide periodontal/gum treatment, preventive services and other oral care. Dental hygienists are autonomous practitioners who work in a collaborative and referral relationship with dentists.
Oral health therapist	✓	Oral health therapists are qualified as *both* a dental therapist and a dental hygienist and provide all the services of both. Like dental therapists and hygienists, they work with dentists and specialists providing orthodontic treatment, specialist periodontal and paediatric treatment, and dental care for other high-needs people.
Dental prosthetist	✓	Dental prosthetists provide assessment, treatment, management and provision of removable dentures and mouth-guards used for sporting activities. With additional education and a written referral from a dentist, they also provide various types of splints, sleep apnoea devices, anti-snoring devices, immediate dentures and additions to existing dentures.

TABLE 15.2	Dental and Oral Health Practitioner Role Descriptions—cont'd	
Role		**Description**
Dental assistant		A dental assistant supports the provision of clinical dental care by preparing patients and assisting dentists, dental specialists, dental hygienists, therapists and oral health therapists in providing care and treatment. They may also carry out reception and administration work and, with additional training, are able to take X-rays and provide oral health education.
Dental technician		A dental technician constructs and repairs dentures and other dental appliances, working closely with a dentist or dental prosthetist and usually having no patient contact.
Specialist areas of dentistry	✓	Registered dental specialists are dentists who have completed additional postgraduate studies and preparation and limit their practice to a specific branch of dentistry, in one of the following areas: dental–maxillofacial radiology, endodontics, oral and maxillofacial surgery, oral medicine, oral pathology, oral surgery, orthodontics, paediatric dentistry, periodontics, prosthodontics, public health dentistry, special needs dentistry, forensic odontology.

✓ indicates those registered for practice with the Australian Health Practitioner Regulation Agency (Dental Board of Australia).
Sources: Adapted from AIHW (2022); Dental Board of Australia (2022).

in education intakes for dentists, and in the immigration of overseas-qualified dentists. This resulted in workforce growth of almost 100% for dentists between 2007 and 2012 with a slower but continued upward trajectory between 2013 and 2021 (AIHW 2022; Health Workforce Australia 2014). Some analysts suggest that there is an over-supply of dentists (arising out of both graduate and immigration pathways) in relation to market demand. There has also been an increase in the number of dental practitioners working part time leading to speculation about unused capacity (DBA 2022; Duckett et al. 2019). However, there are still shortages in public sector settings, unresolved service distribution issues for rural and remote communities, and considerable unmet need in many at-risk population groups, and questionable capacity to address unmet need and improve equity (COAG Health Council 2015; Jean et al. 2020). There have also been changes in the oral health practitioner workforce, although largely related to the phasing-out of dental therapy and dental hygiene courses and their replacement with oral health therapist courses. Workforce modelling for these professions is hampered by a lack of consistent data on their practice activity and of sound evidence to inform modelling for workforce mix (COAG Health Council 2015; Health Workforce Australia 2014).

In 2019, a majority of dentists worked in the private sector (83%), with 42.5% working part-time. A majority of dentists work in major cities, resulting in dentist-to-population ratios of 65 per 100,000 people as compared with 37 per 100,000 people in outer regional areas and 28 per 100,000 people in remote areas. **Dental therapists (DT)** are the only practitioner group who are more prevalent in rural areas with 2.5 per 100,000 people in major cities, and 3.5 per 100,000 and 4 per 100,000 in outer regional and remote settings respectively. **Dental hygienist (DH)** distribution is like that of dentists (5.2 in cities, 2.4 outer regional and 1.2 in remote communities) and oral health therapists range from 6.9 per 100,000 people in cities to 3.4 per 100,000 people in remote settings (AIHW 2022). **Dental prosthetists**, who also mostly work in the private sector (78.2%) and make up about 5% of the dental workforce, have a similar distribution to dentists. In 2019 there were 1267 registered dental prosthetists, with an average ratio of 4.5 per 100,000 people (AIHW 2022). In recent years, the Commonwealth government has put in place some initiatives in an effort to remediate this misdistribution (AGDH 2019) (see Table 15.1). Table 15.3 shows the dental and oral health workforce characteristics for the years 2019–21, and the workforce growth compared with 2012.

Estimating dental technician and dental assistant numbers is difficult as they are not registered practitioners and because very little reliable data is collected other than self-reported census data. There are perceived shortages of dental assistants reported by the professions and the state and territory governments. Dental assistants may undertake Certificate III or IV courses in dental assisting through the **Vocational Education and Training (VET)** sector, although training is

TABLE 15.3   Numbers By Type of Dental Practitioners in Australia

Practitioner Type	Number of Registered Practitioners 2021[a] (% Total Workforce)	Number of Registered (% Total Workforce) in 2012[b]	Practitioner: Population Ratio /100,000[a] (By Location)	% Female[a] (2020)
Dentist	18,587 (74.4%)	14,687 (75.5%)	58.7	43.7
Specialist dentist	1743 (10%)	1330		
Dental therapist	973 (3.2%)	1276 (6.6%)	2.5	95.4
Dental hygienist	1479 (5.9%)	1600 (8.2%)	4.4	93.9
Oral health therapist	2,855 (9.4%)	738 (3.8%)	6.5	87.5
Dental prosthetist	1274 (5.1%)	1161 (6%)	4.5	18.5
TOTAL dental practitioners	24,406	19,462	Growth 2012–2021 = 3900 (20.7%)	52.6
Dental technician		3000		30.7
Dental assistant		19,000		98.2

Sources: a. Dental Board of Australia (2022); AIHW (2022).
b. AIHW (2014).

not currently mandatory and career paths are limited (Health Workforce Australia 2014). Dental technicians undertake workplace-based training or apprenticeships, also completing VET-sector training. There has been considerable growth in the dental technician workforce, with graduate numbers almost doubling between 2007 and 2014.

In recent years there has been an increasing recognition among general health practitioners and others outside the dental sector of the impact of oral disease. Oral disease recognition and referral and preventive advice have been incorporated into the practices of maternal and child health nurses, Aboriginal health workers, community and aged-care nurses, speech pathologists and mental health case workers, among others. The contributions made to oral health promotion and individual care goes largely unmeasured but is an important element of holistic health care and promotion (COAG Health Council 2015; National Advisory Committee on Oral Health 2004). There is also considerable opportunity to develop more holistic approaches to health care through inter-professional practice approaches that integrate oral health and around the common disease risk factors such as diet, smoking, trauma and cancer prevention and through collaborative health promotion approaches.

Dentists and Other Oral Health Practitioners

Dentists, who practise all parts of dentistry, including assessment, diagnosis, treatment, management and preventive services for patients of all ages, are the most readily recognised type of dental practitioner, but not the only one. **Dental prosthetists** work largely from private practices (78.4%) but also in the public sector, providing dentures, mouth guards and other appliances through consulting directly with patients. Dental prosthetists first train as dental technicians to manufacture dentures and dental appliances (through a VET-sector apprenticeship or diploma level qualification), and then complete additional training to enable registration for practice in direct patient care. Tasmania, in 1957, was the first jurisdiction to regulate the practice and title for prosthetists, who in some places are referred to as clinical dental technicians (Australian Dental Prosthetists Association 2022).

In Australia, **dental therapists** have practised for over 50 years, providing diagnostic, preventive, restorative and health promotion services to children and adolescents in a collaborative and referral relationship with dentists. Like their New Zealand counterparts (where they have practised for over 100 years), dental therapists have been responsible for their own diagnosis and treatment planning and have referred to dentists those patients with treatment needs beyond their scope of practice. Dental therapists have been the backbone of school dental services Australia-wide, working in metropolitan, regional, rural and remote settings with some of the population groups with the highest needs, including those with poor access to health services. Until 2000, dental therapists were limited to employment with school dental services, but today they practise in the public and private sectors, community health, hospitals and outreach programs. Likewise, **dental hygienists** have practised in Australia since the early 1970s (internationally for 100 years), providing preventive and periodontal (gum disease) services to people of all ages, mostly in private practice. They have traditionally practised in private practice settings in close collaboration with dentists; however, in recent years they too have moved into all areas that have needs matching their skills. Both types of practitioner originally developed to address areas of dental practice that were not being well served (children and prevention), in collaborative models of care designed to extend the capacity of dentists. More recently, a combination of the two has evolved to produce the **oral health therapist**. Australia currently has approximately 5300 oral health practitioners (see Table 15.3).

Dental therapists and dental hygienists provide primary health care services (dental examinations, diagnosis, treatment planning, preventive, orthodontic and health promotion services), with therapists also providing restorative services (fillings and simple extractions), and hygienists also providing maintenance care for periodontal conditions; these are the most common dental services required in the population. Oral health therapists are able to provide all of these services. Importantly, as autonomous practitioners who collaborate with dentists and refer people with needs beyond their scope of practice to a dentist (or other health practitioner), **oral health therapy practitioners** (dental hygienists, dental and oral health therapists) make an important contribution to the dental and oral health workforce (Case study 15.3). Research over many years has produced evidence that they provide services (within their scope) to the same quality as dentists, reliably recognise the boundaries of their practice and refer, can diagnose and plan treatment care in the most complex patients (including those with complex medical conditions and medications), and provide care that is acceptable to patients (Calache et al. 2009; Dooland 2014; Health Workforce Australia 2011; Hopcraft et al. 2008, 2011; Satur 2002; Satur et al. 2009; Satur & Moffat 2012).

Models of Care for Oral Health Therapy Practitioners

The practice of oral health therapists is situated in a primary health care/public health paradigm that emphasises

---

CASE STUDY 15.3 Oral Health Care in a Remote Aboriginal Community

Debbie is a dental therapist who has worked for 30 years providing remote-area oral health services in remote communities. She provides clinical dental services (check-ups, fillings, extractions and preventive treatments) for 0- to 18–year-olds and oral health promotion from a community-based clinic. She also provides outreach care for smaller, more remote communities, referring back to her own clinic in town for treatment services. Debbie works with the local Aboriginal health workers to ensure that all the eligible children and adolescents in her area receive care, collaborating with community nurses, elders and teachers and referring to a local GP for antibiotics when needed. She manages patients with rheumatic heart conditions and other complex issues locally, using the telephone or Zoom consultations when advice is required. There is a shortage of dentists up north, and a dentist employed by the public sector visits once every 2–3 months to handle cases beyond Debbie's scope of practice.

Mary, a 26-year-old mother of one of Debbie's patients (whom Debbie had routinely treated up until she was 18), presents with toothache – an acute and painful infection with swelling under the area of her lower jaw – asking for help. There is no dentist in the town, and due to staff shortages one will not visit for 6 weeks. The permanent tooth needs extracting (which Debbie was allowed to do up until 1990 before the regulations changed); antibiotics will reduce the infection, but the tooth needs to come out to allow the area to heal properly. Under current regulation and policy, Debbie cannot treat Mary in her clinic, and so Mary is evacuated by air to Darwin to have the tooth extracted at a cost of several thousand dollars.

Case Study Questions

1. What are some of the solutions for a situation like this?
2. Why are there not enough dental practitioners in remote areas?
3. Is this a private or a state/Commonwealth government problem?
4. What are the barriers to oral health for rural and remote residents?

prevention and health promotion, offering the opportunity to re-orient oral health services into more preventive models of care given the appropriate funding models. They graduate 'practice-ready' after completing three-year undergraduate Bachelor's degrees in oral health at university dental or health science faculties and, like dentists, are registered for practice by the Australian Health Practitioner Regulation Agency through the Dental Board of Australia (DBA 2022). Their courses are accredited, again like dentists, by the Australian Dental Council (2020). Where dentists may spend five or even seven years (via graduate-entry models) preparing for practice, oral health therapists offer lower-cost models of care through shorter practice preparation and lower salaries. They are more likely to work in rural and remote settings and outreach programs and offer the opportunity to free up dentists to focus on higher-technology and more complex care.

Oral health therapy practitioners offer considerable scope to extend the capacity of the dental care system by increasing the supply of services, and by working to reduce disease (demand) and extend the reach of public dental services into high-needs populations (supply) through these lower-cost models of care. Research in aged-care settings has shown that dental hygienists can reliably diagnose and plan oral health treatment for dependent people living in residential aged-care settings with high care needs (Hopcraft et al. 2008, 2011), offering the capacity to increase services to an ageing population (see Case study 15.1). Public-sector research has demonstrated that dental therapists can provide restorative care to both children (their traditional patient group) and adults (a more recent development) at the same level of quality and acceptability as dentists (Calache et al. 2009; Satur & Ryan 2014), and many studies have demonstrated their ability to appropriately refer people with needs beyond their scope of practice. Indeed, research over many years in many countries has provided evidence of the quality of care of both dental therapists and dental hygienists (Galloway et al. 2002; Nash et al. 2012; Satur 2002). Increasingly in Australia, they are also working in dental specialist practices including paedodontic, periodontic, prosthodontic and orthodontic practices, and in hospital and special-needs settings including cancer, cleft lip and palate, and HIV specialist units, and in outreach and remote communities.

In traditional private dental practice settings, dentists have been the first provider a patient would see, and they might then be referred to a hygienist or therapist for some components of care although this is changing in some practices. In the public-sector programs and school dental services, dental therapists have traditionally been the first practitioner to examine and treat patients, and only those with needs beyond the therapist's scope would be referred to a dentist. In recent times, many public-sector agencies have moved to utilising the dental or oral health therapist as the primary provider for all patients, with referral to dentists where needed (Teusner et al. 2016). This model offers increased primary prevention for all patients with lower costs of care and uses dentists' higher-level training for more complex care. Indeed, this model was recommended over 30 years ago by the World Health Organization (1990) and has been established as the main model of care in the Netherlands in recent years (Institute of Medicine of the National Academies 2009; den Boer et al. 2020). The real benefit (yet to be realised) would be a reduction in the costs of care and extension of services for high-needs and underserved population groups and patients by enabling practice to top of scope with team dentistry approaches for higher complexity service needs.

In addition to the clinical scope of practice, oral health therapy practitioners undertake preparation in the social sciences, behavioural sciences and health promotion (Australian Dental Council 2022). This preparation is designed to enable interprofessional practice and a focus on the social determinants of health to achieve improved oral health for the community. The vision is that these practitioners represent the capacity to 'un-silo' dentistry and integrate oral health in holistic ways. Collaboration with practitioners in the community, mental health, disability, nursing and welfare sectors is important to improving health generally, and oral health specifically (COAG Health Council 2015). The challenge, as with all health problems, is to re-orient health services and achieve a balance between clinical care and health promotion activity.

Debates Around Oral Health Therapy Practice

There are, of course, some current debates around the practice models of oral health practitioners. Originally, the practice of dental therapists and hygienists was tightly tied to that of dentists, with regulations requiring dentist supervision of their practice. This approach was reinforced by the professionally dominant monopolistic models of dentistry during their years of establishment, and there are discourses from vested interests that would return to these models (ADA 2013, 2018). Many of the arguments applied will be familiar to nurse practitioners. Contemporary health workforce frameworks have now largely been applied to oral health therapy practice, although vestiges of the old rhetoric remain in practice.

One issue held over from past practices relates to the age of people who can receive restorative services from dental and oral health therapists (originally only people over 5 and under 18 years old), arising from old school dental service policies and funding; these underpin understanding among many dentists and remain despite changes to education and national regulation (ADC 2022; Health Workforce Australia 2011; National Advisory Council on Dental Health 2012). There is evidence from Victoria and elsewhere that dental and oral health therapists provide excellent-quality services to preschoolers and adults and can provide comprehensive oral examinations, diagnosis and treatment planning as well as restorative services for people of all ages (Calache et al. 2009; Calache & Hopcraft 2012; Nash et al. 2012). Australian educational settings and dental regulation has accommodated the removal of age limits and the limits on the diagnostic ability of all oral health practitioners, but not everyone in the dentists' profession has recognised and utilised this (DBA 2022; Teusner et al. 2016; Satur 2009). There are still also impediments in state-based legislation around the use of X-ray machines, anaesthesia and medications that limit the ability of oral health practitioners to work and operate practices separately from a dentist.

Despite their autonomous practice, oral health practitioners are in many cases unable to charge directly for their services. Oral health practitioners have not had provider numbers, so their ability to directly bill funding organisations such as insurance companies and Medicare for their services has been problematic. Until recently, all their services were billed under dentists' provider numbers, which imposes a cost layer to billing and creates a bundled service model. As an example, dental therapists, dental hygienists and oral health

therapists can prescribe, interpret and expose X-rays but cannot bill for them – a dentist must sign the prescription and charge for the service. The move by Medicare to enable provider numbers for oral health practitioners for use with the CDBS from 1 July 2022 takes a modest step forward in this space. Some insurance companies have indicated they too will issue provider numbers, however many will not rebate services provided in private practices by dental hygienists or dental and oral health therapists – they must continue to use a dentist's provider number (ADOHTA 2022; Department of Health 2017; DHAA 2019). This results, in many cases, in people receiving services from an oral health therapy practitioner and being charged for those of a dentist. Commonwealth dental services for veterans have also used the same funding models (Department of Veterans' Affairs 2020). A further problem is that this conceals the true data about their contribution to service provision.

Pause *for* Reflection …

Which health practitioners have provider numbers? What would be the benefits of oral health practitioners being able to open their own practices separate from a dentist?

Workforce numbers in the oral health professions are low (around 20% of the dental workforce), and there are arguments to support the notion that increasing the numbers of oral health therapy graduates and decreasing those of dentists to achieve greater numerical parity would offer better service orientation in line with community needs. In our current climate of health sector innovation and reform, oral health therapists, dental therapists, dental hygienists and dental prosthetists offer significant opportunities to improve the way we deliver oral health services and can contribute to increasing access to oral health care, particularly for under-served populations and in the public sector. While the voice of dentists is the loudest and most obvious, the need to consider new ways of providing oral health care means that prevention and health promotion, full utilisation of the skills of the dental workforce, collaborative teamwork and interprofessional practice can re-orient our approaches to oral health and improve access to care.

SUMMARY

- Dental diseases are among the most prevalent and costly in our community.
- The Commonwealth Government funds only around 16% of dental services.
- Only about 45% of Australians have good access to oral health care.

- There is a range of dental practitioners other than dentists.
- There is potential to utilise oral health practitioners much more widely to improve access to care.

REVIEW QUESTIONS

1. Think about the range of dental practitioners and consider why dentists are the most visible. Why do you think the other practitioner types have developed?
2. Why do you think dental and oral health therapists were originally limited to providing fillings for people up to the age of 25? (Note: permanent teeth begin to come through at the age of 6, and by the age of 14 people have most of their permanent teeth.)
3. If 85% of dental services are provided from private practices, how do we ensure the provision of preventive services and health promotion? Will individuals pay for this? What sorts of programs and funding mechanisms do we need to encourage health professionals to provide health promotion services for individuals and communities?
4. How can we increase access to regular dental care for low-income people? Are there better models of care available to address dental diseases?
5. What inter-professional collaborative practice opportunities exist to improve oral health? How could oral health and general health practitioners work together given the barriers imposed by funding and service models?

REFERENCES

Alford, R., 1975. Health Care Politics: Ideological and Interest Group Barriers to Reform. University of Chicago Press, Chicago.

Australian Dental and Oral Health Therapist Association (ADOHTA), 2022. Member Update: Provider Numbers for Oral Health Practitioners, 31 March 2022, ADOHTA. https://www.adohta.net.au/resources/Documents/News/220331%20Joint%20Provider%20number%20member%20update.pdf.

Australian Dental Association (ADA), 2013. Hope for Scope Campaign. ADA, Sydney.

Australian Dental Association (ADA), 2018. ADA, Sydney.

Australian Dental Association (ADA), 2021. Guidelines for teledentistry. https://www.ada.org.au/Covid-19-Portal/Cards/Misc/Critical-Information-For-SA-Members/ADA-Guidelines-for-Teledentistry.

Australian Dental Council (ADC), 2020. Program accreditation standards and competencies. ADC, Melbourne. https://www.adc.org.au/accreditation.

Australian Dental Council (ADC), 2022. Professional Competencies of the Newly Qualified Dental Practitioner. ADC, Melbourne. https://www.adc.org.au/files/accreditation/competencies/ADC_Professional_Competencies_of_the_Newly_Qualified_Practitioner.pdf.

Australian Dental Prosthetists Association (ADPA), 2022. What is a dental prosthetist. ADPA, Melbourne. https://www.adpa.com.au/dentalprosthetistsandyou/what-is-a-dental-prosthetist.

Australian Government Department of Health (AGDH), 2019. Rural Health Multidisciplinary Training (RHMT) Program. https://www.health.gov.au/initiatives-and-programs/rhmt?utm_source=health.gov.au&utm_medium=callout-auto-custom&utm_campaign=digital_transformation.

Australian Institute of Health and Welfare (AIHW), 2014. Dental workforce, 2012. National Health Workforce Series no. 7. Cat. no. HWL 53. AIHW, Canberra.

Australian Institute of Health and Welfare (AIHW), 2018. A discussion of public dental waiting times information in Australia: 2013–14 to 2016–17. Cat. no. DEN 230. AIHW, Canberra. https://www.aihw.gov.au/getmedia/df234a9a-5c47-4483-9cf7-15ce162d3461/aihw-den-230.pdf.aspx?inline=true.

Australian Institute of Health and Welfare (AIHW), 2020a. Health Expenditure Australia 2019–20. Cat. no. HWE87. AIHW, Canberra. https://www.aihw.gov.au/reports/health-welfare-expenditure/health-expenditure-australia-2019-20/contents/about.

Australian Institute of Health and Welfare (AIHW), 2020b. Disparities in potentially preventable hospitalisations across Australia, 2012–13 to 2017–18. AIHW, Canberra.

Australian Institute of Health and Welfare (AIHW), 2021. Cancer data in Australia 2021. Cancer Compendium. Cat. no. CAN 144. AIHW, Canberra.

Australian Institute of Health and Welfare (AIHW), 2022. Oral health and dental care in Australia. Cat. no: DEN 231. AIHW, Canberra.

Australian Institute of Health and Welfare (AIHW), 2022a. Oral health and dental care in Australia. AIHW, Canberra. https://www.aihw.gov.au/reports/dental-oral-health/oral-health-and-dental-care-in-australia/contents/healthy-teeth.

Bacchi, C., 2016. Problematizations in health policy: questioning how "problems" are constituted in policies. Paper presented at the ASSA (Academy of the Social Sciences)-funded Workshop on Understanding Australian Policies on Public Health, Flinders University.

Calache, H., Hopcraft, M., 2012. Provision of oral health care to adult patients by dental therapists without the prescription of a dentist. J. Public Health Dent. 72, 19–27.

Calache, H., Shaw, J., Groves, V., et al., 2009. The capacity of dental therapists to provide direct restorative care to adults. Aust N Z J Public Health 33 (5), 424–429.

Chrisopoulos, S., Harford, J.E., Ellershaw, A., 2016. Oral health and dental care in Australia: key facts and figures 2015. Cat. no. DEN 229. AIHW, Canberra.

Commonwealth of Australia, 2020. Australia's Constitution, AGPS Canberra. https://www.aph.gov.au/About_Parliament/Senate/Powers_practice_n_procedures/Constitution.aspx.

Council of Australian Governments (COAG) Health Council, 2015. Healthy Mouths Healthy Lives: Australia's National Oral Health Plan 2015–2024, prepared by the National Oral Health Monitoring Committee, for AHMAC, Canberra. https://www.health.gov.au/resources/publications/healthy-mouths-healthy-lives-australias-national-oral-health-plan-2015-2024

den Boer, J.C.L., van der Sanden, W.J.M., Bruers, J.J.M. Developments in oral health care in the Netherlands between 1995 and 2018. BMC Oral Health 20, 192 (2020). https://doi.org/10.1186/s12903-020-01174-8.

Dental Board of Australia (DBA), 2020. Adapting to COVID-19: Teledentistry, clinical training, CPD and PII, https://www.dentalboard.gov.au/News/2020-04-22-Adapting-to-COVID19.aspx

Dental Board of Australia (DBA), 2020. Guidelines for scope of practice, AHPRA, Melbourne. https://www.dentalboard.gov.au/Codes-Guidelines/Policies-Codes-Guidelines/Guidelines-Scope-of-practice.aspx.

Dental Board of Australia (DBA), 2022. Registrant data April 2018– March 2022, Ahpra, Melbourne. https://www.dentalboard.gov.au/About-the-Board/Statistics.aspx.

Department of Health, 2017. Guide to the Child Dental Benefits Schedule. Department of Health, Canberra. https://www.health.gov.au/resources/publications/cdbs-guide-to-the-schedule

Dental Hygienists Association of Australia (DHAA), 2019. The power of Provider Numbers, DHAA. https://dhaa.info/common/Uploaded%20files/DHAA/Advocacy/For%20download%20DHAA_Stories_Spread_FIN-Small.pdf.

Department of Veterans' Affairs, 2020. Notes for Dental Service Providers. Australian Government, Canberra. https://www.dva.gov.au/providers/notes-fee-schedules-and-guidelines/notes-providers/notes-dental-service-providers

Dooland, M., 1992. Improving dental health in Australia. Background paper no. 9, National Health Strategy, Department of Health Housing and Community Services, AGPS, Canberra.

Dooland, M., 2014. Revolutionising public dental health, The Health Advocate. Australian Health and Hospitals Association, Canberra.

Duckett, S., Cowgill, M., Swerissen, H., 2019. Filling the gap: A universal dental scheme for Australia. Grattan Institute, Melbourne.

Galloway, J., Gorham, J., Lambert, M., et al., 2002. The professionals complementary to dentistry: systematic review and synthesis. University College London, Eastman Dental Hospital, Dental Team Studies Unit, London.

Health Workforce Australia, 2011. Scope of practice review – oral health practitioners, HWA, Adelaide.

Health Workforce Australia, 2014. Australia's future health workforce – oral health (detailed report). Commonwealth Department of Health, Canberra.

Holden, A., Shaban, R., Spallek, H., 2021. COVID-19 and the dental profession: professional tensions and ethical quandaries; a COVID-19 Sydney policy paper in depth, authored by University of Sydney experts.

Hopcraft, M., Farmer, G., 2021. Impact of COVID-19 on the provision of paediatric dental care: Analysis of the Australian Child Dental Benefits Schedule. M Community Dent Oral Epidemiol. 49 (4), 369–376. doi: 10.1111/cdoe.12611.

Hopcraft, M.S., Morgan, M.V., Satur, J.G., et al., 2008. Dental service provision in Victorian residential aged care facilities. Aust Dent J 53 (3), 239–245.

Hopcraft, M.S., Morgan, M.V., Satur, J.G., et al., 2011. Utilizing dental hygienists to undertake dental examination and referral in residential aged care facilities. Community Dent. Oral Epidemiol. 39 (4), 378–384.

Institute of Medicine of the National Academies (IOM), 2009. The U.S. Oral Health Workforce in the Coming Decade: Workshop Summary. National Academies Press, Washington USA.

Jean, G., Kruger, E., Tennant, M., 2020. Distribution of private dental practices and dentists 2011 and 2018: Analysis by regional area. Aust J Rural Health 28 (5), 453–461.

Lewis, J., 2000. From 'fightback' to 'biteback': the rise and fall of a national dental program. Aust. J. Pub. Admin. 59 (1), 60–72.

Nash, D.A., Friedman, J.W., Mathu-Muju, K.M., et al., 2012. A Review of the Global Literature on Dental Therapists: In the Context of the Movement to Add Therapists to the

Oral Health Workforce in the United States. The Kellogg Foundation, Battle Creek, MI.

National Advisory Committee on Oral Health, 2004. Healthy Mouths Healthy Lives: Australia's National Oral Health Plan 2004–2013. South Australian Department of Health, Adelaide.

National Advisory Council on Dental Health (NACDH), 2012. Report of the National Advisory Council on Dental Health, Commonwealth Department of Health, Canberra.

Nguyen T.M., Tonmukayakul, U., Calache, H., 2021. Dental restrictions to clinical practice during the COVID-19 pandemic: an Australian perspective. JDR Clin Trans Res 6 (3), 291–294. doi: 10.1177/23800844211000341.

Poirier, B., Jensen, E., Sethi, S., 2022. The evolution of the teledentistry landscape in Australia: a scoping review. Aust J Rural Health. doi: 10.1111/ajr.12874.

Parliament of Australia (PoA), 2013. Bridging the dental gap: report on the inquiry into adult dental services, House of Representatives Standing Committee on Health and Ageing, (Chair, J. Hill), Commonwealth of Australia, Canberra.

Productivity Commission, 2017. Introducing competition and informed user choice into human services: reforms to human services. Report no. 85, Canberra. Chapter 12: Public dental services. https://www.pc.gov.au/inquiries/completed/human-services/reforms/report.

Productivity Commission, 2018. Report on government services 2018. Part E, Chapter 10 Primary and community health. https://www.pc.gov.au/research/ongoing/report-on-government-services/2018/health/primary-and-community-health.

Productivity Commission, 2022. Chapter 10: Primary and Community Health in Report on Government Services. https://www.pc.gov.au/research/ongoing/report-on-government-services/2022/health/primary-and-community-health.

Satur, J., 2002. Australian dental policy reform and the utilisation of dental therapists and hygienists, PhD thesis. Deakin University, Melbourne.

Satur, J., Gussy, M., Mariño, R., et al., 2009. Patterns of dental therapists' scope of practice and employment in Victoria, Australia. J Dent Educ 73 (3), 416–425.

Satur, J., Moffat, S., 2012. Chapter 1: History of Oral Health Professions in Australia and New Zealand:1–6, & Chapter 2: Development of oral health therapy:17–26. In: Tsang, A. (Ed), Oral Health Therapy in Australia and New Zealand. Knowledge Books, Sydney.

Satur, J., Ryan, B.M., 2014. Adult dental therapy practice – 20 years in the making. Aust N Z J Dental Oral Health Therapy 2, 1–6.

South Australian Department of Health, 2014. Better oral health in residential care program – Staff Portfolio and Training program, South Australian Department of Health, Adelaide. https://www.sahealth.sa.gov.au/wps/wcm/connect/09fa99004358886a979df72835153af6/BOHRC_Staff_Portfolio_Full_Version%5B1%5D.pdf?MO

D=AJPERES&CACHEID=ROOTWORKSPACE-09fa99004358886a979df72835153af6-nKKIHMM

Spencer, A.J., 2004. Narrowing the inequality gap in oral health and dental care in Australia. Commissioned paper series 2004. Australian Health Policy Institute, University of Sydney.

State Government of Victoria, 2019. Smile Squad Program. https://www.smilesquad.vic.gov.au/.

Teusner, D.N., Amarasena, N., Satur, J., et al., 2016. Dental service provision by oral health therapists, dental hygienists and dental therapists in Australia: implications for workforce modelling. Community Dental Health 33 (1), 15–22.

World Health Organization (WHO), Expert Committee on Educational Imperatives for Oral Health Workforce, 1990. Change or Decay? Educational imperatives for oral health workforce. Report of a WHO Expert Committee, Technical Report Series 794, WHO, Geneva.

FURTHER READING

Council of Australian Governments (COAG) Health Council, 2015. Australian National Oral Health Plan 2015–2024. COAG Health Council, Canberra.

Duckett, S., Cowgill, M., Swerissen, H., 2019. Filling the gap: a universal dental scheme for Australia. Grattan Institute.

Health Workforce Australia (HWA), 2011. Scope of practice review – oral health practitioners, HWA, Adelaide. https://www.yumpu.com/en/document/read/35043590/scope-of-practice-review-health-workforce-australia

House Standing Committee on Health and Ageing, 2013. Bridging the dental gap: report on the inquiry into adult dental services in Australia. Parliament of Australia, Canberra. www.aph.gov.au/parliamentary_business/committees/house_of_representatives_committees?url=haa/dental/report.htm.

National Advisory Council on Dental Health, 2012. Final report of the National Advisory Council on Dental Health. Department of Health, Canberra. https://apo.org.au/node/28453

Productivity Commission, 2017. Introducing competition and informed user choice into human services: reforms to human services. Report no. 85, Canberra. Chapter 12: Public dental services. https://www.pc.gov.au/inquiries/completed/human-services/reforms/report.

ONLINE RESOURCES

ADOHTA – Australian Dental and Oral Health Therapists' Association: https://www.adohta.net.au/.

Dental Hygienists' Association of Australia: https://www.dhaa.info/.

16

Digital Health and the Divide

Sandeep Reddy

KEY LEARNING OUTCOMES

When you finish this chapter you should be able to:
- describe the digital health landscape in Australia
- understand the importance of electronic health records in digital health strategy
- identify various digital health applications to improve health outcomes
- recognise the digital divide separating urban and regional Australia
- examine the role digital health plays in the Indigenous health context in Australia.

KEY TERMS AND ABBREVIATIONS

Australian Digital Health Agency (ADHA)

digital divide

electronic health record (EHR)

mobile-driven health service delivery

My Health Record (MHR)

Medicare Benefits Schedule (MBS)

National Broadband Network (NBN)

Personally Controlled Electronic Health Record (PCEHR)

telehealth

INTRODUCTION

Australians are increasingly spending time online and utilising various forms of digital technology. The Digital Inclusion Index, which considers access, affordability and digital ability, went up from 52.7 in 2014 to 60.2 in 2018 for Australia (Thomas et al. 2018); 80% of Australians now own smartphones and 73% of Australians use the internet to research health issues. The network readiness of Australia was ranked as high as 18 in a list of 139 countries in 2016. As of June 2018, there were 14.7 million internet subscribers in Australia and there were about 27 million mobile handset subscribers (Australian Institute of Health and Welfare (AIHW) 2020). As digital technologies achieve scale, the cost of deploying them has decreased. Organisations that invested early in digital technologies have begun to see the benefits of the investment in the form of labour and process cost savings (Blackburn et al. 2017; Thomas et al. 2018).

DIGITAL HEALTH

The advent of internet and digital technologies has also led to new avenues for engaging patients to adopt healthy lifestyles and to be more involved with health services (Blackburn et al. 2017; Meskó et al. 2017). Coupled with this the proliferation of smart devices that collect health data and delivery of health care through online services has presented new options for treatment and management of diseases. This approach of utilising digital technology to deliver health care so that different points of care are electronically securely connected has been termed digital health (Australian Digital Health Agency (ADHA) 2017). More formally, digital health has been defined as 'the cultural transformation of how disruptive technologies that provide digital and objective data accessible to both caregivers and patients leads to an equal level doctor–patient relationship with shared decision-making and democratization of care' (Meskó et al. 2017, p. 1). Digital health encompasses a range of technologies that can be employed to treat and manage patients while in the process collate and share their information. The discipline includes applications such as mobile health, electronic health records, telehealth, artificial intelligence and wearable devices (AIHW 2020).

Incorporating digital technologies in health care enables automation and simplification of some processes, facilitates better connectivity amongst different parts of the health system and assists in better reporting with the use of advanced analytics (ADHA 2017; Blackburn et al. 2017; National E-Health Transition Authority 2016). Also, the adoption of digital technologies is said to improve access to health care to currently disadvantaged communities by enabling new models of care delivery and improving health literacy (ADHA 2017; Blackburn et al. 2017). These aspects will be explored further into the chapter. It has been stated that digitisation of health care delivery can reduce overall health care expenditure in Australia by 8%–12% and considerably improve the quality of health care by reducing adverse drug events, duplication of tests and re-admissions (Blackburn et al. 2017). On the other hand, movement to digital health can bring problems of its own such as exacerbating access to care for those who do not have access to digital infrastructure (discussed further in a later section), risks to privacy and security of data (Australian Association of Practice Management 2017). While privacy and inappropriate access is a concern even for non-digitally enabled health records, the risks accentuate with a digital health system.

Pause *for* Reflection …

It has been stated that digitisation of health care can reduce health care costs and enable democratisation of care. How do you think this occurs?

ELECTRONIC HEALTH RECORD

Electronic health records (EHRs) are considered to be the flagship application of a digital health strategy. An electronic health record has been described as a longitudinal compilation of health information about individual patients and population stored electronically (Gunter & Terry 2005). National EHRs provide a platform for integrating health care information currently collected through several sources thus enabling

improvement in quality of care. Such health data repositories provide opportunities for research and analysis of the aggregated data such that evidence-based health care strategies can be adopted by governments and health care providers. Also, increased efficiency in health care delivery can be achieved through improved data sharing, reduced medical errors, improved data security, patient empowerment and time saving for staff (ADHA 2017).

In Australia, the National E-Health Transition Authority (NEHTA) was set up in 2005 to implement a national EHR (National E-Health Transition Authority 2016). The other objectives of NEHTA were to hasten the adoption of e-health by delivering required integration infrastructure and health information standards and lead the development of a security framework to enable authorised only access to data. In 2011, the NEHTA initiated a national EHR application termed '**Personally Controlled Electronic Health Record (PCEHR)**' (Morrison et al. 2011; Pearce & Bainbridge 2014). PCEHR was based on a previous 'Better Patient Management' model, which was an Australia-wide secure electronic system for medication management. With PCEHR, patients were to have a secure access portal through which they could view their medical history supplied by various health care providers they had visited. The PCEHR portal would display the patient's health summary, demographic information, medical conditions, medications and allergies (Pearce & Bainbridge 2014). An index and search function would yield a range of personal health care information including referrals, test results and prescriptions (Fig. 16.1).

In 2013, the Australian Government commissioned a review of the progress with the implementation of the PCEHR system (National E-Health Transition Authority 2016). Based on the recommendations from the review, which outlined the need of a dedicated digital health agency to drive the national EHR implementation and strengthen digital health infrastructure in the nation, the 2015–2016 budget allocated funding to establish a national digital health entity (ADHA 2018a). In July 2016, the **Australian Digital Health Agency (ADHA)** commenced operations as a statutory authority reporting to the states and territories health ministers. The ADHA was tasked to improve the health outcomes of all Australians by setting up a national EHR, improving the digital health infrastructure and pursuing the national digital health strategy.

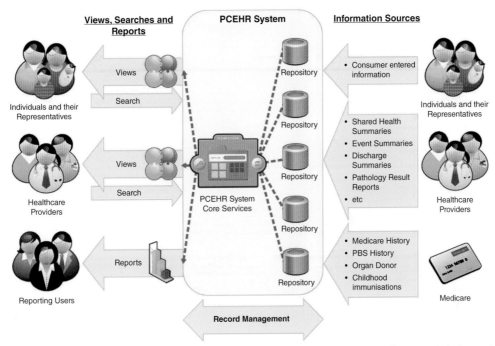

Figure 16.1 PCEHR System. Source: Pearce, C., Bainbridge, M. (2014). A personally controlled electronic health record for Australia. J Am Med Inform Assoc 21 (4), 707–713.

A key objective of the ADHA was to transition the PCEHR to a national **'My Health Record (MHR)'** (National E-Health Transition Authority 2016). The record would by the end of 2018 be created for everyone unless they choose not to do so (Australian Healthcare and Hospitals Association (AHHA) 2018). It was expected that approximately 98% of Australians would have a health record after 2018. An opt-out period would be available for anyone who would not choose to have their medical records saved on the MHR system. This means a child born in 2018 and whose parents have chosen to retain the medical records of the child on the MHR system would potentially many years later have all their health information accessible from one place. The ADHA would partner with the 31 Primary Health Networks and other Healthcare Clinical Information System Providers to source medical information of patients. The MHR is to enable secure health information exchange, better availability and access to prescriptions and medicine information, and drive digital-enabled models of care. Just as with the PCEHR, a shared health summary, event summary, discharge summary, referral letters, and prescription records can be accessed via a

national consumer portal viewed through a compatible web browser (Fig. 16.2).

While many medical, professional and consumer bodies welcomed the introduction of a national EHR system and the opt-out approach bearing in mind the significant delays it took to implement the PCEHR, many quarters of society raised concerns about the opt-out process and privacy aspects of the stored information (ABC Science 2018). The Australian Government and ADHA reacted to the concerns by extending the previously designated period to opt out and by progressing legislative amendments as to who can access the MHR data and highlighting the sophisticated cyber-security protection mechanism and regular audit processes (ADHA 2018b). In November 2018 in Australia more than 700 public hospitals and health services were using the My Health Record system to upload care summaries for patients with a My Health Record (AIHW 2020). Also, over 23 million Australians now have a My Health Record containing relevant clinical information. However, the engagement with My Health Record by patients and their carers is varied due to inadequate computerisation of various clinical practices, and

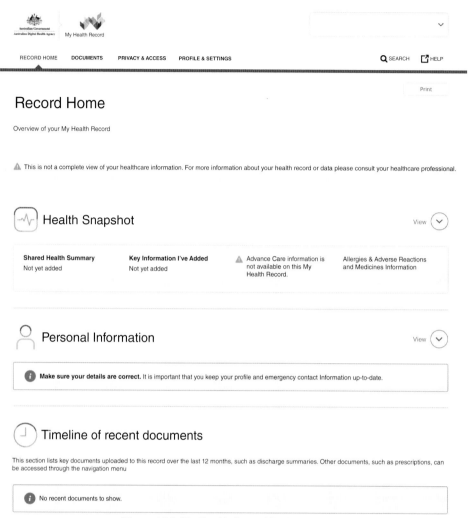

Figure 16.2 My Health Record Patient Portal.

variable user experience for clinicians (Hambleton & Alozios 2019). Yet, with the opt-out approach, it is expected that My Health Record will reach a critical mass and become embedded in routine clinical workflow. Table 16.1 summarises the key digital health developments in the Australian health care system so far.

Bacchi discusses, in her 'What's the problem represented to be' approach, how policies have problem representations contained within them (Bacchi 2016). If we adopt this line of thinking, it is easy to foresee the tensions between the government and the patient community over privacy concerns continue and ongoing amendments or updated policies issued to address these concerns.

Pause *for* Reflection ...
While EHRs have demonstrated improvement in quality of clinical care and communication, some have questioned whether benefits can be realised without related changes in the health system such as introduction of appropriate models of care and adequate funding. There are also barriers such as resistance to adoption of the EHR by clinicians. What other barriers do you foresee with the implementation of a national EHR?

For further demonstration of these points see Case study 16.1.

TABLE 16.1 Major Digital Health Developments in Australia

Year	Major Developments
2000	Aiming to provide a national electronic medical record, the MediConnect initiative is launched.
2004	MediConnect is absorbed into the HealthConnect program with a change in focus to support existing state-based projects.
2005	The National E-Health Transition Authority (NEHTA) is established with a mandate to develop the specifications, standards and infrastructure for an interconnected health sector.
2012	Personally Controlled Electronic Health Record (PCEHR) is launched.
2016	The Australian Digital Health Agency (ADHA) is launched and PCEHR is renamed My Health Record.
2017	ADHA develops the National Digital Health Strategy.
2019	All Australians have a My Health Record, unless they choose not to (opt-out process).

Source: Hambleton, S.J., Aloizos AM, J. (2019). Australia's digital health journey. Med J Aust, 210, S5–S6.

OTHER DIGITAL HEALTH APPLICATIONS IN AUSTRALIA

The national digital health strategy alongside driving the implementation of a national EHR intends to establish digital-enabled models of health care that improve accessibility, quality, safety and efficiency of clinical care. One of the digital health approaches that can enable this in the Australian geographical context is 'telehealth' (Australian Telehealth Society 2017). Telehealth is described as health care delivery or related processes utilising digital technologies to participants separated by distance. Health care delivery is slowly starting to see a shift from traditional face-to-face appointments to remote consultations, which are of lower cost and easier access. Almost every known medical specialty in Australia is now using telehealth approaches (e.g. for further application of these points see Case study 16.2). Of the medical specialties, the image-focused specialties such as radiology, dermatology and pathology have the most mature telehealth applications. Other clinical activities that can be supported by telehealth models include health promotion, diagnosis, treatment and monitoring of chronic conditions, and team-based health care delivery. States and territories in Australia have adopted telehealth programs for many years now with Queensland, Northern Territory and Western Australia having advanced models. Also, the rollout of the **National Broadband Network (NBN)** across

---

CASE STUDY 16.1 Establishing the First Digital Tertiary Hospital in Australia

Digital health care delivery is well established in primary health care settings but not so much in acute care settings. Princess Alexandra Hospital is a major adult teaching hospital in Queensland with 6529 staff and 833 overnight beds (Sullivan et al. 2016). In 2016, the hospital was chosen to become Australia's first tertiary digital hospital. Becoming a digital hospital in this context included establishing an EHR system and enabling integrated digital vital sign monitoring, digital medication management and digital ECG records. The digital implementation process took place over an 18-month period, but the digital conversion occurred rapidly over the last 2 weeks. To achieve the objectives, an implementation team including practising clinicians was established. Large amounts of training (approximately 32,000 hours) was provided to relevant staff including practice of scenarios before and after digitisation occurred. Also, an independent patient safety team was established to monitor adverse events during the course of implementation.

The main technical challenges the implementation team faced included reconciling the legacy and new systems, disruption of normal workflow, slowing down of procedural efficiencies and ensuring clinicians could retrieve significant amounts of clinical data for their patients from the new EHR system (Sullivan et al. 2016). The benefits of the implementation were that patient records were now readily available throughout the hospital, digital recording of vital signs and ECGs were more accessible, there was improved clinical decision support and electronic data audits could now be conducted. It was also found that there was a 50% reduction in the rate of cost growth, a 14% reduction in medication incidents, 17% fewer emergency re-admissions and a 19% reduction in medical imaging (AHHA 2018).

CASE STUDY 16.2   The Royal Institute for Deaf and Blind Children (RIDBC) Teleschool

The RIDBC Teleschool established in 2005 provides education and therapy for children with vision and hearing impairment across regional and remote Australia (Telstra 2017). Research has identified children with such impairments benefit from early intervention and specialist support. The Teleschool utilises various digital technologies to provide high-end and in-home video-conferencing services to involved children and families. RIDBC specialist support involves audiology, speech pathology, occupational therapy, physiotherapy and psychology support. Services from the Teleschool includes assessments, individual sessions, group parent sessions, spoken language development and transition to school support. These services are delivered through a combination of video-conferencing, web-based multimedia programs, mobile applications and face-to-face meetings. Parents have stated the programs offered by the Teleschool have not only benefited their children but also improved their confidence and knowledge of the impairments their children have.

Australia presents a promising opportunity for a broader telehealth network to be achieved. Though, the varied access to appropriate digital equipment amongst health providers to deliver telehealth services means this digital health approach is yet to achieve its full potential (Ellis 2004).

Telehealth had been well established in Australia even before the SARS-CoV-2 pandemic (Taylor et al. 2021). However, the focus was on reducing patients' travel to specialist centres by supporting care in the patient's residence or nearby health facilities. The Australian Government provided payments to specialists as part of the **Medicare Benefits Schedule (MBS)**. There was no funding or support for telehealth delivered by general practitioners (GPs). However, the onset of the pandemic led to the Australian Government introducing temporary MBS telehealth items in 2020 (Desborough et al. 2022). The intention was to reduce the risk of SARS-CoV-2 (COVID-19) transmission and protect patients and health care providers alike. The temporary telehealth support for GPs from the Australian Government has, since January 2022, become permanent with some conditions. Eligible patients can continue to receive telehealth services from GPs, nursing, midwifery, and allied health services where it is considered clinically appropriate. However, 'hotspot' telephone consultations between patients and GPs where prior clinical relationship did not exist are no longer supported by the MBS. To sustain the ongoing use of telehealth, there has been a call to develop the workforce skilled in using telehealth, develop national IT infrastructure to support telehealth, improve interoperability between various patient information systems and integrate telehealth into routine care (Thomas et al. 2020).

Mobile devices are playing a huge role in the digital economy with mobile devices exceeding the human population (Rich & Miah 2014). Consequently, the role of mobile devices and application in health is rapidly increasing. **Mobile-driven health service delivery** can operate where there is no cabled infrastructure. Health and technology entities are increasingly releasing mobile applications whereby an individual patient's health information is collected, recorded and shared with health providers (Meskó et al. 2017; Park et al. 2016). The health data is then used by health providers to variously monitor and manage health conditions. Mobile medical applications, which are defined by the Therapeutic Goods Administration as health-related applications that intend to diagnose or provide therapy, are increasingly used by Australian health care providers in various domains such as preventive health, chronic disease management and mental health (Blackburn et al. 2017) (Case study 16.3 applies in more detail). Mobile health applications have potential to reach vulnerable populations and communities where otherwise other digital technologies cannot be utilised. However, a barrier to wider spread of mobile health is the presence of 'blackspots' (areas with limited or no mobile coverage) (Perlgut 2011; Telstra 2017). While there is a rectification process underway, the vast geographical nature of Australia means there will always be areas where limited mobile coverage abounds.

In the recent period, several COVID-19 related applications have been developed to support contact tracing, surveillance, vaccination, and diagnosis and management amongst other applications (Whitelaw et al. 2020). In Australia, digital technology has been prominent in contact tracing (Goggin 2020; Vogt et al. 2022). Contact tracing is a core public health response to the outbreak of COVID-19. Australia introduced a contact tracing application, based on Singapore's TraceTogether application, called COVIDSafe. The application was

---

CASE STUDY 16.3 Mobile Application to Screen Chronic Diseases

The Brisbane North Primary Health Network (then Metro North Brisbane Medicare Local) launched a mobile application called 'HealthNavigator' in 2014 to provide chronic disease risk assessment, linkage to local general practitioners and access to lifestyle programs and a personalised health report (Seneviratne et al. 2018). The assessments were to be conducted by community health workers or self-administered. The Primary Health Network through an initiative targeted ethnically diverse communities and over a period of 12 months, 2013 assessments were recorded. Of the recorded assessments a total of 41.3% of subjects reported a birthplace outside Australia. Subjects screened by the facilitators were found to have a higher risk of cardiovascular and type 2 diabetes scores compared with the subjects who undertook self-administered assessments. However, there were no significant differences in socio-economic profile of participants screened by facilitated assessments compared with participants undertaking self-administered ones. Evaluation of the mobile application indicates embedding mobile applications in community screening implementation helps with rapid assessments of community risk profiles and translates national guidelines into personalised recommendations.

---

based on a decentralised model using a smartphone proximity tracing approach (Vogt et al. 2022). COVIDSafe would exchange coded information with other smartphone application users via Bluetooth signals and, if a user tested positive, the application would be used by authorities with consent from the user for contact tracing. The costs of developing and operating the COVIDSafe application has been estimated to be over $6 million. However, a subsequent evaluation identified that COVIDSafe had a reduced sensitivity in tracing contacts and was not sufficiently effective to contribute to the public health response to SARS-CoV-2 (COVID-19). This experience indicates effectiveness evaluations have to be integrated into design and implementation of such applications to justify the investment (Vogt et al. 2022).

THE DIGITAL DIVIDE

Australia's growth in overall digitisation is because of increases in digital usage and digital labour. However, the digitisation is uneven across Australia and there has been slow growth in digital infrastructure (Telstra 2017; Willis & Tranter 2006). While the NBN has been the highest profile digital infrastructure program by the government, its aims of connecting all Australians and bridging the **digital divide** has been at best sluggish (Perlgut 2011). The current uneven spread, limitations of technology systems, and access to internet and digital technology has contributed to the digital divide in Australia. National digital connectivity is not only imperative to economic success and positive social dynamics but also important for achieving high-quality health care especially for rural and regional communities and Indigenous Australians (Blackburn et al. 2017; Thomas et al. 2018). Yet, it seems problems lie within the government's current NBN policies and plans where the objective is not so much to improve the bandwidth of internet access but ensure all Australians are connected to broadband internet (Bacchi 2016). This policy may not address the technical requirements for digital health delivery, which relies on large bandwidth and fast internet speeds (ADHA 2017; Australian Telehealth Society 2017; National E-Health Transition Authority 2016).

DIGITAL HEALTH IN RURAL AND REMOTE AUSTRALIA

The degree of remoteness and other geographical and resource indicators impact on the cost and delivery of health services. It has been found rural and remote communities in Australia have lesser access to health services compared to their urban counterparts and consequently face poorer health outcomes (Rural Doctors Association of Australia 2017). Digital technologies have an important role in addressing these gaps by enabling affordable access to health care services. While a digital divide exists between city and country, development of the national digital health strategy and the roll-out of the NBN provides an opportunity to reverse the widening digital divide and aid improved diagnostic, treatment and management of health conditions for rural and remote communities (ADHA 2017; Blackburn et al. 2017).

The national digital health strategy outlines that the digital divide can be addressed through use of appropriate technology and information services to improve access to care and support appropriate models of care, sustainable workforce and collaborative partnerships (ADHA 2017). A pragmatic step is to leverage the existing infrastructure to enhance adoption of digital health technologies to overcome the challenge of distance. Of the technologies, telehealth is a leading option (Australian Telehealth Society 2017). However, the telehealth services have to be designed for the rural consumer with input from clinicians/health care providers for the services to be user appropriate and sustainable (Ellis 2004). Also, digital health care delivery has to consider current technological limitations so appropriate designs are incorporated in delivery. This bespoke approach ensures development of models of care appropriate to the rural and remote setting. The Northern Territory and South Australian health services have actively used telehealth services to increase attendance at their rural and remote clinics, foster collegial decision-making and encourage knowledge sharing between urban and rural clinicians (ADHA 2017; Blackburn et al. 2017).

DIGITAL HEALTH IN THE INDIGENOUS HEALTH CONTEXT

The poorer health status of Indigenous Australians compared with non-Indigenous Australians is well known (Commonwealth of Australia 2017). The 2017 Closing the Gap Prime Minister's report, while outlining the health of Indigenous Australians was slowly improving, noted that the current rate of progress in lessening the gap was insufficient. This gap is exacerbated for Indigenous Australians living in rural and remote areas. In addition to the geographical disadvantage, language and culture can be additional barriers. Studies have identified that digital technologies can be used as a cost-effective approach to overcome Indigenous disadvantage by affirming the Indigenous identity and providing culturally relevant information (Smith & McQuire 2016).

In the context of health, cultural identity is important for Indigenous Australians. Digital technologies have been found to be useful in reinvigorating Indigenous cultural practices (Smith & McQuire 2016). There is potential for the digital infrastructure that is being rolled out in regional and rural areas to build strong health literacy for Indigenous Australians. Digital health services can be used as a creative and cost-effective opportunity to increase engagement of Indigenous Australians through provision of culturally appropriate and evidence-based interventions (Dingwall et al. 2015; Smith & McQuire 2016).

The take-up of the MHR system has the potential to improve Indigenous health outcomes through the process of improved Indigenous health data collection and analysis of the same such that Indigenous health programs can be evidence based and informed by research (ADHA 2017). Further, the national digital health strategy states telehealth could be an important medium in ensuring timely access to health care services for Indigenous Australians enabling early diagnosis and early intervention. In addition, mobile applications have also been found to be effective in improving access to various health services for rural and remote Indigenous Australia (Dingwall et al. 2015). These digital health initiatives incorporating inclusive design principles can be an important factor in closing the health gap for Indigenous Australians.

Pause *for* Reflection ...

The establishment of the Australian Digital Health Agency and the roll-out of the National Broadband Infrastructure present opportunities to increase delivery of health care through digital technologies. However, with poor access to the internet in rural communities and poor health literacy and engagement amongst Indigenous Australians, the digital divide may be harder to address. What measures could the government and health providers adopt to enhance the impact of digital health in these populations?

■ SUMMARY

- Australian organisations and services are increasingly becoming digitised.
- The advent of various digital technologies has presented an opportunity to harness them to deliver health care services.
- Of the various forms of digital health applications being used to deliver health care in Australia are EHRs, telehealth services and mobile health applications.

- The Australian Digital Health Agency is leading the implementation of a national EHR process (MHR) and the national digital health strategy.
- While telehealth had been well established in Australia before the SARS-CoV-2 pandemic, the onset of the pandemic led to increased funding for telehealth.
- While the prevalence of digital infrastructure is increasing, there exists a digital divide between the city

and country populations. The non-uniform spread of digital infrastructure means different digital health delivery models have to be explored.

- Also, there exists a digital health divide between the rest of Australia, and regional and rural communities and Indigenous Australians. Yet, digital health has great prospects in contributing to the health of these disadvantaged communities.

REVIEW QUESTIONS

1. What benefits does incorporation of digital technologies in delivery of health care bring?
2. How do electronic health records increase quality and efficiency in health care delivery?
3. What has led to a digital divide in Australia? How can this be addressed?
4. How can digital health improve the health outcomes of rural and Indigenous Australians?

REFERENCES

ABC Science, 2018. My Health Record opt-out period begins, but privacy concerns remain. https://www.abc.net.au/news/science/2018-07-16/my-health-record-experts-say-its-safe-privacy-concerns-remain/9981658.

Australian Association of Practice Management, 2017. Digital health for better health: the role of practice managers. December, 1–9. AAPM, Melbourne.

Australian Digital Health Agency (ADHA), 2017. Safe, seamless and secure: evolving health and care to meet the needs of modern Australia. National Digital Health Strategy, 1–63. https://conversation.digitalhealth.gov.au/sites/default/files/adha-strategy-doc-2ndaug_0_1.pdf.

Australian Digital Health Agency (ADHA), 2018a. About the Agency. https://www.digitalhealth.gov.au/about-the-agency.

Australian Digital Health Agency (ADHA), 2018b. Opt out of My Health Record. Media release. https://www.digital-health.gov.au/search/query:Opt%20out%20of%20My%20Health%20Record.

Australian Healthcare and Hospitals Association (AHHA), 2018. Digital healthcare. Health Advocate, 1–44. https://ahha.asn.au/system/files/docs/publications/jun2018_tha_web_0.pdf.

Australian Institute of Health and Welfare, 2020. Digital health. AIHW, Canberra. https://www.aihw.gov.au/reports/australias-health/digital-health.

Australian Telehealth Society, 2017. National digital health strategy – a submission to the Australian Digital Health Agency. https://conversation.digitalhealth.gov.au/sites/default/files/2017-05/Australasian%20Telehealth%20Society%20-%20Your%20Health%20Your%20Say%20Submission%202017.pdf.

Bacchi, C., 2016. Problematizations in health policy: questioning how "problems" are constituted in policies. SAGE Open 6 (2), 1–16. doi:10.1177/2158244016653986.

Blackburn, S., Freeland, M., Gartner, D., 2017. Digital Australia: seizing the opportunity from the Fourth Industrial Revolution. Digital Australia, McKinsey. https://www.mckinsey.com/featured-insights/asia-pacific/digital-australia-seizing-opportunity-from-the-fourth-industrial-revolution.

Commonwealth of Australia, 2017. Closing the Gap Prime Minister's report 2017. Commonwealth of Australia, Department of the Prime Minister and Cabinet, p. 112. doi:10.5117/9789053565742.

Desborough, J., Hall Dykgraaf, S., Sturgiss, E., et al., 2022. What has the COVID-19 pandemic taught us about the use of virtual consultations in primary care? Aust J Gen Pract 51 (3), 179–183. doi:10.31128/AJGP-09-21-6184.

Dingwall, K.M., Puszka, S., Sweet, M., et al., 2015. Evaluation of a culturally adapted training course in Indigenous e-mental health. Australas Psychiatry 23 (6), 630–635. doi:10.1177/1039856215608282.

Ellis, I., 2004. Is telehealth the right tool for remote communities? Improving health status in rural Australia. Contemp Nurse 16 (3), 163–168.

Goggin, G., 2020. COVID-19 apps in Singapore and Australia: reimagining healthy nations with digital technology. Media Int Aust 177 (1), 61–75. doi:10.1177/1329878X20949770.

Gunter, T.D., Terry, N.P., 2005. The emergence of national electronic health record architectures in the United States and Australia: models, costs, and questions. J Med Internet Res 7 (1), 1–11. doi:10.2196/jmir.7.1.e3.

Hambleton, S.J., Aloizos AM, J., 2019. Australia's digital health journey. Med J Aust, 210, S5–S6.

Meskó, B., Drobni, Z., Bényei, É., et al., 2017. Digital health is a cultural transformation of traditional healthcare. Mhealth 3, 38. doi:10.21037/mhealth.2017.08.07.

Morrison, Z., Robertson, A., Cresswell, K., et al., 2011. Understanding contrasting approaches to nationwide implementations of electronic health record systems: England, the USA and Australia. J Healthc Eng 2 (1), 25–42.

National E-Health Transition Authority, 2016. Evolution of eHealth in Australia. Achievements, lessons, and opportunities, April, 1–70. https://www.digitalhealth.gov.au/about-the-agency/publications/reports/benefit-and-evaluation-reports/evolution-of-ehealth-in-australia-achievements-lessons-and-opportunities/Evolution of eHealth in Australia_Publication_20160517.pdf.

Park, S., Burford, S., Lee, J.Y., et al., 2016. Mobile health: empowering people with type 2 diabetes using digital tools. News and Media Research Centre, University of Canberra, 1–54. doi:10.1007/978-3-319-12817-7.

Pearce, C., Bainbridge, M., 2014. A personally controlled electronic health record for Australia. J Am Med Inform Assoc 21 (4), 707–713. doi:10.1136/amiajnl-2013-002068.

Perlgut, D., 2011. Digital inclusion in the broadband world: challenges for Australia. In: Communications Policy and Research Forum, pp. 1–13.

Rich, E., Miah, A., 2014. Understanding digital health as public pedagogy: a critical framework. Societies 4 (2), 296–315. doi:10.3390/soc4020296.

Rural Doctors Association of Australia, 2017. Digital health strategy submission, January, 1–16. https://www.rdaa.com.au/documents/item/16.

Seneviratne, M., Hersch, F., Peiris, D.P., 2018. HealthNavigator: a mobile application for chronic disease screening and linkage to services at an urban Primary Health Network. Aust J Prim Health 24 (2), 116–122. doi:10.1071/PY17070.

Smith, K., Chenhall, R., McQuire, S., et al., 2016. Digital futures in Indigenous communities to community hubs. https://www.researchgate.net/publication/306378878_Digital_Futures_in_Indigenous_Communities_From_Health_Kiosks_to_Community_Hubs.

Sullivan, C., Staib, A., Ayre, S., et al., 2016. Pioneering digital disruption: Australia's first integrated digital tertiary hospital. Med J Aust 205 (9), 386–389. doi:10.5694/mja16.00476.

Taylor, A., Caffery L.J., Gesesew, H.A., et al., 2021. How Australian health care services adapted to telehealth during the COVID-19 pandemic: a survey of telehealth professionals. Front Public Health. 26 (9), 648009. doi: 10.3389/fpubh.2021.648009.

Telstra, 2017. Measuring Australia's digital divide: Australian Digital Inclusion Index 2017. https://digitalinclusionindex.org.au/wp-content/uploads/2018/03/Australian-Digital-Inclusion-Index-2017_v2.pdf.

Thomas, J., Barraket, J., Wilson, C.K., et al., 2018. Measuring Australia's digital divide: the Australian Digital Inclusion Index. RMIT University, Melbourne, Australia. https://researchbank.rmit.edu.au/view/rmit:45478.

Thomas, E.E., Haydon, H.M., Mehrotra, A., et al., 2020. Building on the momentum: Sustaining telehealth beyond COVID-19. J Telemed Telecare 28 (4), 301–308.

Vogt, F., Haire, B., Selvey, L., et al., 2022. Effectiveness evaluation of digital contact tracing for COVID-19 in New South Wales, Australia. Lancet Public Health 7, 3, e250–e258.

Whitelaw, S., Mamas, M.A., Topol, E., et al., 2020. Applications of digital technology in COVID-19 pandemic planning and response. Lancet Digital health 2 (8), e435–e440. doi:10.1016/S2589-7500(20)30142-4.

Willis, S., Tranter, B., 2006. Beyond the "digital divide": internet diffusion and inequality in Australia. J Soc 42 (1), 43–59. doi:10.1177/1440783306061352.

FURTHER READING

Rich, E., Miah, A., 2014. Understanding digital health as public pedagogy: a critical framework. Societies 4, 296–315. doi:10.3990/soc4020296.

NEHTA, 2016. Evolution of eHealth in Australia: Achievements, Lessons and Opportunities. National E-Health Transition Authority, Sydney.

Gunter, T.D., Terry, N.P., 2005. The emergence of national electronic health record architectures in the United States and Australia: models, costs, and questions. J Med Internet Res 7 (1), e3.

Willis, S., Tanter, B., 2006. Beyond the 'digital divide': internet diffusion and inequality in Australia. J Soc 42 (1), 43–59. doi:10.1177/1440783306061352.

ONLINE RESOURCES

Australian Digital Health Agency (ADHA), Australia's national digital health strategy: https://www.digitalhealth.gov.au/about-us/strategies-and-plans/national-digital-health-strategy-and-framework-for-action.

17

Australia's Health Workforce

Susan Waller, Keith Sutton and Tony Smith

KEY LEARNING OUTCOMES

When you finish this chapter you should be able to:
- briefly describe the distribution of the health workforce and how it is organised
- explain the roles of health professionals and how they contribute to the health care system
- describe the function of registration and accreditation in the health workforce
- discuss trends and issues that affect the organisation of the health workforce.

KEY TERMS AND ABBREVIATIONS

Aboriginal and Torres Strait Islander
advanced practice
alcohol and other drug (AOD)
allied health professionals (AHPs)
Allied Health Professions Australia (AHPA)
Australian Association of Social Workers (AASW)
Australian College of Nursing (ACN)
Australian Health Practitioner Regulation Agency (Ahpra)
Australian Medical Association (AMA)
Australian Medical Council (AMC)
Australian Nursing and Midwifery Accreditation Council (ANMAC)

Australian Physiotherapy Association (APA)
Australian Psychology Accreditation Council (APAC)
clinical nurse consultant (CNC)
clinical nurse specialist (CNS)
complementary and alternative medicine (CAM)
Department of Veterans' Affairs (DVA)
Dietitians Association of Australia (DAA)
emergency department (ED)
extended scope of practice
fee-for-service
general practitioners (GPs)
interprofessional education and practice
multidisciplinary team (MDT)

National Disability Insurance Scheme (NDIS)
National Rural Health Alliance (NRHA)
non-government organisations (NGOs)
not-for-profit (NFP)
patient services assistant (PSA)
primary care
resident medical officers (RMOs)
scope of practice
secondary care
Speech Pathology Australia (SPA)
technical and further education (TAFE)
tertiary care
value-based health care (VBHC)
Vocational Education and Training (VET)

INTRODUCTION

This chapter describes the health workforce and the contexts in which health professionals work. Sharing some common characteristics and competencies, different health professions have different core or expert knowledge, skills and abilities, complementing each other's roles. While the contexts and the services provided are diverse, they share a common focus on improving the health and well-being of individuals and the population. Optimal health outcomes are achieved when health professionals from different disciplines work together. This was challenged during the SARS-CoV-2 pandemic. Across the world, including in Australia, the health workforce was on the frontline and working to capacity to manage the increased demand for health care.

On the following pages, a broad perspective of the workforce is covered before considering the various practice environments, structural elements, and mechanisms for organising and regulating practice. Potential changes for the future workforce are also presented.

OVERVIEW OF THE AUSTRALIAN HEALTH WORKFORCE

The health workforce includes all those who are employed in providing health and welfare services, in public, government-funded, private and non-government organisations. Increasingly, the health workforce includes people with the experience of living with or caring for someone with a health condition, the latter in either paid or unpaid roles. Volunteers are valued members of the health workforce.

Size and Distribution

More than one million Australians are employed providing health and welfare services (Australian Institute of Health and Welfare (AIHW) 2022). Table 17.1 lists the health professions required by law to be registered by the **Australian Health Practitioner Regulation Agency (Ahpra)** (see link to Ahpra website in Online Resources). The number of practitioners in each profession is based on the annual report of Ahpra for 2020–21,

TABLE 17.1   Practitioners in Regulated Health Professions, 2020–21[†], with Estimated Proportions of Practitioners[‡] in ASGC-RA (2021) Regions, and Proportions in Occupational Sub-groups (Shaded)[§¶]

| Health Profession | Total[†] | APPROXIMATE % OF PRACTITIONERS IN DIFFERENT GEOGRAPHICAL REGIONS[‡] | | | | |
		Major Cities	Inner Regional	Outer Regional	Remote	Very Remote
Allied health						
Aboriginal and Torres Strait Islander health practice	829	18.2	17.4	28.8	15.8	19.7
Chinese medicine practice	4,863	86.4	11.1	2.5	0.0	0.0
Chiropractic	5,968	75.7	18.0	5.3	0.7	0.3
Medical radiation practice	17,844	78.7	15.8	4.9	0.5	0.2
Diagnostic radiography[§]	78.2%					
Nuclear medicine science[§]	7.0%					
Radiation therapy[§]	14.7%					
Occupational therapy	25,632	77.8	15.2	5.9	0.7	0.3
Optometry	6,288	78.5	15.8	5.1	0.4	0.2
Osteopathy	2,951	80.5	19.5	0.0	0.0	0.0
Paramedicine practitioners	21,492	60.9	24.3	11.8	1.8	1.2
Pharmacy	35,262	77.6	15.0	6.2	0.8	0.3
Community pharmacy[¶]	66.7%					
Hospital pharmacy[¶]	21.4%					
Other + non-clinical[¶]	11.9%					

TABLE 17.1   **Practitioners in Regulated Health Professions, 2020–21[†], with Estimated Proportions of Practitioners[‡] in ASGC-RA (2021) Regions, and Proportions in Occupational Sub-groups (Shaded)[§¶]—cont'd**

Health Profession	Total[†]	APPROXIMATE % OF PRACTITIONERS IN DIFFERENT GEOGRAPHICAL REGIONS[‡]				
		Major Cities	Inner Regional	Outer Regional	Remote	Very Remote
Physiotherapy	37,650	80.7	13.6	4.7	0.6	0.3
Podiatry	5,783	76.2	18.0	4.8	0.6	0.4
Psychology	41,817	82.8	12.7	3.8	0.5	0.2
Dental health	24,984	79.5	14.4	5.3	0.6	0.2
Dentists[§]	74.4%					
Dental hygienists/therapists[§]	9.1%					
Dental prosthetists[§]	5.1%					
Oral health therapists[§]	9.4%					
Medical practice	129,066	79.2	13.6	5.8	0.9	0.4
General practitioners[§]	31.0%					
Hospital non-specialists[§]	10.6%					
Specialists[§]	33.5%					
Specialists in training[§]	17.7%					
Other + non-clinical[§]	7.2%					
Nursing and midwifery	458,506	70.3	19.9	8.2	1.0	0.5
Registered nurses[§]	77.5%					
Enrolled nurses[§]	16.2%					
Registered/enrolled nurse & midwife[§]	7.9%					
Nurse practitioners[§]	0.5%					
All health professionals	818,935	73.5	16.3	6.9	1.7	1.6

Abbreviation: ASGC-RA = Australian Standard Geographical Classification – Remoteness Area
Sources: [†] Australian Health Professions Regulation Agency, Annual Report 2020/21; [‡]Estimates based on Australian Government Department of Health (2020) Workforce Data, Summary Statistics; [§]Estimates based on Australian Government Department of Health (2016) Health Workforce Data; [¶]Estimates based on Australian Government Department of Health, Health Workforce Data – 2017 Pharmacy Factsheet.

while the proportions of practitioners in geographical regions and proportions in various occupational sub-groups are based on historical data, as shown. Fig. 17.1 shows the comparative size of the registered professions. The nursing and midwifery workforce is by far the largest, representing some 56% of nationally registered health professionals. Medicine has many specialties, as do other health professions, and makes up just under 16% of the workforce, the remainder being non-nursing and non-medical practitioners in various disciplines. Not shown are the health professions not required to have Ahpra national registration, including audiologists, dietitians, exercise physiologists, social workers and speech pathologists. Reliable data are not available for those occupations, nor for providers of **complementary and alternative medicine (CAM)**.

Table 17.1 illustrates that the proportion of practitioners in the various health professions decreases markedly from 'major cities' through to 'very remote' regions. The exception is the **Aboriginal and Torres Strait Islander** health workforce, which is more evenly distributed across regions, with relatively high proportions in 'remote' and 'very remote' locations compared to other professions. Overall, with some 74% of health professionals practising in 'major cities' and, considering that more than 30% of the Australian population lives

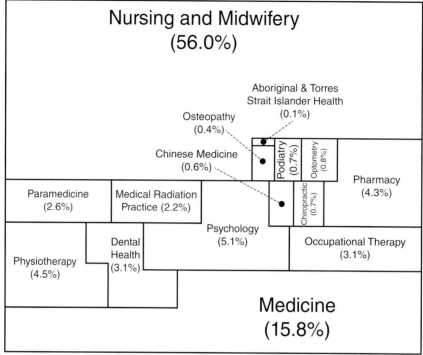

Figure 17.1 Relative size of the workforce in the 15 nationally regulated health professions. *Source:* Australian Health professions Regulation Agency, Annual Report 2020/21.

outside major cities (AIHW 2021), Table 17.1 illustrates the maldistribution of the health workforce between urban compared to rural and remote communities.

ORGANISATION OF THE HEALTH WORKFORCE

This section provides an overview of the workforce across the primary, secondary and tertiary levels of health services. Additional factors that also contribute to workforce organisation are funding, care setting and type of intervention; however, a range of other factors also influence how the health workforce is structured and operates.

Health Care Funding

The Commonwealth and state and territory governments provide most of the funding for health services. Smaller commitments come from private health insurance and direct payments by consumers (gap and **fee-for-service** payments). Commonwealth funding includes the Medical Benefits Schedule (MBS), Pharmaceutical Benefits Scheme (PBS) (see Chapter 7),

Department of Veterans' Affairs (DVA), National Disability Insurance Scheme (NDIS), My Aged Care and grants for Aboriginal and Torres Strait Islander health, primary mental health care and **alcohol and other drug (AOD)** services. State and territory governments fund public health services, including hospitals, mental health, alcohol and drug, dental, community health and preventive health services. Services funded by private health insurance include private inpatient care, dental care, optometry and some other allied health services, as well as some CAM (see Chapter 14).

The majority of health professionals in the public system work in hospitals. States and territories directly manage public health services and contract some service delivery to **non-government organisations (NGOs)** and private providers. Other health professionals operate as private practitioners. Pharmacists are primarily funded via the PBS for handling and dispensing medications. **General practitioners (GPs)**, medical specialists and some **allied health professionals (AHPs)** and nurse practitioners can receive payment through MBS and private health insurance. Dentists are primarily remunerated through private health insurance.

All private health practitioners may also register as providers through other Commonwealth programs and state-based rehabilitation schemes. They may operate as sole providers, or are organised as small businesses or large publicly owned companies. The sector includes both for-profit and **not-for-profit (NFP)** entities where practitioners work on a fee-for-service basis or as salaried employees in both health professional and administrative roles.

Primary and Community Care

Generally, the primary health sector cares for the more common health problems. Consumers can directly access primary and community care without referral. GPs are central to **primary care** (see Chapter 6) and 'gate-keepers' to secondary and tertiary services. They assess, manage and refer patients to other services and practitioners to support diagnosis (pathology and imaging) and treatment (medical specialists and AHPs). Practice nurses in GP clinics provide services such as health screening, immunisations and wound care. GP services are predominantly available on weekdays, with extended hours of service on evenings and weekends. Coordination of after-hours GP services is the responsibility of local Primary Health Networks (PHNs) (see Chapter 6).

Consumers may directly access primary care from AHPs practising privately or in community-based health services. Optometrists and most psychologists and podiatrists operate only in private practice. However, other disciplines (e.g. occupational therapists, physiotherapists and speech pathologists) work in either the public or the private sector, with reduced services available on weekends.

For many people, the first point of primary care is their local pharmacy. The majority of pharmacists either own or work in community pharmacies (Table 17.1). Community pharmacy (see Chapter 26) income is derived from handling and dispensing medications and selling over-the-counter medications and retail products. Many community pharmacists provide vaccinations, including during the SARS-CoV-2 pandemic. Vaccinations and health checks are increasingly part of the pharmacist's role in the community, thus providing greater public access.

Like pharmacists, most dentists are in private practice, although some also service the public sector (see Chapter 15). Publicly funded dental clinics are accessible for people on low incomes and for children, the latter as part of school-based health care. Dental health services commonly employ dental nurses, dental hygienists, and oral health therapists, in both the private and the public sectors.

Providers of CAM are private practitioners and earn income through fee-for-service payments. Reimbursement is possible from private health insurance, though arrangements are limited and the government has restricted rebates for these services (you can read more about their role in Chapter 14).

Secondary Referral Services

Secondary care services manage conditions requiring more specialised care and access is by referral. Specialist medical practitioners (e.g. cardiologists, psychiatrists, etc.) are the main secondary care providers. Medical specialists may be private practitioners who also provide services to public hospitals as visiting consultants or they may be employed as salaried hospital staff specialists.

Diagnostic services, such as pathology and medical imaging, are a component of secondary care and operate in both the public and the private sectors. Referrals are made to specialist pathologists or radiologists from other specialists or GPs, although a limited range of services can be requested by physiotherapists, nurse practitioners, osteopaths, podiatrists, and chiropractors. In medical imaging and pathology, the workforce includes AHPs and nurses, diagnostic radiographers, nuclear medicine scientists, sonographers, medical laboratory scientists, radiology nurses and nurse phlebotomists.

Other services with a specialist focus are mental health and AOD services. Private services are mostly provided by psychiatrists, psychologists and GPs; however, mental health nurses, social workers and occupational therapists are growing components of this sector. Most services are state funded and operate during core business hours; however, some intensive outreach services operate 7 days a week, including 24-hour phone services. Public services may be accessed directly or by referral and community-based services may refer consumers to residential and hospital services.

Community mental health teams include nurses (the largest occupation), psychiatrists, psychologists, occupational therapists and social workers. The NGO-managed psychosocial rehabilitation services workforce includes both degree-qualified health professionals and workers with **Vocational Education and Training (VET)** qualifications. People with a lived experience of mental illness have also become an important part of the mental health workforce and formal qualifications for this role are only now emerging. Most AOD services are delivered by the NFP sector and are principally provided by nurses and VET-qualified practitioners.

Rehabilitation services are provided by AHPs, medical specialists and nurses working in **multidisciplinary teams (MDTs)**. Some AHPs, doctors and nurses undertake advanced training to become specialists in particular aspects of rehabilitation. Rehabilitation services are provided in hospitals, residential and day rehabilitation facilities and increasingly in the home. If unable to manage independent living in the community, individuals may be admitted to a residential care facility.

Funded by the Commonwealth, aged-care services aim to enable older people to remain in their home for as long as they are able, while residential aged care is for those who can no longer live at home. Services range from help in the home with daily tasks and personal care to 24-hour nursing care. Aged-care services are delivered by a range of providers including NFP, private and public-sector organisations. Day-to-day care and support is provided by personal care assistants and enrolled nurses under supervision by registered nurses, while activities are organised by diversional therapists. Allied health and medical services are generally provided by private practitioners in aged care. (See Chapter 8 for more information on aged care.)

Tertiary Referral Services

Tertiary care services are for more complex and / or acute conditions requiring intensive support and treatment. Care is provided in hospitals that integrate general and specialist assessment, treatment and support services. Most staff in hospitals, apart from visiting consultant medical specialists, are salaried employees. They are organised into MDTs. Nurses are the mainstay of hospital care and, working together with **resident medical officers (RMOs)** and other health professionals, care is provided 24 hours a day, 7 days a week.

Commonly, medical specialists admit patients into hospital although in smaller rural hospitals GPs have admitting rights and provide inpatient medical care. Another admission pathway is via the **emergency department (ED)**. This usually involves patients who present to the ED experiencing acute, urgent, painful, disabling, distressing or potentially life-threatening conditions, including trauma (e.g. a motor vehicle accident) and acute illness (e.g. pneumonia). Ambulance service paramedics are usually the first health professionals to respond in out-of-hospital emergencies. They provide immediate care to stabilise or begin treatment of patients at the scene and then transport them to the ED. The majority of paramedics are employed by state ambulance services and their role is outlined in Chapter 25.

Hospital services are organised into wards, departments and specialised units (e.g. coronary care, psychiatric unit, etc.). Health professionals working in these units often undertake advanced training in their field as a prerequisite of their employment. They may be organised into MDTs, working collaboratively, such as in a stroke unit. Allied health, medical imaging, pathology and pharmacy services are usually centralised departments supporting an entire hospital or group of hospitals. Hospitals are dependent upon a range of ancillary services such as patient transport, administration, laundry and maintenance services.

Follow-up care after discharge may involve intensive support within the person's home, which is also known as 'hospital-in-the-home'. People who are terminally ill may be admitted to a palliative care service, at home or in a hospice. These services include specialist doctors, nurses and AHPs, who collaborate to ensure that death is humane and dignified, and that relatives and friends are supported through the process.

Pause *for* Reflection ...

1. Reflect on the varying size and distribution of the registered health professions shown in Table 17.1 and Fig. 17.1 and the implications for health service delivery.
2. Visit the site regarding Allied Health Case Conferencing website of the Department of Health and Aged Care (see Online Resources).
   (a) Explore which case conferences are funded, existing constraints and the patient groups and practitioners involved.
   (b) Identify the professions that are eligible to be reimbursed through the MBS under this provision.
   (c) How might the requirements enhance or hinder interprofessional, collaborative practice?
3. A GP can refer a patient to a physiotherapist, chiropractor, osteopath or exercise physiologist for chronic musculoskeletal conditions. How might the GP choose?

Take your reflections on these questions to the next tutorial class or raise them at your tutorial.

GOVERNANCE AND REGULATION OF THE HEALTH WORKFORCE

The right to practise is governed through processes which accredit educational/training programs and determine who may practise (i.e. registration). Professional associations advocate for their members in relation to those matters.

Education and Accreditation

Most health professional courses have three broad components:

- foundation knowledge about the human body and disease, social and individual determinants of health, and the context of health and illness
- specialist knowledge, skills and attitudes related to practice of specific professions, including observation and simulation
- supervised practice of professional competencies with patients/clients in appropriate settings.

Bodies established by the professions set standards and carry out accreditation reviews. Accreditation standards specify the necessary educational processes, graduate competencies and professional experiences. Accreditation bodies also specify the requirements of obtaining and maintaining accreditation, published as guidelines for universities and other educational providers. When applying for accreditation or renewal, education providers must submit comprehensive documentation on relevant curricula and undergo a review process that usually involves site visits to check staff competencies, facilities, administrative processes, selection procedures, professional placements and governance. Accredited courses are regularly reviewed to ensure standards are maintained and reflect contemporary developments.

Accreditation requirements dictate practice education. For example, currently, student nurses complete 800 hours of clinical practice, while occupational therapy students complete 1000 hours of practice-based education. Accreditation requirements are continuously re-evaluated and evolve under the influence of professional boards in response to developments and demands in the health care system.

Universities and vocational colleges of **technical and further education (TAFE)** must demonstrate that their courses meet specified professional accreditation standards, ensuring graduates are safe and competent to practise. Overall, Ahpra has responsibility for accreditation of programs in the registered professions but can delegate that authority to a committee of the national professional board or to an external body approved by Ahpra. Examples of accrediting authorities include the **Australian Nursing and Midwifery Accreditation Council (ANMAC)**, the **Australian Medical Council (AMC)** and the **Australian Psychology Accreditation Council (APAC)**. In non-registered professions, accreditation is carried out under the auspices of the relevant professional association such as the **Dietitians Association of Australia (DAA)** or **Speech Pathology Australia (SPA)**. Registration and/or licensure to practise requires graduates to provide evidence of having completed an accredited education program.

In October 2018, Ahpra welcomed the release of the Accreditation Systems Review final report (Australian Health Practitioner Regulation Agency (Ahpra) 2018), which led to the establishment of the Health Professions Accreditation Collaborative Forum (see Online Resources). Accreditation authorities have agreed to a common definition of interprofessional education, defined common learning outcomes, and committed to investigate further opportunities for additional interprofessional accreditation practices. These reforms promote requirements for **interprofessional education and practice** to support efficient team-based and coordinated care and are aimed at improved efficiency, safety and quality of care in the Australian health care system.

Registration

Ahpra is the national body that regulates and registers health professionals in Australia. The responsibilities of Ahpra include setting requirements for entry into professions, listing and monitoring who is eligible to practise, determining practice standards, managing complaints, disciplining practitioners where required and providing advice to government on matters relevant to regulation. Each registered profession has its own registration board, which includes experts from the profession, consumers and lawyers. Registration protects individual consumers and the community against sub-optimal health care. For health care workers outside the National Registration and Accreditation Scheme there are codes of conduct managed by state and territory governments, which establish expected standards of care and allow investigation of alleged misconduct.

Professional Associations

With payment of an annual fee, all health professionals can join a professional body or association. Membership is not mandatory, and it is common that a minority, rather than a majority, of practitioners are members of their professional body. Some examples of professional associations are the **Australian College of Nursing (ACN)**, the **Australian Medical Association (AMA)**, the **Australian Physiotherapy Association (APA)** and the **Australian Association of Social Workers (AASW)**. Many professional associations have specialist sub-groups, as well as state and local branches.

Professional associations offer members a range of benefits, such as subscription to a professional journal and newsletter, free career advice and access to 'positions vacant' directories, discounted conference registration and, in some cases, professional indemnity insurance at reduced corporate rates. They promote a sense of belonging, knowledge sharing with peers, and a forum for members to benchmark professional attitudes, opinions and beliefs with those of others. They also provide members with continuing education, which may include access to online, self-directed learning and webinars, as well as face-to-face conferences, symposia or workshops. Through continuing education, professional bodies can influence change and members can maintain currency of practice and thus meet registration requirements.

The collective power of professional associations enables an important advocacy role on behalf of members. The associations also uphold core professional values of the profession and executive members of professional bodies sometimes represent the profession in the public arena. They may influence government policy by lobbying politicians and informing policy debate on behalf of the profession. There is a vested interest in them garnering political support and, if possible, gaining preferential treatment.

Where they have common interests, professional organisations may band together and form alliances. Alliances advocate for members and provide a platform for education and interprofessional collaboration. For example:

- **National Rural Health Alliance (NRHA)** (http://ruralhealth.org.au/about), which currently includes 43 national organisations representing the interests of health professionals, consumers, students and educators in rural and remote areas
- **Allied Health Professions Australia (AHPA)** (https://ahpa.com.au/), which is an alliance of AHP bodies, currently with 21 national allied health associations and a further 14 affiliate members.

Pause *for* Reflection …

1. To understand the governance of your profession visit the Ahpra website and/or your professional association's website. Explore the registration requirements of your profession. Search for the 'code of ethics', 'code of conduct', 'code of practice' or similar. In a few sentences, summarise the key messages of that code.
2. Visit the website of another national board or professional association and explore that profession's governance requirements. In what ways, if any, do they differ from your profession? Why may this be so?

SPECIALISATION, ADVANCED PRACTICE AND EXTENDED SCOPE OF PRACTICE

Health professionals may choose to specialise, which usually requires further study and qualifications in a particular field. Most medical practitioners specialise or sub-specialise. Colleges administer specialist medical education and successful candidates become Fellows of the Colleges. While training, Fellowship candidates work in hospitals or in GP clinics as 'registrars', gaining experience while providing specialist services under supervision.

Some professions, such as dentistry and nursing, have specialties with their own professional sub-groups and certification regulated via national boards. Under state awards, nurses can be employed in roles such as **clinical nurse consultant (CNC)** or a **clinical nurse specialist (CNS)**, providing specialised services in particular fields. Other health professions also have specialties and occupational sub-groups (see Table 17.1), which may require specific qualifications and, though not necessarily marked by industrial award categories, may afford particular memberships and associations.

Overlapping with specialisation and bearing similar characteristics is the concept of **advanced practice** in allied health and nursing. This is 'a state of professional maturity in which the individual demonstrates a level of integrated knowledge, skill and competence that challenges the accepted boundaries of practice' (McGee & Castledine 2003, p. 24). Advanced practitioners are experts in their field, recognised by some professional associations through advanced practitioner membership, and acknowledging the ability to provide more complex clinical services.

The **scope of practice** of health professionals includes a range of fundamental knowledge, skills and abilities. Some competencies are generic and common to all health professions, such as communication and collaborative skills. Other knowledge, skills and abilities are profession specific, and it is these that largely set the boundaries to scope of practice. The Canadian Medical Education Directions (CanMEDS) 2015 Physician Competency Framework (see Online Resources) includes seven practice domains, of which that of 'Expert' defines the particular competencies that graduates are expected to possess and apply in practice (Frank et al. 2015). Each health profession has such a domain of expert knowledge and skills fundamental to their role. With appropriate permission, other professions, including many in Australia, have used the framework to define their own practice requirements. For example, the Australian Physiotherapy Association Competence Framework (version 7.1) (see Online Resources) is based on CanMEDS and affords a comprehensive descriptor of physiotherapy practice domains.

Health professions sometimes extend their scope of practice to adopt knowledge, skills and abilities that traditionally belong in the expert domain of another profession (e.g. nurse practitioners). Where **extended scope of practice** occurs, it is common to find interprofessional tension, as each profession lays claim to legitimacy, authenticity or ownership over the roles or tasks in question, a reality that has been studied in depth for decades (Abbott 1988). Notwithstanding such challenges, new models of care, therapies, procedures and roles, including extended scope of practice, can be safely introduced with guidance by credentialling, competency and capability frameworks (see Online Resources).

Pause *for* Reflection ...

1. Approach a tutor and have a discussion about scope of practice in your profession and how it relates to other professions and practice context.
2. Visit the CanMEDS 2015 website (see Online Resources).
   (a) Open the 'CanMEDS Framework' at the top of the page.
   (b) Open the role of 'Medical Expert', including the table of competencies. Consider how you would reword the statements to reflect your own expert health professional role.

EMERGING TRENDS AND ISSUES IN THE HEALTH WORKFORCE

Australia's population profile is changing (AIHW 2021). One of the challenges in the future is to provide health services for an expanding and ageing population.

Projections are that the proportion of the population aged 65 years and over will increase at a faster rate than that of working age Australians (between 15 and 64 years), thereby widening the gap between the proportion of the population needing care and the proportion in the health care workforce. Using the 'What's the problem represented to be?' (WPR) approach enables practitioners, researchers and policy-makers to critically analyse the implicit assumptions and implications of health policy solutions designed to address complex and challenging issues that will be faced (Bacchi 2016).

The policy shift towards personalised care funding packages (e.g. NDIS, My Aged Care), which aims to ensure consumer involvement in decisions about their health and care needs and choice of provider, is impacting upon how care is organised and delivered. These policy initiatives present individualised funding as the solution to the 'problem' of enabling better outcomes through individuals directing their own care. However, a tension exists between these policy shifts and the capacity of the health workforce to adapt to consumer demands. Care and support roles are changing rapidly as organisations adopt new business models and ways of interacting with consumers in order to remain competitive, flexible and responsive. Implications for the workforce are demonstrated by the increase in casual employment arrangements and, for some AHPs, fixed-term employment contracts in the disability sector.

The health workforce was severely tested during the SARS-CoV-2 pandemic and vulnerabilities in this sector were exposed, with negative impacts on the elderly population, as well as the health workforce. Rationalisation of the workforce in the aged-care sector has contributed to the challenges of increased demand and the need for rapid response during the pandemic. Part of the government response was to introduce the COVID-19 surge health workforce package, intended to clear the backlog of delayed recruitment and streamline entry pathways into the health workforce (see Online Resources). Working with education and accreditation authorities, this included acceleration of training for new clinicians, reviewing the registration process and creating a pandemic sub-register. Some measures continued, such as changes to the MBS to facilitate telemedicine consultations and reforms related to telehealth services.

National and international studies and reports have highlighted the need to change the way health care is delivered. A Grattan Institute report stated that 'too many health professionals squander their valuable skills on work that other people could do' (Duckett et al. 2014, overview p. 3). Some innovations have already occurred but shifting professional boundaries is often fraught, the greatest barrier being issues of professional status and hierarchy (O'Meara et al. 2015) and divergent views concerning role and scope of practice (van Vuuren et al. 2021). Generally, new and evolving roles are negotiated within the context of historical professional boundaries shaped by educational, regulatory and organisational histories; however, as illustrated by the response to the SARS-CoV-2 pandemic, the need to address unanticipated exceptional circumstances can accelerate change.

Technological change is creating greater efficiencies and diversifying roles, tasks and duties. New practices, roles and even entire occupations will develop around large-scale data storage and management. Patients already have an electronic health record, improving the capacity to share data between providers. Problems of distance, geographical remoteness and a lack of health service providers will be increasingly addressed with information technology. Policies being developed to address these challenges represent implicit representations of the universal right to equitable health care. Individual policy initiatives will 'problematise' specific aspects related to access to health care (Bacchi 2016). With local health care coordinators 'on-site', who may be volunteers or assistant practitioners, health professionals can be based remotely from where the care is provided.

Remote robotic surgery using virtual reality is already feasible. It is hard to predict how such technologies will alter future workforce development and clinical practice (Chapter 16 outlines the digital potential).

Models of funding health care may also change. Funding of health care is generally represented as a problem of limited resources allocated according to evidence-based medicine and dedicated to managing increasing need. As referred to by Bacchi (2016), reflecting on the 'problem' implicit in specific policy solutions should form part of the policy development process. For example, **value-based health care** (**VBHC**) is a funding model that balances health care benefit against costs (Teisberg et al. 2020). Providers are held accountable for both quality and outcomes of care and remunerated accordingly. Thus, the best-performing, lowest-cost providers with the highest levels of patient satisfaction are most rewarded. For more information about value-based health care see the link to the Australian Centre for Value-based Health Care under Online Resources. More collaborative models of care will be developed, where consumers access a range of services at a single location. Efficiency and better health outcomes will be achieved with MDTs of health professionals co-located, sharing patients and consulting with each other to diagnose and treat the increasingly common chronic morbidities of ageing. The emphasis will be on keeping people out of hospital, with greater collaborative, interprofessional teamwork to provide community-oriented, home-based care. Case study 17.1 demonstrates some of these points.

CASE STUDY 17.1

Scenario 1

John's wife wheels him into the ED late on Friday evening. A receptionist asks for contact details and John's age (72 years). An ED nurse in the waiting room asks a few more questions. Another nurse wheels John into a cubicle and conducts an assessment. He notes that John has some weakness, is drowsy and cannot speak clearly. He tells John's wife that a registrar will be along shortly.

The registrar completes her own checklist. A stroke possibly accounts for John's presentation. Immediate care is addressed by the registrar. Early next morning John is admitted to the general ward when a patient services assistant (PSA) is available to support his transfer.

Breakfast is delivered. Reviewing the ED notes, a nurse notes difficulty in swallowing. The dietitian on call recommends both nil-by-mouth until John has the consultant review on Monday and a speech pathology assessment; however, these staff members do not work on the weekend.

On Monday morning, the consultant requests a brain CT scan and a chest X-ray, as she is concerned about John's cough and pallor. On Monday afternoon the speech pathologist assesses John and recommends videofluoroscopy. She and a radiographer do this on Tuesday.

John spends 3 weeks in hospital, with aspiration pneumonia and malnutrition. John's stroke is mild. Diabetes is also diagnosed. On discharge, John is referred to a social worker and physiotherapist for ongoing care but is re-admitted to hospital two weeks later after collapsing at home. But it could have been like this …

CASE STUDY 17.1—cont'd

Scenario 2

The admission process is designed around what it is there for, rather than the role of the health professionals. Health care team composition is specific to client groups and their needs. John is stabilised in the ED and then rapidly assigned to the older persons' team, and a range of skills are linked to interprofessional practice at the outset. Dietitians, speech pathologists and radiographers are supported and authorised to work together, guided by person-centred goals and to share specific skills across roles/traditional domains of care. Performance and accountability is both individual and team based. John and his family collaborate with the team to plan his care and discharge.

John recovers at home, supported by the older persons' team care liaison, his GP, a physiotherapist and a diabetes educator. John becomes a volunteer community advocate with the older persons' team.

Case Study Questions

1. In the first scenario, what factors contributed to John's re-admission to hospital?
2. What resources do health care practitioners require to support John in the model of care described in scenario 2?
3. How would interprofessional education during pre-qualification study support a model of interprofessional practice?

A FINAL COMMENTARY

The Australian health workforce is dynamic and must be responsive to change and challenges. Motivation for change can be problematic, intrinsically and extrinsically, including changing patient needs and expectations, implementation of new models of care or funding, dynamics of interprofessional collaboration, and demands of continuing professional education and development, or the unending advance of technology. Mechanisms of health workforce change also include responses to natural disasters and public health emergencies, alongside system reform and quality improvement informed by governmental inquiries and commissions. Health care consumers have greater access to information about their health than ever before, enabling them to have a central role in decision-making, so that patient-centric, rather than profession-centric, care is the optimal practice model. As witnessed during the SARS-CoV-2 pandemic, the lived experience of the majority of the health care workforce may lead to clinician safety being paramount, alongside health care consumer experience in future models of care.

SUMMARY

- The Australian health workforce includes many different occupations, the largest being nursing and midwifery, constituting about 56% of registered practitioners. The various AHPs and medical and dental practitioners make up the bulk of the rest, although there are several other occupations.
- The health workforce is organised around the structural elements of the health care environment, including in primary, secondary and tertiary settings. Health professionals often practise across multiple settings, independently or in teams.
- Health professions are governed and regulated via various mechanisms. Tertiary education and course accreditation are primary means of establishing scopes of practice, which may change with specialisation or advanced and extended roles. Professional bodies have an advocacy as well as a continuing educational role and may influence change.
- Health professional workforce is changing under a variety of influences, not least of which is the rapid growth and ageing of the population, as well as evolving models of care, responses to natural disasters and public health emergencies, and the impact of governmental inquiries and reforms aimed at improving the quality of care.

▌REVIEW QUESTIONS

1. Reflect on the distribution of the health workforce and the potential impact upon access to health care in different communities.

2. Compare the composition of the health workforce in the primary and secondary health sectors. What are the differences and similarities?

3. You are part of a multidisciplinary team. What are the characteristics of the team that will support interprofessional practice?

4. Explore the ways in which the cost of health care is presented through media. What factors influence this public discourse?

5. An interprofessional allied health practitioner has been appointed to work in the ED. What might be the drivers of this new role and appointment?

REFERENCES

Abbott, A., 1988, The System of Professions: An Essay on the Division of Expert Labour. The University of Chicago Press, Chicago.

Australian Bureau of Statistics (ABS), 2021. Australian statistical geography standard – remoteness area (ASGS-RA) edition 3: https://www.abs.gov.au/statistics/standards/australian-statistical-geography-standard-asgs-edition-3/jul2021-jun2026.

Australian Government Department of Health, 2017. Health workforce data – 2017 pharmacy factsheet. https://hwd.health.gov.au/resources/publications/factsheet-alld-pharmacists-2017.pdf.

Australian Health Practitioner Regulation Agency (Ahpra), 2018. Ahpra welcomes release of the accreditation systems review final report. https://www.healthreform.org.au/wp-content/uploads/2018/02/AHCRA-Position-Paper-Workforce-FINAL-DEC-2017.pdf.

Australian Health Practitioner Regulation Agency (Ahpra) and National Boards, 2022. Annual report 2020/21. https://www.ahpra.gov.au/Publications/Annual-reports/Annual-Report-2021.aspx.

Australian Institute of Health and Welfare (AIHW), 2021. Australia's welfare 2021: Profile of Australia's population. AIHW, Canberra. https://www.aihw.gov.au/reports/australias-welfare/profile-of-australias-population.

Australian Institute of Health and Welfare (AIHW), 2022. Workforce – overview. AIHW, Canberra. https://www.aihw.gov.au/reports-data/health-welfare-services/workforce/overview.

Bacchi, C., 2016. Problematizations in health policy: questioning how 'problems' are constituted in policies. Sage Open April–June, 1–16. doi:10.1177/2158244016653986.

Department of Health & Human Services, 2016. Bridging allied health roles for better patient outcomes. Victoria State Government, Melbourne. https://www2.health.vic.gov.au/about/publications/researchandreports/bridging-allied-health-roles-for-better-patient-outcomes.

Duckett, S., Breadon, P., Farmer, J., 2014. Unlocking Skills in Hospitals: Better Jobs, More Care. Grattan Institute, Melbourne.

Frank, J.R., Snell, L., Sherbino, J., 2015. CanMEDS 2015 Physician competency framework. Royal College of Physicians and Surgeons of Canada, Ottawa. http://canmeds.royalcollege.ca/en/framework.

McGee, P., Castledine, G., 2003. Advanced Nursing Practice, second ed. Blackwell Science, Oxford.

O'Meara, P., Stirling, C., Ruest, M., et al., 2015. Community paramedicine model of care: an observational, ethnographic case study. BMC Health Serv Res 16 (1), 39.

Teisberg, E., Wallace, S., O'Hara, S., 2020. Defining and implementing value-based health care: a strategic framework. Acad Med 95 (5), 682–685. doi:10.1097/ACM.0000000000003122.

Van Vuuren, J., Thomas, B., Agarwal, G. et al., 2021. Reshaping healthcare delivery for elderly patients: the role of community paramedicine; a systematic review. BMC Health Serv Res 21, 29. doi:10.1186/s12913-020-06037-0.

FURTHER READING

Australian Healthcare Reform Alliance, 2017. Policy position paper: health workforce. December. https://www.healthreform.org.au/wp-content/uploads/2018/02/AHCRA-Position-Paper-Workforce-FINAL-DEC-2017.pdf.

Recommendations on the Australian Government's Primary Health Care 10 Year Plan, September 2021. Report from the Primary Health Steering Group. https://consultations.health.gov.au/primary-care-mental-health-division/draft-primary-health-care-10-year-plan/supporting_documents/Primary%20Health%20Reform%20Steering%20Group%20%20Recommendations%20September%202021.pdf.

ONLINE RESOURCES

Allied Health Case Conferencing: http://www.mbsonline.gov.au/internet/mbsonline/publishing.nsf/Content/Factsheet-AHCC.

Australia's health is released biennially on the Australian Institute of Health and Welfare website: https://www.aihw.gov.au/reports-statistics/health-welfare-overview/australias-health/overview.

Australian Government Department of Health – Chronic disease management – individual allied health services under Medicare – provider information: http://www9.health.gov.au/mbs/search.cfm?q=allied+health+chronic+disease&Submit=&sopt=S.

Australian Centre for Value-based Health Care is committed to pursuing the creation of a system where health care is funded and delivered with a prime focus on outcomes achieved at an affordable cost for patients and the health system: https://valuebasedcareaustralia.com.au/about/.

Australian Government Department of Health's health workforce data provide resources to investigate the nature of the Australian health workforce: https://hwd.health.gov.au/resources/.

Australian Health Practitioner Regulation Authority (Ahpra) National Boards: http://www.ahpra.gov.au/National-Boards.aspx.

CanMEDS 2015 describes seven characteristics and related competencies expected of physicians. The CanMEDS framework can be downloaded from this website as a pdf file: https://www.royalcollege.ca/rcsite/canmeds-e.

COVID-19 Surge Health Workforce Package: https://www.health.gov.au/initiatives-and-programs/covid-19-surge-health-workforce-package.

Credentialling, competency and capability framework: https://www2.health.vic.gov.au/health-workforce/allied-health-workforce/allied-health-ccc-framework.

Health Professions Accreditation Collaborative Forum is a coalition of the 15 accreditation authorities providing accreditation functions for the National Registration and Accreditation Scheme under the Health Practitioner Regulation National Law: http://hpacf.org.au/.

The APA Physiotherapy Competency Framework v 7.1 (January 2023) is available for download at: https://australian.physio/sites/default/files/APA_COMPETENCE_FRAMEWORK_v7.1_FINAL.pdf

18

Clinical Exercise Physiology in the Australian Health Care System

Steve Selig, Melainie Cameron and Kirsty Rawlings

KEY LEARNING OUTCOMES

When you finish this chapter you should be able to:
- summarise the evolution of clinical exercise physiology practice in Australia
- describe the roles of an Accredited Exercise Physiologist (AEP) and the scope of practice for AEPs
- describe the roles of Exercise & Sports Science Australia (ESSA) and the National Alliance of Self Regulating Health Professionals in the accreditation

of AEPs, and the development of Professional Standards and Code of Professional Conduct and Ethical Practice for AEPs.
- discuss ways in which AEPs and other health professionals collaborate in multidisciplinary service provision
- demonstrate, through the presentation of case material, an understanding of how AEPs practise.

KEY TERMS AND ABBREVIATIONS

Accredited Exercise Physiologist (AEP)

Accredited Exercise Scientist (AES)

Australian Health Practitioner Regulation Agency (Ahpra)

Chronic Disease Management (CDM)

Department of Veterans' Affairs (DVA)

Exercise & Sports Science Australia (ESSA)

National Alliance of Self Regulating Health Professionals (NASRHP)

National Disability Insurance Scheme (NDIS)

INTRODUCTION

In this chapter we describe the scope of practice, education and regulation of **Accredited Exercise Physiologists (AEP)** in Australia. Regulation occurs through a national university course accreditation scheme administered by **Exercise & Sports Science Australia (ESSA)**, which accredits against AEP Professional Standards. We outline the education and development of clinical competencies aligned to the scope of practice of AEPs, summarise where AEPs fit within the health care system, indicate how AEPs may engage in multidisciplinary practice and provide a brief history of the profession. We touch on some evidence supporting the therapeutic

benefits of exercise and conclude by demonstrating these scientific bases for the profession through case examples.

WHAT IS AN ACCREDITED EXERCISE PHYSIOLOGIST?

AEPs are allied health professionals who design and implement individualised exercise and physical activity interventions for people living with acute, sub-acute, and chronic health conditions, disabilities or injuries. **Accredited Exercise Scientist (AES)** is the foundational accreditation for clinical exercise physiology. An AES is trained to provide exercise services for clientele with no overt medical conditions, disabilities or injuries, or work under the guidance of an AEP or other allied health practitioner for the delivery of clinical exercise services.

The primary goals of exercise interventions developed by AEPs are threefold. Firstly, to apply appropriate intensities, volumes and modes of exercise to improve, or at least stabilise, clinical status and alleviate symptoms, while considering client presentations and medical treatments, the available scientific evidence, and the client's individual needs and situation. 'Improvement' in clinical status refers to retarding progression of a condition, or promoting regression of a condition, and these outcomes are known collectively as 'secondary prevention'. Secondly, AEPs work with their clients to improve fitness and function, including the capacity to work or perform activities of daily living (ADLs). The capacity to perform ADLs predicts long-term ability to live independently (Mlinac & Feng 2016). Thirdly, interventions are designed to improve quality of life, including reducing symptoms of depression or anxiety (Kandola et al. 2018; Hallgren et al. 2020) and other co-morbid conditions. A key component of an AEP intervention is to move beyond the often reinforced social construct that an individual is at fault if they have a lifestyle-related disease or are not fit (Bacchi 2016), and identify enablers and barriers to help clients to make long-term lifestyle changes, including addressing social factors (e.g. socio-economic status, family dynamics, social expectations, access to support services, time and availability) and environmental factors (such as urban design, geographic location and accessibility to services), using a person-centred approach to plan an appropriate program that incorporates all of these factors.

For all three of these domains (clinical, functional and psychosocial), there is extensive evidence supporting the efficacy of exercise as a stand-alone (independent) intervention, or combined with other lifestyle interventions such as dietary or mental health interventions across a wide range of pathologies (refer to the seminal review by Pedersen and Saltin (2015)). AEPs contribute extensively to research and knowledge bases regarding the effectiveness of exercise to support the prevention and management of medical conditions, injuries and disabilities. Many AEPs in Australia have contributed to pathology-specific position statements, clinical practice guidelines, and joint position statements with other professions.

REGULATION OF EXERCISE PHYSIOLOGY PRACTICE IN AUSTRALIA

ESSA is the national self-regulating membership body responsible for the accreditation of AEPs. ESSA is a foundation member of the **National Alliance of Self Regulating Health Professions (NASRHP)**, which is committed to providing assurance to consumers, governments and other entities regarding the safety and quality of self-regulating health services, through an evidence-based national framework of regulatory standards. AEPs are required to meet the minimum professional standards as regulated by ESSA, and also adhere to NASRHP standards and requirements pertaining to professional conduct, ethical practice, complaint management and recency of professional practice.

The accreditation of AEPs is restricted to graduates of ESSA-accredited higher education coursework programs. In 2005, just five universities were accredited for clinical exercise physiology; this has increased to 25 universities in 2022, out of a total of 43 public and private universities in Australia. There were approximately 450 AEPs across Australia in 2006 with rapid growth to 4626 AEPs in 2016, and further growth to 6315 AEPs in Australia in 2020 (ESSA 2020).

Professional Standards of an AEP

The professional standards for an AEP are regularly revised by the ESSA Standards Council and are currently composed of four broad standards: Professional Practice, Foundational Knowledge, Assessment and Client Management, and Design and Delivery of Exercise-Based Interventions. Key aspects of AEP practice such as communication, inclusivity and person-centred care are embedded within the standards. Evidence-based practice (EBP) is a core expectation of AEP practice, and ESSA has, for more than two decades, championed the linking of research to practice through its research initiatives, professional development, and national and international conferences. Finally, AEPs must practise in accord with the ESSA Code of Professional Conduct and Ethical Practice.

Historical Perspective

In 2005, the Australian Department of Health released a range of Medicare Australia **Chronic Disease Management (CDM)** items for allied health professionals, including AEPs, to support individuals with one or more chronic disease/s. This change in policy was in response to the increasing incidence, prevalence and costs of managing chronic diseases in Australia, and the perceived lack of ability of individuals to self-manage their chronic conditions without interventions or support (Bacchi 2016; Tuohy 1999). Since 2006, other schemes have been approved for AEPs to provide exercise for individuals with disabilities, individuals injured in motor vehicle accidents or at work, veterans and individuals with private health insurance. Elsewhere in the world there are compensable schemes and professional opportunities for clinical exercise physiologists, however, the breadth and depth of Australian recognition of the AEP as an independent provider of clinical exercise services is without parallel.

From July 2016 to June 2021 the provision of exercise physiology services under the relevant Medicare Benefits Schedule Item number 10953 increased by 20%, compared to only a 0.6% increase in the prerequisite Medicare Benefits Schedule Item Number 721 (preparation by a GP of a GP management plan for a patient with a chronic medical condition) (Australian Government 2022). In total, the number of services provided by AEPs under the Medicare Benefits Schedule (which includes CDM services, Type 2 Diabetes Management services, services provided to Aboriginal and Torres Strait Islander people for CDM and services provided to residents of aged-care facilities) increased by 16% during the same time period (347,915 total AEP services in 2015–16 vs. 402,671 total AEP services in 2020–21). This growth in services aligns with corresponding increases in the number of accredited university courses, new graduates, practising AEPs and full members of ESSA over the past decade. Using Bacchi's 'What's the problem represented to be?' (WPR) framework (Bacchi 2016), it might be argued that this policy response was steeped in the increasing prevalence of lifestyle-related chronic diseases in the Australian population aged 45 years and older, but did not recognise fully the level of service required to support an individual with making significant lifestyle changes (with Medicare sessions limited to five allied health sessions per individual per year). Further, there was no support for changes required in an individual's environment to support lifestyle change, such as a corresponding increase in policy or funding in urban design to support health behaviours, health promotion or health literacy (see Tuohy 1999).

CAREER PATHWAYS FOR EXERCISE PHYSIOLOGISTS IN AUSTRALIA

There are ever-increasing career pathways across a broad range of settings available to AEPs. Opportunities exist within public or private hospital settings (both inpatient and outpatient care), and government-funded community, primary and ambulatory care centres, where AEPs support chronic disease management and lifestyle behaviour change, often within multidisciplinary team environments. Opportunities for AEPs within private-practice settings are increasing with AEPs practising under schemes including Medicare, **Department of Veterans' Affairs (DVA)**, **National Disability Insurance Scheme (NDIS)**, state-based and federal workers' compensation, as well as life and private health insurance. Recent expansions of service offerings include services for clients in oncology, aged care and mental health.

CLINICAL REASONING AND THE MODES OF PRACTICE OF AEPS

AEPs provide their services using a clinical reasoning model (Fig. 18.1) (Maiorana et al. 2018), under which they may receive referrals from other health professionals, including general and specialist medical practitioners. One of the critical elements of this model is that at the point of referral, the referrer transfers the risk of exercise participation to the AEP with the knowledge and consent of the patient. In other words, a referrer such as a general practitioner (GP) is not required to deem that the patient is safe for exercise participation, but rather refers the patient to the AEP and in so doing, knowingly transfers the decision-making regarding the risks and benefits of exercise participation to the AEP. This is distinct from the situation for exercise physiologists in other parts of the world (e.g. UK, USA) where the medical practitioner retains the overall responsibility for the assessment of risk of exercise participation for their patients. In Australia, AEPs are equipped through education and development of clinical competencies to make those decisions independently, triangulating the referral information (presenting medical conditions, treatments and interventions), the patient's story, and the published evidence, with the results of examination, screening and exercise assessments undertaken by the AEP. There are two other elements to referrals from other health professionals to AEPs: (i) the referrer believes that the patient will benefit from exercise or

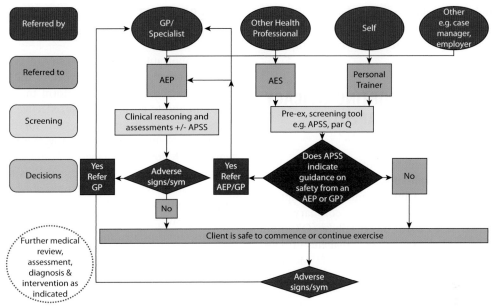

Figure 18.1 Referral, decision, and treatment pathways for AEPs Adapted from Maiorana, A.J., Williams, A.D., Askew, C.D., Levinger, I., Coombes, J., Vicenzino, B., Davison, K., Smart, N.A. & Selig, S.E. 2018. Exercise Professionals with Advanced Clinical Training Should be Afforded Greater Responsibility in Pre-Participation Exercise Screening: A New Collaborative Model between Exercise Professionals and Physicians. Sports Med, 48, 1293–1302.

increased physical activity and (ii) the referrer has discussed with the patient the potential benefits of such a referral to an AEP, and sought and obtained their consent.

AEPs need to collect, record, interpret and report back to the referrer any exercise-related information or data that may contribute to diagnoses, in turn leading to possible changes to treatments, interventions or management strategies. This is just one way in which an AEP may contribute to improvement in a client's clinical status, along with the therapeutic benefits flowing directly from exercise. AEPs collaborate with other health professionals when clients need advice or treatments from other health disciplines or to ensure that their intervention is in line with the client's overall treatment plan, or to clarify any concerns relating to the client's clinical condition or treatments (Fig 18.1) (Maiorana et al. 2018).

LEADING CAUSES OF MORBIDITY AND MORTALITY IN AUSTRALIA

The most recent data from the Australian Institute of Health and Welfare (AIHW) showed that in 2018, 5 million Disability-Adjusted Life Years (DALYs) were lost due to illness or premature death, with the leading contributors to DALYs being coronary heart disease (6.3%), back pain (4.5.6%), other musculoskeletal conditions (4%), dementia (3.85%), COPD (3.5%) and lung cancer (3.19%) (data from AIHW 2021).

There were just over 8400 DALYs lost in 2020 from the SARS-CoV-2 pandemic in Australia; 97% of this disease burden was from fatal cases. This is much lower than the burden due to leading diseases in Australia, however it is anticipated to increase with the number of individuals recovering from COVID-19 and the increase in long COVID cases expected as a result (AIHW 2022). As a result of the SARS-CoV-2 pandemic, ESSA successfully lobbied governments, regulators and funders for the approval of telehealth services across almost all of the pre-existing face-to-face compensable schemes described above. In addition, ESSA has provided professional development and research support for AEPs to provide clinical exercise services to people affected by COVID-19, in particular clients with long COVID who may experience ongoing symptoms including breathlessness and persistent fatigue. Long COVID is broadly associated with cardiac, vascular, respiratory and/or pulmonary sequelae, and people who experience long COVID may benefit from individualised cardiac and/or pulmonary rehabilitation including exercise as a core component (Faghy et al. 2021).

BRIEF EVIDENCE SUPPORTING EFFICACY OF EXERCISE AS A THERAPEUTIC INTERVENTION

Exercise has been shown to confer benefits such as reduced rates of hospitalisation, reduced need for prescribed medications and improvements in symptoms for a long list of conditions including coronary artery disease (Winzer et al. 2018), heart failure (O'Connor et al. 2009; Sagar et al. 2015), type 2 diabetes (T2DM) (Dunstan et al. 2002; Kirwan et al. 2017; McCarthy 2015), cancers including breast, prostate and colorectal cancers (Ballard-Barbash et al. 2012; Cormie et al. 2017; Printz 2020), and depressive and anxiety disorders (Ashdown-Franks et al. 2020; Carek et al. 2011; Hallgren et al. 2020; Rosenbaum et al. 2014; Schuch et al. 2016; Strohle 2009; Stubbs et al. 2017).

> **Pause *for* Reflection ...**
> Consider the challenges that lie ahead for AEPs in a crowded allied health domain, where other professions also provide exercise services. Are there niche areas of expertise and practice that distinguish AEPs from other practitioners?

THE RISK OF ADVERSE SIGNS AND SYMPTOMS DURING EXERCISE: THE 'EXERCISE PARADOX'

The benefits of exercise for clients with a wide range of chronic conditions are undeniable, but there is an acknowledged risk of adverse signs or symptoms, and even (very rarely) sudden cardiac death while clients with chronic conditions are exercising (Franklin et al. 1997). This increased risk during exercise stands in contrast to the reduced risk for the rest of the day and is known as the 'exercise paradox'. AEPs have a primary responsibility to be able to design and implement exercise interventions that are safe during actual exercise participation, yet efficacious in terms of clinical benefits during the 'rest of the day and year'.

ASSESSMENT OF CLIENTS TO INFORM THE EXERCISE PRESCRIPTION

A very important competency of an AEP is the ability to comprehensively assess clients before the commencement of exercise training, to inform the exercise prescription and to ensure it is safe, effective and feasible. Assessments are also valuable tools for documenting changes in client status (e.g. improvement over time or regression following a change in health status) and are repeated at specific time-points, such as following an acute medical event, changes to prescribed medications, interventions, treatments or implantable devices, or following surgery, to ensure the exercise prescription remains appropriate and effective or appropriately modified.

AEPs are competent in designing and/or using established fatigue-, sign-, and symptom-limited incremental exercise tests to assess the risk of participation in exercise, and using the results to prescribe exercise scientifically (Heart Foundation 2019). Incremental test protocols are preferred over single intensity tests such as the Six Minute Walk Test as the former provides a means for establishing safe ranges of exercise intensities and identify any symptom thresholds (Fig. 18.2). Cardiologists and other physicians conducting 'stress tests' often proceed beyond the onset of adverse signs or symptoms and use exercise to provoke signs or symptoms for the purpose of diagnosis. In contrast AEP-led exercise tests are used primarily to determine a safe and effective range of exercise intensities, and these tests are stopped at either fatigue or at the onset of adverse signs or symptoms (Fig. 18.2). Very few clients are referred to AEPs following a recent (and therefore reliable) cardiologist-supervised stress test, thus it is important that AEPs conduct their own exercise assessments for all new clients. Most referrals to AEPs come from general practitioners (GPs) and other health professionals, not cardiologists. It is impracticable, and would cause significant over-servicing, if every client who presented to an AEP for exercise first underwent a cardiologist-supervised stress test (Maiorana et al. 2018).

It is important that AEPs are competent in recognising and taking appropriate and timely (sometimes immediate) action when adverse signs or symptoms arise during exercise. Adverse signs or symptoms may also arise months after the initial assessment, so AEPs need to be vigilant whenever seeing a client, and appropriately

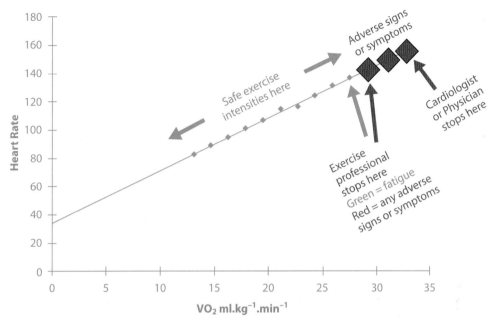

Figure 18.2 Generic model for exercise assessments by AEPs.

report adverse signs or symptoms to the referring health professional (Fig. 18.1) and modify exercise prescription accordingly. This has an additional feed forward benefit for the exercising client who can often return to exercise in better condition than previously, and so derive more benefit from exercise.

MULTIDISCIPLINARY AND INTERPROFESSIONAL PRACTICE: HOW AEPS WORK WITH OTHER HEALTH PROFESSIONALS

Exercise physiologists are not the only allied health practitioners who value the benefits of exercise: dietitians, physiotherapists, podiatrists, diabetes educators, occupational therapists, osteopaths, chiropractors, psychologists and social workers might be expected to encourage patients to exercise, become more active, or maintain ongoing involvement in sport and physical activities. Exercise physiologists are distinguished from their colleagues by their sharp focus on exercise and physical activity as their *primary* clinical intervention, and the detail and depth in which they plan, deliver, monitor, refine and progress exercise with clients. AEPs promote and support lifestyle behaviour change as core

to AEP interventions and understand the influence of complex primary and co-morbidities on clients' safety and capacity to exercise.

Team care may be multidisciplinary (i.e. practitioners from several disciplines each working with an individual patient) or interprofessional (i.e. practitioners working together to determine the most suitable care plan for an individual patient). It might seem intuitively reasonable that multidisciplinary or interprofessional care would serve patients better than single-practitioner care; however, the evidence for this assertion is somewhat mixed. A Cochrane Systematic Review of multidisciplinary rehabilitation for older people with hip fractures found equivocal, mixed and uncertain results (Handoll et al. 2021). When compared with usual care, multidisciplinary care in inpatient settings probably results in fewer cases of 'poor outcome' (i.e. death or deterioration in residential status such that a person would require ongoing institutional care), and multidisciplinary rehabilitation may result in fewer deaths in hospital, but the evidence is equivocal (Handoll et al. 2021). Only three trials compared usual care with multidisciplinary rehabilitation in patients living at home; again the evidence is equivocal. These results speak to the blunt reality of multidisciplinary rehabilitation: that it may be expensive, complex and time-consuming to deliver, and that we cannot be certain whether it delivers substantially improved outcomes.

Naylor and colleagues (2017) conducted a propensity score analysis to explore the value of inpatient rehabilitation following total knee replacement (TKR) surgery in Australia (Naylor et al. 2017). The only significant finding was that at 7 weeks post-surgery, patients discharged to home reported higher quality of life scores than their inpatient counterparts. At 90 and 365 days after surgery, participants in both groups were similar on measures of knee function or general well-being.

The lack of clarity in the research on the comparative efficacy of multidisciplinary care versus solo-practitioner care, and inpatient versus home-based care, also speaks to the reality of AEP work. AEPs can work constructively with other allied health professionals that value

exercise. Sometimes the professional boundaries overlap, and it may be difficult to ascertain which interventions are of most value to patients. AEPs need to be aware of the limitations of their knowledge and skills in any domain and seek help from other practitioners when they approach their own professional boundaries. Unexplored in Naylor and colleagues' study (2017) are the reasons why simpler, home-based rehabilitation appears to afford comparable outcomes to complex, multidisciplinary, inpatient care (Naylor et al. 2017). Regardless, this study serves as a reminder to AEPs not to be seduced by the assumption that complex care delivery is superior, and to ensure that their contributions to any care team serve patients in the first instance.

Case study 18.1 explores interprofessional care involving an AEP.

CASE STUDY 18.1   Cyclist with a Heart Rhythm Disturbance: Interprofessional Care Involving an AEP, GP and cardiologist

Paul is a 51-year-old recreational cyclist with previously high levels of fitness. Recently, Paul had experienced breathlessness, fatigue, light-headedness and feelings of a 'racing heart rate' during and after exercise. Paul's GP referred him to an AEP for an assessment for safety of exercise participation and to design an individualised exercise regimen. Paul's GP had previously prescribed medications to relieve, control and prevent his asthma symptoms, but Paul confessed to being lax with medication compliance. Nevertheless, the AEP assessed his lung function at rest as being adequate, with his large and medium-sized airways both functioning at over 100% of predicted values.

The AEP measured Paul's breathing and monitored his self-reported levels of breathlessness during a fatigue-, sign- and symptom-limited incremental cycle ergometer test. Heart rate and rhythm were monitored using electrocardiography, and haemoglobin oxygen saturation ($HbO_{2sat\%}$) and blood pressure were monitored. Although Paul's lung function fell below predicted values during exercise, $HbO_{2sat\%}$ did not fall and his level of breathlessness was subjectively in line with his level of exertion. At peak exercise, heart rate (HR) reached 98% of age-predicted HR_{peak} and his aerobic fitness was exceptional. The exercise test was uneventful, but at 45 seconds of recovery Paul's HR suddenly accelerated to 252 beats/min for a period of 10 seconds before falling to a near-constant HR of 184 beats/min for the following 3 minutes, and then falling again to a constant 134 beats/min for a further 3 minutes.

Paul was experiencing a post-exercise supraventricular tachycardia (very high heart rate). Attempts at reverting this arrhythmia to normal sinus rhythm using a Valsalva 'straining' manoeuvre failed and the AEP did not want to apply carotid artery massage (which is a method that can interrupt this rhythm disturbance). Fortunately, Paul spontaneously reverted to normal sinus rhythm at 6:50 minutes of passive recovery.

The AEP continued to observe and monitor Paul for a further 20 minutes before permitting him to drive home. Paul was advised to avoid high-intensity exercise until his tachycardia could be followed up. A report on the exercise assessment was provided to the GP within 24 hours. The GP then referred Paul to a cardiologist who subsequently referred Paul to a specialist cardiologist (electrophysiologist) who was able to induce and diagnose the arrhythmia to be dependent on an atrioventricular nodal re-entrant pathway. The pathway was ablated and the arrhythmia was no longer inducible.

Paul then returned to the AEP for a subsequent exercise assessment. His HR and rhythm responses to high-intensity exercise were normal and he was free from symptoms apart from normal fatigue. In the following 12 months, his symptoms did not recur and his anxiety levels concerning participation in high-intensity and high-volume exercise were alleviated. Paul is extremely grateful for the overall services offered by his GP, the AEP and the cardiologists and is now enjoying symptom-free participation in high-intensity cycling.

CASE STUDY 18.1   Cyclist with a Heart Rhythm Disturbance: Interprofessional Care Involving an AEP, GP and cardiologist—cont'd

Case Study Questions

1. Was the exercise test stopped due to breathlessness, fatigue or the arrhythmia?
2. The rhythm disturbance reverted to normal sinus rhythm at just under 7 minutes, and the client never lost consciousness and was unaware of his high heart rate. Do you think that emergency medical services should have been called?
3. How could an AEP deal with poor medication compliance?
4. Imagine this client also had coronary artery disease with exercise-induced chest pain that needed anti-anginal

medication for relief. How could poor asthma management make his chest pain (angina) worse during exercise? Hints: (i) explain how poor asthma management can cause falls in $HbO_{2sat\%}$. (ii) Use the Fick law of the heart to explain why decreased $HbO_{2sat\%}$ can impact negatively on oxygen supply to the heart and therefore make angina worse in individuals with CAD.

5. Referring to Fig. 18.1, comment on the appropriateness of the referral pathways that occurred between the GP, the AEP and the cardiologists.

Pause *for* Reflection …

Consider and discuss each of the following clinical scenarios. Ask where the professional boundaries might be approached, and where AEP practice overlaps with those of practitioners in other disciplines. Identify potential points of dispute with colleagues as well as points of commonality. Consider how the client might be best served in each scenario.

1. Anne had a total hip joint replacement yesterday. The prosthesis is uncemented. Anne needs to be mobilised out of bed as soon as possible to promote bone growth to secure the prosthesis in place. An AEP or a physiotherapist could guide and monitor Anne through this physical activity.
2. Brian has prostate cancer. Because Brian is taking androgen-suppressing medication, his bone density is likely to decline. His oncologist has suggested that he would benefit from an exercise program to maintain his bone mineral density through jumping, skipping and other weight-bearing exercises.

The oncologist values exercise but lacks sufficient time or the skills to plan an exercise intervention, so refers to an AEP to design a suitable program for Brian.

3. Casey has battled with depression for most of her adolescence. Her GP has prescribed antidepressants. Casey declined to see a psychologist because she is concerned about the stigma of mental illness. Her GP recommends that Casey becomes more physically active and refers her to an AEP.
4. Deidre has been discharged home after three weeks in hospital following a fall in which she lacerated her legs, and fractured a wrist and three ribs. A social worker has assessed Deidre as mentally prepared to return home, but highly apprehensive about using the stairs at the front and rear of her Queenslander-style house. The social worker has invited an AEP and an occupational therapist to a case conference to discuss options for Deidre's stair use at home.

SUMMARY

In this chapter, we have considered several factors that affect health service provision by AEPs, including independent roles and collaboration in multidisciplinary teams.

- AEPs design and deliver exercise services with the primary goals to improve the clinical, functional and psychosocial status of clients.
- AEPs accept referrals from medical practitioners and other health professionals and are responsible for assessing and managing the safety of exercise interventions based on a clinical reasoning model.

- Clinical exercise physiology education and accreditation is regulated by ESSA and NASRHP.
- AEPs work broadly across the public and private health care systems and a range of settings to deliver evidence-based exercise interventions.
- It is important that health professionals understand the services provided by other health professionals if interdisciplinary care is to be effective.
- Although there is some overlap of the professional roles of the AEP with those of other allied health

professionals, the sharp focus on exercise and physical activity as their primary clinical interventions, with emphasis on individualised, safe and effective exercise for all clients, distinguishes AEPs from other allied health professions that also value and promote exercise. AEPs are also focused on helping their clients to implement positive long-term health behaviours through counselling and appropriate exercise interventions.

REVIEW QUESTIONS

1. What is an AEP and what does an AEP do?
2. For clients with chronic disease and complex care needs, suggest some common and/or interdisciplinary approaches that dietitians and AEPs may use to improve lifestyle and self-management of clients' health.
3. Imagine you are a health professional in a community health setting. How could you promote increased exercise and physical activity participation in clients with chronic disease and complex care needs?
4. Reflect on the issues relating to the comparative effectiveness of interdisciplinary care, independent care by AEPs and 'usual care' for clients with chronic disease and complex care needs.
5. Compare and contrast the accreditation arrangements for AEPs and dietitians who are accredited via their respective professional associations and NASRHP, to the professions of physiotherapy and occupational therapy accredited via their respective registration boards and the **Australian Health Practitioner Regulation Agency (Ahpra)**.

REFERENCES

Australian Government, 2022. Medicare Australia statistics item report. http://medicarestatistics.humanservices.gov.au/statistics/mbs_item.jsp.

Australian Institute of Health and Welfare (AIHW), 2021. Burden of disease. AIHW, Canberra. https://www.aihw.gov.au/reports-data/health-conditions-disability-deaths/burden-of-disease/overview.

Australian Institute of Health and Welfare (AIHW), 2022. The first year of COVID in Australia: direct and indirect health effects. AIHW, Canberra. https://www.aihw.gov.au/reports/burden-of-disease/the-first-year-of-covid-19-in-australia/summary.

Ashdown-Franks, G., Firth, J., Carney, R., et al., 2020. Exercise as medicine for mental and substance use disorders: a meta-review of the benefits for neuropsychiatric and cognitive outcomes. Sports Med 50, 151–170.

Bacchi, C., 2016. Problematizations in health policy: questioning how "problems" are constituted in policies. SAGE Open, 1–16.

Ballard-Barbash, R., Friedenreich, C.M., Courneya, K.S., 2012. Physical activity, biomarkers, and disease outcomes in cancer survivors: a systematic review. J Natl Cancer Inst 104, 815–40.

Carek, P.J., Laibstain, S.E. Carek, S.M., 2011. Exercise for the treatment of depression and anxiety. Int J Psychiatry Med 41, 15–28.

Cormie, P., Zopf, E.M., Zhang, X., 2017. The impact of exercise on cancer mortality, recurrence, and treatment-related adverse effects. Epidemiol Rev 39, 71–92.

Dunstan, D.W., Daly, R.M., Owen, N., et al., 2002. High-intensity resistance training improves glycemic control in older patients with type 2 diabetes. Diabetes Care 25, 1729–36.

ESSA (Exercise & Sports Science Australia), 2020. Annual report, '20. https://www.essa.org.au/Public/ABOUT_ESSA/Annual_Reports/Public/ABOUT_ESSA/Annual_Reports.aspx?hkey=d06801e4-edbd-4119-ba9e-15758e5f04c3.

Faghy, M.A., Arena, R., Stoner, L., et al., 2021. The need for exercise sciences and an integrated response to COVID-19: A position statement from the international HL-PIVOT network. Prog Cardiovasc Dis 67, 2–10.

Franklin, B.A., Fletcher, G.F., Gordon, N.F., et al., 1997. Cardiovascular evaluation of the athlete. Issues regarding performance, screening and sudden cardiac death. Sports Med 24, 97–119.

Hallgren, M., Kandola, A., Stubbs, B., et al., 2020. Associations of exercise frequency and cardiorespiratory fitness with symptoms of depression and anxiety – a cross-sectional study of 36,595 adults. Ment Health Physical Act 19, 100351.

Handoll, H.H., Cameron, I.D., Mak, J.C., et al., 2021. Multidisciplinary rehabilitation for older people with hip fractures. Cochrane Database Syst Rev 11, CD007125.

Heart Foundation, 2019. A pathway to cardiac recovery: standardised program content for Phase II Cardiac Rehabilitation. https://www.heartfoundation.org.au/getmedia/006fd247-6163-4d04-9b85-9e90a5adbea0/A_Pathway_to_Phase_II_Cardiac_Recovery_(Full_Resource)-(3).pdf.

Kandola, A., Vancampfort, D., Herring, M., et al., 2018. moving to beat anxiety: epidemiology and therapeutic issues with physical activity for anxiety. Curr Psychiatry Rep 20, 63.

Kirwan, J.P., Sacks, J., Nieuwoudt, S. 2017. The essential role of exercise in the management of type 2 diabetes. Cleve Clin J Med 84, S15–S21.

Maiorana, A.J., Williams, A.D., Askew, C.D., et al., 2018. Exercise professionals with advanced clinical training should be afforded greater responsibility in pre-participation exercise screening: a new collaborative model between exercise professionals and physicians. Sports Med 48, 1293–1302.

Mccarthy, M., 2015. Diet and exercise are effective in preventing type 2 diabetes, task force finds. BMJ 351, h3785.

Mlinac, M.E., Feng, M.C. 2016. Assessment of activities of daily living, self-care, and independence. Arch Clin Neuropsychol, 31, 506–16.

Naylor, J.M., Hart, A., Mittal, R., et al., 2017. The value of inpatient rehabilitation after uncomplicated knee arthroplasty: a propensity score analysis. Med J Aust 207, 250–255.

O'connor, C.M., Whellan, D.J., Lee, K.L., et al., 2009. Efficacy and safety of exercise training in patients with chronic heart failure: HF-ACTION randomized controlled trial. Jama 301, 1439–50.

Pedersen, B.K., Saltin, B., 2015. Exercise as medicine – evidence for prescribing exercise as therapy in 26 different chronic diseases. Scand J Med Sci Sports, 25 Suppl 3, 1–72.

Printz, C., 2020. An expanded role for exercise in cancer treatment and survivorship: Backed by a trove of studies regarding the benefits of physical activity for patients with cancer and cancer survivors, researchers have updated exercise guidelines for these groups. Cancer 126, 2731–2732.

Rosenbaum, S., Tiedemann, A., Sherrington, C., et al., 2014. Physical activity interventions for people with mental illness: a systematic review and meta-analysis. J Clin Psychiatry 75, 964–74.

Sagar, V.A., Davies, E.J., Briscoe, S., et al., 2015. Exercise-based rehabilitation for heart failure: systematic review and meta-analysis. Open Heart 2, e000163.

Schuch, F.B., Vancampfort, D., Richards, J., et al., 2016. Exercise as a treatment for depression: A meta-analysis adjusting for publication bias. J Psychiatr Res 77, 42–51.

Strohle, A., 2009. Physical activity, exercise, depression and anxiety disorders. J Neural Transm (Vienna) 116, 777–84.

Stubbs, B., Vancampfort, D., Rosenbaum, S., et al., 2017. An examination of the anxiolytic effects of exercise for people with anxiety and stress-related disorders: A meta-analysis. Psychiatry Res 249, 102–108.

Tuohy, C.H., 1999. Dynamics of a changing health sphere: the United States, Britain, and Canada. Health Aff (Millwood) 18, 114–34.

Winzer, E.B., Woitek, F., Linke, A., 2018. Physical activity in the prevention and treatment of coronary artery disease. J Am Heart Assoc 7.

FURTHER READING

Cameron, M., Hemphill, D., Selig, S., 2011. Clinical Exercise: A Case-Based Approach. Elsevier, Sydney.

Coombes, J., Skinner, T., 2021. ESSA's Student Manual for Health, Exercise and Sport Assessment, second ed. J. Mosby Elsevier, Sydney.

Dietitians Association of Australia (DAA), 2011. Manual for accreditation of dietetic education programs, version 1.2. DAA, Canberra.

ONLINE RESOURCES

Exercise & Sports Science Australia (ESSA), 2021. ESSA annual report 2020: https://www.essa.org.au/Public/ABOUT_ESSA/Annual_Reports/Public/ABOUT_ESSA/Annual_Reports.aspx?hkey=d06801e4-edbd-4119-ba9e-15758e5f04c3.

Australian Government, 2022. Medicare Australia statistics item report: http://medicarestatistics.humanservices.gov.au/statistics/mbs_item.jsp.

Australian Institute of Health and Welfare (AIHW), 2022. Australian Burden of Disease Study 2018: https://www.aihw.gov.au/reports-data/health-conditions-disability-deaths/burden-of-disease/overview.

Australian Institute of Health and Welfare (AIHW), 2022. The first year of COVID in Australia: direct and indirect health effects: https://www.aihw.gov.au/reports/burden-of-disease/the-first-year-of-covid-19-in-australia/summary.

Exercise & Sport Science Australia – professional standards: https://www.essa.org.au/Public/Professional_Standards/The_professional_standards.aspx.

Exercise & Sport Science Australia – position statements: https://www.essa.org.au/Public/Advocacy/Position_Statements/Public/Advocacy/Position_Statements.aspx?hkey=bfe3284e-dfae-4392-877a-b9ab295ea9f7.

Exercise & Sport Science Australia – professional development: https://www.essa.org.au/Public/Professional_Development/ESSA_Professional_Development/Public/Events/Professional_Development_Hub.aspx?hkey=a9d480cf-e846-413d-9e53-e7a0b2a35330.

Exercise & Sport Science Australia/Sports Medicine Australia joint pre-exercise screening tool: https://www.essa.org.au/Public/ABOUT_ESSA/Pre-Exercise_Screening_Systems.aspx.

Changes in Healthcare Professions' Scope of Practice: Legislative Considerations: https://www.ncsbn.org/papers/changes-in-healthcare-professions-scope-of-practice.

Accredited Exercise Scientist Scopes of Practice for the Accredited Exercise Scientist (AES) and the Accredited Exercise Physiologist (AEP): https://www.essa.org.au/Public/Professional_Standards/ESSA_Scope_of_Practice_documents.aspx.

Joint position statements for ESSA, Dietitians Association of Australia (DAA) and Australian Psychological Society (APS): https://www.essa.org.au/Public/Advocacy/Position_Statements.aspx?ss360SearchTerm=position%20statement.

19

Nutrition and Dietetics: Promoting Health for All Australians

Louisa Matwiejczyk, Adeline Lau and Marian McAllister

KEY LEARNING OUTCOMES

When you finish this chapter you should be able to:

- briefly outline the development of nutrition and dietetics as a profession
- describe the range of roles of the dietitian and nutritionist within the Australian health care system
- identify some of the key nutrition disorders and nutrition-related public health issues impacting the health of Australians

- describe how dietitians and nutritionists are involved in interprofessional practice
- identify some of the government policies directing the nutrition and dietetics profession in promoting health for all Australians, including the Australian Dietary Guidelines
- describe how various health reforms have impacted on nutrition-related practice.

KEY TERMS AND ABBREVIATIONS

Accredited Practising Dietitian (APD)
Australian Dietary Guidelines (ADGs)
Australian Health Practitioner Regulation Agency (Ahpra)
Commonwealth Scientific and Industrial Research Organisation (CSIRO)
dietitian
Dietitians Australia (DA)

food insecurity
general practitioners (GPs)
general practitioner management plans (GPMPs)
local government organisations (LGOs)
medical nutrition therapy
national competency standards
non-communicable diseases (NCDs)

Nutrition Society of Australia (NSA)
nutritionist
obesity epidemic
obesogenic environment
public health nutrition
registered nutritionist (RNutr)
social model of health
team care arrangements (TCAs)

INTRODUCTION

Almost all of us are interested in food. We may enjoy selecting food, cooking favourite dishes, and sharing food with family and friends. Many of us also have definite ideas about the types of food we consider crucial in our lives, and, as such, food can play a key role in defining who we are (Germov & Williams 2017; Kokkoris & Stavrova 2021). Food, however, plays a much broader role than the social and cultural practices evident in everyday life. It provides our bodies with nutrients essential for normal functioning and is key to our state of health (Wahlqvist & Gallegos 2020). As early as 400 BCE, the link between food and health was already well known – 'Let food be thy medicine and let thy medicine be food' (Hippocrates 460–377 BCE).

Dietitians and nutritionists are health professionals trained to understand the functions and roles of food in our lives and our communities. These nutrition-related professions use this understanding to enhance individuals, groups and populations' nutritional health by promoting health-enhancing changes to food practices and the food environment (Dietitians Australia 2022a; Nutrition Society Australia (NSA) 2022a).

NUTRITION AND DIETETICS IN AUSTRALIA

A **dietitian** is an allied health professional who is an expert in the nutritional treatment of illness and prevention of disease in individuals and communities. **Accredited Practising Dietitians (APDs)** have completed a minimum 4-year accredited Bachelor's degree in nutrition and dietetics or a relevant undergraduate degree followed by an accredited postgraduate qualification in nutrition and dietetics. APDs have the skills to modify diets to manage various diseases and conditions using **medical nutrition therapy**. The clinical management of patients distinguishes the dietitian from the accredited nutritionist (DA 2022a). An accredited **nutritionist** will be trained in human nutrition, particularly in nutrition public health, health promotion and nutrition communication. Registered nutritionists will not have undertaken the extra coursework, professional practice placements or assessment in medical nutrition therapy and foodservice management. Dietitians may refer to themselves as nutritionists to reflect their broader, non-clinical role, but a nutritionist cannot use the title 'dietitian'.

A nutritionist provides advice on matters relating to food and how it impacts health. In addition, nutritionists design, implement, coordinate and evaluate population-level interventions which promote positive health outcomes through food and nutrition. Other nutrition-related areas nutritionists work in include research, consultancy, work in public health and food-related industries and work as nutrition communicators, nutritionists, food technologists and nutrition scientists (NSA 2022a).

Nutritional and dietetic services are delivered across the health care continuum, from primary prevention and early intervention to managing many diseases. What people eat can increase their risk of developing diet-related conditions such as overweight, obesity and micronutrient deficiencies, and **non-communicable**

diseases **(NCDs)** such as cardiovascular disease, diabetes and some cancers (Afshin et al. 2019). These account for 89% of all deaths in Australia (Wijnen et al. 2022; Australian Institute of Health and Welfare (AIHW) 2020) and 70% of deaths worldwide (World Health Organization (WHO) 2020). Globally, more than 75% of cardiovascular diseases, stroke and diabetes, and 40% of cancers can be prevented or delayed by reducing behavioural risk factors such as poor nutrition, physical inactivity, smoking and harmful alcohol intake (WHO 2020). Dietitians and nutritionists are instrumental in preventing NCDs and treating and supporting people with diet-related diseases and conditions.

NCDs are increasingly prevalent with an ageing population and rising risk factors, including obesity (AIHW 2020a). Many nutrition-related diseases occur later, although food preferences are determined early in life and will track through into adulthood (Haines et al. 2019). This means a 'whole of lifespan' approach is needed, with prevention focused on children and the people who support them, and treatment targeted at adults with NCD risk factors and existing chronic diseases.

Dietetics in Australia

Dietitians Australia (DA) is the peak professional body for dietitians, with more than 7800 members (DA 2022b). Despite the rising prevalence of nutrition-related NCDs and risk factors and the increasing number of dietitians, it remains a small allied health profession comparable to podiatry and optometry (Department of Health 2021). The DA reviewed dietetic university programs to ensure that training meets the **national competency standards** for dietitians in Australia (DA 2021a). Reviewed in 2021, these competency-based standards cover four domains, including practising professionally, positively influencing health, applying critical thinking and integrating evidence into practice, and collaborating with clients and stakeholders (DA 2021a). These domains are described in detail in the standards, and observable or measurable actions support their interpretation to assist in assessing students and dietitians in practice.

Dietitians must graduate from a DA-accredited university program (DA 2022c). Currently, 17 Australian universities offer accredited training programs, including undergraduate (4 years) and postgraduate (18 months–2 years) programs (DA 2022b). Curricula must meet content requirements in biochemistry, human physiology, and food and nutrition science (DA 2022b). Specialist subject areas also include food and nutritional science, medical nutrition therapy, community and **public health nutrition** practice, research skills, communication skills, food service and the sociology of food and nutrition.

Dietitians in Australia can become APDs with the DA after completing a defined and ongoing professional development program and at least one year of mentorship (DA 2022c). APDs are committed to the DA Code of Conduct for dietitians and to undertaking continuing professional development. After at least five years of experience, dietitians can apply to become Advanced APDs by demonstrating expertise in many competencies. Dietitians have progressed to become Fellows of DA (FDA), who are dietitians who are proactive leaders (DA 2022c).

Australian dietetic qualifications are accepted in the UK, some countries in Asia and the Middle East, and some states in Canada (DA 2022c). New Zealand-registered dietitians with an annual practising certificate are also eligible to apply to work in Australia. For accredited dietitians wanting to be recognised as specialists in sports nutrition, Sports Dietitians Australia (Sports Dietitians Australia 2022) offers membership and accreditation options. However, in Australia, dietetic and nutrition practice is not regulated by the government. Reforms implemented through the **Australian Health Practitioner Regulation Agency (Ahpra)** do not include dietitians or nutritionists as nutrition-related activities are not thought to risk harm to the public. Dietetics is a self-regulating profession where the government acknowledges that its members can govern themselves with minimum competency, entry, ongoing education and ethical conduct standards (DA 2022c).

Nutritionists in Australia

Founded in 1975, the **Nutrition Society of Australia (NSA)** was formed by scientists working in nutrition (including physiology, biochemistry, agriculture, medicine, sociology, economics and public health). The NSA comprises qualified practising scientists and educators from diverse backgrounds interested in increasing and communicating nutrition science's scientific value and relevance in Australia. Nutrition is a self-regulated profession, and for nutritionists wanting to be accredited, the Nutrition Society of Australia has developed a voluntary

register of nutritionists (NSA 2022b). This register ensures the quality and safety of practice by approving appropriately qualified individuals who have received an approved level of training and experience. At a minimum, nutritionists have a Bachelor's degree in nutrition to become associate nutritionists. Following three years of relevant experience (or further study), a nutritionist can apply to become a **registered nutritionist (RNutr)**. To maintain this, the RNutr undertakes continuing professional development and must meet minimum competency standards deemed essential by the NSA and the Code of Conduct (NSA 2022b).

Pause *for* Reflection ...

Much of the work delivered by clinically trained dietitians and nutritionists in the community setting may be similar. How might the two roles be differentiated? Can you foresee how these two professions can work in a complementary way in a community-based setting such as community health or a not-for-profit organisation? At what stages of the human lifespan could intervention by a nutritional and dietetic professional benefit?

WHERE DO DIETITIANS AND NUTRITIONISTS WORK?

The nutrition and dietetics workforce works across a range of health settings, including private practice, community health services and government and non-government organisations in metropolitan, rural and remote areas. In addition to providing direct patient care in private and public hospitals, dietitians work in aged-care and disability services. Both nutritionists and dietitians contribute to media and communications, public health policy, food standards, food industry research and education (Allied Health Professions Australia 2022).

Clinical Dietetics

Clinical dietetics usually involves the day-to-day management of clinical conditions such as diabetes, heart disease, cancer, renal disease, gastrointestinal diseases, and other disorders using medical nutrition therapy consistent with the biomedical model of care. Dietitians prescribe individualised and specific dietary regimens that will assist in improving the health of the patient.

They consider the type, amount and consistency of foods in dietary prescriptions and may provide additional high-energy, high-protein supplements to meet nutritional needs. Clinical dietitians often specialise in a particular disorder (e.g. diabetes, renal diseases, liver diseases, eating disorders). They may also become specialists in managing acute care foodservice systems, ensuring quality and efficiency in delivering standard and therapeutic diets. Clinical dietitians work in acute settings such as hospitals, but this work is increasingly provided in community-based settings and private practice with health reform. In hospital settings, the National Safety and Quality Health Standards detail quality standards for improving the quality of care and protecting consumers' health (Australian Commission of Safety and Quality in Health Care (ACSQHC) 2022). This requires implementing comprehensive systems delivering nutrition-related screening and monitoring and evidence-based nutrition care plans complemented with the provision of food and fluids.

Community-Based Dietetics and Nutrition

Community-based dietitians and nutritionists work in primary health care sites such as community health centres, GP Plus Centres, non-government organisations and publicly funded community services such as **local government organisations (LGOs)** in metropolitan, rural and remote areas. Non-government organisations include food relief and welfare services such as Foodbank and philanthropic organisations such as the Heart Foundation and Cancer Council. Community-based dietitians and nutritionists work within a primary health care model or a **social model of health**. Consistent with this approach, community dietitians are increasingly involved in clinical care pathways to assist individual patients re-entering the community from acute care settings and the provision of medical nutrition therapy in community-based services such as Diabetes Australia and aged-care organisations such as Helping Hand Inc.

Dietitians and nutritionists also focus on public health nutrition issues that affect populations, such as the **obesity epidemic**, the food system and climate change or nutritional issues impacting vulnerable subgroups, such as people living in rural and remote areas, people from low socio-economic areas and Indigenous Australians. In a health environment with limited funding and resources, competition for resources between interest groups representing the dominant medically-oriented clinical services and broader public health groups continues to be a feature of the health system. Australia spends less than 1.5% of the national health budget on prevention and relatively insignificant amounts on public health (AIHW 2021a; Shiell & Jackson 2018).

Private Practice

Private practice represents about one-third of total DA membership (Siopis et al. 2020). This increase has been enabled by health reform changes to Medicare which fund more effective partnerships between **general practitioners (GPs)** and private-practice dietitians, especially in chronic disease management through **general practitioner management plans (GPMPs)** and **team care arrangements (TCAs)**. The DA is advocating for further changes in the Medicare Schedule (DA 2021b). If patients have private health insurance, other referral types will be partly funded by these insurers. Private-practice dietitians may work with medical specialists in specialised clinical areas such as radiotherapy and cancer treatment, gastrointestinal disease and weight loss surgery. They may also work as consultants in various settings, including food services, private hospitals and aged-care facilities. There is also an increasing use of telehealth by private-practice dietitians as a flexible and cost-effective option for medical nutrition therapy (Kelly et al. 2020).

Interprofessional Practice and Interprofessional Collaboration

Dietitians and nutritionists work with other health professionals to improve the health care of patients, clients and populations through interprofessional collaboration and interprofessional practice (Schot et al. 2020). For example, within a clinical interprofessional setting, dietitians work closely with speech pathologists, social workers and medical doctors to maximise safe food intake and hydration for people with swallowing disorders. In a community setting, dietitians collaborate with allied health professionals and GPs to support clients with the self-management of their condition. Similarly, nutritionists in LGOs work collaboratively with community development workers, community leaders and the community to plan and implement programs for vulnerable groups. In addition, dietitians and nutritionists work with government and non-government departments and industry to develop policy and population-wide nutrition initiatives in public health.

Case study 19.1 outlines an interprofessional approach for dietetic involvement in the care of a patient admitted to a tertiary hospital. The case study questions ask you to consider what can go wrong in this setting in providing an interprofessional approach to client-centred care.

Other Current and Emerging Areas of Employment for Nutritionists and Dietitians

Government health reform has seen several areas in dietetics grow, such as private practice, services supporting the transition from acute care to home, healthy ageing, disability (particularly with the National Disability

---

CASE STUDY 19.1 Multidisciplinary Care in Nutrition and Dietetics

Shannon is a retired widow living alone with two sons who live interstate. Shannon was diagnosed with type 2 diabetes about five years ago. Shannon has, until recently, enjoyed her weekly swim at the local swimming pool and some gardening work around the house. During the most recent telehealth consult with her regular GP, Shannon was advised to visit the local emergency department (ED) due to a non-healing infected diabetic foot ulcer. Upon presenting to the ED, Shannon was admitted to the surgical ward for wound debridement of a stage 4 infected foot ulcer. Further investigations revealed that Shannon's diabetes control has been sub-optimal, and insulin is started for better glycaemic control.

Shannon's case is discussed at the weekly multidisciplinary team meeting, including medical, nursing and allied health team members. Shannon is feeling very anxious about starting this new insulin regimen and did not know that negligence of diabetes would result in such serious complications. Before discharge, the dietitian gathers information about Shannon's past medical history, weight history, social situation and usual food and beverage intake. Shannon reflects that, since retirement and due to the COVID-19 lockdowns, she had put on quite a bit of weight and could no longer go for weekly swims or move around as much. Shannon also admits to snacking more when lonely, especially during the lockdown period. Shannon also raises concerns about the rising costs of living including increases in fresh food and fuel prices since the COVID-19 lockdowns. As a retiree, Shannon is worried about getting access to affordable healthy fresh food given the ongoing extreme weather events, such as floods and bushfires, causing food supply shortages and higher fresh food prices. In consultation with Shannon and based on Shannon's dietary assessment, the dietitian provides individualised dietary education for improved glycaemic control and a healthy weight. Due to the recent operation, Shannon will have limited mobility until the foot wound has fully healed. During her admission, a social worker also sees Shannon and negotiates additional support for her at home, such as Meals on Wheels or home delivery meal kits and basic cleaning. Shannon is also referred to a physiotherapist to provide some modified home exercises and an occupational therapist to assist with basic activities of daily living when she returns home.

Before discharge, Shannon speaks with the Credentialled Diabetes Nurse Educator and the dietitian to learn more about administering insulin injections and how to prevent and manage hypoglycaemic episodes. Follow-up appointments with the endocrinologist, the Credentialled Diabetes Educator, the GP and a community-based dietitian were scheduled to ensure good continuity of care post-discharge. After the foot wound has completely healed, Shannon will be referred to services provided by her local government organisation (Council), led by a nutritionist, which provides low-cost home-delivered healthy meals, walking groups and socialisation through the community garden programs and an exercise program supported by the exercise physiologist to help with weight management and improve Shannon's diabetes control.

Case Study Questions

1. The scenario described is ideal where the dietitian is a key member of an interprofessional team and the clinical pathway from the acute care setting to the community setting is fluent and effective, and includes services in the community supported by a nutritionist. However, what would be the financial, social and other resource issues that may cause this pathway to be less effective or even ineffective for Shannon's care if she contracted the SARS-CoV-2 virus, requiring hospitalisation with a long recovery time?

2. Do you think the current Australian health care system can efficiently deliver such ideal management from acute to community settings? Consider the reasons for your answer.

3. How different do you think Shannon's care would be if Shannon were an Indigenous woman living in a rural and remote community such as Esperance in Western Australia? How might the interprofessional team be strengthened?

Insurance Scheme), Aboriginal and Torres Strait Islander health, and diet-related NCDs such as diabetes. However, neoliberal government policies and a lack of prioritising preventive and early interventive services have shifted responsibility away from the government to fund nutrition-related services. Significant health reform, coupled with rapid advances in the evidence base and health-related technologies, the impact of the COVID-19 pandemic on the population's nutritional health and the sustainability of our food system and the climate crisis, urgently requires the nutrition and dietetic workforce to expand beyond their traditional roles (Boak et al. 2021; Blair et al. 2021; Willet et al. 2019). Key intersectoral, national and international commissioned expert reports forecast that preventive and well-being management is crucial for improving future nutrition-related health outcomes and for having a sustainable food system, and these reports provide direction for what needs to happen (Australian Academy of Science National Committee for Nutrition 2019; Commonwealth Scientific and Industrial Research Organisation (CSIRO) 2018; EAT-Lancet Commission 2019; Willett et al. 2019). The nutrition and dietetics workforce has significant capabilities from prevention to treatment across the health spectrum. Prevalent issues include overweight and obesity, low health literacy, an unsustainable food system, inequities such as food insecurity, increased incidence of NCDs perpetuated by SARS-CoV-2 virus and a 10-year life expectancy gap between non-Indigenous and Indigenous Australians. In addition, most Australians do not consume core food group foods as recommended in the national dietary guidelines (CSIRO 2018).

Areas of current and emerging employment for nutrition-related professions include:
- government departments, where nutrition-related professionals work to maintain and improve the health of populations, including advising health ministers on appropriate nutrition policy and industry on food regulation and food standards. Examples include front-of-pack labelling, the health star rating of packaged food, the Healthy Food Partnership with the food industry to change their products to be healthier, strategies for a fair and sustainable food system and advocacy for change
- education and research organisations such as universities and the CSIRO, where new discoveries in nutrition and nutrition-related trials, and the need for population-level monitoring and evaluation of food

consumption and nutrition interventions, create many opportunities for nutrition scientists, nutritionists and dietitians
- the food industry, with many opportunities for new, sustainable food product development, innovation, marketing and health promotion
- communication, media and social enterprises where modern technologies such as telehealth, mobile apps and wearables will enable the nutrition and dietetic workforce to develop new roles and work in new sectors while using technology to consult, educate, support and inform the public (Hickson 2018; Kelly et al. 2021). Universal access to the internet by most people for most of their nutrition information, which is predominantly unqualified, and the consequences of the COVID-19 pandemic on how health education is delivered and its impact on NCDs, means that dietetic and nutrition support is imperative (Adamski et al. 2020; Butler & Barrientos 2020; Chung et al. 2021; Kelly et al. 2021).

DIETARY ADVICE IN AUSTRALIA FOR HEALTH FOR ALL

The **Australian Dietary Guidelines (ADGs)** are the national guidelines for healthy eating in Australia (NHMRC 2013a). The ADGs provide evidence-based recommendations that aim to meet the population's immediate dietary needs and prevent chronic disease. Complementing the ADGs is a food selection guide that visually represents the proportion of the five food groups recommended for consumption each day. The Australian Guide to Healthy Eating has been developed for various age groups and specifies daily minimum serves of food from each food group (NHMRC 2013b). The ADGs are currently under review by the National Health and Medical Research Council, and updated guidelines based on the most recent evidence will help to inform current nutrition and dietetic practice (NHMRC 2022).

The 2018 Australian Burden of Disease Study determined that 38% of the disease burden could be prevented if risk factors such as dietary factors were modified. The total burden of disease attributable to all dietary risks was 5.4%, the third most significant risk factor after tobacco use and overweight (including obesity) (AIHW 2021a). Similarly, in 2020 diabetes ranked seventh in Australia's leading causes of death

(ABS 2022). One in twenty (5.3%) people in Australia are diagnosed with diabetes. The incidence increases as people age, increasing to one in five for people aged 75 years and over (19.2%) (ABS 2022). Obesity increases the risk of developing diabetes, with adults with obesity five times more likely to have diabetes (ABS 2018a). Coronary heart disease is the most significant cause of death for Australians (AIHW 2020a). Higher intakes of vegetables and fruit have been linked to lower total and all risk mortality (Wang et al. 2021). However, in Australia, fruit and vegetable consumption is below recommended intakes, with 51.3% of adults reaching the recommended intake of fruit and only 7.5% meeting the recommended intake of vegetables (ABS 2018b). For children, rates are higher, with 73% of children meeting fruit recommendations and 6.0% meeting both the vegetable and fruit recommendations (ABS 2018b).

Australia has some of the most concerning levels of obesity and overweight across the 22 OECD member countries, with the sixth-highest proportion of the population living with overweight or obesity and the fifth highest levels of those living with obesity (AIHW 2020b). Figures show that by the time men and women in Australia are middle-aged, 83% and 74%, respectively, are living with overweight or obesity (AIHW 2020b). Children's levels of overweight and obesity are equally concerning, although levels are plateauing, with 24% of children aged 5–14 years living with overweight or obesity in 2017–18 compared to 23% in 2007–08 (ABS 2019). These figures are alarming when we consider that excessive body weight contributes to chronic diseases, is exceedingly difficult to treat and incurs substantial economic costs in health care and lost productivity (Crosland et al. 2019).

The government has invested considerable public health effort to address the burden of disease, including developing public health national and state-level policies. These statistics, however, suggest that most adults in Australia are unaware of their health condition or do not consider it a problem. This prompts us to consider Bacchi's (2016) proposition of 'What's the problem represented to be?' (discussed in Chapter 1) from the government's perspective and the perspective of those living with these conditions, the public.

An example of a policy that would benefit from an interrogation using Bacchi's (2016) 'What's the problem represented to be?' framework is the ADGs. As a population, we struggle to meet the ADGs. Most adults (94.6%) and children (94%) do not consume enough recommended protective fruit and vegetables, and 33%–41% of total daily energy intake comes from discretionary foods across the age groups (AIHW 2018). Discretionary foods are low in nutrients, but high in energy and fat, added sugar and salt and are a primary contributor to the population's excessive consumption of added sugars, saturated and trans fats and sodium (AIHW 2018). Dietitians and nutritionists have a role in changing this.

Nevertheless, despite government efforts with policy and social marketing messages, the statistics for nutrition-related risk factors and chronic diseases continue to rise (ABS 2022; AIHW 2020a). Deconstructing the ADGs and examining how the underpinning 'problems' are addressed from the perspective of the various levels of government, the public and the food industry is insightful. From the perspective of time-poor parents, particularly mothers, the ADGs are not helpful due to the required planning and time demands to procure and prepare family food to achieve them (Mehta et al. 2020).

Food and Nutrition Policy in Australia

Contemporary dietary advice and nutrition services and interventions provided to the Australian public are directed by national and international nutrition policy. Since 1992, Australia has had a national food and nutrition policy and federal government funding for strategies to reduce obesity and promote preventive health. However, with a change in government in 2013, to one that is neoliberal and favours a small government focusing on the private sector, these policy-driven initiatives were de-funded. Consequently, the states and territories followed by decreasing funding for diet-related initiatives, except for some joint Australian, state and territory government initiatives such as the 'Health Star Rating System' (HSR). The HSR is a voluntary front-of-pack food labelling initiative that complements the Healthy Food Partnership work where the government, the public health sector, and the food industry make positive food-related changes. However, the involvement of multiple levels of government, policy-makers, food industry, legislators, advocacy groups and other stakeholders suggests a tension between interest groups, particularly government, food industry and consumer groups, where change can be perceived as slow based on 'evidence', or threatening. This situation warrants an interrogation of what the problems are represented to be using Bacchi's (2016) framework to provide an understanding of the tensions.

In the face of limited leadership on preventive health, key organisations such as The Obesity Collective (2022) and the Obesity Policy Coalition (2022) emerged, with membership from state governments, industry, academic institutions and community groups lobbying for policy reform and development. After extensive consultation, the federal government has recently released the National Preventive Health Strategy 2021–30 and the National Obesity Strategy 2022–32. Both strategies provide frameworks for action and targets for achievement; however, funding mechanisms and government responsibilities are unclear.

Other examples of policy that involve several stakeholders, including government, private industry and consumers, include the Aged Care Quality Standards and Early Childhood Education and Care National Quality Standards (Aged Care Quality and Safety Commission (ACQSC) 2021; The Australian Children's Education and Care Quality Authority (ACECQA) 2018), which are national benchmarks for the provision of food and nutrition in aged-care facilities and residential care, early childhood education and care services and outside-school-hours services. Similarly, recent changes to the NDIS Practice Standards and Quality Indicators have paved the way for improved nutritional support for people living with a disability, including more comprehensive collaboration between the relevant disciplines (National Disability Insurance Scheme (NDIS) 2021).

Nutrition and dietetic professionals are crucial in developing and implementing national, state and territory policies that provide direction and guidelines for healthy nutrition promotion strategies in everyday practice and to populations.

CURRENT ISSUES IN NUTRITION IN AUSTRALIA

Food System Sustainability and Health, Leaving No One Behind

Several wicked problems challenge Australia in the next two decades, which the nutrition and dietetic workforce are equipped to address. The most pressing problem is that our unsustainable food system perpetuates poor health and exacerbates inequities (Stefanovic 2020). A

decadal plan for the science of nutrition by the Australian Academy of Science provides essential actions needed to ensure Australia's food and nutrition security, improve health and well-being, and reduce environmental impact in the future (Australian Academy of Science National Committee for Nutrition 2019). Internationally, the EAT-Lancet Commission on Food, Planet, and Health has explored whether we can feed a future population of 10 billion people a healthy diet within the capacity of our planet (Willett et al. 2019).

Public health concerns extend to the sustainability of our food supply given food wastage, the challenges of climate warming on our food supply and the demand for food requiring unsustainable food production practices (Willett et al. 2019). These concerns have led to an alternative paradigm for solutions. The ecological paradigm takes a holistic food system literacy approach that considers factors at all levels of influence (Stefanovic 2020). This has implications for the future nutrition and dietetic workforce who, through interprofessional collaboration with experts, industry, scientists, policy-makers and influential stakeholders, including politicians, will contribute to finding solutions to this global issue.

The vulnerability of the global and Australian food system was highlighted by the COVID-19 pandemic. Disruptions to the workforce because of illness and strategies such as lockdowns plunged everyone into food insecurity as supply chains were affected and produce perished because it could not be harvested or processed. Learnings from the impact of COVID-19 on our food system has provided us with insights of what is to come. Our food system both contributes to the climate crisis and is affected by it. Addressing our food system is imperative for the survival of humankind.

Obesity – An Individual's or Government Responsibility?

Contributing to the unsustainability of the food system are overconsumption and the commodification of food, increasing populations' overweight and obesity. The dominant paradigms in the Australian health system addressing the high prevalence of obesity are the medical and behavioural approaches to health care, which promote treating illness and hold individuals responsible for their food behaviour and health (Ralston et al. 2018). Less attention is given to the multitude of social, cultural, structural and environmental factors that influence food choice in Australia and nudge people towards obesity.

This is most evident in the debate surrounding the **obesity epidemic**. Australian culture allows an abundance of cheap high-energy, nutrient-poor, affordable, readily available and heavily marketed foods (Ananthapavan et al. 2020; Rendina et al. 2019). Advertising and marketing abound, promoting the kinds of food not recommended by health authorities, and the location, type and number of takeaway and fast-food outlets allow these high-fat, high-sugar, high-salt food options to become familiar, desirable and all too easily accessible (Ananthapavan et al. 2020; Rendina et al. 2019).

Calls for changes to the **obesogenic environment** started well over a decade ago and continue to attract limited funding. The bulk of public money goes into initiatives to address the problem once it already exists (Ralston et al. 2018). An obesogenic environment refers to a built, physical, social and food environment that encourages overconsumption, unhealthy eating, sedentary behaviour and a lack of physical activity. Limited activity and overconsumption of ultra-processed foods during the COVID-19 pandemic and the syndemic of obesity, undernutrition and climate change are further contributing to the obesity epidemic (Chung et al. 2021; Swinburn et al. 2019). Many dietitians and nutritionists advocate for broader public health initiatives that recognise the influence of social, environmental and cultural factors on food choice and seek to address nutritional health issues more holistically.

Food Insecurity

Paradoxically, while overconsumption of food contributes to Australia's poor health and burgeoning health costs, not having enough food affects many Australians and transcends age, social class and geographical location (Temple et al. 2019). **Food insecurity** is when people do not have physical, social and economic access to sufficient, safe and nutritious food at all times (Gallegos et al. 2017). The cause is multifaceted, relating to individual, social, economic, political and environmental factors. The impact of the COVID-19 pandemic and the ongoing impact of the climate crisis on our food system and food security are both examples of this interrelated complexity. Given that food insecurity has a cultural dimension, it is valuable to examine food security policies against Bacchi's (2016) framework as to what the problem is represented to be and from whose perspective.

Pause *for* **Reflection ...**
Dietitians and nutritionists represent one interest group. What other interest groups have a stake in food consumption?

We are responsible for what we eat and, how much, at an individual level. However, are we? Who is responsible for the proliferation of environmental factors that nudges us to overconsume? Who is responsible for the regulation of these influencing factors? What about children who do not have the knowledge or agency to be responsible for food consumption? Using Bacchi's (2016) model 'What's the problem represented to be?', analyse the ADGs against the six proposed questions or policies (see Chapter 1) developed by welfare groups or the local government addressing food security.

█ SUMMARY

This chapter has outlined key information about the nutrition and dietetic profession in the Australian health care system:

- The roles of dietitians and nutritionists are diverse and include a range of settings, from the clinical biomedical treatment of patients to primary health care and health promotion advocacy work within the health care system.
- Australia's nutrition and dietetics professions have been described as small but growing professions within the allied health sector.

- The primary health issues of concern include non-communicable diseases (NCDs) such as cardiovascular disease, cancer and diabetes, and their risk factors such as obesity. These are all affected by dietary intake and so are an important preventive and treatment focus for the nutrition and dietetic profession, particularly as the significant causes of morbidity and mortality in Australia relate to these conditions.
- The roles of nutritionists and dietitians are evolving as we move through a nutrition transition where our food choices, food consumption patterns and dietary

patterns are changing and need to change in response to factors impacting our food system, such as climate change and pandemics, and advances in technologies and research impacting how we engage with nutrition.

- Key nutrition policies and guidelines that inform nutrition practice in Australia are a specific focus of governments, particularly to create health-promoting food environments and address the growing priority of an unsustainable food system.

REVIEW QUESTIONS

1. Identify where dietitians and nutritionists are employed within the Australian health care system and list the diversity of roles undertaken by nutrition and dietetic professionals.
2. Currently, the number of nutrition and dietetic professionals employed within the community remains small; however, the demand and need for nutrition and dietetic services is increasing. How might the work of dietitians and nutritionists change as they move to create environments that make healthy food choices easier?
3. The last revision of the Australian Dietary Guidelines was in 2013. At the time of writing, it is being currently being reviewed. What factors should the NHMRC and expert panel take into account when revising the guidelines? Has our population changed since 2013? Have factors influencing our food choices

and food consumption patterns changed? Are the public health issues of 2013 still prevalent or have they changed, and to what extent?
4. Outline the structural changes that have been introduced into Medicare that allow dietitians, physiotherapists and others to work with GPs in providing multidisciplinary primary care. Can these changes be explained according to Tuohy's policy development frameworks (see Chapter 1)?
5. Food choices are often seen as individual choices, and there is a belief that individuals should be responsible for changing their behaviours. What structural/environmental factors influence food choices beyond an individual's direct control or behaviours? How do you think policy could respond to addressing these factors affecting food choices?

REFERENCES

Adamski, M., Truby, H., Klassen, K., 2020. Using the internet: nutrition information-seeking behaviours of lay people enrolled in a massive online nutrition course. Nutrients 12 (3), 750.

Afshin, A., Sur, P.J., Fay, K.A., et al., 2019. Health effects of dietary risks in 195 countries, 1990–2017: a systematic analysis for the Global Burden of Disease Study 2017. Lancet 393 (10184), 1958–1972.

Ananthapavan, J., Sacks, G., Brown, V., et al., 2020. Priority-setting for obesity prevention—The Assessing Cost-Effectiveness of obesity prevention policies in Australia (ACE-Obesity Policy) study. PLOS ONE 15 (6), 1–19.

Allied Health Professions Australia 2022. Dietetics. https://ahpa.com.au/allied-health-professions/dietetics/.

Australian Bureau of Statistics (ABS), 2019. Microdata: National Health Survey, 2017–18. Cat. no. 4324.0.55.001. ABS, Canberra.

Australian Academy of Science National Committee for Nutrition, 2019. Nourishing Australia: a decadal plan for the science of nutrition. https://www.science.org.au/

supporting-science/science-policy-and-analysis/decadal-plans-science/nourishing-australia-decadal-plan.

Australian Bureau of Statistics (ABS), 2018a. Overweight and obesity 2017–2018 financial year. ABS, Canberra. https://www.abs.gov.au/statistics/health/health-conditions-and-risks/overweight-and-obesity/latest-release.

Australian Bureau of Statistics (ABS), 2018b. National Health Survey: first results, 2017–18. Cat no. 4364.0.55.001. ABS, Canberra.

Australian Bureau of Statistics (ABS), 2022. Diabetes 2020–2021 financial year. ABS, Canberra. https://www.abs.gov.au/statistics/health/health-conditions-and-risks/diabetes/latest-release.

Australian Children's Education and Care Quality Authority (ACECQA), 2018. National quality standard. https://www.acecqa.gov.au/nqf/national-quality-standard.

Australian Commission on Safety and Quality in Health Care (ACSQHC), 2022. National safety and quality health service standards, second ed, version 2. ACSQHC, Sydney.

Australian Institute of Health and Welfare (AIHW), 2018. Nutrition across the life stages. Cat. no. PHE 227, AIHW, Canberra.

Australian Institute of Health and Welfare (AIHW), 2020a. Burden of disease. AIHW, Canberra. https://www.aihw. gov.au/reports/australias-health/burden-of-disease.

Australian Institute of Health and Welfare (AIHW), 2020b, Overweight and obesity: an interactive insight. Cat. no. PHE 251. AIHW, Canberra.

Australian Institute of Health and Welfare (AIHW), 2021a. Australian Burden of Disease Study 2018: key findings. Australian Burden of Disease Study series 24. Cat. no. BOD 30. AIHW, Canberra.

Australian Government, Aged Care Quality & Safety Commission (ACQSC), 2021. Aged Care Quality Standards. https://www.agedcarequality.gov.au/providers/ standards.

Bacchi, C., 2016. Problematisations in health policy: questioning how "problems" are constituted in policies. SAGE Open, 1–16. doi:10.1177/2158244016653986.

Blair, M., Mitchell, L., Palermo, C., et al., (2021). Trends, challenges, opportunities, and future needs of the dietetic workforce: a systematic scoping review. Nutrition Reviews.

Boak, R., Palermo, C., Gallegos, D., 2021. Towards 2030: Re-imagining the Future of Nutrition and Dietetics in Australia and New Zealand. Report for the Council of Deans of Nutrition and Dietetics, Australia and New Zealand. https://www.dieteticdeans.com.

Butler, M.J., Barrientos, R.M., 2020. The impact of nutrition on COVID-19 susceptibility and long-term consequences. Brain Behav Immun 87, 53–54.

Commonwealth Scientific and Industrial Research Organisation (CSIRO) Futures, 2018. Future of health: shifting Australia's focus from illness treatment to health and wellbeing management. CSIRO, Canberra.

Chung, A., Tully, L., Czernin, S., et al., 2021. Reducing risk of childhood obesity in the wake of Covid-19. BMJ 374.

Crosland, P., Ananthapavan, J., Davison, J., 2019. The economic cost of preventable disease in Australia: a systematic review of estimates and methods. Aust N Z J Public Health 43 (5), 484–495.

Department of Health, 2021. Allied health in Australia, September. Department of Health, Canberra. https://www. health.gov.au/health-topics/allied-health/in-australia.

Dietitians Australia (DA), 2021a. National Competency Standards for Dietitians in Australia. DA, Deakin. https://bit.ly/3DBmcsF.

Dietitians Australia (DA), 2021b. Dietitians Australia priorities for the 2021–22 federal budget. DA, Deakin. https:// treasury.gov.au/sites/default/files/2021-05/171663_ dietitians_australia_supporting_documents.pdf.

Dietitians Australia (DA), 2022a. Dietitian or nutritionist. DA, Deakin. https://dietitiansaustralia.org.au/seeing-dietitian/ what-expect/dietitian-or-nutritionist/.

Dietitians Australia (DA), 2022b, Dietitians Australia annual report 2020–2021. DA, Deakin. https://dietitiansaustralia.org. au/sites/default/files/2022-01/Annual-Report-2020-21.pdf.

Dietitians Australia (DA), 2022c, Credentialing of dietitians. DA, Deakin. https://dietitiansaustralia.org.au/working- dietetics/credentialing-dietitians#How.

EAT-Lancet Commission, 2019. Summary report: healthy diets from sustainable food systems: food planet health. https://eatforum.org/eat-lancet-commission/eat-lancet- commission-summary-report/.

Gallegos, D., Booth, S., Cleve, S., et al., 2017. Food insecurity in Australian households from charity to entitlement. In: Germov, J., Williams, L. (Eds.), A Sociology of Food and Nutrition, fourth ed. Oxford University Press, Melbourne.

Germov, J. Williams, L. 2017. A Sociology of Food & Nutrition: The Social Appetite, fourth ed. Oxford University Press, Melbourne.

Haines, J., Haycraft, E., Lytle, L., et al., 2019. Nurturing children's healthy eating: position statement. Appetite 137, 124–133.

Hickson, M., Child, J., Collinson, A., 2018. Future Dietitian 2025: informing the development of a workforce strategy for dietetics. J Hum Nutr Diet 31, 23–32.

Kelly, J.T., Allman-Farinelli, M., Chen, J., et al., 2020. Dietitians Australia's position statement on telehealth. Nutr Diet 77 (4), 406–415.

Kelly, J.T., Collins, P.F., McCamley, J., et al., 2021. Digital disruption of dietetics: are we ready? J Hum Nutr Diet 34 (1), 134–146.

Kokkoris, M.D., Stavrova, O., 2021. Meaning of food and consumer eating behaviours. Food Qual Prefer 94, 104343.

Mehta, K., Booth, S., Coveney, J., et al., 2020. Feeding the Australian family: challenges for mothers, nutrition, and equity. Health Promot Int 1–8. doi: 10.1093/heapro/daz061.

National Disability Insurance Scheme (NDIS) Quality and Safeguards Commission, 2021. NDIS Practice Standards and Quality Indicators, Version 4. https://www. ndiscommission.gov.au/document/986.

National Health and Medical Research Council (NHMRC), 2013a. Australian Dietary Guidelines. NHMRC, Canberra. https://www.eatforhealth.gov.au/guidelines/australian- guide-healthy-eating.

National Health and Medical Research Council (NHMRC), 2013b. Australian Dietary Guidelines; providing the scientific evidence for healthier Australian diets. NHMRC, Canberra. https://www.nhmrc.gov.au/about-us/ publications/australian-dietary-guidelines.

National Health and Medical Research Council (NHMRC), 2022. Building a healthy Australia, Australian Dietary Guidelines review. https://bit.ly/3uUHf5L.

Nutrition Society Australia (NSA), 2022a. What nutritionists do. https://www.nsa.asn.au/index.cfm//nutrition-study/ what-nutritionists-do/.

Nutrition Society of Australia (NSA), 2022b. About NSA registration. https://www.nsa.asn.au/index.cfm/nsa-registration/about-nsa-registration/.

Obesity Policy Coalition (OPC), 2022. Obesity Policy Coalition – who are we – partners and funders. https://www.opc.org.au/who-we-are/partners.

Ralston, J., Brinsden, H., Buse, K., et al., 2018. Time for a new obesity narrative. Lancet 392 (10156), 1384–1386.

Rendina, D., Campanozzi, A., De Filippo, G., 2019. Methodological approach to the assessment of the obesogenic environment in children and adolescents: A review of the literature. Nutr Metab Cardiovasc Dis 29 (6), 561–571.

Schot, E., Tummers, L., Noordegraaf, M., 2020. Working on working together. A systematic review on how healthcare professionals contribute to interprofessional collaboration. J Interprof Care 34 (3), 332–342.

Shiell, A., Jackson, H., 2018. How much does Australia spend on prevention and how would we know whether it is enough? Health Promot J Austr 29, 7–9.

Siopis, G., Jones, A., Allman-Farinelli, M., 2020. The dietetic workforce distribution geographic atlas provides insight into the inequitable access for dietetic services for people with type 2 diabetes in Australia. Nutri Diet 77 (1), 121–130.

Sports Dietitians Australia, 2022. About us. https://www.sportsdietitians.com.au/about-us/.

Stefanovic, L., Freytag-Leyer, B., Kahl, J., 2020. Food system outcomes: an overview and the contribution to food systems transformation. Front Sustain Food Syst 4, 1–8.

Swinburn, B.A., Kraak, V.I., Allender, S., 2019. The global syndemic of obesity, undernutrition, and climate change: the Lancet Commission report. Lancet 393 (10173), 791–846.

Temple, J.B., Booth, S., Pollard, C.M., 2019. Social assistance payments and food insecurity in Australia: evidence from the household expenditure survey. Int J Environ Res Public Health 16 (3), 455.

The Obesity Collective (TOC), 2022. The Obesity Collective – membership. https://www.obesityaustralia.org/membership.

Wahlqvist, M.L., Gallegos, D., 2020. Food and Nutrition: Sustainable Food and Health Systems, fourth ed. A&U Academic, Sydney.

Wang, D.D., Li, Y., Bhupathiraju, S.N., et al., 2021. Fruit and vegetable intake and mortality: results from 2 prospective cohort studies of US men and women and a meta-analysis of 26 cohort studies. Circulation 143 (17), 1642–1654.

Wijnen, A., Bishop, K., Joshy, G., et al., 2022. Observed and predicted premature mortality in Australia due to non-communicable diseases: a population-based study examining progress towards the WHO 25X25 goal. BMC Medicine 20, 57.

Willett, W., Rockstrom, J., Loken, B., et al., 2019. Food in the anthropocene: the EAT–Lancet Commission on healthy diets from sustainable food system. Lancet Commissions 393 (10170), 447–492.

World Health Organization (WHO), 2020. Non-communicable diseases progress monitor 2020. License: CC BY-NC-SA 3.0 IGO. WHO, Geneva.

FURTHER READING

Brown, J.E., 2020. Nutrition Through THE Life Cycle, seventh ed. Cengage Learning Australia, Melbourne.

Saxelby, C., 2018. Catherine Saxelby's Complete Food and Nutrition Companion: The Ultimate A–Z Guide. Hardie Grant Books, Sydney.

Wahlqvist, M.L., & Gallegos, D. (2020). Food and Nutrition: Sustainable Food and Health Systems, fourth ed. Allen & Unwin, Crow's Nest.

ONLINE RESOURCES

Department of Health and Aged Care – national nutrition policy, laws, programs and initiatives: https://www.health.gov.au/health-topics/food-and-nutrition/what-were-doing.

Dietitians Association of Australia – diet and nutrition health advice, nutrition information and advice written by APDs: https://dietitiansaustralia.org.au/diet-and-nutrition-health-advice.

Eat for Health (national dietary guidelines) – detailed information on the Australian Dietary Guidelines plus advice, tips, resources, recipes and calculators. Extensive scientific background information on each of the guidelines can be found in the Eat for Health educator guide – information for nutrition educators: http://www.eatforhealth.gov.au.

Nutrition Australia – this independent member organisation aims to promote the health and well-being of all Australians and has several resources available: https://nutrition-australia.org/.

20

Health Services Managers in the Australian Health Care System

Joanne Travaglia and Deborah Debono

KEY LEARNING OUTCOMES

When you finish this chapter you should be able to:
- differentiate how the work of managers is understood by two different schools of thought
- describe the roles of health services managers in Australia including a range of professional profiles
- describe the differences and similarities between leadership and management
- identify the role of health services managers in improving quality, safety and equity of health and social care
- outline the competencies required by health services managers.

KEY TERMS AND ABBREVIATIONS

Australasian College of Health Service Management (ACHSM)

Australian Bureau of Statistics (ABS)

Australian Commission on Safety and Quality in Health Care (ACSQHC)

medical rationing

Royal Australasian College of Medical Administrators (RACMA)

social care

INTRODUCTION

Why should a book on the Australian health care system consider managers and management? To put it simply, as Cunliffe (2021: n.p.) claims 'The crucial point is that *what managers do has an impact on people's lives,* on society at large, and on the environment in which we live. And managers like the rest of us are human and fallible'. She goes on to argue that 'managing is a relational, reflexive and moral practice: about who you are and how you relate to others.' This is never more so, we would argue, than in the health (and social) care sectors where people's lives literally depend on the decisions made by managers (and clinicians), as the SARS-CoV-2 pandemic has clearly shown (Parsons & Johal 2020) (more on this issue later in the chapter).

MANAGERS, MANAGEMENT AND ORGANISATIONS

So, what is management and what do managers do? Walshe and Smith (2011) note that there are two distinct schools of thought about these basic questions. The first school of thought is that management is a science, something which can be replicated and evaluated. The second school of thought is that management is an art or a craft, that is, something that is highly individualistic, depending on the person and the context.

Although Walshe and Smith believe the truth is somewhere between the two, it is interesting and useful to consider both perspectives, which they differentiate in the following way.

From the 'management as science' point of view,

... there are knowable facts and provable theories from which we can generalize and develop a codified body of knowledge that managers can then use in their practice ... [and managers] plan, organize, control, communicate and coordinate. Their job is about deploying resources to maximize efficiency and effectiveness in achieving organizational goals.

(Walshe & Smith, 2011, n.p.)

From the 'management as art or craft' perspective,

... there is little in management that is not subjective, open to contestation, dependent on prevailing social and cultural norms. Generalization is highly problematic, there are few if any right or wrong answers, and most practices are contingent and dependent on the situation ... [and managers] communicate, motivate and lead. Their job is fundamentally a social and relational one – about getting things done through other people and so about creating and sustaining organizational environments that enable those things to get done.

(Walshe & Smith, 2011, n.p.)

Pause *for* Reflection ...

Which school of management thought sits most closely with your experience of management?

Can you see value in the other school of thought in general, and as a way of considering the management of health care services in particular?

The reality is that health care systems and services are highly complex organisations, which of course immediately begs the question, 'What is an organisation?' Haveman and Wetts (2019, e12627) define organisations as '... collections of people, material assets, financial resources, and information, whose members have common goals that they cooperate to pursue. ... People create formal organizations when the actions they must undertake to achieve their goals require the joint, sustained, and coordinated efforts of many people'. The more complex an organisation, the more coordination – or management – is required.

MANAGEMENT AND LEADERSHIP

In a previous edition of this book, the authors of this chapter, Maddern et al. (2020, p. 328), noted that:

Authority is part of the job – the manager's mandate to control or coordinate the work of others is included in the position description and often laid out in an organisation chart. It is the organisation that defines and sets the limits of managers' authority, sometimes called delegations. ... Of course, the limits of authority are also set by the laws and regulations of the society and the industry. ... The underlying goal of most organisations can be stated as some version of 'to deliver services or products that meet consumer needs at the required standards and costs'. Government health authorities may define this as 'to provide policy advice and administer programs in accordance with government policies', even this is a specialised version of the general statement. All organisations of any size – rural or metropolitan, network, hospital or community – need managers to coordinate the work ('organise'), to solve problems ('control'), to adapt the organisation to changes in the environment ('plan'), and to enable staff to work collaboratively towards achieving the organisation's goals as effectively as possible ('lead').

The differences between management and leadership is an interesting topic, and one which has generated many publications and much debate. Nienaber (2010, p. 661) reviewed the literature on management and leadership and concluded that 'all of the tasks [he reviewed] fall within the boundaries of management, while leadership tasks overlap with management. Unlike management, leadership has no distinct task that falls exclusively within its boundary.' In other words, a manager has to do everything a leader does, and more. The UK Health Foundation make the distinction between management and leadership in a more pragmatic way (see Table 20.1).

Pause *for* Reflection ...

Reflect on the distinction between management and leadership provided in Table 20.1. Do you think there is a difference between what leaders and managers do in health care? What would this look like in practice? Does it matter? Why?

TABLE 20.1	**Management Versus Leadership**
Management	**Leadership**
Management involves the control, monitoring or organisation of people, processes and systems in order to achieve specific goals. It has been described as consisting of six key tasks: planning, allocating resources, coordinating the work of others, motivating staff, monitoring output and taking responsibility for the process.	Leadership refers to influencing and inspiring others in pursuit of common goals, setting the tone and direction for a group or organisation, and identifying and framing problems for others to solve. In practice, leadership and management are closely interconnected and health care employees at all levels often have to deploy both leadership and management skills in order to carry out their job effectively.

Source: The Health Foundation (2022). Strengthening NHS management and leadership: priorities for reform. https://www.health.org.uk/publications/long-reads/strengthening-nhs-management-and-leadership.

The question of what managers actually *do* is as complicated as the question of what management *is*. Some of the earliest studies of management go back to the start of the 20th century, where Frederick Winslow Taylor (1856–1915) was starting what is known as the school of 'scientific' management, which included people like Henry Ford (inventor of the Model T Ford car), Henry Gantt (inventor of the Gantt chart) and Frank and Lillian Gilbreth (time and motion experts). The people aligned with this school believed that 'improving the practice of management meant making it more scientific' (Kiechel, 2012, p. 65) which in turn meant studying empirically what managers did in order to work out how this could be improved.

The school of scientific management was followed by the administrative school, which included – notably, for our purposes – Henri Fayol (1841–1925), a French mining engineer by training. In his 1916 book on management, Fayol identified the five major functions of management: planning, organising, commanding, coordinating and controlling (now more commonly re-conceptualised as planning, organising, leading and controlling) (Fayol 1916/1949) which you will recognise echo the Health Foundation's definition of health care management outlined in Table 20.1.

More closely aligned to the work of modern health services managers is that of Mary Parker Follett (1868–1933) who was a social worker in the United States in the early 1900s and who put forward many ideas which are still in use in organisations today. These included ideas such as 'win-win' (rather than win-lose) approaches to conflict within organisations, a recognition of the value of diversity for organisations, and the idea that managers should have power 'with' rather than power 'over' the people who work for them (Graham 2003). More recent

leadership theories have emphasised different elements of both managers and organisations, such as the need to manage: culture (Peters & Waterman 1982); strategy (Porter 2008); organisational learning (Senge 2006); and change (Kotter 2007). Goleman has addressed the need for managers to have emotional intelligence, an issue which has gained significant momentum in the health sector (Goleman 1996), while Senge, as well as addressing organisational learning, has advanced the idea of systems thinking for managers (and leaders) that is the ability to perceive the issues that emerge in highly complex, adaptive systems such as health and **social care**.

Pause *for* Reflection ...
How might the characteristics of emotional intelligence – self-awareness, self-regulation, motivation, empathy and social skills – be important for a health care manager to have?

MANAGERS AND MANAGEMENT IN AUSTRALIAN HEALTH CARE

The work of health care managers in Australia is not clearly defined or delineated, although the **Australasian College of Health Service Management (ACHSM)** has produced several sets of health management competencies (which we will discuss later). Much of what we do know about health care management in recent times is from the **Australian Bureau of Statistics (ABS)**. The ABS had identified several different titles/positions for health services managers. These include:
- medical administrator/medical superintendent (including the specialisations of director of clinical services or director of medical services)

- nursing clinical director (including the specialisations of assistant director of nursing, deputy director of nursing and/or executive director of nursing)
- primary health organisation manager
- welfare centre manager (or welfare project manager)
- health and welfare services managers (including director of pharmacy, director of physiotherapy services, director of speech pathology, disability services program manager and/or manager of allied health services).

The ABS states that, in Australia,

... healthcare managers may be expected to undertake the following tasks:
- *providing overall direction and management for the service, facility, organisation or centre*
- *developing, implementing and monitoring procedures, policies and standards for medical, nursing, allied health and administrative staff*
- *coordinating and administering health and welfare programs and clinical services*
- *monitoring and evaluating resources devoted to health, welfare, recreation, housing, employment, training and other community facilities and centres*
- *controlling administrative operations such as budget planning, report preparation, expenditure on supplies, equipment and services*
- *liaising with other health and welfare providers, boards and funding bodies to discuss areas of health and welfare service cooperation and coordination*
- *advising government bodies about measures to improve health and welfare services and facilities*
- *representing the organisation in negotiations, and at conventions, seminars, public hearings and forums*
- *controlling selection, training and supervision of staff*

(Australian Bureau of Statistics (ABS) 2021a, n.p.)

The ABS has a separate category for nurse managers, whom they describe in the following way:

Nurse Managers manage health service units and sub-units of hospitals, aged care and community health care facilities, supervise nursing staff and financial resources to enable the provision of safe, cost-effective nursing care within specified fields or

for particular units, and monitor quality, clinical standards and professional development of nurses. Registration or licensing is required.

(ABS 2021b, n.p.)

A nurse manager might also be called a charge nurse, nurse supervisor or nurse unit manager. Their tasks may include:

- *developing, implementing and monitoring policies and objectives of nursing care as they apply to units, staff and community groups*
- *coordinating the allocation of human and material resources for a health service unit such as recruitment of staff, human resource management, preparation of budgets and fiscal management*
- *monitoring and controlling the performance of nursing and support staff within the unit, and providing leadership*
- *initiating studies to evaluate the effectiveness of nursing services in the unit in relation to objectives, costs and nursing care*
- *promoting working relationships with community agencies and health and education providers*
- *contributing to organisational objectives in relation to quality, safety and risk management*

(ABS 2021b, n.p.)

Three notable absences from the lists of tasks identified for health services managers by the ABS are ensuring patient safety, quality improvement and equity. Yet we know from our own research and from Health Services Management students that many managers are involved in each of these tasks.

Pause *for* Reflection ...
What are some of the similarities and differences in the tasks and responsibilities of nurse managers and other health services managers?

Core Competencies of Health Services Managers

Another source of insight into the tasks of managers are the competency standards set by professional bodies. There are two bodies who directly address health manager competencies – the Australasian College of Health Service Management (ACHSM) and the **Royal Australasian College of Medical Administrators (RACMA)** (which is only for medical doctors). A set of competencies has also been developed for aged-care sector management.

The ACHSM competency frameworks are organised around five domains of practice: (1) Leadership, (2) Health and Health Care Environment, (3) Business Skills, (4) Communication and Relationship Development, (5) Professional and Social Responsibility. Each of these domains is divided into multiple sub-domains with corresponding competency statements. The ACHSM frameworks include 86 competency statements in total (Australasian College of Health Service Management (ACHSM) 2016).

To reinforce our previous statement about what is missing from the ABS definitions of the tasks of health managers, it should be noted that ACHSM has competency statements relating to safety, quality and equity. In relation to safety and quality, ACHSM has a number of different competencies required of health managers, including sub-domains entitled Risk Management and Clinical Governance and Quality and Safety (ACHSM 2016, pp. 10,12,13,16).

While most of the quality and safety competencies are grouped together, there is one notable exception in relation to safety. Under the sub-domain Partnering with Consumers, the ACHSM specifies that a health care manager '2.3.1. Promotes cultural safety and Indigenous rights withrespect to all treaty and/or partnership arrangements' (ACHSM 2016, p. 10).

In relation to equity, ACHSM frames these competencies around partnering with communities starting with 2.3.1 as discussed above, but also including: '2.3.2. Partners with consumers (including family and carers) in the planning, designing and monitoring of care; 2.3.3. Promotes the preferences of both majority and minority communities, particularly Indigenous groups, in relation to health practices and priorities; and 2.4.1. Pursues goals and objectives for improving the health of the community; which demonstrate an understanding of the social determinants of health and of the socioeconomic environment' (ACHSM 2016, pp. 10, 11).

RACMA has what they call a Medical Leadership and Management curriculum. The core of the curriculum competency framework is the role of medical leader, which they define as 'the medical specialist with expertise in health organisation management practice' (Royal Australasian College of Medical Administrators (RACMA) 2011, p. 9). This role is surrounded by six role competencies: medical expert, communicator, advocate, scholar, professional, collaborator and manager. Each role competency is then broken down into key goals. The RACMA framework includes 132 individual enabling competencies and objectives, in total (RACMA 2011).

As with ACHSM, the RACMA competencies indicate the importance of managers' responsibility for both the quality and safety, and equity of care. In relation to equity, RACMA's enabling competencies include some general points, relating to bias and the identification of community needs (RACMA 2011, p. 17).

Pause *for* Reflection ...

Do you agree that health services managers should be responsible for the quality, safety and equity of care? What do you think this responsibility should entail?

Health Services Managers and the Quality and Safety of Care

The quality and safety of health care has been an issue from the inception of the field. The wording of the Hippocratic Oath speaks to the potential for harm caused by health care professionals and interventions (Smith 1996). Although always an issue, the current focus on quality and safety improvement has gained significant momentum since the 1990s when a series of papers was published in Australia and internationally indicating that between 10% and 16% of people who are admitted to hospital experience some form of adverse event, ranging from minor issues to death – many (if not all) of which could have been avoided (Kohn et al. 2000; Wilson et al. 1995). Errors in general take two forms: 'an act of commission (doing something wrong) or omission (failing to do the right thing) that leads to an undesirable outcome or significant potential for such an outcome' (Agency for Healthcare Research and Quality n.d., n.p.). In Australia, health services managers are involved in the monitoring and improving of the safety and quality of care under clinical governance. Clinical governance is an approach to safety and quality which emerged in the UK and which has been taken up by Commonwealth countries around the world. It was first defined in the UK as 'a system through which NHS organisations are accountable for continually improving the quality of their services and safeguarding high standards of care by creating an environment in which excellence in clinical care will flourish' (Scally & Donaldson 1998, p. 62). Clinical governance is of particular importance to health services managers both because it directs strategies and actions meant to identify and respond to risks to quality and safety, and because it is closely aligned to corporate governance, as 'it too is concerned with accountability, effective end results, acceptable resource use and appropriate ways of working and behaving' (Braithwaite & Travaglia 2008, p. 12).

Clinical governance is promoted by

> ... accountability, vigilant governing boards and bodies, a focus on ethics and regulating qualified privilege. It also includes taking steps to institute measures such as continuous improvement, quality assurance, audit, applying standards and ensuring they are met, using clinical indicators, encouraging clinical effectiveness, promoting evidence-based practice, participating in accreditation processes, managing risk, reporting and managing incidents, focusing on patient safety, improving the sharing of information, supporting open disclosure, managing knowledge effectively, obtaining patient consent, providing feedback on performance, promoting continuous education, dealing with complaints effectively, encouraging consumers to participate in decisions affecting their care and credentialling of medical [and other] practitioners.
>
> *(Braithwaite & Travaglia 2008, pp. 12–13)*

Health services managers have a role to play in each of these actions, either directly or in ensuring that they are undertaken by others.

Governing boards and bodies are informed, in part, as to whether their organisation has systems, structures and processes in place to provide safe, high-quality care by accreditation results and reports. Accreditation is a process by which external reviewers assess whether an organisation is compliant with safety and quality standards and the continuous quality improvement strategies in place to achieve safe and high-quality health care. In Australia, the National Safety and Quality Health Service Standards have been developed by the Australian Commission on Safety and Quality in Health Care (ACSQHC). 'All public and private hospitals, day procedure services and public dental practices are required to be accredited to the NSQHS Standards. Many other healthcare facilities will also choose to be accredited in order to improve the safety and quality of health care provision. (Australian Commission on Safety and

Quality in Health Care (ACQSHC) n.d., n.p.). Health services managers at all levels of the organisation are involved in the accreditation process.

Pause *for* Reflection ...
What are some ways in which health care managers might be involved in the accreditation process in health care?

Health Services Managers and the Equity of Care

In the United States the Institute for Health Innovation (IHI) has developed what they originally called the 'triple aim' of health care: improving patient experience, improving population health and lowering per capita costs for health care (Berwick et al. 2008). Since then, they have expanded this to a 'quadruple aim', with the addition of ensuring clinician well-being (Sikka et al. 2015) and finally, in 2021, the addition of health equity has made this a quintuple aim (Nundy et al. 2022). While the quintuple aim originated in the US, it is used in both the UK (Stokes et al. 2021; Wyatt et al. 2020) and Australia (Robertson-Preidler et al. 2017; Whittington et al. 2015).

The classic definition of health equity is from Margaret Whitehead, who wrote that 'Equity in health implies that ideally everyone should have a fair opportunity to attain their full health potential and, more pragmatically, that no one should be disadvantaged from achieving this potential, if it can be avoided' (Whitehead 1992, p. 433) which should translate into 'equal access to available care for equal need, equal utilization for equal need, equal quality of care for all' (Whitehead 1992, p. 434). The link between equity and quality improvement in health care, as envisaged by the quintuple aim approach, has been described in the following way: 'The pursuit of health equity ought to be elevated as the fifth aim for health care improvement, purposefully including with all improvement and innovation efforts a focus on individuals and communities who need them most' (Nundy et al. 2022, p. 521). A key role for health services managers in the pursuit of equity is ensuring that health care resources are equitably distributed (Lane et al. 2017), an issue which came to the fore during the SARS-CoV-2 pandemic, and that good governance, including transparency and participation in health systems decision-making, is maintained (Labonté 2010).

When thinking about health equity and disadvantage, we must consider the impact of colonisation on the health of Aboriginal and Torres Strait Islander people (see Chapter 10). There is essentially no aspect of the health of Aboriginal and Torres Strait Islander people that is not affected by colonisation. Through setting priorities for the organisation to meet the needs for Aboriginal and Torres Strait Islander people, the governing body in an organisation can direct resources to improve care (The Wardliparingga Aboriginal Research Unit of the South Australian Health and Medical Research Institute 2017). Because of the ongoing inequity experienced by Aboriginal and Torres Strait Islander people, the **Australian Commission on Safety and Quality in Health Care (ACSQHC)** has defined, within the National Safety and Quality Health Service Standards, six actions to meet the needs of Aboriginal and/or Torres Strait Islander people. Health care managers play a pivotal role in enabling and enacting the six actions proposed by the ACSQHC (The Wardliparingga Aboriginal Research Unit of the South Australian Health and Medical Research Institute 2017). These six actions are:

- partnering with communities
- governance and identifying priorities
- implementation and monitoring in partnership with Aboriginal and/or Torres Strait Islander people
- cultural awareness and cultural competency
- welcoming environment
- identifying people of Aboriginal and Torres Strait Islander origin.

Pause *for* Reflection ...

Can you think of specific examples of activities health managers might undertake for each of the six actions proposed by the ACSQHC to meet the health needs of Aboriginal and Torres Strait Islander people?

Health Services Managers and COVID-19

Throughout this chapter there have been references to the impact of the SARS-CoV-2 pandemic on health care in general, and on health services managers in particular. This is because, unlike any other event in recent history, the pandemic began to reveal very early on both the underlying weaknesses in health care systems around the world, and the differential impact on vulnerable groups.

The complexities of the pandemic are beyond the scope of this chapter (and indeed this book), but it is impossible to write a chapter about the management of health services in the 21st century without its consideration. What the SARS-CoV-2 pandemic highlighted was exactly how organised (or not) health care services and systems were for the almost inevitable eventuality of a pandemic, remembering of course that the SARS-CoV-2 pandemic was preceded relatively recently by several other serious coronavirus outbreaks, including MERS and SARS (Khan et al. 2020). The impact of COVID-19 has been immense, and health care services have scrambled to take care of a rapidly increasing number of patients, while at the same time facing reductions in the number of staff, as health care workers (and/or their families) themselves became ill and died (Bandyopadhyay et al. 2020; Chutiyami et al. 2022). This perfect storm tested systems, managers, leaders and workers to their limits, and in many cases beyond (see Case study 20.1).

As Chen and McNamara (2020, p. 1) argue, 'the current public health crisis has exposed deep cracks in social equality and justice for marginalised and vulnerable communities around the world'. The impact of COVID-19 also brought to the fore accusations of discrimination and, in particular, ageism (Lichtenstein 2021) and ableism, as services scrambled to decide how to allocate dwindling resources (known as **medical rationing**). Ethicists have pointed out both during and after the height of the outbreak that this principle was not the only approach possible to deciding the distribution of resources. As Paton (2020, p. 1) argued:

The guiding principles of the pandemic have emerged, in one form or another, to favour fairness, especially with regard to allocating resources and prioritizing care. However, fairness is not equivalent to equity when it comes to healthcare, and the focus on fairness means that existing guidance inadvertently discriminates against people from ethnic minority backgrounds ... [as a result there is a need to include and understand] the relationship between ethnicity and health, in any ethical and clinical guidance for care during the pandemic. ... To do otherwise ... would be actively choosing to allow a proportion of the British population to die for no other reason than their ethnic background.

Similar arguments were made about the way in which medical rationing was employed or discussed, particularly early on, in relation to people with disabilities. Cieza et al. (2021) note that denial of COVID-19

CASE STUDY 20.1   Management Case Study: Leadership and Management in a Time of Crisis

Most people in our community believed that the public health intervention in response to the SARS-CoV-2 virus began on the 25th of January 2020, when the first case was identified in Australia. However, there is a 700-year history and knowledge set that has actually been brought to bear in the response around the world to pandemics.

What COVID-19 meant for the ambulance service was that for weeks and weeks and weeks on end (particularly with the Delta variant), there were long delays for people needing to access care and a huge workload for our staff. Our paramedics were really stretched to the limits of what they were able to tolerate. This is the point where there needs to be a transition from management to leadership.

One of the things that has become clear over the last two years is that as a manager/leader you do not have the luxury of making decisions in the way that you have historically done it – you cannot wait until you are absolutely sure and have absolutely all the data and absolutely all of the evidence. You must make decisions when they are needed. You then have to be able to defend those decisions objectively to another person knowing that you made them with the best information available at the time, even if the decision turned out to be wrong. The virus has adapted, it has changed and mutated into at least four entirely different variants, each impacting the community in entirely different ways. The problem is, you usually do not know what that impact is going to be until after the wave has hit you, and that was very difficult for people to adjust to psychologically.

Probably the most important things a leader can do need to occur before the crisis. It is really to do with the organisational culture and it is about determining what sort of culture your leadership team is going to have and expect from those around them, from the outset. Every organisation has its espoused values within health. For us, collaboration, openness, respectfulness and empowerment are our espoused values. Every leader needs to ask the question, 'What are values in use?' What do we really value here – what do our organisational behaviours, policies, processes and structures demonstrate we value? It is the role of the executive to continuously push the organisation by their own behaviours to meet the values that are espoused. If you wait until a crisis you have already missed the boat. So, the key to our ability to respond to COVID-19 actually began years ago when we embedded the organisational culture we wanted. We determined not just by what we said, but how we interacted with each other as a group that we were going to live our values so that everybody else could see what we valued and replicate that in the workplace. And it is a continual battle every single day to project those values. You have to go back to the basics. You have to decide, first and foremost, what the principles are that we are going to achieve. You have to very clearly lay out your core objectives and it has to be a small number of objectives. For us it was about keeping the workforce safe and doing the best by the community, and representing good value to government.

Acknowledgement: Adapted from a seminar presentation by Adjunct Associate Professor Dr Dominic Morgan, Commissioner and Chief Executive, NSW Ambulance, 2022.

Case Study Questions

1. What are the main issues identified in the case study?
2. What is organisational culture and why is it considered important?
3. What is the role of managers and leaders in relation to organisational culture?
4. If you were a health care manager or leader, how and when might you prepare your organisation for a crisis?

treatment based on disability was seen in many countries, including the United Kingdom and the United States. Many health care managers were asked to make and enact decisions that were, for them, morally distressing.

While Australia never reached the stage of services in the rest of the world where patients had to be either turned away or left to die because of a lack of resources including ventilators and staff, we still had mini-crises around issues such as the availability of vaccines. Our health care systems, managers and staff were also stressed and stretched by the pandemic. Health care worker stressors 'centred on paucity of, or changing, evidence, leading to absence of, or mistrust in, guidelines; unprecedented alterations to the autonomy and sense of control of clinicians; and deficiencies in communication and support' (Broom et al. 2022, p. 75). The same study also found a number of protective factors for health care workers, which included 'the development of clear guidance from respected clinical leaders or recognized clinical bodies, interpersonal support, and strong teamwork, leadership, and a sense of organizational preparedness' (Broom et al. 2022, p. 75). You will recognise many of these factors from the list of the tasks and or competencies of health services managers identified by the ABS, ACHSM and RACMA.

> **Pause *for* Reflection ...**
> How do fairness and equity differ? What role do health care managers play in relation to fairness and equity? Refer to Chapters 5, 9 and 29 to remind yourself of these definitions and concepts.

▌ SUMMARY

In this chapter, we have outlined these points:
- What managers do has an impact on people's lives, on society at large, and on the environment in which we live.
- There are two schools of thought about what managers do: 'management as science' and 'management as an art or craft'.
- Health care management is complicated because health care is a complex system.
- Managers and leaders have different roles and require different yet similar skills.

- The 'quintuple aim' identifies five elements needed to achieve health transformation and realise better health and improved economy. The five elements of the quintuple aim are improved patient experience, better patient outcomes, lower costs, health care staff well-being and health equity.
- Managers have an important role to play in all of these elements, the safety, quality and equity of care.
- Managers need a strong ethical framework.

▌ REVIEW QUESTIONS

1. What are some of the responsibilities of health care managers?
2. What is the difference between a manager and a leader?
3. Do you agree with medical rationing?

4. How are managers involved in improving safety, quality and equity in health and social care?
5. How has the SARS-CoV-2 pandemic highlighted the importance of health care managers with a strong ethical framework?

REFERENCES

Agency for Healthcare Research and Quality, n.d. Glossary: error. https://psnet.ahrq.gov/glossary-0#glossary-heading-term-73780.

Australasian College of Health Service Management, 2016. Master Health Service Management Competency Framework. Australasian College of Health Service Management, Sydney.

Australian Bureau of Statistics (ABS), 2021a. 1342 Health and welfare services managers. ANZSCO – Australian and New Zealand Standard Classification of Occupation. https://www.abs.gov.au/statistics/classifications/anzsco-australian-and-new-zealand-standard-classification-occupations/2021/browse-classification/1/13/134/1342.

Australian Bureau of Statistics (ABS), 2021b. 2543 Nurse managers. ANZSCO – Australian and New Zealand Standard Classification of Occupation. https://www.abs.gov.au/statistics/classifications/anzsco-australian-and-new-zealand-standard-classification-occupations/2021/browse-classification/2/25/254/2543.

Australian Commission on Safety and Quality in Health Care. (n.d.). The National Safety and Quality Health Service Standards (NSQHS). https://www.safetyandquality.gov.au/standards/national-safety-and-quality-health-service-nsqhs-standards/assessment-nsqhs-standards.

Bandyopadhyay, S., Baticulon, R.E., Kadhum, M., et al., 2020. Infection and mortality of healthcare workers worldwide from COVID-19: a systematic review. BMJ Glob Health 5 (12), e003097.

Berwick, D.M., Nolan, T.W., Whittington, J., 2008. The triple aim: care, health, and cost. Health Affairs 27 (3), 759–769.

Braithwaite, J., Travaglia, J.F., 2008. An overview of clinical governance policies, practices and initiatives. Aust Health Rev 32 (1), 10–22.

Broom, J., Williams Veazey, L., Broom, A., et al., 2022. Experiences of the SARS-CoV-2 pandemic amongst Australian healthcare workers: from stressors to protective factors. J Hosp Infect 121, 75–81.

Chen, B., McNamara, D.M., 2020. Disability discrimination, medical rationing and COVID-19. Asian Bioeth Rev 12 (4), 511–518.

Chutiyami, M., Bello, U.M., Salihu, D., et al., 2022. COVID-19 pandemic-related mortality, infection, symptoms, complications, comorbidities, and other aspects of physical health among healthcare workers globally: An umbrella review. Int J Nurs Stud 104211.

Cieza, A., Kamenov, K., Al Ghaib, O.A., et al., 2021. Disability and COVID-19: ensuring no one is left behind. Arch Public Health 79 (1), 148.

Cunliffe, A.L., 2021. A Very Short, Fairly Interesting and Reasonably Cheap Book About Management, third ed. SAGE, London.

Fayol, H., 1916 (1949). General and Industrial Management. Pitman, London.

Goleman, D., 1996. Emotional Intelligence: Why it Can Matter More than IQ. Bloomsbury, London.

Graham, P., 2003. Mary Parker Follett prophet of management. Beard Books, Washington, D.C.

Haveman, H.A., Wetts, R., 2019. Organizational theory: from classical sociology to the 1970s. Sociol Compass 13 (3), e12627.

The Health Foundation, 2022. Strengthening NHS management and leadership: priorities for reform. https://www.health.org.uk/publications/long-reads/strengthening-nhs-management-and-leadership.

Khan, S., Siddique, R., Ali, A., et al., 2020. The spread of novel coronavirus has created an alarming situation worldwide. J Infect Public Health 13 (4), 469–471.

Kiechel, W., 2012. The management century. Harv Bus Rev 90 (11), 62–75.

Kohn, L.T., Corrigan, J.M., Donaldson, M.S., 2000. To err is human: building a safer health system. National Academy Press, Washington, D.C.

Kotter, J., 2007. Leading change: why transformation efforts fail. Harv Bus Rev 86, 97–103.

Labonté, R., 2010. Health systems governance for health equity: critical reflections. Revista de salud pública 12, 62–76.

Lane, H., Sarkies, M., Martin, J., et al., 2017. Equity in healthcare resource allocation decision making: a systematic review. Soc Sci Med 175, 11–27.

Lichtenstein, B., 2021. From "coffin dodger" to "boomer remover": outbreaks of ageism in three countries with divergent approaches to coronavirus control. J Gerontol Series B 76 (4), e206-e212.

Maddern, J., Cahill Lambert, A., Dwyer, J., 2020. Health care managers in a changing system. In: Willis, E., Reynolds, L., Rudge, T. (Eds.), Understanding the Australian Health Care System, fourth ed. Elsevier Health Sciences, Sydney, pp. 327–343.

Nienaber, H., 2010. Conceptualisation of management and leadership. Manag Decis 48 (5), 661–675.

Nundy, S., Cooper, L.A., Mate, K.S., 2022. The quintuple aim for health care improvement: a new imperative to advance health equity. JAMA 327 (6), 521–522.

Parsons, J.A., Johal, H.K., 2020. Best interests versus resource allocation: could COVID-19 cloud decision-making for the cognitively impaired? J Med Ethics 46 (7), 447–450.

Paton, A., 2020. Fairness, Ethnicity, and COVID-19 ethics: a discussion of how the focus on fairness in ethical guidance during the pandemic discriminates against people from ethnic minority backgrounds. J Bioeth Inq 17 (4), 595–600.

Peters, T., Waterman, R., 1982. In Search of Excellence. Harper & Row, New York.

Porter, M.E., 2008. The five competitive forces that shape strategy. Harv Bus Rev 86 (1), 25–40.

Robertson-Preidler, J., Anstey, M., Biller-Andorno, N., et al., 2017. Approaches to appropriate care delivery from a policy perspective: a case study of Australia, England and Switzerland. Health Policy 121 (7), 770–777.

Royal Australasian College of Medical Administrators, 2011. Curriculum document. Royal Australasian College of Medical Administrators, Malvern, Victoria.

Scally, G., Donaldson, L.J., 1998. The NHS's 50 anniversary. Clinical governance and the drive for quality improvement in the new NHS in England. BMJ 317 (7150), 61–65.

Senge, P.M., 2006. The fifth discipline: the art and practice of the learning organization. Currency.

Sikka, R., Morath, J.M., Leape, L., 2015. The quadruple aim: care, health, cost and meaning in work. BMJ Qual Saf 24 (10), 608–610.

Smith, D.C., 1996. The Hippocratic Oath and modern medicine. Journal of the history of medicine and allied sciences 51 (4), 484–500.

Stokes, J., Shah, V., Goldzahl, L., et al., 2021. Does prevention-focused integration lead to the triple aim? An evaluation of two new care models in England. J Health Serv Res Policy 26 (2), 125–132.

Walshe, K., Smith, J., 2011. Healthcare management, third ed. McGraw-Hill Education, London.

The Wardliparingga Aboriginal Research Unit of the South Australian Health and Medical Research Institute, 2017. National Safety and Quality Health Service Standards user guide for Aboriginal and Torres Strait Islander health. Australian Commission on Safety and Quality in Health Care, Sydney.

Whitehead, M., 1992. The concepts and principles of equity and health. Int J Health Serv 22 (3), 429–445.

Whittington, J.W., Nolan, K., Lewis, N., et al., 2015. Pursuing the triple aim: the first 7 years. Milbank Q 93 (2), 263–300.

Wilson, R.M., Runciman, W.B., Gibberd, R.W., et al., 1995. The quality in Australian health care study. Med J Aust 163 (9), 458–471.

Wyatt, D., Lampon, S., McKevitt, C., 2020. Delivering healthcare's 'triple aim': electronic health records and the health research participant in the UK National Health Service. Sociol Health Illn 42 (6), 1312–1327.

FURTHER READING

Itchhaporia, D., 2021. The evolution of the quintuple aim. J Am Coll Cardiol 78 (22), 2262–2264. doi:10.1016/j.jacc.2021.10.018.

Nundy, S., Cooper, L.A., Mate, K.S., 2022. The quintuple aim for health care improvement: a new imperative to advance health equity. JAMA 327 (6), 521–522. doi:10.1001/jama.2021.25181.

Whitehead, M., 1991. The concepts and principles of equity and health. Health Promot Int 6, (3), 217–228. doi:10.1093/heapro/6.3.217.

ONLINE RESOURCES

Mate, K., 2022. On the Quintuple Aim: Why Expand Beyond the Triple Aim? Institute of Health Improvement: https://www.ihi.org/communities/blogs/on-the-quintuple-aim-why-expand-beyond-the-triple-aim.

The following link provides numerous resources, including videoed interviews with leaders in the field of patient safety, about the importance of clinician well-being and joy at work: https://www.ihi.org/Topics/Joy-In-Work/Pages/default.aspx.

Royal Australasian College of Medical Administrators (RACMA), a specialist medical college that provides education, training, knowledge and advice in medical management: https://racma.edu.au/.

Australasian College of Health Service Management ('The College'), the peak professional body for health managers in Australasia, which brings together health leaders to learn, network and share ideas. https://www.achsm.org.au/about-us.

A brief video describing the role of medical and health services managers can be found at: https://www.youtube.com/watch?v=jmh01pXYn5I.

21

The Medical Profession in Australia

E Michael Shanahan

KEY LEARNING OUTCOMES

When you finish this chapter you should be able to:
- understand how the profession of medicine in Australia is organised, funded and delivered
- understand the training pathways to becoming a medical practitioner in Australia
- understand what it means to be a medical professional and how this notion is evolving and changing over time
- understand current issues regarding the medical workforce and how this impacts on the delivery of good health care in Australia.

KEY TERMS AND ABBREVIATIONS

Australian Commission on Safety and Quality in Health Care (ACSQHC)
Australian Health Practitioners Regulation Agency (Ahpra)
Australian Medical Council (AMC)
bulk-billing
code of conduct

constructivist learning
contextual learning
continuing professional development (CPD)
corporatised
economic rationalism
evidence-based practice
fee-for-service
gap fee

National Safety and Quality Health Service (NSQHS)
neoliberalism
proceduralist
programmatic assessment
reflective learners
registered medical officer (RMO)
trainee medical officer (TMO)

INTRODUCTION: WHAT IS A MEDICAL PRACTITIONER?

While acknowledging that in Australian Indigenous culture there is a long tradition of the delivery of medical care, this chapter will focus on the practice of medicine in Australia provided by those practitioners educated in the 'Western' practice of medicine. Medicine in Australia has been practised by individuals trained in this manner since the beginning of white settlement in the latter part of the 18th century, with the arrival of several doctors on the first fleet in 1788 (Lewis 2014).

Modern medical training in Australia has its roots in what is considered to be largely Western European traditions. In the early 19th century qualified doctors practising in Australia were graduates from (mainly) British medical schools, with Australian apprentices being sent to Britain to obtain formal qualifications. The first medical school in Australia was established in 1862 at the University of Melbourne but it wasn't until 1900 that the *Medical Practitioners (Amendment) Act 1900* (Act No 33 1900) was passed. It imposed penalties on persons using titles including Surgeon or Physician if they were not appropriately registered (Lewis 2014).

The Australian Bureau of Statistics (ABS) Standard Classification of Occupations defines medical practitioners as individuals who diagnose physical and mental illnesses, disorders and injuries, provide medical care to patients and prescribe and perform medical and surgical treatments to promote and restore good health (Australian Bureau of Statistics (ABS) 2006). A medical practitioner (as defined by the *Health Practitioner Regulation National Law Act 2009*) is an individual who is registered with the Medical Board of Australia. The Medical Board acts under the umbrella of the **Australian Health Practitioners Regulation Agency (Ahpra)**, which is responsible for a suite of health practitioner registration authorities. The role of the Medical Board is to maintain the medical register and decide the requirements for registration and to approve accredited programs of study as providing qualifications for registration. The **Australian Medical Council (AMC)** is the organisation charged by the Medical Board with the responsibility to approve and reaccredit programs licensed to deliver medical education. Students successfully undertaking such programs can then be registered as medical practitioners in Australia.

The AMC also set the standards for medical practitioners trained outside Australia who wish to work in Australia. Those international medical graduates wishing to work in Australia usually have to undergo assessments arranged by the AMC and undertake a period of supervised work prior to achieving full registration.

MEDICAL EDUCATION IN AUSTRALIA

Prior to the mid 1860s all legitimate medical practitioners in Australia had undertaken their assessments and licensure through medical schools and colleges outside of Australasia, mainly in Britain. From the 1860s medical schools began to develop in Australia. By 1900 there were three schools (Melbourne, Sydney and Adelaide) with a further five schools added until the mid 1960s (Geffen 2014). Medical education in Australia until the 1960s followed in the tradition of medical education on the model of Flexner, namely an undergraduate pre-clinical education followed by a period of clinical immersion. Since the mid 1960s there has been a steady expansion in the numbers and types of medical schools. Since 2000, in response to perceived current and future shortages of medical practitioners in Australia, there has been a rapid expansion in the number of medical schools and students. Currently there are 21 medical schools in Australia (see Table 21.1).

TABLE 21.1 **Medical Programs in Australia 2021**		
Medical School	**Year Opened**	**Current Enrolment (2022)**
University of Melbourne	1862	1417
University of Sydney	1883	1117
University of Adelaide	1885	1003
University of Western Australia	1956	880
University of Tasmania	1965	609
Monash University	1958	2014
The University of NSW	1960	1674
Flinders University	1974	713
Newcastle University	1978	975
Deakin University	2008	582
Griffith University	2004	874

Continued

TABLE 21.1   Medical Programs in Australia 2021—cont'd

Medical School	Year Opened	Current Enrolment (2022)
University of Wollongong	2006	328
University of Notre Dame (Sydney and Fremantle)	2008	893
Bond University	2005	768
Australian National University	2004	409
James Cook University	2000	1126
University of Queensland	1936	1448
Western Sydney University*	2007	649
Curtin University	2017	403
Macquarie University	2018	232
Charles Sturt University*	2021	43

Source: Medical Deans Australia and New Zealand.
*Joint program between WSU and CSU.

In 2021 there were over 18,000 students enrolled in medical school in Australia, which represents an increase of approximately 100% since the year 2000. At the end of 2020, 3656 medical students graduated from Australian medical schools. Female graduates made up 52.8% of the cohort. Commencement into medical schools in Australia in 2022 is projected to be 4065. There are 412 Aboriginal and Torres Strait Islander students enrolled in Australian medical schools, an increase of over 40% since 2016 (Medical Deans Australia and New Zealand 2020).

Medical education has also changed markedly since the 1960s. The majority of medical students in Australia are now in postgraduate programs (Medical Schools Outcomes Database 2017). The style of education delivery has moved from traditional lecture format to more modern adult learning approaches emphasising **constructivist learning**, collaborative and **contextual learning** approaches. The aim of developing self-directed learners, with emphasis on **reflective learners** capable of developing into self-correcting practitioners, is now emphasised. To facilitate this, forms of **programmatic assessment** for learning are increasingly underpinning the assessment processes in medical courses as traditional formal examination-based assessments are becoming less central to student progress. What continues to be central to medical education, however, is the clinical immersive experience with its cognitive apprenticeship-style learning approaches, underpinned by increasingly sophisticated forms of workplace-based assessments.

Increasingly, the process of medical education is seen as a continuum where skills are developed over many years from novice to expert, with the medical school providing only the first step in the process. Medical school graduate students obtain provisional registration with the Medical Board (internship). They then generally enter training programs run by the medical colleges in order to differentiate into various areas of speciality (including family medicine or 'general practice'). During this period of a medical practitioner's training they generally work under supervision in hospital or community-based employment and are known as **trainee medical officers** (**TMOs**), either **registered medical officers** (**RMOs**) or registrars. Usually the term 'registrar' is reserved for the more senior TMOs, but the meaning of this title is not defined and does not imply any particular level of qualification such as passing a specialist examination.

Developing into an independent medical practitioner takes many years of training. Beyond internship, further training generally takes a minimum of 4–6 years, depending on the trainee's progress and the speciality pathway chosen. Additionally, because of a bottleneck at the level of entering programs, a doctor might wait for several years (generally undertaking RMO or 'service' positions) prior to being accepted in the program of their choice. Their progress can be further impeded by their success or otherwise with the rigorous exams (set by the colleges) that they are required to pass. Following the completion of their training program if an individual wishes to work in a staff position in the public or academic environment, often a higher degree (such as a PhD) is undertaken. This may take a further 3–5 years to complete. Therefore, it is not uncommon for specialists to have taken 20 years or more to complete the training process from the commencement of medical school to working as an independent consultant. The personal and community investment in the training of these individuals is considerable. Following the completion of their formal education, all medical practitioners now undertake some form of **continuing professional development (CPD)**, again usually under the umbrella of their specialist colleges. The maintenance of professional education is now mandated by Ahpra and the continued medical registration of the practitioner is dependent on being part of a continued education program.

THE MODERN MEDICAL PROFESSIONAL

The medical profession is often seen as the archetypical professional group (Willis 1989). But what does being a medical professional mean in the 21st century? Generally, the understanding of being a professional implies a control over one's work (Freidson 1970). According to Freidson, elements of being a professional include having a strong service ethic, having a professional monopoly over an area of knowledge and having autonomy of practice (including a capacity to set one's own price for one's work). The responsibility to self-regulate is also said to be central to the idea of being a professional.

In modern medical practice a number of these concepts no longer hold true, or are under significant threat. Nonetheless at many levels the modern medical practitioner would identify as a professional and would be regarded as such by the majority of the community in Australia.

Pause *for* Reflection ...

So, how does this development of a professional identity come about, and what does it mean to be a medical professional in Australia?

Professionalism is a required core competency for medical practitioners. Increasingly, the development of a medical professional identity among medical students is considered to be a central task of medical schools (Byyny 2015). The development of a true professional identity involves the development of a mindset and attitude which transcends rules and means an individual will seek to do 'the right thing' in a situation whether or not they have previously encountered it. The fully formed professional is habitually faithful to professional values in highly complex situations. Sustaining professionalism is considered to be a complex adaptive problem that defies easy definition and where the rules are constantly changing (Lucey 2015). It involves a deep understanding of ethics, the law and community values as well as high-level interpersonal skills. Despite the difficulties, most medical schools in Australia have developed, or are developing, an explicit thread of professionalism within their curriculum (Parker et al. 2008). These curricula are sometimes supported by explicit codes of conduct and mechanisms to correct aberrant behaviour (including progression impediment), with the ultimate sanction being exclusion from the medical school. Although a separate **code of conduct** for Australian medical students has yet to be developed, a number of these codes do exist around the world (e.g. UK, Ireland). A code of conduct for doctors that describes what is expected of all doctors registered to practise medicine in Australia has been developed by the Australian Medical Council (2009). In addition, the Medical Board of Australia produces a document called 'Good medical practice: a code of conduct for doctors in Australia' (Medical Board of Australia Ahpra 2009). So, what are the fundamental principles expounded by these curricula and the doctors' code of practice? Byyny (2015) has recently outlined these principles as follows:

- Adhere to high ethical standards: do right, avoid wrong and do no harm.
- Subordinate your own interests to your patients.
- Avoid business, financial and organisational conflicts of interest.
- Honour the social contract you have undertaken with patients and communities.
- Understand the non-biologic determinants of poor health and the economic, psychological, social and cultural factors that contribute to health and illness.
- Care for patients who are unable to pay, advocate for the medically underserved.
- Be accountable, both ethically and financially.
- Be thoughtful, compassionate and collegial.
- Continue to learn, increase your competence and strive for excellence.

- Work to advance the field of medicine, and share knowledge for the benefit of others.
- Reflect dispassionately on your own actions, behaviours and decisions to improve your knowledge, skills, judgement, decision-making, accountability and professionalism.

All modern Australian medical practitioners would be expected to adhere to these standards. The standards would also be part of every medical curricula in the country, and indeed in most medical courses in the world. They are certainly explicitly articulated in the code of conduct produced by the AMC.

> **Pause *for* Reflection ...**
> In an era of tight resource allocation where do some of the tensions lie in medical practice? How does a practitioner provide the best care for their individual patient while balancing this against the need to conserve the community resources?

What about the sociological view of medical professionalism? How well do these ideas hold up when considering medical practice in Australia? Willis argues that a number of challenges to the profession since the 1960s have radically reshaped the concept of professionalism as relating to the medical profession. These include challenges to medical dominance posed by **neoliberalism** and **economic rationalism**, a growth in consumerism and associated litigiousness, the change from a cottage industry basis to mass marketing as medicine has become industrialised, the rise of complementary medicine and the changing roles of health care professionals (Willis 2006).

1 The Concept of Autonomy of Practice

Increasingly medicine is not being practised in the autonomous way it once was. Practice guidelines and restrictions on prescribing (often because of cost to the community or considerations of patient safety) are part of every medical practitioner's way of life. Guidelines are promulgated in the interests of safety and consistency of practice and are often developed under the guise of 'evidence-based practice'. There is however, considerable push back on these guidelines with the increasing understanding that the evidence base upon which they are derived can be flimsy and the application of population-based evidence to the individual circumstance contains a flawed logic (Lenzer 2013). There is clear evidence that

the application of practice guidelines among experienced medical practitioners is at best limited (Mafi et al. 2013). Nonetheless, the push for such guidelines is continuing and likely to increase, especially when they can be used for cost containment. There are a number of other restrictions on the autonomy of medical practice becoming obvious in daily medical practice. Some of these are generated by directives from the **Australian Commission on Safety and Quality in Health Care** (**ACSQHC**) who audit medical practice against the **National Safety and Quality Health Service** (**NSQHS**) standards. These processes are often seen as burdensome but are the reality of modern medical practice.

The rollout of electronic medical records and electronic prescribing also has the potential to limit the autonomy of medical practice. While on balance these developments are seen to be advantageous in terms of patient safety, they also hold the potential to restrict the ordering of what might be considered to be unnecessary tests or 'off-label' medical prescribing. ('Off-label' is the term used when medication is prescribed for indications other than those approved by the Pharmaceutical Benefits Scheme.)

2 The Notion of Self-Regulation

Increasingly in Australia the idea that professions can be self-regulating has been disabused. The primary regulatory authorities for the medical profession, Ahpra and the Medical Boards, have significant community, non-medical representation. With respect to currency of practice, although the maintenance of professional education continues to be delivered by the profession through the colleges, this is now linked to the practitioner's registration though the Medical Board. Medical practitioners are subject to audit with respect to their education through both their colleges and Ahpra.

3 The Notion of Price Setting

The remuneration of medical practitioners in Australia is complex and many models exist (see below). Suffice to say that for many practitioners (such as those on public salaries) there is no possibility of setting a price directly for the service provided. For others there is still (theoretically) considerable autonomy, although there are many practical restrictions on setting very high fees. For some in the profession however, this remains a jealously guarded right and privilege.

4 The Notion of a Monopoly of a Body of Knowledge

Increasingly medical knowledge in itself is becoming widely accessible. Almost universal access to computers with increasingly sophisticated search engines and diagnostic algorithms means the role of the doctor as the repository of medical knowledge is rapidly declining (Ieraci 2018). What it is increasingly being replaced with is the ability to apply this knowledge to the individual's situation. This can only come with the perspective that experience brings, and demands the development of high-level communication and cognitive skills. Technical skills (such as surgical skills) are also being facilitated with (but not replaced by) robotics. These changes are being reflected in the changing content of medical school curricula and training programs. Despite the prediction of some futurists, the likelihood of the profession of medicine being replaced by artificial intelligence remains low.

5 A Strong Service Ethic

Although most medical practitioners have a strong service ethic in the sense of considering the primacy of their patient's needs, increasingly the implications of this commitment are being seen by the profession as potentially unhealthy for the individuals in the system. Long hours of work and the personal psychological toll of many years of training and the burden of medical responsibility have seen individuals pay a heavy price. Suicide rates in the medical profession (including among junior medical staff and medical students) exceed the national average. There is considerable discussion about how this might be addressed (beyondblue 2013), but possible solutions may include reducing the hours of work and increasing the flexibility of work practice. There is evidence that this is starting to occur (Munir 2018).

Pause *for* Reflection …

Given these increasingly tight restrictions on medical practice how well does the concept of 'medical dominance' hold true in this century?

Case study 21.1 describes the ways in which medical practitioners work interprofessionally and collaboratively.

CASE STUDY 21.1

Medical practitioners often work interprofessionally and collaboratively. One example is a multidisciplinary ward round in a hospital setting. Another more complex example would involve altering work roles and processes to improve the overall delivery of care.

Some of the reasons why medical professionals work interprofessionally include changing population demographics and the increasing burden of chronic diseases; the increasing complexity of knowledge and skills required to provide holistic care; increasing specialisation in the professions; and the pursuit of continuity of care in the movement of continuous quality improvement (Nancarrow 2013).

There are three types of interprofessional collaboration interventions that medical professionals can be involved in: education-based, practice-based and organisational-based. However intuitively appealing they seem, measuring the effectiveness of the intervention is challenging due to their conceptual nature (Reeves 2017).

The Australian Teamwork Study (Black et al. 2013) is an example of interprofessional collaboration in a primary care general practice setting. It was an education and practice-based intervention which involved a team-based approach in the management of chronic diseases. This structured intervention used non-GP staff in a GP practice to measure the quality of care for patients living with diabetes and cardiovascular disease. GPs and non-GP practice staff (administrative and nursing staff) were educated in 11 elements known to contribute to enhanced teamwork for chronic care management. These elements included structured appointment systems; patient disease registers; recall and reminders; patient education; planned care; practice-based linkages; roles, responsibilities and job descriptions; communication and meetings; practice billing; record keeping and quality. The practices were supported by several follow-up visits, regular telephone and email support, and the provision of resource manuals and workbooks.

In measuring the effectiveness of the intervention, the study wanted to see if there was an improvement in the processes such as changes in team roles and also to patients' outcomes. The study findings were a little disappointing in that they showed that teamwork improved, however there was no improvement in the patients'

Continued

THE MEDICAL WORKFORCE IN AUSTRALIA

There were 129,066 medical practitioners registered with the Medical Board in 2020–21; just over 400 doctors per 100,000 population (Medical Board of Australia 2021). The number of doctors registered has grown consistently at a rate of 3.9% from 2005–15 reflecting the significant increase in the numbers of medical student places in Australia from around the year 2000. The percentage of women as a total of the workforce continues to increase, reflecting the increase in the percentage of women in medical schools over the last two decades. In 2016–17, women made up 42% of the workforce and by 2020–21 this had risen to 44.8%. In addition, women made up over half of all clinician specialists in training. Women now make up 40% of the specialist workforce (up from 20% ten years previously) though major disparities still exist in some groups such as surgery. The average hours of work for medical practitioners in Australia is 41 hours per week. The largest proportion of clinicians are specialists (35%) followed by general practitioners (31.1%), specialists in training (16%) and hospital non-specialists (12%) (Australian Government Department of Health 2021).

Under-Serviced Groups

Estimates of the numbers of doctors identifying as Indigenous vary but may be around 400. This is an approximate doubling since 2004, but estimates suggest approximately 10 times that number would be required if the proportion was to reflect the numbers of Indigenous people in the community. In 2021, over 400 medical students identified as Indigenous.

Major cities continue to have the highest rate of supply of registered medical practitioners with the supply of medical practitioners overall lowest in remote/very remote areas. In 2020 only 1345 medical practitioners were registered and employed in remote or very remote areas. Paradoxically, the supply of general practitioners in remote/very remote areas was the highest per capita (136 FTE per 100,000) but the Australian Institute of Health and Welfare (AIHW 2022) caution against suggesting this reflects adequate servicing, pointing out that service delivery models vary radically in urban compared with remote areas. Of the non-clinician medical practitioners, the majority worked in areas of medical administration (1490 or 34.6%), research (24.5%) or teaching (AIHW 2015).

EMPLOYMENT AND REMUNERATION

Traditionally in Australia employment levels in registered medical practitioners have been very high. The employment arrangements and subsequent remuneration vary widely as would be expected given the enormous variety in medical practice and the complexities of delivering a medical service in a country such as Australia. As in many countries, various blends of 'public' and 'private' employment arrangements exist in medicine. Many practitioners derive their employment from a mixture of these arrangements. At one end of the 'public' spectrum are doctors fully employed by the state and remunerated via a fixed salary. This tends to be more the case with provisionally registered doctors and doctors in training. At the other end of the spectrum are doctors working fully 'in private'. These doctors set their own fee schedules and are paid '**fee-for-service**'. The majority of these services, however, are still heavily underwritten by the public purse through the Medicare system. Those working in such arrangements have the opportunity to 'bulk-bill' their patients and receive the fee determined by the item number attached to that service. Item number schedules are a hybrid of time-based and service-based items. Many practitioners charge above the scheduled fee, and the patient then encounters a 'gap fee' at the point of delivery (the gap being the difference between the fee charged and the Medicare rebate). Increasingly general practitioner services are becoming **corporatised**, where individual practitioners allow a company to take over the running of the 'business' of medicine and the doctors simply contract themselves to the organisation and receive a proportion of the takings that they generate (Erny-Albrecht & Bywood 2016).

The federal government uses various levers to try to control costs in the health care system. Among the most unpopular with the medical profession has been a freeze on Medicare rebates. This has had a negative effect on doctors' remuneration and led to much debate about doctors ceasing **bulk-billing** services. The logical effect of this behaviour is to cost shift the price of service delivery into pockets of patients.

There is considerable debate in the medical political literature about the most appropriate way to work, and of the various incentives that drive practice behaviours. For example, it is often stated that '**proceduralists**' are relatively well remunerated for the performance of individual procedures, potentially encouraging them to perform more procedures than may be otherwise considered medically necessary. Good examples of this in the Australian system include knee arthroscopy and shoulder ultrasound (Awerbach 2008; Harris et al. 2018). Despite the ongoing debates and tensions, doctors are still among the best remunerated occupational groups in Australia today.

THE PUBLIC VIEW OF THE MEDICAL PROFESSION

Despite the occasional political portrayal of medical practitioners working in their own self-interest, confidence in the profession remains high. Most Australians visit their doctors each year (ABS 2013) and most surveys put medical practitioners at or near the top of trustworthiness and satisfaction, with 90% of the community trusting doctors. Patient complaints to Ahpra and disciplinary actions against medical practitioners remains low with 5% of practitioners having complaints made about them in 2020–21 resulting in 0.4% having their registration suspended or cancelled (Ahpra 2021). This would suggest the commitment to the social contract between doctors and the community (part of being a professional) continues to be central to how doctors deliver their community responsibilities.

CURRENT AND FUTURE CHALLENGES

No doubt the single biggest challenge facing medical practice in recent times is the SARS-CoV-2 pandemic. While pandemics are not new, the current pandemic has had a profound impact on the way medicine has been practised in Australia and indeed around the world. Some of the significant challenges faced by doctors include the problem of providing an adequate medical service delivery in the face of staff and equipment shortages, increased demand, anxious and frustrated patients, rapidly changing conditions and government directions including temporarily halting non-urgent service delivery. COVID-19 has forced many doctors to employ telephone and telehealth models of care (see Chapter 16). This approach may be adequate for some services but is clearly unsatisfactory for many. COVID-19 has also profoundly impacted upon the teaching and training of medical students and junior doctors, particularly in the clinical environment.

The medical profession in the 21st century faces extraordinary challenges to achieve its primary role of delivering quality medical care to the Australian community. An almost inexorable increase in medical costs coupled with rising community expectations of care and improving technical ability to increasingly prolong life, make for a perfect storm with respect to resource allocation. The profession itself needs to be nimble enough to meet changing community expectations, and continue to redefine and reshape what it means to be a medical professional. Educational institutions likewise need to be flexible enough to recognise and lead the changes. New technologies and artificial intelligence will certainly continue to redefine the role of a doctor. The maldistribution of medical services in particular with a relative lack of service to rural and remote Australia continues to be a major issue. Inequities in health care outcomes among Indigenous Australians and those of poorer socio-economic status remain as major challenges to a fairer Australia in which the medical profession has a major role to play. Nonetheless the profession has shown itself to be robust and highly adaptable to changing environments and circumstances. There is every indication that new generations of Australian medical practitioners will have the skill and courage to continue with the necessary reforms to meet these and future challenges.

SUMMARY

This chapter outlines what it means to be a medical practitioner in Australia in the 21st century. It discusses the pathway practitioners take to become doctors, and then some of the responsibilities they have when practising medicine. The chapter also describes the concept of medical professionalism and how this has changed since the turn of the century. The demographics of the Australian medical workforce is briefly outlined, and some of the contemporary challenges facing current and future practice in Australia are discussed.

REVIEW QUESTIONS

1. Outline the pathway for a medical practitioner to become a fully registered independent doctor. Do you think the community can continue to afford such a lengthy pathway, and how might the same outcome be achieved in a lesser time period?

2. A significant maldistribution of medical services still exists in Australia. How might this issue be addressed effectively?

3. Do you think that the continued development of artificial intelligence will make the role of the doctor largely redundant? If not, why not?

4. Over the last decade, the Commonwealth Government offered a number of 'bonded' places to medical students to enter medical schools around Australia. Apply Bacchi's approach to try to examine why this policy was developed

REFERENCES

Ahpra, 2022. Annual report 2021/22. https://www.ahpra.gov.au/Publications/Annual-reports/Annual-Report-2022.aspx.

Australian Bureau of Statistics (ABS), 2006. Australian and New Zealand standard classification of occupations. Cat. No. 1220.0. ABS, Canberra.

Australian Bureau of Statistics (ABS), 2013. 4839.0 Patient experiences in Australia: summary of findings 2012–13. ABS, Canberra. http://www.abs.gov.au/ausstats/abs@.nsf/Lookup/4839.0main+features32012-13.

Australian Commission on Safety and Quality in Health Care, 2018. The National Safety and Quality Health Service (NSQHS) Standards. https://www.safetyandquality.gov.au/our-work/assessment-to-the-nsqhs-standards/.

Australian Institute of Health and Welfare (AIHW), 2015. Medical practitioners workforce 2015. AIHW, Canberra. https://www.aihw.gov.au/reports/workforce/medical-practitioners-workforce-2015/contents/how-many-medical-practitioners-are-there.

Australian Institute of Health and Welfare (AIHW), 2022. Rural and remote health. AIHW, Canberra. https://www.aihw.gov.au/reports/rural-remote-australians/rural-and-remote-health.

Australian Government Department of Health, 2021. Summary statistics, medical profession. https://hwd.health.gov.au/resources/data/summary-mdcl.html.

Australian Medical Council, 2009. Good medical practice: a code of conduct for doctors in Australia. https://www.medicalboard.gov.au/Codes-Guidelines-Policies/Code-of-conduct.aspx.

Awerbach, M., 2008. The clinical utility of ultrasonography for rotator cuff disease, shoulder impingement syndrome and subacromial bursitis. Med J Aust 188 (1), 50–53.

beyondblue, 2013. National mental health survey of doctors and medical students. October. https://www.beyondblue.org.au/docs/default-source/research-project-files/bl1132-report—-nmhdmss-full-report_web.pdf?sfvrsn=4.

Black, D.A., Taggart, J., Jayasinghe, U.W., et al., 2013. The Teamwork Study: enhancing the role of non-GP staff in chronic disease management in general practice. Aust J Prim Health 2013, 19, 184–189.

Byyny, R.L., 2015. Medical Professionalism: Best Practices. Alpha Omega Alpha Honor Medical Society, California.

Erny-Albrecht K, Bywood P., 2016. Corporatisation of general practice – impact and implications. PHCRIS Policy Issue Review. Primary Health Care Research & Information Service, Adelaide. https://dspace.flinders.edu.au/xmlui/bitstream/handle/2328/38389/phcris_pub_8460.pdf?sequence=1&isAllowed=y.

Freidson, E., 1970. Profession of medicine: a study of the sociology of applied knowledge. University of Chicago Press, Chicago.

Geffen, L., 2014. A brief history of medical education and training in Australia. MJA 201 (1), S19–S22.

Harris, I., O'Connor, D., Buchbinder, R., 2018. Needless procedures: knee arthroscopy is one of the most common but least effective surgeries The Conversation, 13 September.

https://theconversation.com/needless-procedures-knee-arthroscopy-is-one-of-the-most-common-but-least-effective-surgeries-102705.

Ieraci, S., 2018. Redefining the physician's role in the era of online health information. MJA 209 (8), 340–341.

Lenzer, J., 2013. Why we can't trust clinical guidelines. BMJ 346, f3830.

Lewis, M.J., 2014. Medicine in colonial Australia 1788–1900. MJA 201 (1), S5–S10.

Lucey, C.R., 2015. The problem with professionalism. In: Byyny R.L., Papadakis, M.A., Paauw, D.S. (Eds), Medical Professionalism: Best Practices. Alpha Omega Alpha Honor Medical Society, California, pp. 9–21.

Mafi, J.N., McCarthy, E.P., Davis, R.B., et al., 2013. Worsening trends in the management and treatment of back pain. JAMA Intern Med 173(17), 1573–1581. doi:10.1001/jamainternmed.2013.8992.

Medical Board of Australia, 2021. Annual report 2020/21. https://www.medicalboard.gov.au/News/Annual-report.aspx.

Medical Board of Australia Ahpra, 2020. Good medical practice: a code of conduct for doctors in Australia. October. https://www.medicalboard.gov.au/Codes-Guidelines-Polcies/Codes-of coduct.aspx.

Medical Deans Australia and New Zealand, 2020. Student statistics report 2020. https://medicaldeans.org.au/md/2021/11/MDANZ-Student-Statistics-Report-2020.pdf.

Medical Schools Outcomes Database National Report, 2017. Medical Deans Australia and New Zealand, Sydney. https://medicaldeans.org.au/data/?md_year=2018&data_type+Enrolments&country+AU&student=total&preview=.

Munir, V., 2018. MABEL: Doctors shouldn't work in excess of 50 hours per week. MJA insight issue 6. https://www.doctorportal.com.au/mjainsight/2018/6/mabel-doctors-shouldn't-work-in-excess-of-50-hours-per-week/.

Nancarrow, S., Booth, A., Ariss, S., et al., 2013. Ten principles of good interdisciplinary team work. Hum Resour Health 11, 19. http://www.human-resources-health.com/content/11/1/19.

Parker, M., Luke, H., Zhang, J., et al., 2008. The "pyramid of professionalism": seven years of experience with an integrated program of teaching, developing, and assessing professionalism among medical students. Acad Med 83 (8), 733–41. doi:10.1097/ACM.0b013e31817ec5e4.

Reeves, S., Pelone, F., Harrison, R., et al., 2017. Interprofessional collaboration to improve professional practice and healthcare outcomes review. Cochrane Database Syst Rev 6(6), CD000072. doi:10.1002/14651858.CD000072.pub3.

Shot, E., Tummers, L., Noordengraaf, M., 2020. Working on working together. A systematic review on how healthcare professionals contribute to interprofessional collaboration. J Interprof Care 34 (3), 332–342. doi:10.1080/13256 1820.2019.1636007.

Willis, E., 1983 (revised ed. 1989). Medical Dominance. Allen and Unwin, Sydney.

Willis, E., 2006. Introduction: taking stock of medical dominance. Health Sociol Rev 15 (5) 421–431.

FURTHER READING

Dent, J.A., Harden, R.M., 2013. A Practical Guide for Medical Teachers, fourth ed. Churchill Livingstone Elsevier.

Groopman, J., 2007. How Doctors Think. Houghton Mifflin.

Tai-Seale, M., Olson, C., Li, J., et al., 2017. The practice of medicine. Health Aff (Millwood) 36 (4), 655–662.

ONLINE RESOURCES

To search for Australian medical colleges, go to Ahpra's Approved Programs of Study page: https://www.ahpra.gov.au/education/approved-programs-of-study.aspx.

22

Midwifery in Australia

Kathleen Baird, Vanessa Scarf and Melanie Briggs

KEY LEARNING OUTCOMES

When you finish this chapter you should be able to:
- define the role and scope of a midwife in Australia
- understand the legal and regulatory frameworks underpinning midwifery
- appreciate the drive to reform maternity services in Australia

- understand the arrangement and costing models of maternity care
- appreciate the history and the importance of birthing on country for First Nations women.

KEY TERMS AND ABBREVIATIONS

Australian College of Midwives (ACM)

Australian Institute of Health and Welfare (AIHW)

Australian Health Practitioner Regulation Agency (Ahpra)

caesarean section (CS)

continuity of midwifery care (CoC)

Organisation for Economic Co-operation and Development (OECD)

Medicare Benefits Schedule (MBS)

midwifery group practice (MGP)

Nursing and Midwifery Board of Australia (NMBA)

Pharmaceutical Benefits Scheme (PBS)

professional indemnity insurance (PII)

woman-centred

INTRODUCTION

Australia is regarded as a safe country in which to have a baby; it compares well on the global stage in regard to measures of safety and quality of care. Yet there remains a need for continued improvement and reform in the maternity sector (Council of Australian Governments (COAG) 2019). The aim of any maternity service should be to deliver high-quality, safe care, however, it is also important that maternity care services are designed to be inclusive, collaborative, equitable and woman centred, established within a continuity of care model.

Maternity services in Australia are currently delivered through a mix of public and private services. The planning and delivery of maternity services is primarily agreed upon by individual states and territories through publicly funded care models, with the Commonwealth providing national direction and supporting efforts to improve care and outcomes (Department of Health 2018). While women have some choice around the model of maternity care they receive during their pregnancy, this very much depends on where they live and their social and personal circumstances.

This chapter will discuss the design of current maternity services, maternity regulation and education, maternity reform agenda, current maternity models of care and the drive for woman-centred midwifery continuity of care. It will also highlight the requirement to design and deliver a maternity model of care that is acceptable by First Nations women and their families.

MATERNITY CARE IN AUSTRALIA

In 2020, there were 294,369 births registered, a decrease of 3.7% from 2019 (**Australian Institute of Health and Welfare (AIHW)** 2021). The birth rate in Australia has seen a steady decline from 64.6 per 1000 women in 2009 to 57.6 in 2019. The fertility rate of women aged 20 to 24 years saw the largest decline, with the most pronounced decline among women aged 15 to 19 years where the fertility rate decreased by nearly two-thirds (to 7.8 per 1000 women). In contrast, the fertility rate of women aged 40 to 44 years almost tripled to 15.2 per 1000 women, while women aged 30 to 34 years continue to have the highest fertility rate (110 babies per 1000 women), followed by women aged 25 to 29 years (79.7 babies per 1000 women) (Australian Bureau of Statistics (ABS) 2022).

In Australia, the average maternal age of a first-time mother increased from 27.9 in 2009 to 29.4 in 2019 (AIHW 2021). The proportion of young mothers (under 20 years of age) decreased from 4.0% in 2009 to 1.9% in 2019. The rate of young First Nations mothers (under 20 years of age) also decreased from 20% in 2009 to 11% in 2019 (AIHW 2021). However, despite the overall improvements in infant and child mortality over the last two decades, babies born to First Nations mothers, including low birthweight, preterm births and perinatal deaths, continue to be higher than the general population (AIHW 2021b).

The rate of stillbirth in Australia decreased from 3.8 per 1000 births in 2000 to 2.6 per 1000 births in 2019, and the rate of neonatal deaths in Australia has decreased from 2.9 per 1000 live births in 2000 to 2.4 per 1000 live births in 2019. Perinatal mortality rates were higher among women experiencing most disadvantage, including babies born to women aged 20–24 and 40 years of age and over, Aboriginal and Torres Strait Islander women, women living in very remote areas and the most disadvantaged areas of Australia (see Fig 22.1) (AIHW 2021).

There continues to be a disparity between babies born to Aboriginal and Torres Strait Islander women and non-Indigenous women. During 2016–18, the perinatal death rate among babies to Aboriginal and Torres Strait Islander women was 14.8 per 1000 births compared to 8.5 per 1000 births among babies born to non-Indigenous women. While the disparity between Indigenous and non-Indigenous Australians continues to exist, there has been a marked decline in the perinatal mortality rate for First Nations Peoples. Between 1998 and 2018 there was

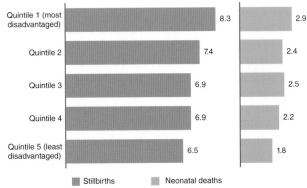

Notes:
1. The rate is the number of deaths per 1000 births. Stillbirth and perinatal mortality rates were calculated using total births (live births and stillbirths). Neonatal mortality rates were calculated using live births.
2. Relative disadvantage is expressed in 5 quintiles, each representing approximately 20% of the population, and the quintiles are assigned using the ABS SEIFA IRSD 2016 scores applied to Statistical Areas Level 2 (SA2) of mother's area of usual residence.
3. Only includes records where mother's usual residence is an Australian state and/or territory (excluding 'Other territories').

Figure 22.1 Perinatal Morality Rates by Socio-Economic Status.

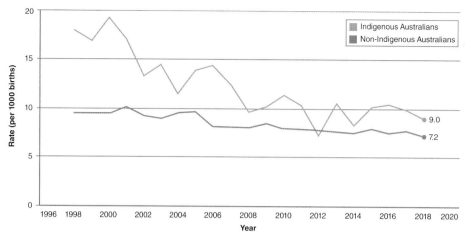

Figure 22.2 Perinatal Morality Rates – Indigenous and Non-Indigenous Women. *Source*: Australian Institute of Health and Welfare & National Indigenous Australian Agency, Perinatal Mortality, 2021.

a decrease of 55% in the perinatal mortality rates from 18 to 9 per 1000 births representing a decline of 0.5 per 1000 births each year (see Fig 22.2).

In 2020, 97% of all births in Australia took place in a hospital setting, 75% occurred in a public hospital, 2.3% at a birth centre, 0.3% at home and 0.6% elsewhere (AIHW 2021a). In 2019, almost two in three women (64%) in Australia experienced a vaginal birth, while the remainder (36%) had a **caesarean section (CS)** birth. Australia has seen a steady increase in the caesarean section rate over the last two decades, and Australia's rate of 34 per 100 live births is higher than the **Organisation for Economic Co-operation and Development (OECD)** average of 28 per 100 live births (OECD 2019). The increasing age of first-time mothers and subsequent risks of obstetric complications is the reason commonly put forward to explain the rise in CS rates in Australia. The higher rates of CS birth for privately funded women compared with publicly funded women is commonly attributed to differences in the populations. Women having a CS birth in a private hospital are more likely to be older and less financially disadvantaged (Australian Commission on Safety and Quality in Health Care 2017).

MIDWIFERY REGULATION AND EDUCATION AND THE SCOPE OF THE MIDWIFE

Midwives in Australia are academically prepared to practise across the full scope of midwifery practice, to work in partnership with women and provide care from preconception (prior to pregnancy) or early pregnancy, to birth and until the baby is 6 weeks old. Midwifery care is provided by midwives in several settings, including public and private health services or in a woman's home. All midwives in Australia are accountable for the care they provide to women and their infant(s) regardless of the setting. It is the responsibility of the midwife to ensure all decisions, recommendations and options of care are focused on the need and safety of the woman and her infant/s (Nursing and Midwifery Board of Australia (NMBA) 2017/2021).

Midwifery in Australia is recognised as a distinct profession, separate from nursing, governed by education and regulation. Underpinning midwifery is a wellness model by way of a 'with-woman' emphasis. While midwives promote normal midwifery care, they are also trained to identify and care for women experiencing variations from normal, in collaboration with other health professionals.

Midwifery is regulated by the **Australian Health Practitioner Regulation Agency (Ahpra)** by means of the **Nursing and Midwifery Board of Australia (NMBA)**. All midwives must be registered with the NMBA and meet the NMBA's registration standards to be able to practise in Australia. The NMBA regulates midwives and students of midwifery by setting the national standards of practice, codes and guidelines for midwives. The standards include five core registration standards, required under the Health Practitioner Regulation National Law (the National Law) and other profession-specific registration standards. These standards, codes and guidelines provide midwives, employers and the public with information about the minimum standards required to practise as a midwife in Australia. Importantly, the NMBA protects the public by ensuring only suitably qualified competent midwives are registered to practise in Australia.

The title of 'midwife' is protected under the *Health Practitioner Regulation National Law Act 2009*. To practise as a registered midwife in Australia, a midwife must have completed an approved course in midwifery at university and the course of study must be approved by the NMBA. The approved program of study must be reassessed every five years by the NMBA. Professional standards characterise and specify the conduct and practice of midwives and include codes of conduct, standards for practice and codes of ethics. To remain registered as a midwife, there is a requirement for all midwives to undertake 20 hours of continuing professional practice a year. An endorsed midwife who holds an endorsement for scheduled medicines is required to complete an additional 10 hours CPD per year relating to their context of practice, prescribing and administration of medicines, consultation and referral.

The Department of Health and Aged Care (2021a) defines a midwife's scope of practice as:

- *providing health support, care and advice to women before conception, and during labour, birth and the postnatal period*
- *promoting natural childbirth and identifying complications for the woman and her baby*
- *consulting with other health professionals and referring to medical care or other health professions when required*
- *implementing emergency measures.*

In 2021, there were approximately 6500 midwives with a midwife-only registration and 28,800 midwives with dual registration (nurse and midwife) (Department of Health and Aged Care 2021b). The number of midwives with a midwife-only registration has seen a steady increase from 3402 in 2016 to 4982 in 2020. Likewise, midwives with a dual registration have seen a decrease in numbers from 23,377 in 2016 to 21,256 in 2020 (Department of Health and Aged Care 2021b). Of the midwifery workforce in Australia, 87.6% has an Australian qualification with 77.7% of practising midwives born in Australia. Only 1.3% of the midwifery workforce identify as Aboriginal and/or Torres Strait Islander. A total of 70.1% of the midwifery workforce practise in metropolitan areas and 98.7% of the midwifery workforce is female, with an average age of 47.3 years. In 2019, 10,005.9 FTE (full-time equivalent) midwives worked in the public sector with 2409.6 working in the private sector (Department of Health and Aged Care 2022).

MIDWIFERY EDUCATION

In Australia there are various education routes leading to the registration of a midwife. They include:

- Bachelor of Midwifery: a full-time three-year undergraduate degree program
- Bachelor of Nursing and Midwifery: a four-year dual nursing and midwifery undergraduate program
- Graduate Diploma of Midwifery: a postgraduate program for registered nurses who wish to pursue a career in midwifery, usually over 12–18 months
- Master of Midwifery: may or may not lead to registration as a midwife, it is usually 2 years in length, depending on the university.

Once registered, midwives can obtain an additional endorsement to their registration that allows them to prescribe certain medications. Endorsed midwives can apply to Medicare for a Medicare provider number and/or a **Pharmaceutical Benefits Scheme (PBS)** provider number, allowing them to provide services eligible for a Medicare rebate enabling them to be recognised as an eligible midwife. Currently in Australia there are certain requirements in the Registration Standard for Eligible Midwives (NMBA 2017/2021), including:

- midwifery experience that constitutes the equivalent of three years' full-time post initial registration as a midwife
- current competence to provide pregnancy, labour, birth and postnatal care to women and their infants (the continuum of midwifery care)
- participation in an additional 20 hours per year of continuing professional development (total of 40 hours) relevant to the continuum of midwifery care
- successful completion of an NMBA-approved professional midwifery practice review program for midwives working across the continuum of midwifery care (to be conducted every three years)
- formal undertaking to complete, within 18 months of recognition, an accredited and approved program of study determined by the Board to develop midwives' knowledge and skills in prescribing.

For the midwife to provide services and receive a Medicare provider number, a midwife must be self-employed and working in private practice, have professional indemnity insurance (PII) and have a collaborative arrangement with a medical practitioner. The collaborative arrangement is a legislated requirement and includes the ability of the midwife to consult with an obstetric medical practitioner who provides obstetric services, or a medical practitioner employed or engaged by a hospital and authorised by the hospital to participate in a collaborative arrangement (Department of Health 2012).

The Health Practitioner Regulation National Law (the National Law) was enacted in each state and territory of Australia in 2009 and 2010. The goal of the National Law was to create a national registration and accreditation scheme for registered health practitioners (the National Scheme). Following the introduction of the Health Practitioner Regulation National Law all midwives, regardless of their place of work, are required to have PII. Employed midwives are usually appropriately covered by their employer for any duties or activities that the midwife will carry out as part of their role. This is not the case for endorsed midwives in private practice. Currently there is only one available provider of indemnity insurance, which is a Commonwealth-supported scheme that provides cover for pregnancy, labour and birth, and postnatal care. However, it does not provide cover for homebirth. Under section 283 of the National Law, there is exemption from PII arrangements for midwives practising private midwifery who provide intrapartum services for women planning to have a homebirth (NMBA 2016).

Pause *for* Reflection …

Barriers to Private Midwifery Practice

There continue to be barriers for midwives who wish to work in private midwifery in Australia. These barriers include:

1. the requirement to have the equivalent of three years full-time practice prior to being eligible for endorsement to prescribe medicines
2. the requirement for a collaborative arrangement between a midwife and a medical practitioner
3. acceptance of the exclusion from the government-sponsored PII scheme for homebirth.

In other countries such as New Zealand and the United Kingdom these exemptions do not exist for midwives who wish to enter into private practice, so why do you think they exist in Australia?

National Midwifery Guidelines for Consultation and Referral

The aim of the National Midwifery Guidelines for Consultation and Referral (edition 4) (ACM 2021) is to facilitate collaboration between midwives and doctors in the care of individual women through guidance about consultation and referral indications to support integrated maternity care. They were developed by the **Australian College of Midwives (ACM)** and endorsed by the Royal Australian and New Zealand College of Obstetricians and Gynaecologists, and state and territory governments. The purpose of the guidelines is to foster a collaborative, multidisciplinary approach to the provision of maternity care across Australia. The guidelines provide clear guidance to midwives across all practice contexts regardless of the setting they work in and ensure maternity services provide collaborative, safe, quality and evidence-based midwifery care to women, babies and their families (ACM 2021).

REFORM OF AUSTRALIAN MATERNITY SERVICES

The National Maternity Services Plan (Australian Health Ministers' Advisory Council 2011) provided a strategic framework to guide policy and program development for maternity services from 2010 to 2015. The Plan identified actions under the four priority areas of Access, Service Delivery, Workforce and Infrastructure to improve women's access to maternity services and service delivery. The Plan was extended until 30 June 2016. In 2017, the Australian Health Ministers' Advisory Council (AHMAC) agreed to develop a National Strategic Approach to Maternity Services (NSAMS). Following several public and professional consultations a national strategy document titled *Woman-Centred Care: Strategic Directions for Australian Maternity Services* was endorsed by the Council of Australian Governments (COAG) in 2019. The purpose of the strategy was to provide a national strategic direction to support Australia's maternity care system and enable improvements aligned with contemporary practice and evidence (Commonwealth of Australia 2019). The plan recognises that women are the decision-makers in their care and maternity care should reflect their individual needs.

The strategy is centred around four main values: safety, respect, choice and access. The values are underpinned by 12 principles for woman-centred maternity care and apply to all health care professionals involved in providing maternity care to the woman and her family (Commonwealth of Australia 2019) (see Fig 22.3). The strategy is unable to influence private obstetric care, or private midwifery practice.

Fig. 22.3 gives visual representation of the purpose, values and principles outlined in the document. The inner ring represents the purpose of the document and is surrounded by the values. The rays represent the principles and the outer ring represents the respectful maternity charter: the universal rights of childbearing women.

Maternity care is a national priority. Other policy documents focusing on maintaining a high standard of maternity care in Australia include the Clinical Practice Guidelines: Pregnancy Care Guidelines (Department of Health 2020). The guidelines detail specific approaches to pregnancy care for a range of groups, with a focus on improving the experience of antenatal care for Aboriginal and Torres Strait Islander women, migrant and refugee women, and women with severe mental illness (Department of Health 2020). The Midwife Standards

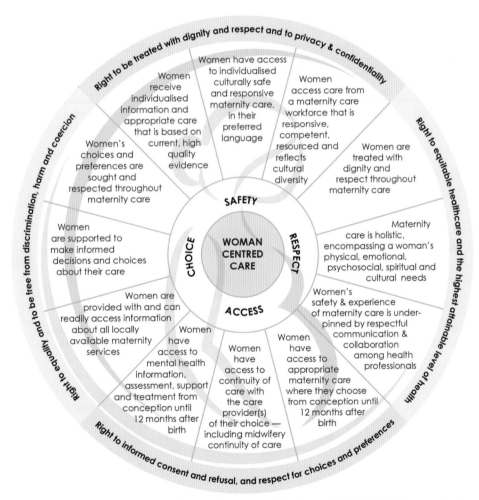

Figure 22.3 Woman-Centred Care. *Source*: Commonwealth of Australia (2019), Woman-centred care: Strategic directions for Australian maternity services. COAG Health Council, Canberra.

for Practice (NMBA 2018) define **woman-centred care** as follows:

> *Woman-centred care recognises the woman's baby or babies, partner, family and community, and respects cultural and religious diversity as defined by the woman herself, it should consider the woman's individual circumstances and aim to meet the woman's physical, emotional, psychosocial, spiritual and cultural needs.*

Many Australian women face social disadvantage, and often experience difficulties in accessing health services. As a result they experience worse health and psychosocial outcomes in pregnancy and birth. Woman-centred care should be built on a reciprocal partnership through effective communication, enabling individual decision-making and self-determination supporting the woman to care for herself and her family (NMBA 2018, p. 9).

MODELS OF MATERNITY CARE

The provision of maternity care can be classified by its model of care. Donnolley et al. (2017) identified eleven models of care in operation in Australia (see Table 22.1) however, while these models exist in all states and territories, there is jurisdictional variation in availability of access for women and midwives to some birth settings and hospital visiting arrangements. Hospital antenatal outpatient clinics have a variety of organisational structures and are most commonly staffed by midwives who

TABLE 22.1   Models of Maternity Care and Proportion of Women who Engage in the Models

Model of Care	Definition	Percentage
Public hospital maternity care	Antenatal care is provided in hospital outpatient clinics (either onsite or in community-based clinics) by midwives and/or doctors. This may include specific clinics such specialist obstetric clinics, but also includes midwife-led outpatient clinics. Care is multidisciplinary where required.	40.8
Midwifery group practice caseload care	Antenatal, labour and postnatal care is provided by a known primary midwife (CoC) through a public hospital. Where available, women can choose to give birth at home (publicly funded homebirth), in a birth centre or in the hospital birth unit.	15.1
Shared care	Antenatal care is provided by a community-based care provider (accredited GP and/or midwife) in collaboration with hospital outpatient maternity clinics.	14.6
Private obstetrician care	Antenatal care is provided by a private specialist obstetrician. Women give birth in either a private or public hospital by the private specialist obstetrician in collaboration with hospital midwives.	10.5
Public hospital high risk maternity care	Antenatal care is provided in a public hospital specialist high-risk maternity outpatient service (including obstetric, maternal-fetal medicine, renal, endocrine etc) in collaboration with midwives.	4.8
General practitioner obstetrician care	Antenatal care is provided by a GP obstetrician, women give birth in a public or private hospital under the care of the hospital-based midwives and the GP obstetrician. This is a common model of care in rural areas.	4.1
Remote area maternity care	Antenatal care is provided by remote area midwives (or nurses), which may be in collaboration with a remote area doctor (this may include fly-in-fly-out or by telehealth). Women are often required to relocate to a regional or metropolitan hospital to give birth, where they are cared for by hospital midwives and doctors.	3.0
Combined care	Antenatal care is provided in the community by a private maternity service provider (midwife and/or doctor). Women give birth in hospital and are cared for by hospital midwifery and medical staff.	2.7

TABLE 22.1 Models of Maternity Care and Proportion of Women who Engage in the Models—cont'd

Model of Care	Definition	Percentage
Private midwifery care	Antenatal, intrapartum and postnatal care is provided by a privately practising midwife or group of midwives. A collaborative arrangement with a doctor is established in the event of identified risk factors. Antenatal, intrapartum and postnatal care is provided in a range of settings including the home and in a public hospital where there is an arrangement for visiting rights allowing continuity of care. Otherwise, upon transfer to hospital, the care is handed over to hospital staff.	2.2
Team midwifery care	Antenatal, labour and postnatal care is provided by a small team of midwives (no more than eight) through a public hospital.	1.8
Private obstetrician and private midwife joint care	Antenatal care is provided by the privately practising midwife and obstetrician in the collaborative practice. Women give birth in a public or private hospital under the care of the private midwife and/or doctor, in collaboration with the hospital staff.	0.4

Source: Australian Institute of Health and Welfare (AIHW) (2021a). Australia's mothers and babies Summary Report. AIHW, Canberra. https://www.aihw.gov.au/reports/mothers-babies/australias-mothers-babies/contents/about; Donnolley, N.R., Chambers, G.M., Butler-Henderson, K.A., et al. (2017). More than a name: Heterogeneity in characteristics of models of maternity care reported from the Australian Maternity Care Classification System validation study. Women Birth 30(4), 332–341.

provide the bulk of the antenatal care for women with a healthy pregnancy. Close collaboration with the obstetric staff in these clinics allows for ease of referral if any complication arises. Other options available to women in the public hospital setting are obstetric outpatient clinics, specialist obstetric clinics and high-risk obstetric services, which include maternal-fetal medicine specialists and other specialties such as renal and endocrine. These services are available in large centres, requiring women in rural areas with existing health issues or who develop complications during their pregnancy to travel or transfer to a maternity hospital away from their home.

To engage in pregnancy care through the private sector, women must obtain a referral from a general practitioner (GP) to see a private obstetrician. Costs associated with this model include reimbursement through private health insurance and out-of-pocket costs for women. Women who engage a midwife in private practice are able to redeem a Medicare rebate for their antenatal care and pay out-of-pocket for other services provided by the midwife including birth and postnatal care.

CONTINUITY OF MIDWIFERY CARE

Continuity of midwifery care enables women to develop a relationship with the same caregiver(s) throughout pregnancy, birth and the postnatal period. A Cochrane review of midwife-led continuity of care models including 15 randomised controlled trials involving 17,674 mothers (Sandall et al. 2016) found that women who received midwife continuity of care were more likely to experience a spontaneous vaginal birth, less likely to have an epidural, less likely to have a premature birth and stillbirth, and rated midwife-led continuity of care highly. Despite the overwhelming evidence which demonstrates the positive outcomes for both women and their babies when they receive continuity of midwifery care, in Australia, progress to universally introduce this model of care continues to be slow. Primarily, midwifery continuity of care in Australia has been largely focused on women at low risk of complications (Beckmann et al. 2012; Homer et al. 2001; McLachlan et al. 2015), with appropriate referral and collaboration, studies of midwife-led models of care have shown benefits to women of all risk profiles (Allen et al. 2019; Lewis et al. 2016; Tracy et al. 2013; Turnbull et al. 2009). The first Australian National Report on Models of Care confirmed just how few women can access continuity of care models of midwifery care with only 15% of pregnant women receiving continuity of midwifery care (AIHW 2021c).

FUNDING AND COSTS

Australian governments, both state and federal, fund and support universal access to health care through the taxation-funded Medicare system, which is delivered via public and private services. At the federal level, Medicare subsidises GP and medical specialist consultations, pharmaceuticals, tests and public hospitals, as well as an increasing number of other health professionals (Duckett & Willcox 2015) including endorsed midwives. State and territory governments are responsible for operating public hospitals and receive funding through activity-based funding (ABF), a mechanism by which hospitals are recompensed for the number and acuity of patients that are treated in a public hospital. Other contributions come from Medicare, non-government organisations, individuals and private health insurers. This complex funding structure can result in cost-shifting between levels of government; for example, GP antenatal shared care may be encouraged by health services to ease the burden in metropolitan public hospital antenatal clinics. GP shared care can, however, be a way of receiving continuity of carer, particularly for women in rural settings (Hoang et al. 2014).

Studies from Australia evaluating the cost of models of midwifery care have demonstrated lower costs for women in midwifery-led models compared with standard hospital care for women in all risk categories (Homer et al. 2001; Rowley 1995). More recently, the M@ngo Study evaluated the cost associated with midwifery group practices, which had caseloads of high- and low-risk women and found a cost saving of (AU)$566.74 for women managed in the **midwifery group practice (MGP)** model of care (Tracy et al. 2013). Similarly, when comparing a 'standard primipara' (a term used to describe a woman pregnant with her first baby, between the ages of 20 and 34, free of obstetric and medical complications and carrying a singleton pregnancy in the cephalic presentation) across three models of care – MGP, standard hospital care and private obstetric care – costs were $1300–$1500 lower for women in the MGP group than women cared for by a private obstetrician or in the standard hospital care group (Tracy et al. 2014).

Women from remote areas in Australia are usually required to relocate to a metropolitan centre close to their due date, which disrupts families and separates women from their support networks at a time of great need. A study by Gao et al. (2014) compared the cost of midwifery group practice and the usual-care model (local health centres, usually in remote locations, delivered by midwives, Aboriginal Health Workers (AHW), District Medical Officers (DMO) and 'fly-in fly-out' specialist obstetricians). Notwithstanding the increase in cost for antenatal and postnatal care, infant readmission and travel, there were significant savings in birthing costs and fewer catastrophic outcomes for infants born vaginally, which saved on special care nursery costs resulting in a cost saving of $703 per mother–infant episode.

Pause *for* Reflection …

Access to Continuity of Midwifery Care for All Australian Women

We know that midwifery continuity of care models produce improved clinical outcomes for women and babies, cost savings for the health system and high maternal satisfaction with care. Yet there continue to be barriers to accessing midwifery continuity of care in Australia, with approximately only 15% of women having access to midwifery group practice.

Using the guidelines by Bacchi (2012) consider the current policies governing the implementation of continuity of midwifery care in Australia.

1. What factors hinder the expansion of midwife-led models of care?
2. How can maternity services reform to enable universal access for all women to access continuity of midwifery care?

MATERNITY CARE DURING THE SARS-COV-2 PANDEMIC

Australia, like many countries around the world, has felt the impact of the SARS-CoV-2 pandemic. In 2020, during the peak of the pandemic, the provision of maternity care changed considerably to reduce the risk of transmission of the virus. Regardless of state or territory, all Australians including pregnant women were encouraged to stay at home during peak transmission times to reduce the risk of transmission. Service interruptions during this time affected the ability of pregnant women to attend face-to-face antenatal care appointments in person and most antenatal interaction occurred via telehealth (AIHW 2021d). Women did not only encounter restricted face-to-face appointments during the antenatal period, but most hospitals placed restrictions during labour, birth and in the postnatal period. This included most hospitals limiting the presence of support persons, often restricting this to one

CASE STUDY 21.1 South Coast Women's Health and Welfare Aboriginal Corporation Waminda: Developing the Waminda Balaang Healing Framework

Most of the care that I provide is in the woman's home, in community or in a clinical setting and is dependent on the woman's place of choice. The care is not only clinically focused but is fluid and embeds cultural practices and protocols at its core for wellness. Being an Aboriginal midwife, I am fortunate to work at the South Coast Women's Health and Welfare Aboriginal Corporation Waminda where women and their Aboriginal families are at the centre of our model of care and are supported by a diverse range of programs that focus on meeting the social and emotional needs of the woman and her family. Below is an example of how a culturally embedded practice is being used in conjunction with Western clinical tools.

Preparing culturally for birth is one of, if not the most, important aspect of pregnancy care that I provide. Ensuring women are grounded and connected spiritually, emotionally and physically and are well informed of their choices using the best available evidence. Many of the women I provide care for unconsciously carry intergenerational trauma as well as intergenerational strengths. For these women who carry trauma, they can be emotionally effected and may result in having a high Edinburgh

Depression Scale (EDS) score, for example. Within our service we conduct the EDS early in pregnancy and more frequently if practical, however, I also go out on country, conducting bunaan (ceremony) with the woman, whilst holding the space for her to release and reflect on negative thoughts, feelings, trauma, strengths, family, kinship systems, language and culture, using the Waminda Balaang Healing Framework. This framework was developed by the women of Waminda and is used as a self-assessment tool that enables the woman to identify her own connection to culture and build on her strengths in preparation for birth.

**Melanie Briggs, Waminda Midwife
and Birthing on Country Advocate**

Case Study Questions

1. Why is it important to consider the emotional, social and cultural well-being of First Nations women during pregnancy?
2. Why do you think the Waminda Balaang Healing Framework is successful and what lessons can we learn from the framework that could be implemented in other areas?

person only. Early research suggests the changes implemented by health services due to the pandemic have had a profound impact on pregnant women and their maternity journey and experience (Sweet et al. 2022). A national survey across Australia involving 3364 participants found women felt distressed and alone due to the public health restrictions on limited visitors. Women were required to navigate the rapid and significant changes to their care pathway and were often expected to coordinate their own care. Equally, some women also reported some benefits to the restrictions including more time for rest, and privacy allowing for the establishment of breastfeeding and bonding with their baby (Wilson et al. 2021). Long-term outcomes of the restrictions introduced are yet to be fully explored.

BIRTHING ON COUNTRY AND PROVIDING CULTURAL MATERNITY CARE

The initiation of human existence and birthing lies in the hands of the oldest living culture on earth, First Nations women in Australia. For thousands of years women would birth on their traditional homelands,

surrounded by women and children using traditional medicines for pregnancy, labour, birth and postpartum. First Nations women have roles in community, and some of these roles include caring for bindjal (pregnant) balaang (women) on (ngura) country as well as being knowledge holders and lore keepers of traditional customs for women's business. First Nations midwifery has a wider scope of practice, where care includes cultural, spiritual and emotional well-being, while including family in the planning of pregnancy, labour, birth, postpartum and parenting. Case study 22.1 provides an example of the implementation of a culturally appropriate maternity model of care for First Nations women living on the South Coast of New South Wales. Similar models are being introduced with encouraging outcomes in other states and territories in Australia.

THE FUTURE OF AUSTRALIAN MATERNITY SERVICES

Underpinning the capacity of any maternity service is the need to provide consistently safe, high-quality maternity care, and although Australia is one of the safest places to be born, there are many challenges to overcome to meet the provision of a woman-centred quality maternity service. Australia continues to see rising intervention rates in childbirth with a national caesarean rate of 34%, three times the rate recommended by the World Health Organization. (World Health Organization 2021). Increasing continuity of midwifery care models may be one way to reduce the rising intervention rate.

If we are truly to address the ever-increasing high rates of intervention, then midwives must have the freedom to work to the full scope of their practice and provide woman-centred care.

Australian maternity services must also continue to make every effort to address the needs of First Nations women, women from culturally and linguistically diverse (CALD) backgrounds, socially disadvantaged women, and women living in rural and remote areas.

SUMMARY

This chapter has provided a brief overview of midwifery in Australia. The following points illuminate the current position and tensions of midwifery in Australia.

- Inequality in maternal and newborn outcomes between First Nations women and other Australians remains and must be addressed by increasing the First Nations midwifery workforce and delivering culturally safe care.
- Midwifery continuity of care models produce improved clinical outcomes for women and babies and cost savings for the health system, and result in high maternal satisfaction with care, yet only 15% of Australian women are able to access this model of care. Every effort should be made to facilitate women's access to this model.
- Intervention rates continue to rise with a current caesarean rate of 34%, however, this increased rate of intervention has not resulted in an improvement in perinatal morality.
- The scope of the midwife in Australia meets the international definition of a midwife, yet there is a requirement for midwives to have 3 years full-time practice prior to be eligible for endorsement to prescribe medicines.

REVIEW QUESTIONS

1. There continue to be social and birthing inequalities between Australia's First Nations women and other Australians. To address this there needs to be an investment in growing the First Nations midwifery workforce and changes to maternity provision to ensure they feel culturally safe. What structures do you think need to be put in place to allow this to happen?
2. Australia's complex funding structure contributes to the restriction of midwifery models of care. This is particularly evident in rural and remote areas of the country. Using the guidelines by Bacchi (2012) discussed in Chapter 1, critique the evidence around models of care and consider how we advocate for a change in the funding structure.
3. Midwifery in Australia is legally recognised as a profession separate from nursing; however, culture change within health services is needed to allow for the full utilisation and acknowledgement of midwives as the primary care providers for childbearing women and their families. How do we advocate for and promote midwifery as a separate profession?
4. Describe the various models of maternity care (see Table 22.1) and consider the scope of practice of the midwife in each model.

REFERENCES

Allen, J., Kildea, S., Tracy, M., et al., 2019. The impact of caseload midwifery, compared with standard care, on women's perceptions of antenatal care quality: Survey results from the M@NGO randomized controlled trial for women of any risk. Birth 46(3), 439–449. https://doi.org/10.1111/birt.12436.

Australian Bureau of Statistics (ABS), 2022. Births Australia. ABS, Canberra. https://www.abs.gov.au/statistics/people/population/births-australia/latest-release#national.

Australian College of Midwives (ACM), 2021. National Midwifery Guidelines for Consultation and Referral, fourth ed. https://www.midwives.org.au/Web/Shop/ACM-Shop-Clinical-Items.aspx.

Australian Commission on Safety and Quality in Health Care, 2017. Second Australian Atlas of Healthcare Variation, Women's Health and Maternity. https://www.safetyandquality.gov.au/our-work/healthcare-variation/atlas-2017/atlas-2017-3-womens-health-and-maternity.

Australian Health Ministers' Advisory Council, 2011. National maternity services plan. Commonwealth of Australia, Canberra.

Australian Institute of Health and Welfare (AIHW), 2021a. Australia's mothers and babies Summary Report. AIHW, Canberra. https://www.aihw.gov.au/reports/mothers-babies/australias-mothers-babies/contents/about.

Australian Institute of Health and Welfare (AIHW), 2021b. Pregnancy and birth outcomes for Aboriginal and Torres Strait Islander women 2016–2018. Cat. No. IHW 234. AIHW, Canberra.

Australian Institute of Health and Welfare (AIHW), 2021c. Maternity care in Australia: first national report on models of care. AIHW, Canberra. https://www.aihw.gov.au/getmedia/fca695dd-c549-4306-ab08-29c5bdd1e908/Maternity-care-in-Australia-first-national-report-on-models-of-care-2021.pdf.aspx?inline=true

Australian Institute of Health and Welfare (AIHW), 2021d. Antenatal care during COVID-19. AIHW, Canberra. https://www.aihw.gov.au/reports/mothers-babies/antenatal-care-during-covid-19/contents/antenatal-care-and-covid-19.

Australian Institute of Health and Welfare (AIHW) & National Indigenous Australian Agency, 2021. Aboriginal and Torres Islanders Health Performance Framework, Perinatal mortality. https://www.indigenoushpf.gov.au/measures/1-21-perinatal-mortality#.YepMWoTs2zw.mailto.

Bacchi, C., 2012. Introducing the 'What's the problem represented to be?' approach. In: Bletsas, A., Beasley, C. (Eds.), Engaging With Carol Bacchi: Strategic Interventions and Exchanges. University of Adelaide Press, Adelaide. https://www.adelaide.edu.au/carst/docs/wpr/wpr-summary.pdf.

Beckmann, M., Kildea, S., Gibbons, K., 2012. Midwifery group practice and mode of birth. Women Birth 25 (4), 187–193. https://doi.org/10.1016/j.wombi.2011.11.001.

Council of Australian Governments (COAG), 2019. Woman-centred care: Strategic directions for Australian maternity. COAG Health Council, Canberra.

Department of Health, 2012. Collaborative arrangements for participating midwives and nurse practitioners. https://www1.health.gov.au/internet/main/publishing.nsf/Content/midwives-nurse-pract-collaborative-arrangements.

Department of Health, 2018. Strategic Directions for Australian Maternity Services, (Draft for consultation paper 2) Australian Health Ministers Advisory Council. Canberra, Department of Health.

Department of Health, 2020. Clinical Practice Guidelines: Pregnancy Care. Department of Health, Canberra.

Department of Health and Aged Care, 2021a. About nurses and midwives. Australian Government, Canberra. https://www.health.gov.au/topics/nurses-and-midwives/about#:~:text=A%20midwife's%20scope%20of%20practice,the%20woman%20and%20her%20baby.

Department of Health and Aged Care, 2021b. Health Workforce Data. Australian Government, Canberra. https://www.health.gov.au/resources/apps-and-tools/health-workforce-data.

Department of Health and Aged Care, 2022. National Health Workforce Dataset. https://hwd.health.gov.au/resources/information/nhwds.html.

Donnolley, N.R., Chambers, G.M., Butler-Henderson, K.A., et al., 2017. More than a name: Heterogeneity in characteristics of models of maternity care reported from the Australian Maternity Care Classification System validation study. Women Birth 30 (4), 332–341.

Duckett, S., Willcox, S., 2015. Australian Health Care System, fifth ed. Oxford University Press.

Gao, Y., Gold, L., Josif, C., et al., 2014. A cost-consequences analysis of a Midwifery Group Practice for Aboriginal mothers and infants in the Top End of the Northern Territory, Australia. Midwifery 30 (4), 447–55.

Hoang, H., Le, Q., Ogden, K., 2014. Women's maternity care needs and related service models in rural areas: A comprehensive systematic review of qualitative evidence. Women Birth 27 (4), 233–241.

Homer, C., Davis, G., Brodie, P., et al. 2001. Collaboration in maternity care: a randomised controlled trial comparing community-based continuity of care with standard hospital care. BJOG 108 (1), 16–22. https://doi.org/10.1111/j.1471-0528.2001.00022.x.

Homer, C.S., Matha, D.V., Jordan, L.G., et al. 2001. Community-based continuity of midwifery care versus standard hospital care: a cost analysis. Aust Health Rev 24 (1), 85–93.

Lewis, L., Hauck, Y., Crichton, C., et al. 2016. An overview of the first 'no exit' midwifery group practice in a tertiary maternity hospital in Western Australia: Outcomes, satisfaction and perceptions of care. Women Birth 29 (6), 494–502. https://doi.org/10.1016/j.wombi.2016.04.009.

McLachlan, H., Forster, D., Davey, M., 2015. The effect of primary midwife-led care on women's experience of childbirth: results from the COSMOS randomised controlled trial. BJOG 123 (3), 465–474. https://doi.org/10.1111/1471-0528.13713.

National Health Workforce Dataset (NHWDS), 2021. Nurses and midwives 2016–2019. http://hwd.health.gov.au.

Nursing and Midwifery Board of Australia, 2016. Registration Standard: Professional Indemnity Insurance Arrangements. Nursing and Midwifery Board of Australia, Canberra.

Nursing and Midwifery Board of Australia, 2017/2021. Safety and quality guidelines for private practising midwives.

Nursing and Midwifery Board of Australia, Canberra. (updated, November 2021).

Nursing and Midwifery Board of Australia, 2018. Midwife Standards for Practice 2018. Nursing and Midwifery Board of Australia, Canberra.

Organisation for Economic Co-operation and Development (OECD), 2019. SF2.3: Age of mothers at childbirth and age-specific fertility. Paris: OECD. http://www.oecd.org/els/soc/SF_2_3_Age_mothers_childbirth.pdf.

Rowley, M.J., Hensley, M.J., Brinsmead, M.W., et al., 1995. Continuity of care by a midwife team versus routine care during pregnancy and birth: a randomised trial. Med J Aust 163 (6), 289–293.

Sandall, J., Soltani, H., Gates, S., et al. 2016. Midwife-led continuity models versus other models of care for child-bearing women. Cochrane Database Syst Rev (4): CD004667.

Sweet, L., Wilson, A.N., Bradfield, Z., 2022. Childbearing women's experiences of the maternity care system in Australia during the first wave of the COVID-19 pandemic. Women Birth 35 (3), 223–231. doi:10.1016/j.wombi.2021.08.010.

Tracy, S., Hartz, D., Tracy, M., 2013. Caseload midwifery care versus standard maternity care for women of any risk: M@NGO, a randomised controlled trial. Lancet 382 (9906), 1723–1732. https://doi.org/10.1016/s0140-6736(13)61406-3.

Tracy, S.K., Welsh, A., Hall, B., et al., 2014. Caseload midwifery compared to standard or private obstetric care for first time mothers in a public teaching hospital in Australia: a cross sectional study of cost and birth outcomes. BMC Pregnancy Childbirth 14 (1), 1–9.

Turnbull, D., Baghurst, P., Collins, C., et al., 2009. An evaluation of midwifery group practice. Part 1: clinical effectiveness. Women Birth 22, 3–9.

Wilson, A.N., Sweet, L., Vasilevski, R.M., 2021. Australian women's experiences of receiving maternity care during the COVID-19 pandemic: A cross-sectional national survey. Birth. doi:10.1111/birt.12569.

World Health Organization (WHO), 2021. WHO Statement on caesarean section rates. https://www.who.int/news-room/questions-and-answers/item/who-statement-on-caesarean-section-rates-frequently-asked-questions.

FURTHER READING

Asefa, A., Semaan, A., Delvaux, T., Huysmans, E., Galle, A., Sacks, E., ... & Benova, L. (2022). The impact of COVID-19 on the provision of respectful maternity care: Findings from a global survey of health workers. Women and Birth 35 (4), 378–386.

Hickey, S., Couchman, K., Stapleton, H., et al., 2019. Experiences of health service providers establishing an Aboriginal-Mainstream partnership to improve maternity care for Aboriginal and Torres Strait Islander families in an urban setting. Eval Program Plann 77, 101705.

Sandall, J., Soltani, H., Gates, S., et al., 2016. Midwife-led continuity models versus other models of care for childbearing women. Cochrane Database Syst Rev (4).

Seijmonsbergen-Schermers, A.E., Van Den Akker, T., Rydahl, E., et al., 2020. Variations in use of childbirth interventions in 13 high-income countries: A multinational cross-sectional study. PLOS Med 17 (5), e1003103.

ONLINE RESOURCES

Birthing on Country Centre of Excellence: https://www.birthingoncountry.com/centre-for-research-excellence.

Australian College of Midwives: https://www.midwives.org.au/.

Australian Institute of Health and Welfare Mothers and Babies Report: https://www.aihw.gov.au/reports/mothers-babies/australias-mothers-babies/contents/about.

Australian Nursing and Midwifery Council Professional Standards: https://www.anmac.org.au/standards-and-review.

Ahpra Nursing and Midwifery Board of Australia: https://www.nursingmidwiferyboard.gov.au/.

23

Nursing in Australia

Sarah Wise and Christine Duffield

KEY LEARNING OUTCOMES

When you finish this chapter you should be able to:

- describe the differences between the three levels of licensed nurse, and unlicensed health workers
- demonstrate an understanding of nursing supply problems in Australia
- identify how scope of practice varies according to the level of nurse, the individual and the context
- demonstrate an understanding of the evolving nature of the nursing-medical boundary, and the constraints placed on nurse practitioners
- outline the importance of regulated nurse staffing to patient and resident safety and quality of care.

KEY TERMS AND ABBREVIATIONS

Australian Health Practitioner Regulation Agency (Ahpra)
Australian Medical Association (AMA)
Australian Nursing and Midwifery Accreditation Council (ANMAC)
enrolled nurse (EN)

general practitioner (GP)
International Council of Nurses (ICN)
Medicare Benefits Schedule (MBS)
nurse practitioner (NP)
Nursing and Midwifery Board of Australia (NMBA)

personal care worker (PCW)
Pharmaceutical Benefits Scheme (PBS)
practice nurse
registered nurse (RN)
residential aged-care facility (RACF)
unlicensed health worker

INTRODUCTION

Nursing is by far the largest health profession in Australia, comprising more than half of the professional health care workforce performing a wide range of roles in health, aged care and other settings. Nurses work autonomously and collaboratively within the interprofessional team, initiating some duties independently as well as performing tasks delegated from other professionals, primarily doctors and other nurses. From the earliest times, nursing sought to establish itself as a distinct profession, separate from and equal to medicine (Larson 1977). In establishing their own professional mandate, nursing's leaders were concerned the profession should not become a diluted version of medicine nor subservient to it, particularly in light of the historic gender segregation of the two professions (Davies 1996). In doing so, nursing has established itself as the patient's advocate within the health system with an ethos of enablement, as this statement from the **International Council of Nurses (ICN)** (2022) illustrates:

The unique function of nurses in caring for individuals, sick or well, is to assess their responses to their health status and to assist them in the performance of those activities contributing to health or recovery or to dignified death that they would perform unaided if they had the necessary strength, will, or knowledge, and to do this in such a way as to help them gain full or partial independence as rapidly as possible. Within the total health care environment, nurses share with other health professionals ... the functions of planning, implementation, and evaluation to ensure the adequacy of the health system for promoting health, preventing illness, and caring for ill and disabled people.

The chapter will describe nursing as a licensed profession with different levels of educational attainment, experience and autonomy, nursing's place in the health workforce and challenges for the supply and demand for nurses. The concept of scope of practice will be explored, with a focus on interprofessional issues at the boundary between nursing and medical practice. The chapter concludes with a discussion of the role and controversies of nurse staffing regulations for safe, quality care in health and aged care.

NURSING AS A LICENSED PROFESSION

Nursing is a licensed profession under the *Health Practitioner Regulation National Law Act 2009* (Ahpra 2022a). Professional regulation is administered by the **Nursing and Midwifery Board of Australia (NMBA)**, one of fifteen national boards supported by the **Australian Health Practitioner Regulation Agency (Ahpra)**. Together, the national boards and Ahpra provide independent registration and accreditation to ensure only suitably trained, competent and ethical health practitioners are licensed to practise under a protected professional title (Ahpra 2022b).

Protection of title means only licensed professionals can perform certain jobs. As Freidson (2001, p. 56) explains, 'Should consumers or managers wish to have the tasks connected with those [professions] performed, they are not free to employ any willing worker, or to themselves train workers for the purpose. Instead they must use bona fide members of the [profession]'. There are three protected nursing titles: **nurse practitioner (NP)**, **registered nurse (RN)** and **enrolled nurse (EN)** differentiated by their qualifications, level of functioning and professional accountability as defined by legislation and standards set by the NMBA (Table 23.1). Collectively, NPs RNs, and ENs are 'licensed nurses'.

An RN is authorised to practise without supervision and is accountable and responsible for the nursing care they provide, and for their decisions to delegate tasks to ENs and **unlicensed health workers** (NMBA 2020). Nurse practitioners are distinguished from RNs by their legal mandate to autonomously diagnose, prescribe and refer within their scope of practice, that is for the patients and conditions they are educated and competent to manage (Scanlon et al. 2016). Enrolled nurses are educated in educational institutions other than universities. They practise under the supervision (direct and indirect) of an RN (or NP) and are directly accountable for their own actions.

In addition to licensed nurses, there is a growing group of unlicensed health workers who are increasingly forming part of the nursing team in aged care (e.g. **personal care workers**) and in hospitals (e.g. Assistant in Nursing). Official training of unlicensed health workers is traditionally short and does not have to meet national standards, and so they do not register with the NMBA. Unlicensed workers are not responsible for overall patient care and should only undertake routine tasks that do not involve clinical decision-making (e.g.

TABLE 23.1 **Nursing Roles – Regulation and Qualifications**			
	Protected Title	**Registration with NMBA**	**Minimum Qualifications**
Nurse practitioner	Yes	Registered nurse with additional endorsement	An RN plus Master's degree and 5000 hours of supervised practice (Department of Health and Aged Care 2021a)
Registered nurse	Yes	Registered nurse	Bachelor of Nursing
Enrolled nurse	Yes	Enrolled nurse	Diploma of Nursing (Enrolled Nurse)
Unlicensed health worker	No	None	None, Certificate III or IV as determined by employer

personal care). However, the line between *routine* tasks and the more advanced technical and decision-making tasks which should remain with licensed nurses can be unclear (Duffield et al. 2019). Moreover, supervision arrangements in some aged-care settings call into question who is responsible for overall care. In hospitals, an unlicensed worker's tasks should be delegated from a licensed nurse who is responsible for supervising their work (NMBA 2013). However, in **residential aged-care facilities (RACFs)** supervision may be indirect (i.e. the licensed nurse may not be present) while there may be no supervision by a licensed nurse at all in aged care delivered at home (Wise 2020).

The NMBA develops and enforces codes of conduct, standards of practice and codes of ethics for each level of licensed nurse that include the principle that nurses engage with people as individuals in a respectful way, foster open, honest and compassionate professional relationships, and adhere to privacy and confidentiality obligations. There are specific expectations set for culturally safe practice for Aboriginal and/or Torres Strait Islander people (NMBA 2018). Nurses apply for an annual practising certificate to ensure that each nurse practises within their scope, is of sound health and good character (e.g. they have not committed a criminal offence, or had limits placed on their practice), have undertaken the mandated hours of continuing professional education, and hold professional indemnity insurance (Ahpra 2015; NMBA 2016b, 2016c).

The NMBA is also responsible for accrediting the programs and providers of nurse education (under the **Australian Nursing and Midwifery Accreditation Council (ANMAC)**), assessment of competencies of overseas-trained nurses who wish to register to practise in Australia, and adjudication of cases of unsafe practice or unprofessional conduct.

THE NURSING WORKFORCE

Nursing is by far the largest health profession in Australia, and worldwide. Table 23.2 shows that nurses comprise half of the professional health care workforce registered and employed in Australia, more than three times the size of the medical workforce. As of 30 September 2021 there were 2227 endorsed nurse practitioners in Australia (NMBA 2021).

The majority (61%) are employed in hospitals, followed by RACFs (14%), community health care services

TABLE 23.2 Health Professionals Registered and Employed in Australia, 2020

	Headcount	Percentage of Health Professionals
Registered nurses	271,009	42%
Enrolled nurses	52,342	8%
Midwives*	26,238	4%
Medical practitioners	105,293	17%
Allied Health Professionals	187,597	29%
Total	642,479	100%

* Includes dual registered RNs and midwives ($n=21,256$)
Source: National Health Workforce Dataset (NHWD 2020). Summary statistics.
https://hwd.health.gov.au/resources/dashboards/nhwds-summary-metrics.htm

(7%) and general practice (4%) (NHWD 2020). Nurses also work in other settings such as schools, correctional facilities and the defence force. A total of 92% are employed in clinical roles with the remainder using their clinical experience to work as managers, in teaching and education, or research (NHWD 2020).

Australia has a high number of nurses for the size of its population. There are 121.5 nurses per 10,000 of the population in Australia compared to an average of 107.7 per 10,000 in other high-income countries (e.g. in Europe and North America). In contrast, low-income (e.g. in central Africa) and lower-middle income countries (e.g. in south-east Asia) have only 9.1 and 16.7 nurses per 10,000 respectively (WHO 2020).

However, Australia's geographical vastness presents distinct challenges for supply of nurses. Table 23.3 shows the number and density (per 10,000 of the population) of nurses and midwives (separate data are not available) using the Modified Monash Model, a classification of geographical remoteness (Department of Health and Aged Care 2021c). There are *fewer* nurses per 10,000 population in metropolitan areas (122.5) (i.e. major cities) than in remote (135.8) and very remote areas (130) (e.g. in Aboriginal and Torres Strait Islander community health centres in Central Australia). 'Large rural towns' have the highest number of nurses per 10,000 (152.4) since they often have a small hospital

TABLE 23.3 Distribution of FTE Nurses and Midwives by Modified Monash Model, 2019

Modified Monash Model	FTE	FTE Per 10,000 Population
MM1— Metropolitan	222,666	122.6
MM2 – Regional centres	30,221	136.4
MM3 – Large rural towns	24,025	152.5
MM4 – Medium rural towns	10,898	113.2
MM5 – Small rural towns	11,196	64.3
MM6 – Remote communities	3,839	135.8
MM7 – Very remote communities	2,764	130.0
Australia	303,723	121.5

FTE (full-time equivalent) based on 38 hours per week
Source: National Health Workforce Dataset (NMBA 2019).

and a residential aged-care facility that service a vast catchment area. However, the higher number of nurses per 10,000 population in rural and remote areas does not translate into better access to care, since people must travel long distances to their nearest health facility, with specialist care often only available in metropolitan and large regional centres.

The nursing workforce in Australia is large and growing. Figure 23.1 shows that young people are entering the profession in unprecedented numbers. In 2019, Australia produced the highest number of nursing graduates in the OECD, for the size of its population (more than twice the average) (OECD 2020). At the same time, there has been an increase in the proportion of graduates not employed as an RN within six months of qualifying, and a decline in secure, ongoing employment for those who do (Doleman et al. 2022). The underemployment of graduate nurses is surprising given labour market analysis by the Australian Government, which finds RNs to be the second most 'in-demand' occupation in the whole economy, after unlicensed health workers for aged and disability care (National Skills Commission 2021). Demand for RNs may be high but employers do not necessarily have the budget for supported graduate nursing positions (involving additional training and supervision requirements), or to offer them ongoing employment (Doleman et al. 2022). Moreover, most universities are located in major cities and graduates usually want to work in the health facilities where they trained, exacerbating the shortage of nurses in rural and regional areas.

Figure 23.1 also illustrates the problem of nurse retention, with employment levels dropping across the life course from younger, to older age groups. The challenges of balancing the long and unsocial hours of shift

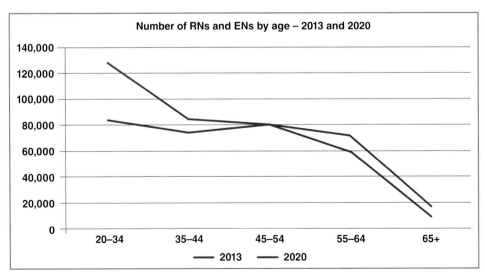

Figure 23.1 Age Composition of the Nursing Workforce *(n)*. Data from NHWD (2020). National Health Workforce Dataset 2020. Australian Government, Canberra.

work with family life, along with high workloads, stress and responsibilities which are often not commensurate with salaries, drive many nurses to leave the profession (Moloney et al. 2018). During the COVID-19 pandemic, many countries (including Australia) implemented policies to make it easier for nurses who had recently left the profession to return to work, to assist with mass vaccination and deliver frontline care. Despite this short-term increase in supply, initial analysis suggests working through the pandemic will cause many nurses to leave the profession early due to ill-health and burnout (Buchan et al. 2022).

> **Pause** *for* **Reflection ...**
> Australia can attract people to study nursing at university, but it is difficult to retain them in the long-term. The ability to increase pay is limited due to pressured public finances. What else could be done to encourage nurses to: (a) stay in the profession, and (b) move to regional and remote areas where they are needed?

SCOPE OF NURSING PRACTICE

So far, we have described the different levels of nursing, and nurses' education, regulation and where they work. The ICN definition of nursing provided at the beginning of this chapter gives a broad description of the *function* of nursing roles but not specifically what they *do* day-to-day. Unlike some jurisdictions in the United States and Canada where individual tasks are regulated and tied to specific roles (Dower et al. 2013), in Australia only the prescription and supply of medications are regulated by state and territory laws. All other clinical tasks are regulated through the more flexible concept of scope of practice:

> *Scope of practice is that in which nurses are educated, competent to perform and permitted by law. The actual scope of practice is influenced by the context in which the nurse practises, the health needs of people, the level of competence and confidence of the nurse and the policy requirements of the service provider.*
>
> *(NMBA 2016a)*

A *profession's scope of practice* includes the roles, functions, responsibilities, activities and decision-making capacities that members of that profession are *generally* educated, competent and authorised to perform. There are tasks common to most nurses' scope of practice such as taking and recording a patient's blood pressure, but what they do with that information depends on their level of education, registration and where they work: an NP, RN or EN will interpret and act upon a blood pressure reading in different ways. An *individual's scope of practice* is based on that person's specific experience and education, and the context in which they work. The onus is on the nurse to judge which patients, conditions and tasks are within their scope of practice based on their own education, knowledge, competency, experience and lawful authority (NMBA 2008). Nurses' scope of practice, the training they receive, the skills and tasks they acquire, and career progression are greatly influenced by policy and practice in their workplace (Djukic & Kovner 2010).

A 3-year Bachelor of Nursing degree and general registration with the NMBA allows a graduate nurse to enter any field (except midwifery). Nurses may also undertake workplace training and postgraduate education to gain qualifications in a clinical speciality but, unlike doctors, nurses cannot register as specialists (Ahpra 2018). The titles clinical nurse consultant (CNC) and clinical nurse specialist (CNS) are used for RNs practising for some years in a clinical speciality (with CNCs considered to be practising at an advanced level). Role responsibilities and educational requirements vary between states, and titles are not protected by the NMBA.

Scope of practice encompasses activities beyond direct care tasks such as giving medications or performing wound care. Nurses spend a high proportion of their time communicating with patients and relatives, coordinating the interprofessional team and ensuring that patients transition safely through the health system (Wise et al. 2020).

Nurses are the 'glue' that hold the health system together, requiring clinical judgement, excellent communication and negotiation skills, knowledge of individual patients and the complex health system (Wise et al. 2022). Allen (2014) describes this essential function as the 'invisible work of nurses' since it goes largely unrecognised. It also often involves nurses challenging the traditional hierarchy and doctors' decisions, without formal authority to do so (Wise et al. 2022).

INTERPROFESSIONAL ISSUES AT THE NURSING-MEDICAL BOUNDARY

Scope of practice ties each profession to a set of tasks, but these ties are not absolute or permanent (Abbott

1988). The evolution of professional scopes of practice at the nursing-medical boundary is demonstrated by a long-term trend of the shifting of tasks from doctors to nurses. As early as the 1950s, Hughes et al. (1958) observed that as medical science advances and demand for health care rises, doctors learn new techniques and continue to reorganise their work by delegating tasks to others, especially nurses.

Evaluation studies confirm a trend of RNs undertaking increasingly complex medical tasks over time (Djukic & Kovner 2010). Nurses have long been involved in wound care, and for many years have undertaken laceration repair (Middleton 2006). Once only performed by doctors, venepuncture and the insertion and removal of peripheral and central venous access devices increasingly became part of everyday nursing practice (Dougherty & Lamb 2009) and specially trained RNs are now performing diagnostic gastrointestinal endoscopy and flexible sigmoidoscopy (Duffield et al. 2017). Internationally, reforms have allowed RNs to prescribe medications, albeit with greater constraints on their autonomy than doctors. In Australia RNs cannot legally write a prescription, but in some workplaces they may be permitted to initiate and administer medications in limited circumstances by following a protocol (Ecker et al. 2020; Ladd & Schober 2018).

Nurses' increased involvement in medical tasks is frequently described as 'blurring' the boundaries between the two professions. The NP role is at the forefront of this trend, since it challenges medicine's long-standing monopoly over the right to diagnose and determine treatments. Nurse practitioners' responsibilities include advanced patient assessment, diagnosis and management of diseases, referral, prescribing, and the ordering and interpretation of diagnostic investigations for the patient population or conditions within their scope of practice (Scanlon et al. 2018). While sharing these tasks with the medical profession, NPs do not regard themselves as 'mini-doctors' but retain the core nursing values, especially enabling patients in their care (Jennings et al. 2015). A study comparing the tasks of NPs and doctors performing similar roles in an Australian emergency department found NPs spent a significantly higher proportion of their time on patient communication: educating them about their condition and providing information and resources to support their ongoing care and treatment (Wise et al. 2020).

Nurse practitioners have the potential to fill critical service gaps in primary care where they could be proactive in managing chronic disease and reducing hospital admissions, especially in remote and rural Australia where there is a chronic shortage of **general practitioners (GPs)** (AIHW 2018). However, progress in this area has been slow because the **Australian Medical Association (AMA)** has opposed NPs' access to the **Medicare Benefits Schedule (MBS)** and **Pharmaceutical Benefits Scheme (PBS)**, the principal method of reimbursement in primary care (Harvey 2011; Schadewaldt et al. 2016). When the first Australian NP was licensed and employed in outback New South Wales in 2001, they were not permitted to obtain MBS provider or PBS prescriber numbers so patients had to pay the full cost of fees, medications and any services to which they were referred (Harvey 2011).

From 2010 NPs working in private practice can obtain provider and prescriber numbers but, in a concession obtained by the Australian Medical Association (AMA), they must be in a 'collaborative arrangement' with a named doctor (Schadewaldt et al. 2016). Despite ample evidence of NPs providing safe and cost-effective primary care in other countries (Traczynski & Udalova 2018) and the requirement to collaborate forming part of every profession's code of conduct, the AMA argued that collaborative arrangements were needed to provide 'an overarching quality framework to preserve patient safety and ensure that medical practitioners are not left out of the loop' (AMA 2010, p. 3). The fee-for-service MBS funding model means there is no financial incentive for a GP to engage an NP in a collaborative arrangement. Many GPs employ a **practice nurse** who, under delegated medical authority, performs tasks such as pap smears, Chronic Disease Management, immunisations and wound care. In this delegation model, the GP collects the MBS fee for services provided by the practice nurse.

The collaborative arrangement concession achieved by the AMA might be viewed as the medical profession closing the primary care market to competition from independent NPs (Larson 1977). Moreover, the MBS rebate set for NPs (i.e. MBS items 82200-82215) is around half that for GPs, and less than that received by allied health providers such as audiologists and physiotherapists. Nurse practitioners are also not permitted to refer patients for basic diagnostic imaging such as X-ray and ultrasound under the MBS, so patients would have to pay the full cost of services.

For these reasons, NPs predominantly work as salaried employees in public hospitals where they do not require provider or prescriber numbers to work to their full scope of practice. The largest group works in emergency departments, where they commonly order diagnostic imaging. Despite the AMA's lobbying to restrict NPs' practice in primary care, the vast majority of Australian NPs feel supported and respected by the doctors in their workplace (Scanlon et al. 2018).

Pause *for* Reflection …

Over several decades, there has been a concerted media campaign and lobbying waged by what Tuohy (1999, p. 15) refers to as 'professional collegial institutions' such as the AMA against nurses working in the NP role. These institutions argue that patients would be put at risk from a health care system that 'fragmented care'. To what extent is current policy surrounding NPs a product/outcome of the market? To what extent is it a product/outcome of contestation with professional collegial institutions such as the AMA?

NURSE STAFFING AND PATIENT SAFETY

The financial sustainability of health care is one of the most significant challenges facing governments, with increasing demand and rising costs threatening to undermine stretched public finances. Health care is a labour-intensive industry therefore staffing accounts for the majority of health care expenditure. As the largest item in the staffing budget, nursing is continually subjected to budgetary constraints, often despite increasing workloads. Cuts to nurse staffing can be made by reducing the number of nurses and/or by 'diluting' the skill mix, that is substituting RNs with cheaper unlicensed health care workers.

However, there is a large body of research demonstrating that increasing the number of patients each RN must look after negatively impacts the quality and safety of patient care, including missed care, hospital-acquired infections and falls (McHugh et al. 2021). Poor nurse staffing is also associated with negative outcomes for nurses themselves, including burnout, job dissatisfaction and intentions to leave their current role (Aiken et al. 2012).

Unlike many countries, nurse staffing in most Australian public hospitals is regulated by legislation (Van den Heede et al. 2020). Often referred to generically as 'ratios' (i.e. the number of patients per nurse), nursing unions have negotiated different arrangements for regulating workload in each state. These specify *minimum* staff levels using traditional ratios (Queensland), the number of nurses per 20 patients on a ward (Victoria), or the of number of nursing hours per patient day (New South Wales), as well as skill mix requirements (i.e. the proportion of care provided by RNs). In all jurisdictions these standards vary according to the acuity and dependency of patients on the ward, and time of day (staffing is generally permitted to be lower on night shifts).

The principle that nurse staffing influences patient safety is well-established but the use of regulation to manage workloads remains controversial since there is no research evidence to support the optimal number and mix of staff (Van den Heede et al. 2020). Regulations can also be inflexible, take crucial decisions away from nurse managers and lead to *minimum* rather than *optimal* staffing. In addition, key drivers of nursing workload such as the 'invisible work' of coordination, and the turnover and the mix of patients coming through the ward are not captured by measures based on patient numbers (Duffield et al. 2020). Staffing regulations represent a compromise between nurses and their unions, management and government budget-holders but have led to Australian public hospitals enjoying some of the highest levels of nurse staffing in the world. This stands in sharp contrast to the situation in aged care where a voluntary approach to safe staffing prevailed for many years.

Evidence garnered by the Royal Commission into Aged Care Quality and Safety (https://agedcare.royal-commission.gov.au/) revealed that since minimum staff standards were dropped in the early 2000s, staffing levels and skill mix in residential aged care have declined in absolute terms, and relative to the rising health *and* social needs of an older and more clinically complex population. Government funding, and therefore the staffing of the aged-care sector, has been based on the notion that it provides 'social care' not 'health care'. This has allowed the workforce to become dominated by unlicensed **'personal care workers' (PCWs)**, only 66% of whom in residential aged care and 60% in home care have a relevant care qualification (usually Certificate III) (Department of Health and Aged Care 2021b). More than half of Australian aged-care residents (57.6%) are living in facilities with 'unacceptable' staffing with questionable supervision arrangements (Eagar

CASE STUDY 23.1   Residential Aged-Care Facilities (RACFs)

Mark is an endorsed NP with 15 years emergency department experience. He is now employed by the community health unit of a large hospital to provide acute clinical services to older people living in RACFs located in the local health district. He routinely sees residents who would not otherwise have access to timely primary care. A typical day may require Mark to assess, diagnose and treat minor illnesses or injuries including infections, wounds and mental health episodes.

Mark has MBS and PBS provider numbers as he has a collaborative arrangement with a doctor in the community health unit. He performs wound care, diagnoses minor illness and determines appropriate treatments, writes prescriptions, orders pathology and refers to other providers. However, residents can experience delays in receiving necessary diagnostic imaging tests as current MBS rules do not enable NPs to initiate simple imaging like X-rays and ultrasound that are normally subsidised in primary care. This leads to an unnecessary duplication of services, requiring either a second attendance by a GP or, worse, an unnecessary transfer to an emergency department.

Some residents do not have access to a regular GP for comprehensive medical assessments or team care arrangements, including accessing allied health services.

Those residents do not have their chronic health conditions proactively assessed and managed for early signs of deterioration, increasing the incidence of acute events and hospitalisation, and reducing their overall quality of life. The ongoing care of residents with dementia is also a concern. Residents and RACF staff have asked Mark to expand his services to provide chronic care and dementia care including comprehensive health assessments, Chronic Disease Management, cognitive and behavioural management for dementia and case conferences.

Case Study Questions

1. What are the problems that the NP is assisting with?
2. Why would a hospital provide an acute clinical service for residents when aged care is not a state responsibility?
3. Which other roles (health professionals and others) would the NP have to work with to ensure patients receive the acute care they need?
4. What would the NP and their employer have to consider when responding to the RACF's request to expand services into chronic and dementia care?
5. How might demand for the NP service change if the RACF increased their RN staffing?

---

et al. 2019). Moreover, the MBS does not adequately remunerate GPs to visit RACFs or older people at home, or to coordinate with aged-care staff while the MBS constrains NPs in the services they can provide. Limited access to RNs, GPs and NPs potentially leaves aged-care residents and those receiving care at home with no skilled 'eyes' overseeing their care and their potential deterioration, and can lead to avoidable hospital admissions. (See Case study 23.1.)

The SARS-CoV-2 pandemic highlighted an aged-care system struggling to meet the health needs of vulnerable Australians. Even where sufficient personal protective equipment was available, PCWs were not trained in how to use it (Royal Commission into Aged Care Quality and Safety 2020). A national survey of nurses (including unlicensed health workers) across health and aged care found those working in RACFs reported the highest proportion of COVID-19 infections; they were also the most concerned about COVID-19 related risks to their personal and mental health, and about job security and financial hardship. They also reported the highest levels

of workplace demands, exhaustion, more symptoms of depression, anxiety, and stress and the lowest level of job satisfaction (Adelson et al. 2021).

The Royal Commission made numerous recommendations to improve staffing in aged care but the government only accepted some of these. From 2022 a new funding model called the Australian National Aged Care Classification more closely ties funding to the clinical needs of residents and from October 2023 minimum staffing standards will be reintroduced. All RACFs must provide minimum care minutes per day and have an RN onsite for at least 16 hours per day (Department of Health and Aged Care 2022). There will be more funding for GPs to provide care to aged-care residents, and training for PCWs but no mandated minimum qualifications and there are no proposals to regulate staffing in the home care sector, where many more people receive services. These measures will improve safety for residents and working conditions for staff, but are likely to fall short of what is required for a high-quality aged-care system that meets both health *and* social needs.

SUMMARY

- The nursing workforce is large and diverse, and demand is increasing. More people are joining the profession than ever before but there are challenges in supplying nurses outside metropolitan areas. The pay and conditions of nursing work also make it difficult to retain nurses over the life course.
- Each individual nurse must determine which activities fall within their scope of practice based on their registration, education, experience and where they work. Much of nurses' work expands beyond direct clinical care, incorporating the 'invisible work' of communication and coordination of the interprofessional team to ensure patients' transitions safely through the health system.
- The boundary between nursing and medicine is always evolving. The NP role challenges medicine's long-standing monopoly over the right to diagnose and determine treatments. However, the medical profession has lobbied to constrain NPs' ability to receive rebates for their services limiting their ability to fill critical service gaps in primary and aged care.
- The number and mix of nursing staffing has a major impact on patient and resident safety, and nurse job satisfaction. Staffing is regulated in many public hospitals but not in aged care for many. Funding models based on providing 'social care' ignored the rising health needs of older people allowing the workforce to become dominated by unlicensed workers with limited supervision and training.

REVIEW QUESTIONS

1. What advantages and disadvantages can you see in allowing individual nurses to judge their own scope of practice?
2. Why are nurses well-placed to coordinate patients' care, and what challenges might they face communicating and taking action within an interprofessional team?
3. Nurse practitioners in hospitals generally enjoy good working relationships with the doctors they work with, yet at a policy level the medical profession seeks to exclude them from working independently in primary care. Can you explain the difference between these two positions?
4. Why does using a high proportion of unlicensed health workers have a negative impact on the quality of patient/resident care and on the job satisfaction of nurses?
5. Carol Bacchi (2012, 2016) has developed six questions we can use to ask what is the 'real' problem (see Chapter 1). Using her framework, analyse the problem of funding aged care as social care only or clinical care only. How can we rethink this 'problem'?

REFERENCES

Abbott, A. 1988. The system of the professions: an essay on the expert division of labor. University of Chicago Press, Chicago.

Adelson, P., Fish, J., Peters, M., 2021. COVID-19 and workforce wellbeing: A survey of the Australian nursing, midwifery, and care worker workforce. A report prepared for the Australian Nursing and Midwifery Federation., University of South Australia, Adelaide.

Ahpra, 2015. Registration standard: criminal history. https://www.nursingmidwiferyboard.gov.au/Registration-Standards/Criminal-history.aspx.

Ahpra, 2018. Glossary, Australian Health Practitioner Regulation Agency.

Ahpra, 2022a. Legislation, Australian Health Practitioner Regulation Agency. https://www.ahpra.gov.au/about-ahpra/what-we-do/legislation.aspx.

Ahpra, 2022b. Who we are, Australian Health Practitioner Regulation Agency. https://www.ahpra.gov.au/about-ahpra/who-we-are.aspx.

Australian Institute of Health and Welfare (AIHW), 2018. Survey of Health Care: selected findings for rural and remote Australians. AIHW, Canberra. https://www.aihw.gov.au/reports/rural-remote-australians/survey-health-care-selected-findings-rural-remote/contents/summary.

Aiken, L.H., Sermeus, W., Van den Heede, K., et al., 2012. 'Patient safety, satisfaction, and quality of hospital care: cross sectional surveys of nurses and patients in 12 countries in Europe and the United State. BMJ (Clinical Research Ed.) 344, e1717-e.

Allen, D., 2014, The Invisible Work of Nurses: Hospitals, Organisation and Healthcare. Routledge, Abingdon.

Australian Medical Association (AMA), 2010. Collaborative Arrangements: What You Need to Know. AMA, Canberra.

Bacchi, C., 2012. Introducing the 'What's the problem represented to be?' approach. In: Bletsas, A., Beasley, C. (Eds.), Engaging With Carol Bacchi: Strategic Interventions and Exchanges. University of Adelaide Press, Adelaide, pp. 21–24. https://www.adelaide.edu.au/carst/docs/wpr/wpr-summary.pdf.

Bacchi, C., 2016. Problematizations in health policy: questioning how "problems" are constituted in policies. Paper presented at the ASSA (Academy of the Social Sciences)-funded Workshop on Understanding Australian Policies on Public Health, Flinders University.

Buchan, J., Catton, H., Shaffer, F.A., 2022. Sustain and Retain in 2022 and Beyond. The Global Nursing Workforce and the COVID-19 Pandemic. Internation Council of Nurses & International Centre on Nurse Migration.

Davies, C., 1996. The sociology of professions and the profession of gender. Sociology 30 (4), 661–78.

Department of Health and Aged Care, 2021a. About nurses and midwives. Australian Government, Canberra.

Department of Health and Aged Care 2021b, 2020. Aged Care Workforce Census. Australian Government, Canberra. https://www.health.gov.au/topics/nurses-and-midwives/about.

Department of Health and Aged Care, 2021c. Modified Monash Model. Australian Government, Canberra. https://www.health.gov.au/health-topics/rural-health-workforce/classifications/mmm.

Department of Health and Aged Care, 2022. Residential aged care funding reform. Australian Government, Canberra. https://www.health.gov.au/topics/aged-care/aged-care-reforms-and-reviews/residential-aged-care-funding-reform.

Djukic, M., Kovner, C.T., 2010. Overlap of registered nurse and physician practice: implications for U.S. Health Care Reform. Policy Polit Nurs Pract 11 (1), 13–22.

Doleman, G., Duffield, C., Li, I.W., et al., 2022. Employment of the Australian graduate nursing workforce: A retrospective analysis. Collegian 29 (2), 229–35.

Dougherty, L., Lamb, J., 2009. Intravenous Therapy in Nursing Practice. John Wiley & Sons.

Dower, C., Moore, J., Langelier, M., 2013. It is time to restructure health professions' scope-of-practice regulations to remove barriers to care. Health Affairs 32 (11), 1971–6.

Duffield, C., Chapman, S., Rowbotham, S., et al., 2017. Nurse-performed endoscopy: implications for the nursing profession in Australia. Policy Polit Nurs Pract 18 (1), 36–43.

Duffield, C., Roche, M.A., Wise, S., et al., 2020. Harnessing ward-level administrative data and expert knowledge to improve staffing decisions: A multi-method case study. J Adv Nurs 76 (1), 287–96.

Duffield, C., Twigg, D., Roche, M., et al., 2019. Uncovering the disconnect between nursing workforce policy intentions, implementation, and outcomes: lessons learned from the addition of a nursing assistant role. Policy Polit Nurs Pract 20 (4), 228–38.

Eagar, K., Westera, A., Snoek, M., et al., 2019. How Australian residential aged-care staffing levels compare with international and national benchmarks. Centre for Health Service Development, Australian Health Services Research Institute, University of Wollongong, Canberra.

Ecker, S., Joshi, R., Shanthosh, J., et al., 2020. Non-medical prescribing policies: a global scoping review., Health Policy 124 (7), 721–6.

Freidson, E., 2001. Professionalism. The Third Logic. University of Chicago Press, Chicago.

Harvey, C., 2011. Legislative hegemony and nurse practitioner practice in rural and remote Australia. Health Sociol Rev 20 (3), 269–80.

Hughes, E.C., MacGill Hughes, H., Deutscher, I., 1958. Twenty Thousand Nurses Tell Their Story. J.B. Lippincott Company, Philadelphia.

International Council of Nurses, 2022. Nursing definitions. https://www.icn.ch/nursing-policy/nursing-definitions.

Jennings, N., Clifford, S., Fox, A.R., et al., 2015. The impact of nurse practitioner services on cost, quality of care, satisfaction and waiting times in the emergency department: a systematic review. Int J Nurs Stud 52 (1), 421–35.

Ladd, E., Schober, M., 2018. Nurse prescribing from the global vantage point: the intersection between role and policy. Policy Polit Nurs Pract 19 (1–2), 40–9.

Larson, M.S., 1977. The Rise of Professionalism. A Sociological Analysis. University of California Press, Berkeley.

McHugh, M.D., Aiken, L.H., Sloane, D.M., 2021. Effects of nurse-to-patient ratio legislation on nurse staffing and patient mortality, readmissions, and length of stay: a prospective study in a panel of hospital. Lancet 397 (10288), 1905–13.

Middleton, R., 2006. Suturing as an advanced skill for Registered Nurses in the emergency department. Aust J Rural Health 14 (6), 258–62.

Moloney, W., Boxall, P., Parsons, M., et al., 2018. Factors predicting Registered Nurses' intentions to leave their organization and profession: a job demands-resources framework. J Adv Nurs 74 (4), 864–75.

National Skills Commission, 2021. The state of Australia's skills 2021: now and into the future. Australian Government, Canberra.

NHWD, 2020. National Health Workforce Dataset 2020. Australian Government, Canberra.

Nursing and Midwifery Board of Australia (NMBA), 2008. Code of Professional Conduct for Nurses in Australia. NMBA, Melbourne.

Nursing and Midwifery Board of Australia (NMBA), 2013. Scope of nursing practice decision making framework. NMBA, Melbourne.

Nursing and Midwifery Board of Australia (NMBA), 2016a. Registered Nurse Standards for Practice. NMBA, Melbourne.

Nursing and Midwifery Board of Australia (NMBA), 2016b. Registration Standard: Continuing Professional Development. NMBA, Melbourne. https://www.nursing-midwiferyboard.gov.au/Registration-Standards/Continuing-professional-development.aspx.

Nursing and Midwifery Board of Australia (NMBA), 2016c. Registration Standard: Professional Indemnity Insurance Arrangements. NMBA, Melbourne. https://www.nursingmidwiferyboard.gov.au/Registration-Standards/Professional-indemnity-insurance-arrangements.aspx.

Nursing and Midwifery Board of Australia (NMBA), 2018. Professional Standards. NMBA, Melbourne. https://www.nursingmidwiferyboard.gov.au/Codes-Guidelines-Statements/Professional-standards.aspx.

Nursing and Midwifery Board of Australia (NMBA), 2019. Nurses and Midwives 2019 Factsheet. NMBA, Melbourne.

Nursing and Midwifery Board of Australia (NMBA), 2020. Decision-making framework for nursing and midwifery. NMBA, Melbourne. https://www.nursingmidwiferyboard.gov.au/codes-guidelines-statements/frameworks.aspx.

Nursing and Midwifery Board of Australia (NMBA), 2021. Registrant data. Reporting period: 1 July 2021 to 30 September 2021. NMBA, Melbourne.

OECD, 2020. Nursing graduate. Organization for Economic Development. https://www.oecd-ilibrary.org/content/data/c54611e3-en.

Royal Commission into Aged Care Quality and Safety, 2020. Aged care and COVID-19: a special report, O/N H-985234. Commonwealth of Australia, Canberra.

Scanlon, A., Cashin, A., Bryce, J., et al., 2016. The complexities of defining nurse practitioner scope of practice in the Australian context. Collegian 23 (1), 129–42.

Scanlon, A., Murphy, M., Tori, K. et al., 2018. A national study of Australian Nurse Practitioners' organizational practice environment. J Nurse Pract 14 (5), 414–8.e3.

Schadewaldt, V., McInnes, E., Hiller, J.E. et al., 2016. Experiences of nurse practitioners and medical practitioners working in collaborative practice models in primary healthcare in Australia – a multiple case study using mixed method. BMC Family Practice 17 (1), 99.

Traczynski, J., Udalova, V., 2018. Nurse practitioner independence, health care utilization, and health outcome. Journal of Health Economics 58, 90–109.

Tuohy, C.J., 1999. Accidental Logics: The Dynamics of Change in the Health Care Arena in the United States, Britain, and Canada. OUP, New York.

Van den Heede, K., Cornelis, J., Bouckaert, N., et al., 2020. Safe nurse staffing policies for hospitals in England, Ireland, California, Victoria and Queensland: A discussion paper. Health Policy 124 (10), 1064–73.

World Health Organization (WHO), 2020. State of the world's nursing 2020: investing in education, jobs and leadership. World Health Organization, Geneva.

Wise, S., 2020. Staffing policy in aged care must look beyond the number. Aust Health Rev 44 (6), 829–30.

Wise, S., Duffield, C., Fry, M. et al., 2020. Clarifying workforce flexibility from a division of labor perspective: a mixed methods study of an emergency department team. Hum Resour Health 18 (1), 17.

Wise, S., Duffield, C., Fry, M.. et al., 2022. 'Nurse' role in accomplishing interprofessional coordination: lessons in 'almost managing' an emergency department team. J Nurs Manag 30 (1), 198–204.

FURTHER READING

Allen, D., 2007. What do you do at work? Profession building and doing nursing. Int Nurs Rev 2 54 (1), 41–48.

Chiarella, M., Currie, J., Wand, T., 2020. Liability and collaborative arrangements for nurse practitioner practice in Australia. Aust Health Rev 44 (2), 172–7.

Eagar, K., Westera, A., Kobel, C., 2020. Australian residential aged care is understaffed. Med J Aust, 212 (11), 507–508.e1.

Gardner, G., Duffield, C., Doubrovsky, A., et al., 2017. The structure of nursing: a national examination of titles and practice profiles. Int Nurs Rev 64 (2), 233–241.

Needleman, J., 2017. Nursing skill mix and patient outcome. BMJ Quality & Safety 26 (7), 525–8.

ONLINE RESOURCES

Australian College of Nursing: https://www.acn.edu.au/.

Nursing and Midwifery Board of Australia: https://www.nursingmidwiferyboard.gov.au/.

National Health Workforce Dataset: https://www.aihw.gov.au/about-our-data/our-data-collections/national-health-workforce-dataset.

24

Occupational Therapy

Sandra Mortimer and Ellice Willcourt

KEY LEARNING OUTCOMES

When you finish this chapter you should be able to:
- describe occupation and its relationship to health and well-being
- describe the scope and organisation of occupational therapy in Australia
- describe the application of occupational therapy across the life-span and in different contexts
- describe the range of roles that occupational therapists may undertake within the Australian health care system
- reflect on the likely impact of contemporary trends and health issues on the future profile of occupational therapy.

KEY TERMS AND ABBREVIATIONS

Alzheimer's disease
American Occupational Therapy Association (AOTA)
Australian Health Practitioner Regulation Agency (Ahpra)
client-centred practice
continuing professional development (CPD)

National Disability Insurance Scheme (NDIS)
occupation
occupational engagement
occupational justice
occupational therapist (OT)
Occupational Therapy Australia (OTA)

Occupational Therapy Board of Australia (OTBA)
speech pathologist (SP)
spinal cord injury
World Federation of Occupational Therapists (WFOT)

INTRODUCTION

This chapter will introduce the concepts and practice of occupational therapy in Australia. To be able to understand what occupational therapy is, you first need to understand the meaning of the term 'occupation'. This is what most clearly differentiates the **occupational therapist (OT)** from other members of an interprofessional health care team. The initial section of this chapter will discuss the concept of occupation. The second part will then outline how occupation is related to health and well-being and therefore applied as therapy, particularly in an Australian context.

OCCUPATION AND OCCUPATIONAL ENGAGEMENT

Occupation is defined as 'everyday personalized activities that people do as individuals, in families, and with communities to occupy time and bring meaning and purpose to life' (**American Occupational Therapy Association (AOTA)** 2020, p. 79). You can see by this definition that it is much broader than 'work', which is so often what people associate with occupation. Occupation in this context encompasses everything we want and need to do. What we do, and how and why we do these things, has a significant impact on our health and well-being.

Occupational therapy is about 'achieving health, well-being, and participation in life through engagement in occupation' (AOTA 2020, p. 5). Occupational therapy intervention focuses on supporting clients, who may be individuals, groups or populations, to engage in the occupations of everyday life that support them to live meaningful lives (AOTA 2020). It is important to keep in mind that what is 'meaningful' needs to be defined by the client. To do this, OTs need to be able to understand the barriers and facilitators to occupational engagement. **Occupational engagement** is the 'performance of occupations as the result of choice, motivation, and meaning within a supportive context and environment' (AOTA 2020, p. 5).

Occupational therapists use occupation as a therapeutic tool. The occupations that people choose to undertake often reflect and shape their current and future identity (Forsyth et al. 2019). Think about an occupation you enjoy and how you feel when you do it. Think about how that occupation reflects your sense of self and how this may have changed over time. Think back to living in lockdown as a response to the SARS-CoV-2 pandemic and all the ways your daily occupations were changed. Occupations are central to a person's sense of competence and have value and meaning to that individual (AOTA 2020). Engaging in occupations can influence mood, emotions, physical and cognitive capacities.

Pause *for* Reflection ...

Read the following and reflect on the influence of meaningful occupation.

Picture Maggie, a 76-year-old woman with **Alzheimer's disease** who has been living in a nursing home for 3 months following the death of her husband. She has become less and less responsive to her children, the staff and her surroundings. She sits day after day slumped over in her wheelchair.

The OT talks with Maggie's children to see what occupations have been important in her life, and discovers that Maggie used to love music and dancing. She danced as a young child right through to her 30s, and then was involved in teaching children. She loved musicals and was always singing, listening to music, working on routines and sewing costumes.

The OT suggests they bring in some examples of her former interests and start talking with Maggie

about this. The OT explains how we experience our occupations through a range of our senses and how this may help Maggie access her memories. Her children bring in photos, trophies, music, ballet costumes, Maggie's old sewing box and, becoming very creative, a pair of old, smelly tap shoes. They spread these around Maggie and gently talk to her about what they have found, showing her the items and allowing her to feel them and experience them. Slowly but surely, Maggie begins to respond and starts to talk about her dancing days as she handles the costumes and shoes. She shows interest in her environment, notices the photos and starts to smile. She then looks up at her daughter and smiles at her.

Occupational engagement is highly individualised. One person may categorise ironing as work, another as a domestic chore and yet another may find it relaxing and calming. When OTs work with clients, they identify and analyse the individual elements of each occupation and consider how these support or hinder occupational engagement, the impact this has on the client's health and well-being, and their ability to participate in life as they would wish to. They match this with their understanding of the client as a whole and the factors that may impact on that person's occupational choices. These factors may include the client's values, beliefs and spirituality, body functions and body structures. The final element that OTs consider is the environmental factors that influence occupational engagement. These include physical, social and attitudinal contexts (AOTA 2020). A consideration of culturally relevant occupations is particularly important. Context and environment influence how and when an occupation is carried out. As an example, think about the occupation of swimming. You could swim in many different environments such as the beach, a river, a public indoor pool, a private backyard pool. How might these different places influence the way you swim? An indoor pool can be used any time of the year regardless of the weather. Taking a swim with friends to cool down in summer in a backyard pool is very different to swimming laps for fitness in an indoor public pool.

Pause *for* Reflection ...

Consider how your understanding about occupation has changed since reading the above. Can you see how it encompasses much more than 'work'?

IMPACT OF OCCUPATION ON HEALTH AND WELL-BEING

As well as the definitions of health already considered in this book, occupational therapy considers health as a resource to allow people to engage in meaningful occupation.

Active engagement in meaningful occupation generally promotes and maintains health and well-being. There are cases, however, where active engagement in occupation can be harmful to health and well-being – for example, addictive occupations such as gambling. Another example is professional musicianship. The occupation of rehearsing and performing with a violin at a professional level requires the musician to hold certain parts of their body (trunk, neck, shoulders) in sustained and often awkward positions while other body parts (fingers, wrists) are engaged in fast and repetitive movements for long periods of time. The focus and concentration required to play at this level means that musicians often lose track of time. They enter a state of 'flow' which has been defined as a rare, focused state of consciousness (Csikszentmihalyi 1993). This is usually considered to be a health-enhancing state, but a study of professional musicians by Guptill (2012) drew attention to the negative effects that 'flow' can have on health. Even though these musicians experienced pain and physical injury as a result of their playing, many of them still reported an enhanced sense of well-being because the occupation was so valued, reflected their sense of identity and positively influenced their mood and emotional state (Guptill 2012). It is also important to consider that sometimes occupations that are more traditionally considered 'unhealthy' or illegal can still add meaning and purpose to someone's life (Kiepek et al. 2019). Some examples of these may be graffitiing, smoking or substance use. Occupational therapists consider that health is enhanced when people can participate in a range of occupations that match their needs, values, interests and capacities. These occupations form a pattern that supports occupational or life balance (Matuska & Barrett 2019), which in turn supports health and well-being. This highlights the importance of understanding an occupation and taking into consideration the person's perspective, particularly around the value or meaning of the occupation.

> **Pause *for* Reflection ...**
> Consider the range of occupations you engage in that hold meaning and value to you. What impact do these have on your health and well-being?

Supportive environments also play a crucial role in maximising participation, health and well-being. Occupational therapists consider the social determinants of health and understand that these influence opportunities to participate in occupations. This applies across all ages but can be highlighted when considering learning and development outcomes for young children. Children learn and develop from a context of safe and secure relationships and opportunities to engage in core occupations such as playing. When working with a child presenting with a developmental delay, an OT will strive to understand the broader social, cultural and environmental influences that may be impacting on this child and family, such as access to safe and secure environments, safety, adequate shelter and food, parental well-being and mental health and financial security. The OT will be mindful of these when planning therapeutic interventions (see Case study 24.1 later in the chapter as an example).

OCCUPATIONAL SCIENCE

Occupational science offers a knowledge base that supports occupational therapy practice with a focus on analysing and optimising knowledge about occupation (Wright-St Clair & Hocking 2019). It is important for OTs to understand people as occupational beings and to understand how occupation can influence a person's life both positively and negatively. As already discussed in this book, efficiency, effectiveness and equity are core drivers for health system performance, and in challenging economic environments there is increasing pressure from health services and other employers to apply evidence and demonstrate value.

OCCUPATIONAL JUSTICE

Occupational therapists also focus on the social justice agenda previously discussed in this book by considering human rights from an occupational perspective. The **World Federation of Occupational Therapists (WFOT)** *Position statement on human rights* (2019a) endorses the United Nations' (1948) *Universal declaration of human rights* and adds a perspective in relation to human occupation and participation that recognises people's rights to participate in meaningful occupations consistent with their culture, context and values. **Occupational justice** 'is concerned with enabling, mediating and advocating for environments in which all people's opportunities to engage in occupation are just, health-promoting and meaningful' (Hocking 2017, p. 33).

A model of occupational justice described by Townsend and Wilcock (2004) highlights the need to consider and protect people's different priorities, needs and capacities and how they are expressed through what they do. Occupational rights include the right to:

- participate in a range of occupations for health, development and social inclusion
- make choices and share decision-making in daily life
- experience meaning and enrichment in one's occupations
- receive fair privileges for diverse participation in occupations (Wilcock & Hocking 2015, p. 407).

This approach expands possible occupational therapy intervention from an individual clinical role to one of working with people, populations, and communities to advocate for and enact change at a policy or program level to address issues of occupational injustice. This is where an understanding of Bacchi's (2009) 'What's the problem represented to be' (WPR) approach to policy analysis can support occupational therapy practice. Core to this approach is the underlying assumption that a policy sets out to address a problem but that this presumed 'problem' is often implicit and unexamined (Bacchi 2009). Policies 'make a "problem" exist as a particular type of "problem"' (Bacchi 2009, p. 263). Unless we carefully examine how these problems are constructed, we risk missing key information, perspectives or considerations that may be shaping the 'solutions'. The WPR process provides the mechanism to do this by examining policies through a series of six questions, outlined in Chapter 1, that critically examine how problems are thought about and acted upon rather than accepting the problem as a given. Bacchi challenges us to move the focus from '"problem" solving to "problem" questioning' (Bacchi 2009, p. vii) to enable more nuanced considerations. There is emerging research applying the WPR model directly to clinical practices (Mortimer 2021) to support clinicians to critically reflect on their practices and the outcomes for their clients. Critical reflection enables OTs and other health professionals to consider the broader social and political structural factors that influence their practice (Bay et al. 2019). This can be a very helpful tool to support OTs working across all areas of practice but especially with an occupational justice lens.

Occupational deprivation is one outcome of occupational injustice and is defined as 'a state of prolonged preclusion from engagement in occupations of necessity and/or meaning due to factors which stand outside of the control of the individual' (Whiteford 2000, p. 305). Alex's situation as described in the following *Pause for reflection* is an example of occupational deprivation.

Pause *for* Reflection ...

Alex is a 28-year-old man who has experienced significant mental health concerns over the past seven years which affect his motivation and concentration. He has been receiving medication through his general practitioner but needs allied health assistance to help him meet his goals. He currently lives at home with his parents but would like to move out of home and find employment. He is entitled to OT services through the **National Disability Insurance Scheme (NDIS)**, however, he has been waiting for 8 months for his funding to be approved. In the meantime, he sits at home, smoking cigarettes and watching television. Imagine how Alex's daily life and the occupations he wants and needs to do are affected by these circumstances. How does this impact on his occupational rights?

- This is an example of occupational injustice. In this case, access to occupational therapy services is impacted by long wait times. AOTA is very aware of these challenges and has been actively involved in advocating for access to OTs within mental health and, more broadly, raising practice issues with the NDIS. See current issues on the **Occupational Therapy Australia (OTA)** website: https://otaus.com.au/media-and-advocacy/current-issues.
- Consider how application of Bacchi's six questions could support understanding of the factors influencing Alex's care and outcomes.

OCCUPATION AS THERAPY

The use of occupation as therapy has been recorded since ancient times, with noted Greek and Roman physicians such as Hippocrates and Celsus advocating their use. A more organised form of occupational therapy emerged around 200 years ago within large mental asylums. People with mental illnesses were managed by being sent to asylums and essentially incarcerated, often with the use of shackles or other restraints. Key European physicians including Philippe Pinel (often referred to as the 'father of modern psychiatry') transformed

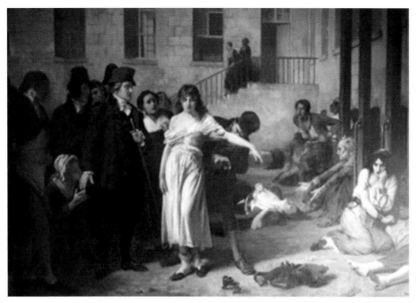

Figure 24.1 Pinel A La Salpêtrière By T. Robert-Fleury, 1896 *Source*: Public domain.

these large asylums by removing inmates' chains and providing them with a daily structure that involved regular occupations including physical exercise, work, music, reading and farming. This change was evocatively captured by French painter Robert-Fleury in 1896 (Fig. 24.1).

From the late 1800s, occupation began to be used more in deliberately therapeutic ways, individualised to each patient and conceptualised scientifically within contemporary journals. Like many other allied health professions, however, the first formal occupational therapy educational programs emerged around World War I, with large numbers of war-wounded personnel requiring rehabilitation. From that point on, occupational therapy began to expand to focus increasingly on aspects such as physical recovery and function using occupation in addition to mental health. World War II saw the development of the first Australian occupational therapy educational program in Sydney in 1942 (Bearup 1996).

HOW OCCUPATIONAL THERAPY IS ORGANISED IN AUSTRALIA

Educational programs for occupational therapy are at Bachelor's or Master's degree level in Australia. Some

countries, such as the USA, now require a Master's or a Doctoral degree as a minimum qualification for practice. Programs in Australia need to be accredited by the Occupational Therapy Council to ensure graduates have the knowledge, skills and attributes required to practise (Occupational Therapy Council 2018). OT programs are required to ensure graduates meet the required competency standards for OT practice (Occupational Therapy Board of Australia 2018). An essential part of this accreditation is the requirement that occupational therapy students must have a minimum of 1000 hours of fieldwork practice in their course.

Occupational therapy is a registered profession, so to be able to practise as, and call yourself, an OT you must be registered with the **Australian Health Practitioner Regulation Agency (Ahpra)**. The **Occupational Therapy Board of Australia (OTBA)** works under the auspices of Ahpra to set standards, regulate therapists and manage complaints against therapists. In December 2021, there were 27,666 registered OTs in Australia (Ahpra 2022). Occupational therapy students are also registered by Ahpra and have similar requirements to other therapists around aspects such as health (i.e. fitness to practise) and character (in particular, criminal history). One of the key registration requirements for

OTs is the need to demonstrate the completion of **continuing professional development (CPD)** activities to renew their registration annually. OTBA requires OTs to complete at least 20 hours of targeted education each year (OTBA 2021). Many people may consider that when they graduate with a university degree, they would have covered what there is to know about their professional area. However, as outlined in Chapter 1, patient safety and quality in health care have become increasingly important public issues. Health professionals need to continue to develop their knowledge and skills to ensure client safety and best practice; the CPD requirements are an example of how this need has been translated into the *Health Practitioner Regulation National Law*. Another example of ensuring public safety is the requirement for qualified OTs to continue to meet the competency standards throughout their careers. These competency standards focus on four conceptual areas of occupational therapy practice: professionalism, knowledge and learning, occupational therapy process and practice, and communication. Each of these is supported by practice behaviours which address specific core competencies (OTBA 2018).

In addition to the registration authority in Australia, OTs also have a professional association, Occupational Therapy Australia (OTA), which operates to promote occupational therapy and support members. Professional associations are organised and operated by members of the profession and are therefore different to the legal authority of the registration boards. OTA is the peak professional body representing the interests of OTs and advocating for the profession. It is also a major provider of CPD, including national and state conferences. The association has an official journal, the *Australian Occupational Therapy Journal*, which is one of the key internationally recognised journals in the profession. OTA also provides practical support to members, such as a mentoring program for new therapists and access to professional indemnity insurance (OTA 2022).

WFOT is the key international body for occupational therapy and sets minimum standards for occupational therapy educational programs which are used as part of course accreditation in Australia. WFOT enables consistent standards for OTs across the world. The federation is recognised by the United Nations and regularly collaborates with other key international bodies such as the World Health Organization (WHO) in key projects around occupation and well-being (WFOT 2019b).

OCCUPATIONAL THERAPY PRACTICE IN AUSTRALIA

Occupational therapists in Australia work with people across all age groups, from newborn babies to those very senior in years. Most OTs (89%) work as clinicians. Other roles include administration, education, research and project work (Department of Health 2020). OTs work across many settings, including hospitals, community health services, private practices, rehabilitation centres, schools, aged-care facilities and people's homes or workplaces. In 2019 the most common area of practice was paediatrics, followed by rehabilitation and then aged care with more that 75% employed within metropolitan areas (Department of Health 2020). In response to the SARS-CoV-2 pandemic, OTs have adapted their practice models to provide more telehealth services. Telehealth enables OTs to offer services to people who are experiencing access issues due to factors such as illness, social isolation or location.

Occupational therapists frequently work with individuals, but may also work with groups of people or with organisations to enhance their occupational engagement. As an example of working with all of these, an OT may provide a service for an *organisation*, such as an industrial workplace, providing *education groups for workers* around body mechanics with the aim of reducing manual-handling injuries. The people that OTs work with may be called by various terms relevant to their setting, such as 'student', 'worker', 'patient' or 'consumer', but typically OTs identify those they work with as *clients* (AOTA 2020). The term 'client' raises a central aspect for OTs: **client-centred practice**. At the heart of occupational therapy is the collaboration between the client and the therapist in setting goals that are meaningful and relevant to the client (Schell et al. 2019). This requires excellent communication skills (Taylor 2020). WFOT (2012, para 1) describes occupational therapy as 'a client-centred health profession concerned with promoting health and well-being through occupation. The primary goal of occupational therapy is to enable people to participate in the activities of everyday life'. The three areas that OTs focus on to achieve this goal include aspects of the *person*, the *occupation* and the *environment*, and occupational therapy intervention is built around these aspects.

This focus has meant that occupational therapists are well placed to respond to the daily living challenges related to living with SARS-CoV-2. SARS-CoV-2 continues to cause disruption to daily life, impacting on people being able to engage in their everyday occupations (Mynard 2020). Consider all the ways your occupations have been disrupted through the SARS-CoV-2 pandemic. How has this impacted on you, your occupations and environment? You may have felt socially isolated or lacking in motivation. Your eating habits may have changed, and you may have lost or gained weight. You may not have been able to do the things that mattered to you such as going to work or seeing your family and friends. You may not have been able to access essential services such as supermarkets, gyms or your general practitioner. This may have impacted on your physical or mental health and sense of well-being. OTs have supported their clients to adapt to these changes and have changed the way they deliver service (e.g. telehealth). This has been enabled by changes to funding and service delivery models.

As a further example of how OTs consider the person, occupation and environment, consider Tom, who sustained a **spinal cord injury** following a car accident. The OT assesses *personal factors* that are impacting on his occupational engagement. In this case, the injury has fully severed the connections between Tom's brain and spinal cord, meaning that there is a total loss of sensation in his legs and lower trunk and he is unable to move his lower limbs. One of Tom's key goals is to regain mobility. The OT works with Tom to strengthen his upper limbs to compensate for the loss of lower-limb function, so that he can transfer from chairs and beds using his arms instead. Strengthening his upper limbs also prepares Tom for using a wheelchair to mobilise.

Using a wheelchair is an example of how an OT may modify an *occupation* to enable engagement in daily life tasks. The OT carefully measures Tom for a wheelchair, taking into account his specific interests and lifestyle. For example, does the wheelchair need to be lightweight and able to be dismantled easily to go into a car? Given Tom's lack of sensation, he is at risk of skin breakdown. To address this the OT needs to provide appropriate pressure-relieving cushions as part of the wheelchair provision, and will also teach Tom routine movements to ensure that the blood flow to the areas he is sitting on is maintained.

The OT also considers the *environment* in which each occupation will be taking place:
- What are Tom's home and workplace like?
- Is access possible or are modifications to the environment needed, such as ramps at entrances?

This example shows a range of interventions that an OT may use when considering the person, occupation and environment, and their interaction. Now that Tom can mobilise, the OT can work with him to support occupational engagement in his priority areas of work, study and socialising.

The number of OTs has grown substantially over the last decade. OTBA (2022) data confirm the number of registered OTs increased by 43% from 2013 to 2021. Historically, OTs in Australia have been mainly employed by government or non-government agencies. However, with the introduction of the NDIS, more OTs are working in private practice. Key private-practice areas include working with children, work injury prevention and management, mental health, home modifications, driver assessment, hand therapy, rehabilitation and disability. The increase in private practice reflects the changes to funding streams. As outlined in Chapter 1, Tuohy (1999) points out that the health reform agenda continues to shape the mix of private versus public provision of health care. For example, prior to the implementation of the NDIS, disability providers were mostly block-funded with government funding being given to key agencies to provide set services. Under the NDIS, funding is individualised and goal-based (see Chapter 12).

Increasing delivery of services through programs like the NDIS potentially offers clients more choice in health practitioners. However, it may also lead to more fragmented care. OTs frequently work with other health professionals in an interdisciplinary team, as outlined in Chapter 1. Private practice can potentially make this harder and requires considerable effort by practitioners to ensure that intervention is coordinated for their clients. Case study 24.1 highlights the role of occupational therapy and how interdisciplinary practice is important in meeting the needs of clients.

CASE STUDY 24.1 Providing Occupational Therapy in an Interdisciplinary Context

Jacob is 2 years old and has been referred to an early childhood development team by his mother, Ruth, because he is not yet talking. Ruth and Jacob meet with two members of the interdisciplinary team, an OT and a **speech pathologist (SP)**. After a brief time where they play together, getting comfortable in the play space, the role of the service and the purpose of this initial meeting are explained.

The OT talks with Ruth and takes an in-depth developmental, medical and occupational history of Jacob and his family. She gains a sense of what has happened in this boy's life to date, and how this might be impacting on his learning and development. She establishes a relationship with Ruth that honours and respects Ruth's role as the expert in Jacob's life, and begins to build a therapeutic partnership that will underpin future interventions. She also gains a sense of the environments in which Jacob interacts (home, child care, etc.) and how these may influence his development. The questions she asks help to establish a sense of how considerations of safety, employment and financial security, nutrition, physical activity and sleep may be influencing health and well-being for this boy and his family. She also gains a sense of how Ruth is feeling and what support or challenges she has in her role as his mother and in any other key roles she plays.

During this time, the SP plays with Jacob and gains a sense of his capacities and challenges. The OT and SP then swap over and the SP develops her connection with Ruth, explaining what she has noticed about Jacob's play and communication and checking whether this is typical for him. She then asks specific questions about Jacob's speech and language development while the OT interacts with Jacob and gains a sense of his fine and gross motor skills, play styles and preferences, and sensory responses.

Once the initial information is gathered, the OT and SP discuss with Ruth their observations and any recommendations that could be put into action straight away, and together develop a therapy plan. Following the session, the SP and OT write a summary which captures the family's circumstances as well as their combined assessment of Jacob's speech and language skills, fine and gross motor skills, concentration and attention, sensory responses, play styles and skills, and how he responds to his mother, the therapists and the therapy environment. This information is discussed at the weekly interdisciplinary team meeting, which includes the OT, SP, child psychologist, social worker, physiotherapist and dietitian. Jacob and his family's needs are prioritised and a service plan is agreed on. A copy of this is sent to Ruth.

Case Study Questions

1. What are the advantages for Ruth and Jacob of this interdisciplinary approach?
2. Why is it important to consider the client's goals when developing a therapy plan?
3. How does this interdisciplinary approach strengthen the occupational therapy approach and reduce costs and waiting times for occupational therapy specifically and the health service as a whole?
4. What might be some challenges of working in an interdisciplinary team?

▍SUMMARY

This chapter has provided information on the occupational therapy profession, including an in-depth understanding of occupation and how its therapeutic use underpins occupational therapy. In particular:

- Occupations are activities that hold meaning and value for people. Occupation influences people's health and well-being and shapes identity.
- Occupational science is the study of human occupation and all its complexity.
- Occupational justice considers issues of rights, equity and justice from an occupational point of view, and contributes another perspective to contemporary local and global health issues.
- Occupational therapy has developed from its early days in large mental health asylums to a progressive profession working across many sectors and undertaking many roles.

- Educational programs within Australia are at Bachelor's or Master's degree level.
- Occupational therapy is a registered profession under Ahpra, and therapists are required to undertake regular continuing professional development.
- OTA operates as the peak body representing occupational therapists across the country.
- OTs work in a client-centred framework, and specifically consider aspects of the person, the occupation and the environment in their assessment and therapy.
- The number of occupational therapy positions has grown considerably over the past decade. Therapists are increasingly finding employment in private practice, mainly because of different funding streams becoming available.

REVIEW QUESTIONS

1. Define 'occupation' and describe how it influences health and well-being.
2. Explain how occupational science relates to occupational therapy.
3. Why do registration boards, and many professional associations, require health professionals to provide evidence of continuing professional development?
4. Where do occupational therapists generally work, and how is this changing? What are the factors that

are driving this? Apply Bacchi's analysis discussed in Chapter 1 and work through the six questions when considering how the NDIA policy is impacting on the delivery of health care services.

5. Consider Tom from the example earlier and the way OT services may change based on current COVID-19 restrictions.

REFERENCES

Australian Health Practitioner Registration Authority, 2022. Annual report 2021/22. https://www.ahpra.gov.au/Publications/Annual-reports/Annual-Report-2022.aspx.

American Occupational Therapy Association, 2020. Occupational therapy practice framework: domain and process, fourth ed. Am J Occup Ther, 7 4(Suppl. 2). https://doi.org/10.5014/ajot.2020.74S2001.

Bacchi, C., 2009. Analysing Policy: What's the Problem Represented To Be? Pearson, Australia.

Bay, U., Haynes, A., Western, D., 2019. Thinking what we do: reflexively testing post-structural theoretical concepts with social work practitioners and fieldwork educators. Soc Work Edu 38 (7), pp. 1–13. https://doi.org/10.1080/02615479.2019.1586868.

Bearup, C,. 1996. Occupational Therapists in Wartime. Australian Association of Occupational Therapists, Adelaide.

Csikszentmihalyi, M., 1993. Activity and happiness: toward a science of occupation. J Occup Sci 1 (1), 38–42.

Department of Health, 2020. Occupational therapists. Department of Health, Canberra. https://hwd.health.gov.au/resources/publications/factsheet-alld-occupational-therapists-2019.pdf

Forsyth, K., Taylor, R.R., Kramer, J.M., et al., 2019. The model of human occupation. In: Schell B.A.B., Gillen, G. (Eds), Willard and Spackman's Occupational Therapy, thirteenth ed. Wolters Kluwer, Philadelphia, pp. 601–621.

Guptill, C., 2012. Injured professional musicians and the complex relationship between occupation and health. J Occup Sci 19 (3), 258–270.

Hocking, C., 2017. Occupational justice as social justice: the moral claim for inclusion. J Occup Sci 24 (1), 29–42. doi:10.1080/14427591.2017.1294016.

Kiepek, N.C., Beagan, B., Rudman, D.L., et al., 2019. Silences around occupations framed as unhealthy, illegal, and deviant. J Occup Sci 26 (3), 341–353.

Matuska, K., Barrett, K., 2019. Patterns of occupation. In: Schell B.A.B., Gillen, G. (Eds), Willard and Spackman's Occupational Therapy, thirteenth ed. Wolters Kluwer, Philadelphia, pp. 212–222.

Mortimer, S., 2021. Examining health care practices for young children with complex feeding difficulties and their families: What's the problem represented to be? DPH thesis, Flinders University, College of Medicine and Public Health. https://theses.flinders.edu.au/view/53743409-a03b-4b48-bfc4-705e9f5a2e44/1

Mynard, L., 2020. The new normal: navigating everyday life during COVID-19. Occupational Therapy Australia. https://otaus.com.au/publicassets/97c2319e-0bc0-ea11-9434-005056be13b5/The%20New%20Normal_ebook_Final.pdf

Occupational Therapy Australia, 2022. About the association. https://www.otaus.com.au/about/about-ota.

Occupational Therapy Board of Australia, 2021. Continuing professional development. https://www.occupationaltherapyboard.gov.au/Registration-Standards/Continuing-professional-development.aspx

Occupational Therapy Board of Australia, 2022. Statistics. https://www.occupationaltherapyboard.gov.au/About/Statistics.aspx

Occupational Therapy Board of Australia, 2018. Australian occupational therapy competency standards 2018. https://www.occupationaltherapyboard.gov.au/codes-guidelines/competencies.aspx.

Occupational Therapy Council of Australia, 2018. Accreditation standards for Australian entry-level occupational therapy education programs. https://www.occupationaltherapyboard.gov.au/Accreditation.aspx.

Schell, B., Gillen, G., Coppola, S., 2019. Contemporary occupational therapy practice. In: Schell, B.A.B., Gillen, G. (Eds), Willard and Spackman's Occupational Therapy, thirteenth ed. Wolters Kluwer, Philadelphia, pp. 56–70.

Taylor, R.R., 2020. The intentional relationship: occupational therapy and use of self, second ed. F.A. Davis, Philadelphia.

Townsend, E, Wilcock, A.A., 2004. Occupational justice and client centred practice: a dialogue in progress. Can J Occup Ther 71 (2), 75–87.

Tuohy, C., 1999. Accidental Logics: the Dynamics of Change in the Health Care Arena in United States, Britain and Canada. OUP, New York.

United Nations (UN), 1948. Universal declaration of human rights. UN, Geneva. https://www.un.org/en/universal-declaration-human-rights/index.html.

Whiteford, G., 2000. Occupational deprivation: global challenge in the new millennium. Br J Occup Ther 63 (5), 200–204.

Wilcock, A.A., Hocking, C., 2015. An occupational perspective on health, third ed. SLACK Incorporated, Thorofare NJ.

World Federation of Occupational Therapists, 2012. Definition of occupational therapy, https://wfot.org/about/about-occupational-therapy.

World Federation of Occupational Therapists, 2019a. Position statement on human rights. https://wfot.org/resources/occupational-therapy-and-human-rights.

World Federation of Occupational Therapists, 2019b. Partners. https://www.wfot.org/about/partners.

Wright-St Clair, V., Hocking, C., 2019. Occupational science: The study of occupation. In: Schell B.A.B., Gillen, G. (Eds), Willard and Spackman's Occupational Therapy, thirteenth ed. Wolters Kluwer, Philadelphia, pp. 124–139.

Brown, T., Bourke-Taylor, H., Isbel, S., et al., 2021. Occupational Therapy in Australia: Professional and Practice Issues, second ed. Allen & Unwin, Sydney.

Burnett, S., 2018. Personal and social contexts of disability: implications for occupational therapists. In: Pendleton, H., Schultz-Krohn, W. (Eds), Pedretti's Occupational Therapy: Practice Skills for Physical Dysfunction, eighth ed. Elsevier Mosby, Missouri, pp. 71–91.

FURTHER READING

American Occupational Therapy Association, 2020. Occupational therapy practice framework: domain and process, fourth ed. Am J Occup Ther 74 (Suppl. 2), 7412510010. https://doi.org/10.5014/ajot.2020.74S2001.

ONLINE RESOURCES

Occupational Therapy Australia – the peak body representing occupational therapists in Australia – includes information for students to learn more about the profession: https://www.otaus.com.au.

Mynard, L., 2020. The new normal: navigating everyday life during COVID-19. Occupational Therapy Australia. https://otaus.com.au/publicassets/97c2319e-0bc0-ea11-9434-005056be13b5/The%20New%20Normal_ebook_Final.pdf.

Occupational Therapy Board of Australia – the regulatory board for occupational therapy in Australia has statistics on registered therapists, plus the guidelines and standards that are required to be met: https://www.occupationaltherapyboard.gov.au.

World Federation of Occupational Therapists – information about occupational therapy internationally: https://www.wfot.org.

25

Paramedicine and the Health Care System

Alan Morrison and Louise Reynolds

KEY LEARNING OUTCOMES

When you finish this chapter you should be able to:
- describe how the introduction of the National Registration and Accreditation Scheme regulates paramedicine practice
- discuss the nature of the work of paramedics including workload, funding and skills
- evaluate the impact of the SARS-CoV-2 pandemic on out-of-hospital care delivery in meeting service user demands and community expectations.

KEY TERMS AND ABBREVIATIONS

ambulance services
Australian Health Practitioner
　Regulation Agency (Ahpra)
community paramedicine
emergency department (ED)

extended care paramedic (ECP)
intensive care paramedic (ICP)
National Registration and
　Accreditation Scheme
　(NRAS)

Paramedicine Board of Australia
　(PBA)
protected title
ramping
surge workforce

INTRODUCTION

In this chapter we will describe the inclusion of paramedics as part of the National Registration and Accreditation Scheme (NRAS) as the 15th health professional group. As of 1 December 2018, 'paramedic' is a protected title, which means that only those who are registered with the Paramedicine Board of Australia can identify themselves as a paramedic. Registered paramedics are required to meet the standards, codes and guidelines set by the Board.

Paramedicine practice continues to evolve with an increasing body of research evidence that defines the nature of the work and its impact on health outcomes. Paramedics have been on the frontline during the SARS-CoV-2 pandemic, providing both urgent and primary out-of-hospital care. This has seen an enhanced recognition of paramedicine as an important contributor to the health system and patient outcomes that will endure post the pandemic.

TRANSITION TO NEW AND EMERGING ROLES – THE NATIONAL REGISTRATION AND ACCREDITATION SCHEME

What is Paramedic Regulation?
The **National Registration and Accreditation Scheme** (**NRAS**) commenced in Australia in 2010 with the establishment of 10 national boards, with a further four professional boards added in 2012 (Bennett et al. 2018). The primary purpose of the NRAS is to protect the health and safety of the public by making sure 'that only

registered health practitioners who are suitably trained and qualified to practise in a competent and ethical manner are registered' (**Australian Health Practitioner Regulation Agency (Ahpra)** 2022). The NRAS ensures that all regulated health professionals are registered against consistent, high-quality, national professional standards and can practise across state and territory borders without having to re-register in each jurisdiction. The addition of paramedics to the NRAS has its basis in these objectives.

The addition of paramedicine as the 15th profession to the NRAS began following a 2015 agreement by the Council of Australian Governments Health Council (federal, state and territory health ministers) to move towards paramedic registration. A subsequent federal parliamentary Senate Committee report recommended the addition of paramedicine to the NRAS citing the complexity of paramedic practice, alignment with other professions included in the NRAS and the 'desirability of nationally consistent professional standards for paramedics' (Commonwealth of Australia 2016; Bennett et al. 2018). The Health Council took the decision to include paramedicine in the NRAS on the 7 October 2016 (Commonwealth of Australia 2017).

The **Paramedicine Board of Australia (PBA)** was appointed on 19 October 2017 and commenced work with Ahpra to facilitate the regulation of paramedicine. The stated functions of the Paramedicine Board, consistent with the objective and principles of the NRAS, are:

- registering paramedics and students
- developing standards, codes and guidelines for the paramedic profession
- handling notifications, complaints, investigations and disciplinary hearings
- assessing overseas-trained practitioners who wish to practise in Australia; and
- approving accreditation standards and accredited programs of study.

(Paramedicine Board of Australia 2022a)

Paramedicine commenced participation in the NRAS on 1 December 2018 following the passing of the *Health Practitioner Regulation National Law and Other Legislation Amendment Bill 2017* (the National Law) in all Australian states. From that date, 'paramedic' was a **protected title** under the National Law and anyone wanting to be identified as a paramedic needed to meet the standards, codes and guidelines set down by the PBA.

Responsibilities of Regulated Paramedics

So, what does this mean for paramedics and their practice? Paramedicine's addition to the NRAS may be considered by some as due recognition of paramedicine's status as a health profession and its contribution to the effectiveness of the health care system in the provision of care to the community (Paramedics Australasia 2011). Whilst this perspective may be valid as an incidental outcome, it risks minimising the primary objective of health practitioner regulation, that is, the protection of the health and safety of the public, as opposed to promoting the interests or status of a profession.

There is, however, a relationship between professionalism and regulation that places a priority on public safety and impacts on one's practice as a registered health practitioner. Townsend and Luck (2019) identify that the National Law contains 'principles and objectives that are consistent with the notion of professionalism' (p. 3) and in that context the necessity of putting the patient's interests first. As registered health professionals, paramedics have a personal responsibility to make the well-being and needs of their patient their first concern, practising safely and competency whilst delivering care within an ethical framework (Paramedicine Board of Australia 2018, p. 5). This personal responsibility extends to 'maintaining a high level of professional competence and conduct' (Paramedicine Board of Australia 2018, p. 5). Whilst historical employer–employee governance requirements remain applicable for paramedics within their employment relationship, regulation within the NRAS represents an additional layer of personal regulatory responsibility directed towards the public good (Townsend & Luck 2019). For a more detailed discussion about this relationship see Townsend and Luck (2019).

The Paramedicine Board of Australia has made these regulatory responsibilities explicit through the publication of Registration Standards, the Code of Conduct and the Professional Capabilities for Registered Paramedics. They give guidance to paramedics on professional practice in the context of pursuing public safety. Registration standards describe what is required to gain and maintain registration. The Code of Conduct provides guidance on how to practise effectively within an ethical framework. The Professional Capabilities describe the generic 'knowledge, skills and professional attributes needed for safe and competent practice of paramedicine in Australia' (Paramedicine Board of Australia 2021, p. 2). The legal right to claim the protected title 'paramedic' is based on attaining registration with the Paramedicine Board and maintaining an ongoing, demonstrated commitment to upholding these standards. It is important that paramedics have a working understanding of these documents and apply them to their clinical practice.

Professional Identity

Understanding these intersecting regulatory and professional responsibilities goes to the heart of what it means to be a paramedic. How paramedics view themselves can influence their approach to practice impacting on patients and themselves. In further defining paramedicine, a recent four-stage Delphi process by Williams et al. (2021) involved a panel of Australian and international experts who developed this broad definition of paramedicine as currently practised:

> Paramedicine is a domain of practice and health profession that specialises across a range of settings including, but not limited to, emergency and primary care. Paramedics work in a variety of clinical settings such as emergency medical services, **ambulance services**, hospitals and clinics as well as non-clinical roles, such as education, leadership, public health and research. Paramedics possess complex knowledge and skills, a broad scope of practice and are an essential part of the healthcare system. Depending on location, paramedics may practice under medical direction or independently, often in unscheduled, unpredictable or dynamic settings.
>
> **(Williams et al. 2021, p. 3568)**

Pause *for* Reflection ...

How accurate does the Williams et al. (2021) definition reflect Australasian paramedicine practice? Is it practical or beneficial to have a universal definition which encompasses all the variations in practice? Why or why not?

The changing nature and complexity of paramedic work has already been identified as a key driver for the inclusion of paramedicine in the NRAS. Paramedics working in traditional state jurisdictional ambulance services encounter an increasing case load extending beyond just emergency presentations. McManamny et al. (2021) highlight research indicating a greater role for paramedics in providing health care, which can

occur in and outside of the traditional ambulance services. This reflects changing community perceptions of paramedics and the care they provide through ambulance services (Eaton et al. 2021).

In continuing the discussion of identity, Furness et al. (2021, p. 135) derived six archetypes from the literature representing common perceptions of paramedics, however they recognise it is unclear which ones still currently inform identity and which don't. Furness et al. (2021) advocate further exploration of what it means to be a paramedic with paramedics themselves to enhance their evolving understanding of practice and positively impacting undergraduate education, practice frameworks and practitioner well-being. How paramedics view themselves, their sense of identity, is important to how they practise.

In this context the regulatory and professional responsibilities implicit in being a registered health professional are fundamental to formulating a contemporary professional identity, placing the patient at the centre of practice. Identity narrowly derived in a traditional conception of paramedic as emergency service worker, or first responder, runs the risk of dismissing whole cohorts of patients (especially socially disadvantaged and low-acuity patients) as 'non-paramedic' patients (O'Meara & Duthie 2018, p. 366). This may result in paramedic failure to exercise their responsibility of making the patient's need their first priority. This can have negative consequences for the well-being of the patient and consequently the paramedic if they have failed in their obligations to the patient. Identity more broadly based in self-awareness as a registered health practitioner specialising in paramedicine is more likely to result in a paramedic realising their regulatory and professional responsibilities with presumably better outcomes for patients.

PARAMEDICINE PRACTICE WITHIN THE HEALTH CARE SYSTEM

Australians trust, have confidence in, and are satisfied with the care provided by paramedics in this service-provision context (Productivity Commission 2021).

Demographics

With over 21,000 registered paramedics in Australia (Paramedicine Board of Australia 2022b), nearly half are females (46.1%) (Box 25.1). Over 80% of all registrants

BOX 25.1 Paramedicine Demographics

- 21,492 registered paramedics
- 80% of all registered paramedics are located in NSW, Victoria and Queensland
- 46.1% of registered paramedics are female

are in the eastern states of Australia: NSW, Victoria and Queensland (Paramedicine Board of Australia 2022b).

Of the approximately 21,000 registered paramedics, over 16,000 of them work in jurisdictional ambulance services (Productivity Commission 2021). However, Paramedicine Board of Australia data (Paramedicine Board of Australia 2022b) does not tell us in which sector the registered paramedic is located. It can be assumed that paramedics are predominantly employed by a jurisdictional state-based ambulance service, however, there are other sectors that employ paramedics, such as the defence forces, private non-emergency patient transport (NEPT), and industrial and aeromedical retrieval services, as well as new and emerging roles in primary care, community health and palliative care.

Some Australian ambulance services supplement their workforce with volunteers or community first responders in rural and remote regions. There are over 8000 ambulance volunteers predominantly in Western Australia, South Australia and Victoria (Productivity Commission 2021). This workforce is unregistered (Paramedicine Board of Australia 2022a).

In the late 1990s, there was a transition from ambulance service vocational programs to higher education pre-employment education. This transition took some time, where today, the primary pathway to gaining employment as a paramedic is the completion of a university degree. Interestingly, internationally there is a still a debate as to paramedics needing a university degree to gain employment (Ludwig 2018).

Pathways into a paramedic university degree with the completion of vocational study are still available at some universities in some states. For example, in Victoria, completing a Diploma can lead into a degree program (see Victoria University) and in Western Australia, there is currently a hybrid program in which student paramedics are employed by the ambulance service (St John WA 2022).

From 2019–20 data there were 8507 paramedic students across Australia and New Zealand (CAA 2020)

enrolled in Paramedicine Board of Australia approved programs (see Box 25.2). The accreditation ensures that standards are met in being able to graduate students who will be eligible for registration (Paramedicine Board of Australia 2021).

Currently, with the number of graduating students and the current national attrition rate of 2.7% for paramedics leaving the workforce there is an oversupply of paramedics competing for employment with jurisdictional ambulance services (Paramedicine Board of Australia 2022b). Most students aspire to gain employment with their local jurisdictional ambulance service (Devenish et al. 2020). What this means is that many newly graduated students may seek employment with another service, such as international services like the National Health Service in the UK (Devenish et al. 2015).

Having explored the emerging identity and scope of paramedicine practice, it is important to situate the practitioner and practice within the health care system. The majority of paramedics are currently employed by Australian and New Zealand jurisdictional ambulance services. These blend the best elements of the Franco-German ('stay and stabilise') and the Anglo-American ('load and go') models of service delivery. Depending on the clinical presentation of the case, suitably qualified and skilled paramedics are deployed to a case, which is typified as: 'the right paramedic to the right patient at the right time'.

This is a rationalising of resources based on clinical need which is assessed through (telephone) triage process. Based on a Franco-German model, the higher level of care is brought to the patient, which is evident by having retrieval services especially in rural and remote regions. In comparison, the Anglo-American model focuses on assessing the patient, making a clinical decision based on their presentation and determining the most appropriate care pathway. This may or, in some cases, may not mean transporting them to a hospital. The clinical decision-making and determining the care pathway process means matching patient need and transferring care to another clinician or service such as a general practitioner (GP) or hospital at home. The care of the paramedic is then discharged when the patient's care needs have been met. When compared to the Franco-German model, in Australia and New Zealand crewing is almost exclusively paramedics rather than physicians (medical doctors).

BOX 25.2   Australian and New Zealand University Providers of Paramedic Programs

New Zealand
Auckland University of Technology: http://www.aut.ac.nz/
Whitireia Community Polytechnic: http://www.whitireia.ac.nz/

Australian Capital Territory (ACT)
Australian Catholic University (ACT, VIC, QLD, NSW): http://www.acu.edu.au/

New South Wales (NSW)
Charles Sturt University: http://www.csu.edu.au/
Western Sydney University: https://www.westernsydney.edu.au/

Queensland (Qld)
Central Queensland University: http://www.cqu.edu.au/
Griffith University: http://www.griffith.edu.au/
Queensland University of Technology: http://www.qut.edu.au/
University of Queensland: http://www.uq.edu.au/
University of Southern Queensland: https://www.usq.edu.au/
University of Sunshine Coast: http://www.usc.edu.au/

South Australia (SA)
Flinders University: http://www.flinders.edu.au/

Tasmania (Tas)
University of Tasmania (TAS, NSW): http://www.utas.edu.au/

Victoria (Vic)
Federation University Australia: http://federation.edu.au/
LaTrobe University: http://www.latrobe.edu.au/
Monash University: http://www.monash.edu.au/
Victoria University: http://www.vu.edu.au/

Northern Territory (NT)
Charles Darwin University: https://www.cdu.edu.au/

Western Australia (WA)
Curtin University: https://www.curtin.edu.au/
Edith Cowan University: http://www.ecu.edu.au/
University of Notre Dame: https://www.notredame.edu.au/

Working Life

Once graduated, paramedics work across a variety of settings. The Productivity Commission (2021) reports the number of incidents, responses and patients transported by jurisdictional ambulance services. From Table 25.1, you can see in this practice context that from the number of incidents, there may be more than one ambulance responding to the case. Attending an incident, you can see not all patients are transported to hospital. This confirms the shift in the focus to out-of-hospital care, away from emergency response work to being able to refer patients to other care pathways.

Many Australians think that ambulance services are funded by Medicare (Hunter 2021; Services Australia 2021), however this is not the case. Only two states in Australia (Queensland and Tasmania) provide government cover for ambulance costs, which means there needs to be a form of insurance to cover potential costs.

Funding of ambulance services comes from direct government grants, transport feeds and subscriptions, not Medicare. As you can see in Table 25.2, ambulance service operations cost multi-billion dollars. When you look at ambulance service annual reports, the biggest expense is staff salary and wages.

TABLE 25.1   Australian Ambulance Services Incidents, Responses and Transported Patients in 2020

	Incidents	Responses	Patients	
Emergency	1,482,121	2,003,475	Transported	3,297,822
Urgent	1,406,855	1,717,994	Not transported	451,674

Source: Adapted from Productivity Commission (2021). Report on government services. Chapter 11. https://www.pc.gov.au/research/ongoing/report-on-government-services/2021/health/ambulance-services.

TABLE 25.2 **Financial Reporting of Australian Ambulance Services**

	NSW	Vic	Qld	WA	SA	Tas	ACT	NT	Aust
Government grants	873.4	875.8	834.3	159.8	160.5	94.1	63.4	34.2	3 095.4
Transport fees	222.0	213.1	56.8	127.0	117.2	9.6	7.7	3.0	756.3
Subscriptions and other income	15.6	99.7	14.3	41.2	41.2	4.6	–	1.3	217.9
Total revenue	1 111.0	1 188.6	905.4	328.0	318.9	108.3	71.0	38.6	4 069.7

Source: Adapted from Productivity Commission (2021). Report on government services. Chapter 11. https://www.pc.gov.au/research/ongoing/report-on-government-services/2021/health/ambulance-services.

Occupational Hazards

Because of the nature of out-of-hospital treatment, paramedics are subject to significant stressors and potential hazards. Paramedics, depending on their practice context, can attend to people in distress or agitation, having to make clinical decisions for patients experiencing critical presentations (Arial et al. 2011; Holland 2011; LeBlanc et al. 2011; Shepherd & Wild 2014; van der Ploeg & Kleber 2003). Because of these factors, paramedics have one of the highest rates of burnout compared with other health professions (Lawn et al. 2020; LeBlanc et al. 2011).

Compounding the psychological stressors, professions such as paramedicine, which involve close contact with clients or patients, are at greater risk of being exposed to client-initiated workplace violence (Brough 2005). This includes intimidation, sexual harassment (Independent Inquiry 2021), and verbal, physical and sexual abuse. In both international and Australian studies it has been found that around 80% of paramedics have experienced a form of workplace violence, most predominantly verbal abuse (Boyle et al. 2007; Boyle & McKenna 2017). Paramedics working during the SARS-CoV-2 pandemic have experienced significant mental and physical health challenges (Petrie et al. 2022; Smallwood et al. 2021a; Smallwood et al. 2021b).

Pause *for* Reflection ...

During the SARS-CoV-2 pandemic, some jurisdictional ambulance services became innovative and introduced virtual care (telehealth) to facilitate secondary triage and delivery of alternative care pathways. These have now become established as a permanent mode of service delivery for appropriate patient presentations. What do you think are some of the benefits and limitations of this innovation for health service delivery, the workforce and the community?

THE FUTURE OF HEALTH CARE NEEDS – PARAMEDICINE MOVING BEYOND URGENT CARE

This discussion has identified the role of paramedics and paramedicine practice as both a health and emergency service. The blurring of these boundaries makes it challenging to shift from being a 'treat and transport' service for 'crisis, emergency and disasters' now to 'out-of-hospital, mobile primary care provider'.

This shift was evident during the SARS-CoV-2 pandemic, which saw changes in workload demand (Lavigne et al. 2021). Demand for services were from those populations made vulnerable by the system, such as people living with mental health disorders, due to shortfalls and difficulty in accessing care in the community-based care model such as general practitioners (Lavigne et al. 2021).

With the increased demand for jurisdictional ambulance service responses, the follow-on effect was **ramping**. Only 25% of the 23,000 Australians who attend a public **emergency department (ED)** on any one day arrive by ambulance (AIHW 2020). The volume of patients attending a public ED means a chain reaction or flow-on effect can occur, say during winter. This effect causes ramping, which occurs when no suitable ED bed is available for a patient who arrives by ambulance at hospital, preventing them from being transferred from ambulance care to the ED (Gaughan et al. 2018; Hammond et al. 2012; Honeyfind et al. 2018). With the paramedic still delivering treatment to the patient on board, the ambulance, is forced to wait outside the ED until such time as the patient can be accommodated and assessed by hospital staff.

A root cause analysis might identify that ramping is due to an ageing population, increases in co-morbid chronic conditions, changes in family structures and social support, pricing (free service), reduced access to other primary health care services (such as after-hours GP services), increased health awareness and changes in community expectations, and lack of alternative services (Gaughan et al. 2018; Honeyfind et al. 2018; Livingston et al. 2007; Lowthian et al. 2011).

Changes to service delivery, with **extended care paramedics (ECP)** or community paramedics, has seen primary care being delivered to patients for ongoing treatment of chronic diseases such as diabetes, and respiratory or cardiovascular conditions (Duckett et al. 2013). This type of care model has been used elsewhere in the world, such as in North America (Bigham et al. 2013; O'Meara 2014; O'Meara et al. 2015), facilitated by telehealth technology (Choi et al. 2016) for some time. Evidence suggests that community paramedics are effective in reducing ED presentations (Lurie et al. 2021) with the goal of **community paramedicine** to fill the gaps in the health care system (Wingrove 2011).

Pause *for* Reflection …

Nationally and internationally, paramedicine has evolved to include general primary care and specialist services such as mental health, cardiac, stroke and palliative care. Examples include Ambulance Victoria mobile stroke response and mental health (PACER), while the UK National Health Service implemented 'falls truck', who were able to assess and refer 'elderly fallers'. What, if any, are the tensions for targeting resources?

Current and Future Employment Opportunities

In response to increased demand for services during the SARS-CoV-2 pandemic, several ambulance services enacted **surge workforce** strategies. This involved recruitment of additional graduates, above attrition rates, for paramedic roles as well as paramedic students for various support roles. As of 2021, there were nearly 1500 student paramedics employed by ambulance services (Productivity Commission 2021). Student support roles involved a limited scope of practice, usually as assistants to paramedics. Paramedics and paramedic students have also been actively sought by health departments as vaccinators at vaccination hubs. Opportunities for employment also emerged in primary care and residential aged-care contexts.

The medium- to long-term impact of these surge strategies remains to be seen. For jurisdictional ambulance services, a return to pre-pandemic demand with a now enhanced substantive workforce may see recruitment return to addressing attrition, which may remain low. However, even pre-pandemic demand was challenging service delivery capacity. This demand along with an enhanced understanding of paramedicine's contribution to the health care system may result in increased employment opportunities in the coming years. In addition, demand is recognised as having an impact on the workforce due to fatigue (Rees et al. 2021), which may also result in enhancements to the workforce. The emergence of paramedicine as a registered health profession is anticipated to result in new employment opportunities as paramedics continue to be recognised as capable of filling identified gaps in the provision of care and the health professional workforce.

Case study 25.1 outlines an example of the work of paramedics as they engage in patient care.

CASE STUDY 25.1

Dorothy is an 84-year-old female living independently at home, with some supported care through her local council's Home and Community Care program. She has a number of chronic conditions such as atrial fibrillation, hypertension and hyperlipidaemia. These are well managed by her local GP and medication. Dorothy is a widow and her family lives interstate.

Dorothy is an avid gardener and has had a fall in her backyard. Wearing her personal safety alarm, on a necklace pendant, she activates it by pressing the button. This raises the alarm to the state ambulance service, which dispatches a nearby crew to Dorothy's house.

Initially, the paramedic crew couldn't locate Dorothy and notify the Communication Centre to contact the police, as they may have to break into her house. However, part of the conditions of her personal alarm subscription was the installation of key in a locked box in a location recorded on the ambulance service computer system. This information was relayed to the attending crew who were able to gain access into the property once the police were in attendance.

Dorothy was found in the rear garden complaining of pain to her left hip. The paramedic crew assessed her injuries and made a provisional diagnosis of fractured neck of femur. Along with splinting, posturing and initial pain

CASE STUDY 25.1—cont'd

relief, the paramedic crew prepared Dorothy for transport to the local public hospital's ED. However, the pain relief offered by the paramedic crew was not sufficient to ease Dorothy's pain, so the crew called for **intensive care paramedic (ICP)** backup. The ICP who attended was able to give her a different type of analgesia which was more effective in relieving her pain.

The paramedic crew handed over care to the ED triage registered nurse. After a period of time, Dorothy was transferred to ward where she underwent surgery for a hip replacement. After a week, she was transferred by non-emergency ambulance to a rehabilitation hospital for ongoing treatment to help her regain her mobility.

Once she was discharged home, Dorothy had some ongoing issues with the surgical wound on her hip, which remained problematic in terms of healing. As part of her discharge planning, Dorothy had in-home support from the Royal District Nursing Service for her wound management. As it was after hours and her GP clinic was closed, the RDNS RN rang the ambulance service as he was concerned about the condition of the wound heading into a weekend. In response to information provided by the

RN, the call taker in the Communications Centre despatched an extended care paramedic (ECP) to assess Dorothy. The ECP was able to assess and treat her wound with some other medications and made a referral that Dorothy follow up with her GP the next day.

Case Study Questions

1. What important information about Dorothy's social situation would the paramedic provide in the initial handover to the registered nurse at the ED triage? Why would this be important for noting by the hospital?
2. Identify the various points where Dorothy's care has been transferred. At these points, consider the type of information that is being transferred. Does this information match with Dorothy's care needs?
3. Consider the types of other care providers that paramedics may come into contact with, such as the Royal District Nursing Service in caring for elderly people for an ageing population and older people living in their homes. Identify five other providers that paramedics may come into contact with in relation to Dorothy's situation.

SUMMARY

This chapter has described the current reforms for paramedics and out-of-hospital care. Paramedics have been included as a registered health profession with the NRAS, are university educated and participate in research. Paramedics have been on the frontline of the SARS-CoV-2 pandemic, which has seen a considerable strain on the health care system. This has resulted in an increased recognition of the role and value of paramedics in providing health care to the community. They have continued to demonstrate their capabilities and are being utilised to address service provision and workforce gaps, including community-based primary health care services through expanding their scope of practice.

REVIEW QUESTIONS

1. What is the primary objective of health practitioner regulation for paramedics under the National Registration and Accreditation Scheme?
2. What are the implications of registration for practising as a paramedic?
3. What, if any, are the potential or future roles for graduate paramedics outside of jurisdictional ambulance services?
4. During the SARS-CoV-2 pandemic, ambulance services introduced virtual care (telehealth) consultations. Do you think this innovation in service meets the expectation of the public when they call for an ambulance?
5. Extended care paramedics in community roles are 'filling gaps' in providing out-of-hospital care. What do you see as some of the drivers for paramedics becoming involved in these areas of care provision?

REFERENCES

Arial, M., Wild, P., Benoit, D., et al., 2011. Multi-level modelling of aspects associated with poor mental health in a sample of prehospital emergency professionals. Am J Ind Med 54, 847–857.

Australian Health Practitioner Regulation Agency (Ahpra), 2022. Regulatory principles for the National Scheme. https://www. Ahpra.gov.au/About-Ahpra/What-We-Do/Regulatory-principles.aspx.

Australian Institute of Health and Welfare (AIHW), 2020. Australia's health 2020: in brief. Australia's health series no. 17. Cat. no. AUS 232. AIHW, Canberra.

Bennett, B., Carney, T., Chiarella, M., et al., 2018. Australia's National Registration and Accreditation Scheme for Health Practitioners: a national approach to polycentric regulation? Sydney Law Rev 40, 159–181.

Bigham, B.L., Kennedy, S.M., Drennan, I., et al., 2013. Expanding paramedic scope of practice in the community: a systematic review of the literature. Prehosp Emerg Care 17 (3), 361–372.

Boyle, M., Koritsas, S., Coles, J., et al., 2007. A pilot study of workplace violence towards paramedics. Emerg Med J 24, 760–763.

Boyle, M., McKenna, L., 2017. Paramedic student exposure to workplace violence during clinical placements – a cross-sectional study. Nurse Educ Prac 22, 93–97.

Brough, P., 2005. Workplace violence experienced by paramedics – relationship with social support, job satisfaction, and psychological strain. Australas J Disaster Trauma Stud 2005–2, 1–11.

Choi, B.Y., Blumberg, C., Williams, K., 2016. Mobile integrated health care and community paramedicine: an emerging emergency medical services concept. Ann Emerg Med, 67 (3), 361–366.

Commonwealth of Australia, The Senate, Legal and Constitutional Affairs References Committee, 2017. Establishment of a national registration system for Australian paramedics to improve and ensure patient and community safety. https://www.aph.gov.au/Parliamentary_Business/Committees/Senate/Legal_and_Constitutional_Affairs/Paramedics/Report.

Commonwealth of Australia (Department of Health), 2017. Establishment of a national registration system for Australian paramedics to improve and ensure patient and community safety. https://www.health.gov.au/resources/publications/establishment-of-a-national-registration-system-for-australian-paramedics-to-improve-and-ensure-patient-and-community-safety.

Council of Ambulance Authorities, 2020. Annual report 2019–2020. https://www.caa.net.au/annual-reports.

Devenish, S., Clark, M., Fleming, M., et al., 2015. Australian paramedic graduates transitioning into UK NHS ambulance services: what are the potential challenges? J Paramed Pract 7 (10), 492–498.

Devenish, S., Rolley, A., Long, D., 2020. Investigating career intentions of undergraduate paramedic students studying in Queensland, Australia. Australas J Paramed, 17.

Duckett, S., Breadon, P., Ginnivan, L., 2013. Access all areas: new solutions for GP shortages in rural Australia. Grattan Institute, Melbourne

Eaton, G., Wong, G., Tierney, S., 2021. Understanding the role of the paramedic in primary care: a realist review. BMC Medicine 19 (1), 1–14.

Furness, S., Hanson, L., Spier, J., 2021. Archetypal meanings of being a paramedic: a hermeneutic review. Australas Emerg Care 24 (2), 135–140.

Gaughan, J., Kasteridis, P., Mason, A., et al., 2018. Waits in A&E departments of the English NHS, 2018 International Health Congress, St Hugh's College Oxford University, 28th–30th June 2018. http://www.globalhealthcongress.org/.

Hammond, E., Shaban, R.Z., Holzhauser, K., et al., 2012. An exploratory study to examine the phenomenon and practice of ambulance ramping at hospitals within the Queensland Health Southern Districts and the Queensland Ambulance Service. Queensland Health & Griffith University, Brisbane. http://www.griffith.edu.au/__data/assets/pdf_file/0011/389567/Ambulance-Ramping-Study.pdf.

Health Practitioner Regulation National Law and Other Legislation Amendment Bill 2017 (The National Law) [NSW]. https://www.parliament.nsw.gov.au/bills/Pages/bill-details.aspx?pk=3448.

Holland, M., 2011. The dangers of detrimental coping in emergency medical services. Prehosp Emerg Care 15 (3), 331–337.

Honeyford, K., Bottle, A., Aylin, P., 2018. ED attendances: an overlooked performance metric? A statistician's perspective 2018 International Health Congress, St Hugh' College Oxford University, 28th–30th June 2018. http://www.globalhealthcongress.org/.

Hunter, C., 2021. Ambulance cover in Australia. https://www.finder.com.au/health-insurance/ambulance-cover.

Independent Inquiry, 2021. https://www.humanrights.vic.gov.au/static/0cfed5e5830ef5b0ec6b31e1f3ae63ef/Resource-Ambulance_Victoria_Independent_Review_Workplace_Equality-Volume_1_Full-Document-v2.pdf.

Lavigne, T., De Tavernier, B., Van Regenmortel, N., et al., 2021. Effect of the first wave of the Belgian COVID-19 pandemic on physician-provided prehospital critical care in the city of Antwerp (Belgium). Prehosp Disaster Med 1–7.

Lawn, S., Roberts, L., Willis, E., et al., 2020. The effects of emergency medical service work on the psychological, physical, and social well-being of ambulance personnel: a systematic review of qualitative research. BMC Psychiatry 20 (1), 1–16.

LeBlanc, V.R. Regehr, C., Birze, A., et al., 2011. The association between posttraumatic stress, coping, and acute stress responses in paramedics. Traumatology 17 (4), 10–16.

Livingston, C., Condron, J., Dennekamp, M., et al., 2007. Factors in ambulance demand: options for funding and forecasting. The Australian Institute for Primary Care, Faculty of Health Sciences, Latrobe University, Victoria.

Lowthian, J.A., Jolley D.J., Curtis A.J., et al., 2011. The challenge of population ageing: accelerating demands for emergency ambulance services by older patients 1995–2015. Med J Aust 194 (11), 574–578.

Ludwig, G., 2018. EMS: do you need a college degree to be a paramedic? Firehouse 1, September. https://www.firehouse.com/careers-education/article/21013720/do-you-need-a-college-degrees-to-be-paramedic-firehouse-gary-ludwig.

Lurie, T., Adibhatla, S., Andhavarapu, S., et al., 2021. 163 Study design influences effect size: systematic review and meta-analysis of mobile integrated health community paramedicine programs' effect on emergency department visits. Ann Emerg Med 78 (4), S66.

McManamny, T.E., Dwyer, R., Cantwell, K., et al., 2021. Emergency ambulance demand by older adults from rural and regional Victoria, Australia. Australas J Ageing 41 (1), e74–e81. doi:10.1111/ajag.12960.

O'Meara, P., 2014. Community paramedics: a scoping review of their emergence and potential impact. Int Paramed Pract 4 (1), 5–12.

O'Meara, P., Stirling, C., Ruest, M., et al., 2015. Community paramedicine model of care: an observational, ethnographic case study. BMC Health Services Research 16 (1), 39.

O'Meara, P., Duthie, S., 2018. Paramedicine in Australia and New Zealand: a comparative overview. Aust J Rural Health 26(5), 363–368.

Paramedicine Board of Australia, 2018. Code of conduct (interim). https://www.paramedicineboard.gov.au/Professional-standards/Codes-guidelines-and-policies/Code-of-conduct.aspx.

Paramedicine Board of Australia, 2021. Professional capabilities for registered paramedics. https://www.paramedicineboard.gov.au/Professional-standards/Professional-capabilities-for-registered-paramedics.aspx).

Paramedicine Board of Australia, 2022a. Functions of the Board. https://www.paramedicineboard.gov.au/About.

Paramedicine Board of Australia, 2022b. Statistics. https://www.paramedicineboard.gov.au/News/Statistics.aspx.

Paramedics Australasia, 2011. The forgotten health profession: a commentary highlighting the omission of paramedics and paramedic services from national health care policy considerations. https://apcollege.edu.au/pdf/media-other/PA-ForgottenProfession-single-page.pdf.

Petrie, K., Smallwood, N., Pascoe, A., 2022. Mental health symptoms and workplace challenges among Australian paramedics during the COVID-19 pandemic. Int J Environ Res Public Health 19 (2), 1004.

Productivity Commission, 2021. Report on government services. Chapter 11. https://www.pc.gov.au/research/ongoing/report-on-government-services/2021/health/ambulance-services.

Rees, N., Smythe, L., Hogan, C., et al., 2021. Paramedic experiences of providing care in Wales (UK) during the 2020 COVID-19 pandemic (PECC-19): a qualitative study using evolved grounded theory. BMJ Open 11, e048677. doi:10.1136/bmjopen-2021-048677.

Services Australia, 2021. Health care and Medicare. https://www.servicesaustralia.gov.au/health-care-and-medicare?context=60092.

Shepherd, L., Wild, J., 2014. Cognitive appraisals, objectivity and coping in ambulance workers: a pilot study. Emerg Med J 31, 41–44.

Smallwood, N., Karimi, L., Pascoe, A., et al., 2021. Coping strategies adopted by Australian frontline health workers to address psychological distress during the COVID-19 pandemic. Gen Hosp Psychiatry 72, 124–130.

Smallwood, N., Karimi, L., Bismark, M., et al., 2021. High levels of psychosocial distress among Australian frontline healthcare workers during the COVID-19 pandemic: a cross-sectional survey. Gen Psychiatry 34 (5).

St John Ambulance Western Australia, 2016. Direct Entry Ambulance Paramedic. https://stjohnwa.com.au/changelives/employment#current.

Townsend, R., Luck, M., 2019. Applied Paramedic Law, Ethics and Professionalism: Australia and New Zealand. Elsevier Health Sciences.

van der Ploeg, E., Kleber, R.J., 2003. Acute and chronic job stressors among ambulance personnel: predictors of health symptoms. Occup Environ Med 60(Suppl 1), i40–i46.

Williams, B., Beovich, B., Olaussen, A., 2021. The definition of paramedicine: an international Delphi study. Journal of Multidisciplinary Healthcare 14, 3561.

Wingrove, G., 2011. International roundtable on community paramedicine. Australas J Paramed 9 (1). http://ro.ecu.edu.au/jephc/vol9/iss1/1.

FURTHER READING

Pap, R., Stephenson, M., Simpson, P.M., et al., 2023. [In Press] Acceptability of Australian prehospital care quality indicators: an explanatory sequential mixed methods study. Paramedicine.

Shannon, B., Baldry, S., O'Meara, P., et al. 2023. The definition of a community paramedic: an international consensus. Paramedicine 20 (1), 4–22.

Williams, B., Beovich, B., Olaussen, A., 2021. The definition of paramedicine: an international delphi study. J Multidiscip Healthc 14, 3561–3570.

ONLINE RESOURCES

Ahpra Paramedicine Board of Australia: https://www.para-medicineboard.gov.au/.

Australasian College of Paramedicine: https://paramedics.org/.

Council of Ambulance Authorities: https://www.caa.net.au/.

Productivity Commission Report on Government Services, Chapter 11 Ambulance Services: https://www.pc.gov.au/ongoing/report-on-government-services/2023/health/ambulance-services.

26

The Pharmacist's Unique Contribution to Australia's Health System

Stephen Carter

KEY LEARNING OUTCOMES

When you finish this chapter you should be able to:
- describe the key activities of pharmacists
- understand the unique contribution of community pharmacies to the health system, which includes the judicious sale of medicines and the provision of health services
- explain the extent to which pharmacists collaborate with other members of the health care system
- using Tuohy's model of accidental logics, discuss how the Australian health system could make the most use of pharmacists' unique skillset.

KEY TERMS AND ABBREVIATIONS

community pharmacy
Community Pharmacy Agreement (CPA)
consultant pharmacist
consumer[1]
customer
home medicines review (HMR)
medication reconciliation
medicines

minor ailment
National Medicines Policy (NMP)
patient
Pharmaceutical Benefits Scheme (PBS)
Pharmaceutical Society of Australia
Pharmacy Guild of Australia

Quality Care in Pharmacy Program (QCPP)
quality use of medicines (QUM)
residential aged-care facility (RACF)
residential medication management review (RMMR)

INTRODUCTION

This chapter provides an introduction to the profession of pharmacy. It describes the various roles of pharmacists currently working in Australia and shows how these roles are being developed, regulated and funded. It briefly touches on the history of the profession, and discusses how many pharmacists look towards a future that makes more use of their unique skills.

---

[1]The use of the terms **consumer**, **customer** and **patient** overlap considerably in regards to pharmacy.

WORKPLACE AND FUNDING

While pharmacists work in a range of settings, the majority of pharmacists in Australia are employed within community pharmacies (Australian Government Department of Health 2019). While being private businesses, the most important source of funding for pharmacists in community pharmacies is the **Pharmaceutical Benefits Scheme** (**PBS**). While the funding model for PBS medicines includes payments for some other services, most of the income received is for dispensing medicines. The payments are made under agreements between pharmacists and the

TABLE 26.1   Proportion of Australian Pharmacists Working in Various Settings

Setting	Percentage
Community pharmacy	63.2%
Hospital	22.5%
Community health care service	2.7%
Medical centre	2.3%
Other private practice	1.6%
Educational facility	1.4%
Other government department or agency	1.3%
Pharmaceutical manufacturing	1.0%
Other commercial	0.8%
Residential health care facility	0.8%
Defence force	0.8%
Wholesale pharmacy	0.6%
Correctional services	0.4%
Aboriginal and Torres Strait Islander health service	0.2%
Other – not stated	0.2%

Source: Adapted from National Health Workforce Data Sets, 2019 (Australian Government Department of Health 2019).

Commonwealth, through **Community Pharmacy Agreements (CPAs)**, renegotiated every five years. The second most frequent setting is within the hospital sector, where funding is made through state government health budgets. Other places of work include clinical and non-clinical settings, each with a unique funding model (see Table 26.1).

WHAT DO PHARMACISTS DO?

Pharmacists are the health professionals involved in the safe custody, preparation, dispensing and provision of medicines, together with systems and information to assure quality of use (Pharmaceutical Society of Australia 2017). So, before describing the roles of pharmacists it is helpful first to carefully consider what **medicines** are and how the supply of medicines is regulated.

MEDICINES, PEOPLE AND HEALTH SYSTEMS

Medicines are used to alleviate symptoms and/or to maintain health and well-being. They form the basis for the treatment of many acute and most chronic diseases.

They are widely used in Australian society, particularly among older consumers. The most recent national telephone poll demonstrated that, among persons aged 50 years and older, almost 90% had taken a medicine in the last 24 hours (Morgan et al. 2012). Furthermore, many are using a lot of medicines. A recent analysis of medicines dispensed under the PBS estimated that on a typical day in 2018, 49% of those who had medicines dispensed were taking 5 or more a day and 26% were using more than 10 a day (Wylie et al. 2020). Medicines can make a significant contribution to the health and welfare of our society. It is difficult now to imagine a world without penicillin, painkillers, vaccinations and a plethora of other substances. Medicines are so important that the World Health Organization (WHO) maintains an Essential Medicines List, which sets out those medicines that it considers are necessary for basic health systems (World Health Organization (WHO) 2021). The main problem with medicines is that not only do they help, they also have the potential to cause harm. It was Paracelsus who wrote: 'All substances are poisons; there is none which is not a poison. The right dose differentiates a poison from a remedy'. The potential for harm from medicines is highlighted in that, within Australia, 2.5% of all hospital admissions are attributable to problems with medicines, half of which are considered avoidable (Lim et al. 2022). The competing tensions of Australia's need to use valuable medicines yet avoid medication-related harm is reflected in Australia's adoption of a **National Medicines Policy (NMP)** in 2000, which was reviewed for the first time in 2021 (Australian Government Depart of Health and Ageing 2022). The NMP's central objectives are to ensure:

- timely access to the medicines that Australians need, at a cost individuals and the community can afford
- medicines meeting appropriate standards of quality, safety and efficacy
- quality use of medicines
- maintaining a responsible and viable medicines industry.

Pause *for* Reflection …

Have you ever noticed how older family members use quite a few medicines? Have you talked with them about that? Do you think their medicines use is influenced by a high level of collaboration in the health system? It would be useful to apply Bacchi's 'What is the problem represented to be?' (the WPR approach, see Chapter 1) when thinking about how the role of the pharmacist is evolving under the NMP.

The laws regarding how medicines are stored and supplied are under the jurisdiction of the states and territories. For example, in NSW there is a *Poisons and Therapeutic Goods Act 1966* and its associated *Regulations*. Some medicine products are considered relatively safe and may be sold in any location (i.e. these are not scheduled). Medicine products categorised in the 'Schedules' represent a more significant risk to the consumer because of their inherent potency or because the quantity within the pack represents problems if taken in excessive doses and/or for an extended time (Box 26.1).

ROLES OF THE PHARMACIST

First and foremost, the general public tends to view pharmacists' work through the lens of the supply function. Supplying medicines is a key role for pharmacists in community pharmacies, in hospitals and throughout the distribution chain. The pharmacist needs to ensure that the medicines are supplied in accordance with professional standards and the law and transported and stored to protect the physical and chemical properties of the medicines. In the next few sections, we deal with the supply functions of dispensing prescription medicines and providing medicines 'over the counter'.

Dispensing Medicines

To the general public, the dispensing of medicines on receipt of a prescription is probably the most familiar role of pharmacists. When dispensing, the pharmacist ensures that the supplied medicine is prescribed legally, accurately reflects the prescriber's intentions, and is consistent with the needs and safety of the patient. In order to reduce the risk of treatment-caused harm, pharmacists need to implement good systems, with continuous quality improvement coupled with a professional and patient-centred approach to dispensing. Most Australian community pharmacies subscribe to the **Quality Care in Pharmacy Program (QCPP)** (a quality insurance program) because the PBS provides practice incentives, which depends on maintaining QCPP accreditation. This requires each pharmacy to allocate sufficient resources, including an adequate number of pharmacists, technicians/assistants, appropriate technology, well-designed work-flow, a private or semi-private area to consult with patients and of course sufficient stock. Maintaining quality services during the SARS-CoV-2 pandemic required much adaptation to service delivery (Lubi et al. 2021).

Prescriptions Require Review

It should be noted that, when dispensing prescriptions, it is not sufficient for the pharmacist to simply follow the instructions of the prescriber. Whenever a medicine is dispensed, the pharmacist is obliged to review the prescription, based on the information available to them. Using the dispensing history and information gleaned from interviewing the patient, the pharmacist needs to make several judgements regarding the appropriateness of each prescription.

These judgements of appropriateness include consideration of:
- dose, frequency and length of treatment
- whether the medicine is suitable for the condition prescribed
- the patient's past history of adverse events
- potential drug–drug interactions and drug–disease interactions
- practicality of the prescribed regimen and the likelihood of being adherent to the regimen, and
- patient preference.

If the pharmacist considers that the medicine may have a preventable adverse effect on the patient, it is the responsibility of the pharmacist to intervene and converse with the prescriber. Once the pharmacist is comfortable with the prescription, the product is prepared, labelled and handed or delivered to the patient. There are certain circumstances that should prompt the pharmacist to initiate patient counselling proactively. Such circumstances may include when a new medicine is prescribed, when there is a change in the dose or frequency of administration, when the brand of medicine has changed or when the medicine is known to be particularly problematic (Pharmaceutical Society of Australia 2019).

It is perhaps not surprising that the most common reason for contact between pharmacists and medical practitioners is to sort out prescribing problems. The topic of these conversations tend to focus on administrative errors, but clinical issues are discussed at times (Zielińska-Tomczak et al. 2021). Pharmacists tend to feel some anxiety about contacting medical practitioners about prescribing errors, as they are also required to maintain good working relationships (Basak et al. 2015). Setting up truly collaborative practice between GPs and community pharmacists is thus challenging and requires paying greater attention to, and facilitating better use of, technology to improve documentation and communication practices (Sim et al. 2020).

Collaborating to Manage the Opiate Crisis

An example of where more collaborative practice between patients, prescribers and dispensers has potential to improve patient outcomes is managing the so-called worldwide 'opiate crisis' (Jayawardana et al. 2021). Historically, injected heroin was the most frequently used opiate, but this has been replaced by prescribed medicines such as morphine, codeine and oxycontin. Pharmacists feel great pressure during dispensing of opiates to avoid supplying inappropriately and tend to feel like 'gate-keepers' (Vadiei et al. 2022).

Yet collaboration is tricky. Historically, medical practitioners and pharmacists do not share a common data-sharing system. This means that neither has been able to view what has already been prescribed by other doctors and dispensed in other pharmacies. The MyHealthRecord (MHR) is designed to help overcome this, but many people have opted out of MHR and the data about medicines is made available after a delay (of up to 30 days). The Australian Government has recently enabled a national *real-time* monitoring system for opiates and this is being progressively rolled out across the states and territories. In Victoria, where the system is mandatory, it has been reported that there was a 25% reduction in the proportion of people taking a high-risk prescription opioid medication within the first 6 months of implementation (Paola 2020). Evaluation of the programs will consider the impact on consumers who genuinely require larger

quantities such as those being treated for cancer, and also that patients are not subject to stigma during challenging conversations (Haines & Prathivadi 2021).

Compounding

Prior to the 1950s, the majority of prescriptions were not available from wholesale manufacturers. Virtually all prescription medicines were prepared by the pharmacist according to formulae with individual ingredients using ancient techniques. Since the 1950s, however, this type of dispensing fell into decline as the 'evidence-based' pharmaceutical industry took over.

However, not all medicines, particularly creams, ointments and washes, were able to be prepared in the variety of strengths and combinations which were demanded of, for example, dermatologists. Filling this gap in need, the art and science of compounding has recently undergone a minor resurgence, especially in **community pharmacies**. Australia ensures that compounding is a key component of undergraduate training (Kosari et al. 2020). While many hospitals provide specialised compounding services, quite a number of community pharmacies focus on this area in order to customise formulations to meet the specific needs of the patient and/or doctor. However, it is not possible to compound medicines with the same level of quality control and scrutiny as commercial medicines. The Pharmacy Council of New South Wales, the state government body that regulates pharmacies, has recently increased its surveillance of pharmacists in response to an increasing number of consumer complaints about compounded medicines (Pharmacy Council of New South Wales 2019).

Pharmacists in Community Pharmacies

While a significant component of community pharmacy work is dispensing medicines, the community pharmacist is also often the first health professional that patients see for **minor ailments**. Pharmacists must be good communicators as the diagnostic role of the pharmacist does depend on performing physical examinations. Pharmacists (or their delegated assistants) are therefore expected to initiate a dialogue with their **customers** in order to ensure that the patient is provided with optimal care. The **Pharmaceutical Society of Australia** has developed and refined professional practice standards (the Standards) (Pharmaceutical Society of Australia 2017), which, among other things, provide pharmacists with guidance regarding the sale of medicines for minor ailments. Recall that many medicines can be sold without involving pharmacists (see Box 26.1). The Standards include structured protocols of how pharmacists' delegated assistants should manage consultations with patients, and under what circumstances the assistant should refer the patient to the pharmacist. If the medicine is a 'scheduled medicine' this means that, in order for the medicine to be sold, this dialogue is expected to occur regardless of whether the customer self-selects or requests a treatment for a symptom. The patient should receive instructions for use that are practical and should be provided with sufficient information to allow them to use the medicines wisely. The pharmacist also has a professional obligation to refer a patient to another health provider if he/she believes that that is in the interests of the patient. In this way, community pharmacies also provide a 'triage' service.

The general public values having direct access to pharmacists working in community pharmacies, particularly as a source of prescription and non-prescription medicines information and to help people with selection of non-prescription medicines (Carter et al. 2021). Here, it should be noted that the lack of privacy within community pharmacies has long been recognised as a potential communication barrier. However, lack of privacy is just one communication barrier faced by pharmacists, as they balance patient expectations while ensuring patient safety. To some extent, the community pharmacy's capacity to act professionally is being undermined by modern trends in consumerism, corporatisation and mercantilism of pharmacy (Ilardo & Speciale 2020). An increasing body of work is exploring the use of simulated patients (like mystery shoppers) to provide structured feedback to pharmacists (Collins et al. 2021). The feedback can assist pharmacists to act professionally while managing patient expectations and improving patient safety. There is scope for these methods to be included in quality assurance processes (see QCPP, above).

Pause *for* Reflection …

An area where pharmacists have had their scope of practice reduced in recent years is in the supply of codeine-containing analgesics. Prior to 2018, low-strength codeine (≤ 15 mg) was available without prescription by consulting with a pharmacist. Noting that internationally, codeine was the most widely consumed opiate analgesic and responsible for

misuse, dependence and harms, the Australian Government re-scheduled codeine in February 2018 to be prescription-only. An analysis of telephone call data collected by the NSW Poisons Information Centre concluded that this strategy reduced use and harm with no evidence for substitution with high-strength codeine products or other pharmaceutical opioids (Cairns et al. 2020). Do you ever recall that codeine was available over the counter? If we go back to 2010, these medicines were available in pharmacies in pack sizes of 100 without the requirement to speak to a pharmacist. How do you feel about the change to prescription-only?

Payments for the Triage Role

Within Australian community pharmacies, the vast majority of pharmacists' consultations are not paid for by governments. In addition, community pharmacies have generally not charged their customers for these relatively informal consultations. They have relied on the income derived from the mark-up from the sale of medicines, subsidised by the dispensing of prescriptions. While this strategy has worked well over the past, falling remuneration from PBS dispensing reminds pharmacists of their unfunded contribution to the health system. Internationally, health systems are exploring ways with which to remunerate pharmacists for their contribution to the health system, through funding structured minor ailments services. Australian research shows that a trial of a minor ailments service conducted among 30 pharmacies in Sydney was cost-effective (Dineen-Griffin et al. 2020). That study concluded that if pharmacists were remunerated at the award rate, there would be an overall reduction in costs to the health system, through reduced Medicare rebates and fewer hospital emergency department presentations. Here it is important to note that pharmacists cannot claim for any services through the Medicare Benefits Schedule (MBS), regardless of whether the service is provided in a community pharmacy or medical practice.

Communicable Diseases and Vaccination

To some extent, the public health impact of community pharmacies has been clearer since the SARS-CoV-2 pandemic, where pharmacists have had a key role in maintaining the supply of critical medicines, administering vaccines and supplying Rapid Antigen Tests. Pharmacists must be especially accredited to do vaccination and do so in a private space. Yet, prior to 2014, pharmacists were prevented from administering any vaccinations, despite the fact this had been common practice in other countries. While it is currently challenging to estimate the public health impact of pharmacists administering COVID-19 vaccinations, the impact is clearer in regards to influenza. For example, the recently improved influenza vaccine coverage is partly attributed to pharmacies (and nurse administered vaccines in the workplace) (Trent et al. 2021).

Pause *for* Reflection ...

During the early days of pharmacist-provided vaccination there were numerous press releases from the medical practitioner groups such as the Australian Medical Association (AMA) and the Royal Australian College of General Practitioners (RACGP) who advocated against this for influenza (Dow 2018), and then recently for COVID-19 (Clun 2020). As Rachel Clun highlights, this is an example of the so-called 'turf-wars'. The Australian Government's approach to setting fees for COVID-19 vaccination services is interesting, as it pays GP practices considerably more than community pharmacies for the same services. The fee disparity has been attributed as the main reason why half of NSW's pharmacy network opted out of paediatric COVID-19 vaccinations by February 2022, as reported by ABC NEWS (Jones 2022). How do you think the Australian Government should manage the payment of fees to different health professionals for the same service?

Hospital Pharmacy

Hospital pharmacists are involved in a range of activities aimed at improving the **quality use of medicines (QUM)** within the hospital and beyond. Some of the activities are quite specialised. Pharmacists, particularly senior pharmacists, may work on medicine and therapeutics committees where they have a role in advising the hospital on which medicines should be included on lists of medicines that are readily available in the hospital. The benefits of having these 'formularies' are that they can decrease errors and reduce costs. Pharmacists contribute to the evaluation of new and expensive medicines that specialist medical practitioners wish to use. Hospitals are often the site where clinical trials are conducted and pharmacists are often involved in this area of research.

Focus on Clinical Activities in Hospital Pharmacy

Hospital pharmacists may be involved in a broad range of clinical activities. In hospitals, pharmacists tend to have access to the complete patient record. Records include diagnoses, reasons for admission, pathology reports, and medical and paramedical opinions. Pharmacists may have direct contact with the patient and their caregivers, who report that pharmacists help them with information to help avoid side effects (Loo et al. 2021). The close proximity to other health professionals working on ward rounds facilitates interprofessional communication. Multidisciplinary teams typically consult with pharmacists for opinions on the most appropriate and cost-effective medicines and combinations of medicines to use, the best method to administer the medicines, the optimal doses and timing of doses and ways to monitor for adverse effects.

The focus on clinical activities makes hospital pharmacy a very attractive career option for pharmacy interns, despite the high level of competition for positions. The competition is thought to be high because graduating pharmacy students perceive that the role of the hospital pharmacist is particularly patient focused and that their skills can have a direct contribution to patient care. In addition, the level of remuneration for pharmacists employed in hospitals tends to be higher than for those employed in community pharmacies (Professional Pharmacists Australia 2021).

An emerging role for hospital pharmacists is to work within accident and emergency departments. Here the pharmacist performs **medication reconciliation** using a systematic process to obtain an accurate and complete list of all medications taken prior to admission to hospital. Evidence suggests that having pharmacists perform medication reconciliation reduces the chances of medication errors (Ciapponi et al. 2021). Medication reconciliation is recommended by the Australian Commission on Safety and Quality in Health Care whenever patients are transferred between settings, both within the hospital and in the transition between hospital and the home or **residential aged-care facility (RACF)**.

Medication Management Reviews by Consultant Pharmacists

Quite a number of pharmacists work independently of community or hospital pharmacies, providing medication management review services. Medication management reviews are funded by the Commonwealth under the Community Pharmacy Agreements and in RACFs are called **residential medication management reviews (RMMRs)**. The pharmacist collaborates with nursing and support staff, medical practitioners and the community pharmacist who supplies the residents' medicines. The RMMR aims to ensure that residents are receiving appropriate medication therapy, including monitoring. A similar service is available for people living at home called **home medicines review (HMR)**.

An RMMR and/or an HMR is initiated with a request from the patient's GP to a pharmacist, who may be their preferred community pharmacist or a **consultant pharmacist** who works independently. The pharmacist generally visits the patient and caregiver(s) at their home for an extended interview regarding medication management issues. Following the visit, the pharmacist sends a written report documenting medication review findings and recommendations to the GP, who then formulates a revised medication management plan with the patient. Pharmacists who perform RMMR and HMR must be accredited by an approved credentialling body.

Pharmacists in Residential Aged-Care Facilities

Pharmacists have a key role in improving medication safety within RACFs. Here, pharmacists may provide RMMR and other services designed to improve the quality use of medicines (QUM). A QUM service has a focus on improving the quality use of medicines by influencing practices and procedures. When performing QUM services, the pharmacist provides medication advisory activities, quality assurance and continuous improvement activities and education for nursing and support staff.

Reducing Sedative Prescribing in Residential Aged-Care Facilities

An area of particular focus on both RMMR and QUM activities in aged-care facilities is to reduce the overall use of medicines that are particularly harmful for the oldest old. One class of medicines that are potentially harmful include antipsychotic medications that are used to manage behavioural and psychological symptoms of dementia. The Royal Commission into Aged Care Safety and Quality (The Commission) highlighted increasing consumers' and health professionals' concerns about the overuse of these medicines to control behaviour. The Commission made a range of recommendations relevant to the role of pharmacists. Several recommendations were designed to broaden access to medication review services, such as making RMMR mandatory on entry to the facility. The Commission also recommended that by 2024, pharmacists (along with other allied health professionals) should be employed by each facility. Here it is worth noting that embedding pharmacists onsite in RACFs has been advocated for by the Pharmaceutical Society of Australia, and particularly after the successful completion of a pilot trial (McDerby et al. 2020). Yet, the **Pharmacy Guild of Australia** submission to The Commission argued against embedding pharmacists, stating that community pharmacists already provide services and that such a proposal would result in duplication.

Pharmacists in Medical Centres

An interesting development in the career options for Australian pharmacists is working onsite in general practices (Sudeshika et al. 2021). In this role, pharmacists have clinical roles in performing medication reviews and supporting GPs with prescribing advice. Collaboration with doctors and practice nurses is facilitated and leads to significant health care improvements for patients (Shaw & Couzos 2021). GP practice pharmacists also provide non-clinical roles, similar to the work in RACFs. Here pharmacists may conduct prescribing audits (otherwise known as medicines use reviews) with feedback to prescribers (see Case study 26.1). Embedding pharmacists results in patients having fewer medication-related problems (Benson et al. 2018). At present, the biggest barrier to having more pharmacists working in GP practices is the lack of a sustainable funding mechanism (Sudeshika et al. 2021).

TOWARDS PRESCRIBING

Many allied health professionals are legally allowed to prescribe medicines. It has been a tenet of our health system that, for most prescription medicines, there is value in separating the role of prescribing from the act of dispensing of a medicine. Given some pharmacists now work in non-supply roles, such as residential care facilities and medical practices, the notion that non-dispensing pharmacists could prescribe has begun to emerge in Australia. In the United Kingdom, pharmacists are able to prescribe with various levels of autonomy, ranging

CASE STUDY 26.1 Interprofessional Practice

Consider the following situation. Chelsea is a non-dispensing pharmacist who works within a medical practice. Each week Chelsea conducts medicines use reviews. How that works is that she picks a therapeutic area and (1) audits the GPs' prescribing practices within that therapeutic area, and (2) provides a short education session on the topic to the GPs and practice nurses. This week, Chelsea has been focusing on osteoporosis. Osteoporosis is a chronic bone disease which needs to be treated for years to help reduce the risk of fractures.

One of the patients identified is Janet, a 68-year-old patient with osteoporosis, thyroid insufficiency, hypertension and nerve pain. Janet had a prescription for Denosumab injection issued 8 months ago and there is a record of it being administered by the practice nurses. However, Denosumab needs to be administered every six months and she has not had another dose. This means that she is 2 months' overdue. This is important because stopping this medicine (without replacement) puts her at risk of vertebral fractures. During her regular GP consultation, Janet explained to the GP that she doesn't really think that having the injection is worth it. The GP asks Janet if she would like to speak to the pharmacist about the injection. Janet agrees and immediately afterwards has a consultation with the pharmacist, Chelsea. Chelsea and Janet talk for some time about osteoporosis and Denosumab. Chelsea uses motivational interviewing to uncover that Janet is quite concerned about a very rare side effect whereby dental problems can cause an alarming jaw disease. Chelsea also mentions to the GP that Janet is using a medicine called Amitriptyline for nerve pain, which can lead to falls

(and increases the chance of a fracture). The GP, Chelsea and Janet discuss this. The GP arranges for the practice nurse to assist Janet with a dental check-up and then implements the pharmacist's recommendation for a slow withdrawal of Amitriptyline.

It would be interesting to use Tuohy's 'accidental logics' (see Chapter 1) to explore how the non-dispensing pharmacist working in medical centres remains unfunded by the Commonwealth, while funding is provided for those working in aged care. Perhaps this has arisen from the principle of 'separation of prescribing from dispensing', a phrase coined as early as 1921 (Braithwaite 1921). It means that the prescriber cannot be the dispenser (except under limited circumstances). This two-step process is meant to promote safety and to minimise opportunity for commercial incentives to drive prescribing behaviours. Matching the two-step process, Commonwealth funding for community medical services is made through the MBS while funding for dispensing is made through the PBS. As the role of the pharmacist has expanded to include non-dispensing services provided in the community and in aged care, funding has been made available through the PBS (using Community Pharmacy Agreements), not under the MBS. Perhaps as a sign of things to come, the federal budget for 2022 has allocated $345 million over 4 years to provide onsite pharmacists to address the poor medication practices uncovered in The Royal Commission Report (mentioned above). That funding is not provided through either the PBS or the MBS. It will be interesting to see how the funding of non-dispensing pharmacists in medical practices is resolved.

from prescribing under direct supervision by a medical practitioner to fully independent prescribing within their clinical specialty. Currently, the Pharmacy Board of Australia state that there is no national regulatory barrier to pharmacists prescribing under supervision, within an arrangement referred to as 'collaborative healthcare

environment' (Pharmacy Board of Australia 2019). What such arrangements refer to is yet to be worked through. Nevertheless, there are significant barriers at the state and territory levels. It is difficult to gauge the appetite that the health system has for autonomous prescribing by pharmacists in Australia at this stage.

SUMMARY

The emerging role of pharmacists as members of the health care team is at a critical stage in history. Australian pharmacists and the health system in general will benefit by finding new and equitable ways to make better use of pharmacists' unique skills. When

reviewing the content of this chapter, we can reflect on how:

- consumers, governments and other third-party payers may not have formed clear expectations about the emerging role of the clinical pharmacist

- the Pharmaceutical Society of Australia advocates that pharmacists should be provided with Medicare provider numbers for payments through the MBS, similar to most other health professionals

- pharmacists working within medical practices, clinics and residential care facilities will become more commonplace.

REVIEW QUESTIONS

1. Describe the range of activities that a community pharmacist provides within a community pharmacy.
2. Compare the opportunities for interprofessional collaboration with other members of the health care team for hospital pharmacists with those of a community pharmacist.
3. Considering the training and skills of pharmacists, and reflecting on your own experience with pharmacists, to what extent are Australians making the most use of pharmacists' expertise?
4. How could we use Carol Bacchi's model to redefine the problem of sedative use in residential aged-care facilities?

REFERENCES

Australian Government Depart of Health and Ageing, 2022. Review of the National Medicines Policy – Consultation on the draft of the National Medicines Policy. https://www.pbs.gov.au/info/news/2022/02/review-of-the-national-medicines-policy-consultation.

Australian Government Department of Health, 2019. Pharmacists factsheet. https://hwd.health.gov.au/resources/publications/factsheet-alld-2019.html.

Basak, R., Bentley, J.P., Mccaffrey, D.J., et al., 2015. The role of perceived impact on relationship quality in pharmacists' willingness to influence indication-based off-label prescribing decisions. Soc Sci Med 132, 181–189.

Benson, H., Lucas, C., Benrimoj, S.I., et al., 2018. Pharmacists in general practice: recommendations resulting from team-based collaborative care. Aust J Prim Health 24, 448–454.

Braithwaite, J.O., 1921. The separation of prescribing and dispensing. Lancet 197, 459.

Cairns, R., Schaffer, A.L., Brown, J.A., et al., 2020. Codeine use and harms in Australia: evaluating the effects of rescheduling. Addiction 115, 451–459.

Carter, S.R., Ng, R., El-den, S., et al., 2021. A patient-reported experience measure for community pharmacy including development of a short-form: the perceived service quality scale. Res Social Adm Pharm 18 (8), 3369–3378. doi:10.1016/j.sapharm.2021.11.011.

Ciapponi, A., Fernandez Nievas, S.E., Seijo, M., et al., 2021. Reducing medication errors for adults in hospital settings. Cochrane Database Syst Rev 25 11(11): CD009985. doi:10.1002/14651858.CD009985.pub2.

Clun, R., 2020. Turf war: pharmacists will deliver COVID-19 vaccine despite GP concerns. Sydney Morning Herald, 9 December. https://www.smh.com.au/politics/federal/turf-war-pharmacists-will-deliver-covid-19-vaccine-despite-gp-concerns-20201207-p56ldv.html.

Collins, J.C., Chong, W.W., De Almeida Neto, A.C., et al., 2021. The simulated patient method: design and application in health services research. Res Social Adm Pharm 17, 2108–2115.

Dineen-Griffin, S., Vargas, C., Williams, K.A., et al., 2020. Cost utility of a pharmacist-led minor ailment service compared with usual pharmacist care. Cost Eff Resour Alloc 18, 24.

Dow, A., 2018. Pharmacists and doctors trade jabs over the best time to get flu shot. Sydney Morning Herald, 29 March. https://www.smh.com.au/healthcare/pharmacists-and-doctors-trade-jabs-over-the-best-time-to-get-flu-shot-20180328-p4z6ne.html.

Haines, S., Prathivadi, P., 2021. Evaluation of Australian prescription drug monitoring programs need a holistic approach. Aust J Prim Health 27, 354–356.

Ilardo, M.L., Speciale, A., 2020. The community pharmacist: perceived barriers and patient-centered care communication. Int J Environ Res Public Health 17, 536.

Jayawardana, S., Forman, R., Johnston-Webber, C., et al., 2021. Global consumption of prescription opioid analgesics between 2009–2019: a country-level observational study. eClinicalMedicine, 42.

Jones, A., 2022. NSW pharmacists pull out of COVID vaccinations and free RATs amid payment battle. ABC News, 10 February. https://www.abc.net.au/news/2022-02-10/pharmacist-pay-disparity-child-vaccination/100800400.

Kosari, S., Buss, V.H., Peterson, G.M., et al., 2020. Evaluation of pharmaceutical compounding training in the Australian undergraduate Pharmacy curricula. Pharmacy 8, 27.

Lim, R., Ellett, L.M.K., Semple, S., et al., 2022. The extent of medication-related hospital admissions in Australia: a review from 1988 to 2021. Drug Safety.

Loo, J., Greaves, G., Lewis, P.J., 2021. Exploring patients' pharmacy stories: an analysis of online feedback. Int J Clin Pharm 43, 1584–1593.

Lubi, K., Sepp, K., Rass, H., et al., 2021. A qualitative study of the challenges in rearranging community pharmacy service provision during the COVID-19 public health emergency: the prism of social practice theory. Public Health in Practice 2, 100212.

McDerby, N., Kosari, S., Bail, K., et al., 2020. Residential aged care pharmacist: an australian pilot trial exploring the impact on quality use of medicines indicators. Medicines 7.

Morgan, T.K., Williamson, M., Pirotta, M., et al., 2012. A national census of medicines use: a 24-hour snapshot of Australians aged 50 years and older. Med J Aust, 196, 50–53.

Paola, S. 2020. It's already making a difference. Aust J Pharm 101, 20–22.

Pharmaceutical Society of Australia, 2017. Professional practice standards version 5. http://www.psa.org.au/supporting-practice/professional-practice-standards/version-4.

Pharmaceutical Society of Australia, 2019. Dispensing practice guidelines. https://www.psa.org.au/wp-content/uploads/2019/06/5574-PSA-Dispensing-Practice-guidelines_FINAL.pdf.

Pharmacy Board of Australia, 2019. Pharmacist prescribing – position statement. https://www.pharmacyboard.gov.au/news/professional-practice-issues/pharmacist-prescribing-position-statement.aspx.

Pharmacy Council of New South Wales, 2019. Think before you compound that medicine. https://www.pharmacy-council.nsw.gov.au/think-you-compound-medicine.

Professional Pharmacists Australia, 2021. Community and hospital pharmacists employment and remuneration report. https://members.professionalsaustralia.org.au/documents/ppa/2021Community_and_Hospital_Pharmacists_Remuneration_Report.pdf.

Shaw, C., Couzos, S., 2021. Integration of non-dispensing pharmacists into primary healthcare services: an umbrella review and narrative synthesis of the effect on patient outcomes. Aust J Gen Pract 50, 403–408.

Sim, T.F., Hattingh, H.L., Sunderland, B., et al., 2020. Effective communication and collaboration with health professionals: a qualitative study of primary care pharmacists in Western Australia. PLOS ONE 15, e0234580.

Sudeshika, T., Naunton, M., Deeks, L.S., 2021. General practice pharmacists in Australia: a systematic review. PLOS ONE, 16, e0258674.

Trent, M.J., Salmon, D.A., MacIntyre, C.R., 2021. Pharmacy, workplace or primary care? Where Australian adults get their influenza vaccines. Aust N Z J Public Health 45, 385–390.

Vadiei, N., Eldridge, L.A., Meyerson, B.E., et al., 2022. "The gatekeepers in prevention": community pharmacist perceptions of their role in the opioid epidemic. Subst Abus 43, 319–327.

World Health Organization, 2021. WHO model list of essential medicines 22th list. http://www.who.int/medicines/publications/essentialmedicines/en/.

Wylie, C.E., Daniels, B., Brett, J., et al., 2020. A national study on prescribed medicine use in Australia on a typical day. Pharmacoepidemiol Drug Saf 29, 1046–1053.

Zielińska-Tomczak, Ł., Cerbin-Koczorowska, M., Przymuszała, P., et al., 2021. How to effectively promote interprofessional collaboration? A qualitative study on physicians' and pharmacists' perspectives driven by the theory of planned behavior. BMC Health Services Research 21, 903.

FURTHER READING

International Pharmaceutical Federation (FIP), 2020. Transforming the global pharmaceutical workforce. https://www.fip.org/workforce.

ONLINE RESOURCES

Royal Commission into Aged Care Quality and Safety: https://agedcare.royalcommission.gov.au/.

Australian Commission on Safety and Quality in Healthcare – medication safety: http://www.safetyandquality.gov.au/our-work/medication-safety/.

Australian Government Department of Health and Aged Care – What we're doing about medicines: https://www1.health.gov.au/internet/main/publishing.nsf/Content/New-7th-Community-Pharmacy-Agreement.

Seventh Community Pharmacy Agreement: https://www.health.gov.au/resources/publications/budget-2020-21-improving-access-to-medicines-seventh-community-pharmacy-agreement.

Pharmaceutical Society of Australia: http://www.psa.org.au/.

Pharmacy Board of Australia: http://www.pharmacyboard.gov.au/.

Pharmacy Guild of Australia: http://www.guild.org.au/.

Society of Hospital Pharmacists of Australia: http://shpa.org.au/.

27

Health Profession Regulation: The Case of Physiotherapy

Matthew Sutton

KEY LEARNING OUTCOMES

When you finish this chapter you should be able to:

- describe the roles and purpose of the physiotherapy profession
- describe a brief history of the physiotherapy profession in Australia
- outline the various clinical fields in which physiotherapists work in the Australian health care system and the career structure in the public and private sectors
- define the roles of the relevant regulatory and professional bodies for the physiotherapy profession in Australia
- describe the requirements for registration as a physiotherapist
- discuss the advantages and ways in which physiotherapists may work in a multidisciplinary environment
- discuss the challenges facing the physiotherapy profession and the opportunities for further development
- discuss future directions for the practice of physiotherapy.

KEY TERMS AND ABBREVIATIONS

Australian Health Practitioner Regulation Agency (Ahpra)
Australian Physiotherapy Association (APA)
Australian Physiotherapy Council (APC)

Chronic Disease Management (CDM)
continuing professional development (CPD)
emergency department (ED)
extended-scope physiotherapist (ESP)

interprofessional practice (IPP)
Physiotherapy Board of Australia (PBA)
primary-contact practitioners (PCPs)
team care arrangement (TCA)
World Physiotherapy

INTRODUCTION

Founded in 1951, **World Physiotherapy** (formally World Confederation for Physical Therapy) is recognised as the global body that represents the profession of physiotherapy. It provides the following definition of the roles of physiotherapy:

Physical therapy [physiotherapy] is services provided by physical therapists to individuals and populations to develop, maintain and restore maximum movement and functional ability throughout the life-span. The service is provided in circumstances where movement and function are threatened by ageing, injury, pain, diseases, disorders, conditions and/or environmental factors and with the understanding that functional movement is central to what it means to be healthy.

(World Physiotherapy 2019, p. 1)

The terms 'physical therapy' and 'physiotherapy' are used interchangeably and are dependent on the country of practice. In Australia, the term 'physiotherapy' is the accepted nomenclature for the profession.

The profession of physiotherapy focuses on the assessment and management of human movement and function. Physiotherapists have a role across the entire life-span, from neonatal intensive-care units working with premature babies through to assisting function and quality of life in elderly and palliative care environments at the end of life. Physiotherapists work across a range of health care settings, with the primary aim of improving the quality of life of the people, or clients, they are treating.

HISTORY

The physiotherapy profession has evolved significantly over time. Physiotherapy in Australia developed from a massage-based profession established by the formation of the Australasian Massage Association in 1906 (McMeeken 2017). This became recognised as the professional body for physiotherapists, and in 1938 became the **Australian Physiotherapy Association (APA)**. The role of the physiotherapist has evolved, largely in relation to societal demands, with the title 'physiotherapist' being adopted in the mid 1920s. The World Wars (1914–18 and 1939–45) resulted in mass casualties returning from service, requiring a greater emphasis on rehabilitation following injury. In between these wars, the poliomyelitis epidemic resulted in a further demand for the services of physiotherapists (McMeeken 2014). The role of the physiotherapist has been shaped in more recent times by the emphasis on evidence-based practice (EBP), as well as the rise in prevalence of chronic diseases such as osteoarthritis, diabetes and cardiorespiratory conditions.

One of the most significant events in the physiotherapy profession in Australia occurred on 14 August 1976 (Chipchase et al. 2006) – the establishment of primary-contact status. This allowed people to be treated by a physiotherapist without needing a referral by a doctor and provided the profession with significantly increased autonomy. Australia was the first country to enact this change, which resulted in significantly greater autonomy for the profession.

REGISTRATION PATHWAY AND REQUIREMENTS

The first university course to provide an educational pathway for the physiotherapy profession was established in 1938. This was a 3-year Diploma program (Forster 1969). World Physiotherapy has since established the minimum duration of education required to become a physiotherapist to be 4 years. Australia has incorporated this guideline into all national curricula, and all physiotherapy Bachelor's programs are now of 4 years equivalent duration. In the late 1990s, the APA endorsed the introduction of graduate-entry physiotherapy programs (Chipchase et al. 2006). These programs are typically 2 years in duration for a Master's degree and 3 years for a Doctoral degree qualification. There are currently 24 universities across Australia offering physiotherapy programs, with undergraduate, graduate-entry masters and Doctoral programs available (**Australian Health Practitioner Regulation Agency (Ahpra)** 2022).

In Australia, the professional title of 'physiotherapist' is protected by legislation. This means that only those that have graduated from an accredited program can bestow this title upon themselves. Additionally, in order to practise as a physiotherapist, registration must be renewed annually. To maintain registration, physiotherapists must participate in ongoing education, referred to as **continuing professional development (CPD)**. The minimum requirement for CPD is 20 hours per year of relevant educational activities.

Despite registration being a nationally administered process, legislation remains state/territory based. Legislation provides the framework by which physiotherapists are able to practise. For example, according to most state legislation in Australia, physiotherapists are able to use acupuncture as a treatment. However, there are other treatments that are prohibited by legislation. For example, physiotherapists are unable to prescribe medications in Australia.

RELEVANT PROFESSIONAL AND REGULATORY BODIES

Physiotherapy accreditation and registration are overseen by the **Australian Physiotherapy Council (APC)** and the Australian Health Practitioner Regulation Agency (Ahpra). The **Physiotherapy Board of Australia (PBA)** is one of the most important regulatory organisations for the physiotherapy profession and exists as a sub-branch of Ahpra. The role of the PBA is to administer and manage the registration of physiotherapists and students and develop the code of conduct by which registered physiotherapists must abide as part of professional practice. This code is based on the four ethical principles of autonomy, beneficence (providing a positive health outcome), non-maleficence (doing no harm) and justice. It is also the role of the PBA to manage complaints and notifications made against physiotherapists. Further detail on the roles of the PBA can be found online.

The APA is the national professional body that represents physiotherapists and plays a key role in advocating for the rights and progression of the physiotherapy profession. While membership of the APA is voluntary, it plays an important role in the establishment of CPD programs. The APA has national special-interest groups – for example, cardiorespiratory, palliative care, disability, women's, men's and pelvic health, mental health, musculoskeletal and neurology. A full list of the special-interest groups is available via the APA website.

Pause *for* Reflection …

As you can see, physiotherapists do much more than manage musculoskeletal disorders. Were you aware the profession was involved in the management of a range of other conditions and populations such as managing incontinence, helping people with respiratory problems or helping to allow people to stay in their own homes as they age? If you were a physiotherapist, what area would interest you to practise in? Consider either the types of conditions you would like to treat (e.g. musculoskeletal, respiratory, neurological), or what populations (paediatric or aged care, for example).

CURRENT STATUS OF PHYSIOTHERAPY

Physiotherapists most commonly pursue a pathway into clinical practice. There are three core clinical areas in which entry-level Australian physiotherapists are commonly trained: musculoskeletal, neurological and cardiorespiratory physiotherapy. However, physiotherapists also develop expertise in many other areas such as the APA national specialty areas listed above. Physiotherapists work in private, public and non-government organisations (NGOs) or community organisations and across rural, regional and metropolitan settings.

The introduction of Ahpra in 2010 enabled for the first time the collection of reliable demographic and epidemiological data across Australia for the profession of physiotherapy. In 2014, Health Workforce Australia (HWA 2014) released a report providing the most detailed and accurate information on Australia's physiotherapy workforce ever seen up until this time. Since then, the National Health Workforce Data Set (NHWDS) has provided this information through a combination of survey and registration renewal data. These data showed that in 2019 there were 34,844 registered physiotherapists, with 29,508 of these currently in paid employment as physiotherapists. A snapshot of the profession showed the following facts for the workforce in 2019:

- 81% worked in metropolitan areas
- 64% were female
- average age was 38 years
- 0.7% identified as Aboriginal and/or Torres Strait Islander
- 72% were born in Australia.

The clinical workforce had seen a yearly compound growth rate of 6%, since 2015 with an increase of just under 6000 physiotherapists in that five-year period (Australian Government 2019). Of the entire physiotherapy workforce, 92% worked primarily in a clinical role, with 53% of these reporting their principal scope of practice as musculoskeletal, followed by 15% working in aged care.

There has been a trend of increased participation in the private workforce, with a corresponding decrease in the public sector. In 2019, 72% of the workforce was working in the private sector, with 28% working in the public sector. From 2015 to 2019, this represents a reduction of just under 3% of the workforce reporting working in the public sector, with a corresponding increase in private-sector participation of nearly 3% (Australian Government 2019).

WORKING IN THE PUBLIC HEALTH CARE SYSTEM

Physiotherapists working in the public health care system in Australia do so predominantly in a hospital environment. This provides the opportunity to work across a range of clinical areas. In the hospital setting, early-career physiotherapists will gain experience in the core clinical areas of musculoskeletal, cardiorespiratory and neurological physiotherapy and may also be introduced to other areas such as paediatrics, orthopaedics, gerontology and women's health. It is through this pathway that many physiotherapists develop a broad range of skills and gain experience in a variety of clinical areas.

Physiotherapists in the public system may also work in primary care as community-based physiotherapists. In these roles, they may work in a community health service or supported residential facility (SRF), or visit people's places of residence to assist with optimising functional abilities and quality of life.

While the physiotherapy profession has a national registration structure, public salaries and awards are state/territory based. These are negotiated between employers and the relevant unions through the enterprise bargaining process, which occurs around every 3 years. Although wages and conditions differ across states and territories, there exist some general consistencies. The first band or grade of physiotherapists generally has less than 4–5 years of post-registration clinical experience and works across a range of clinical areas. Physiotherapists working in the second band are starting to develop expertise in a particular clinical area and are expected to work with less direct supervision. It is not uncommon for second-band physiotherapists to also continue to work in a range of fields. Band three physiotherapists are considered to have developed expertise in their clinical area and provide supervision to staff and consultation in this area. More recently, with the development of advanced-practice and extended scope of practice roles, physiotherapy is seeing the development of clinical roles in bands four and five, when previously these bands were largely restricted to management positions.

WORKING IN THE PRIVATE HEALTH CARE SYSTEM

The majority of physiotherapists working in the private sector do so in private-practice clinics as **primary-contact practitioners (PCPs)**, predominantly in the area of musculoskeletal physiotherapy (Australian Government 2019). Other clinical specialties in which physiotherapists work privately include women's health, paediatrics and aged care. Physiotherapists also work in private hospitals and undertake occupational health roles for private companies.

Private-practice physiotherapists regularly treat people without first getting a referral from a doctor. This model provides a significant degree of autonomy, but it carries a greater degree of risk. For example, many people will see a physiotherapist for lower-back pain without first visiting their local doctor. In an extremely small percentage of people, lower-back pain may be caused by a serious health condition such as cancer, an aortic aneurysm or a deep infection. Consequently, physiotherapists must have adequate training and expertise to be able to recognise signs of serious pathology and refer to a doctor or **emergency department (ED)** for appropriate management. Additionally, physiotherapists need to have the expertise to identify other serious pathologies such as fractures after trauma – for example, an ankle injury sustained while playing sport. To facilitate this, physiotherapists are able to order X-rays that are partly funded by the federal government through Medicare.

So who pays for services provided by the private health sector? For physiotherapists, this is no different to many other health care professionals: they use a fee-for-service system. The fees charged by physiotherapists are largely driven by market forces. In contrast to the Australian Medical Association (AMA), the APA does not provide a recommended fee schedule. Comcare, the national work health and safety and workers' compensation authority, provides a guide for the rates to be charged for physiotherapy services, with significant variation from state to state. For example, an initial consultation in South Australia is $85, however, in the Northern Territory it attracts $121–$151 (Australian Government 2021). If users have private health insurance cover, they will be reimbursed a percentage of the total fee. Since 2000, many private practices have become 'preferred providers' for private health insurers. In return for the private health insurer recommending the services of a particular practice, the user will pay a smaller gap between the consultation fee and the rebate from the insurer. It is worth noting that 'preferred-provider' status is not directly related to the quality of care provided, but simply a willingness of the practice to be contractually obliged to reduce fees for any members of that particular private insurance company. There has been considerable debate within the profession regarding the advantages of being involved in such a system, as while it potentially increases the number of people seen by a practice it also reduces revenue per customer. The APA has concerns that such preferred-provider arrangements will potentially lead to an imbalance of power between small physiotherapy practices and private health insurers in Australia. The insurance company, not the physiotherapist, sets the fees and potentially reduces revenue per client. Additionally, there is no obvious justifiable reason for assigning a higher rebate to preferred providers with respect to either improved health outcomes or greater clinical expertise. This practice also has the potential to drive prices down across the entire industry in order for practices to compete at a financial level. Consequently, physiotherapy practices are investing in other means to improve services. It is now not uncommon for practices to have purpose-built gymnasiums, including aquatic physiotherapy facilities. Physiotherapy practice business models have also undergone significant change in this time. Historically, private practices were largely managed by a sole practitioner but Australia has seen the emergence of franchise-style practices over the last 10 to 15 years.

Third-party funders are often a significant source of revenue for physiotherapy private-practice clinics and organisations. These are funded by either the state in the case of compensable clients, such as Workcover and compulsory third-party (CTP) insurance, or the federal government for Department of Veterans' Affairs (DVA) and the National Disability Insurance Scheme (NDIS). These all have very different funding models and fee structures. Additionally, these schemes in general do not recognise any additional career development or education a clinician has undertaken, such as a postgraduate Master's degree, when setting fee structures.

In 1999, the federal government, via Medicare, introduced the Enhanced Primary Care (EPC) scheme in recognition of the increased prevalence of chronic disease. This was renamed the **Chronic Disease Management (CDM)** schedule in 2005. Through this scheme, private-practice physiotherapists were able to receive funding for services from the federal government for the first time. A GP is required to initially assess a client with a chronic condition such as diabetes or osteoarthritis and implement a **team care arrangement (TCA)**, which may include services from a physiotherapist or other allied health professional. To be eligible for a TCA, at least three health care professionals (including the GP) need to be involved in the management of the client. A maximum of five visits to allied health professionals in a single year is funded. The health care and funding model that provides the framework for managing this increasing population has not evolved in over 15 years. There was an increase of 240% in the number of physiotherapy consultations providing musculoskeletal services to older adults from 2009 to 2018 (Orrock et al. 2020) indicating a strong demand for this service.

In 2015–16 there were over six million allied health consultations provided under this scheme, of which 31% were provided by physiotherapists, second only to podiatrists (41%) (Duckett 2018). While this scheme was widely acknowledged as a positive step towards addressing chronic disease through a multidisciplinary approach, there has been criticism that the number of visits funded is insufficient to significantly improve health outcomes in a population with complex health needs (Mitchell et al. 2017). This can be illustrated by considering an elderly person with both diabetes and osteoarthritis. There is strong evidence to support interventions provided by physiotherapists, occupational therapists (OTs), dietitians, podiatrists and exercise physiologists (Gwynne-Jones et al. 2018; Jayakumar 2019; O'Leary et al. 2018). However, with only a total of five visits allowed in a single year across all allied health professionals, there would obviously be considerable rationalisation of which services to select. Indeed, the client might be able to see a physiotherapist only once or twice under such circumstances. A therapist's ability to provide a meaningful and effective intervention may be impaired, potentially compromising the patient outcome.

Pause *for* Reflection ...

As we have seen, physiotherapists working in private practice attract their clients from a variety of sources and schemes, including privately insured clients, third-party compensable schemes and as part of a team care arrangement (TCA), funded directly through Medicare. Consider two clients both seeing a physiotherapist due to chronic lower-back pain. One is funded by a third-party insurer and eligible for an indeterminate number of consultations, and one is funded by a TCA and only able to see you on one or two occasions as they are also seeing a dietitian. As the physiotherapist, would this influence how you manage the client? If so, how and why?

INTERPROFESSIONAL PRACTICE – THE ROLE OF PHYSIOTHERAPY

There is growing acknowledgement within the health care sector of the importance of effective interprofessional teams to deliver high-quality care. As a result, there is increasing emphasis on physiotherapists working in interprofessional models of care, alongside doctors, nurses and other allied health professionals. **Interprofessional practice (IPP)** is 'the process in which different professional groups work together to positively impact health' (Zwarenstein et al. 2009, p. 2). As its name suggests, a multidisciplinary team is one in which a number of health care professionals are involved in a client's care. The distinction for an interprofessional collaborative model of care is that this involves a model in which all health professionals associated with a client's care work collaboratively, with effective communication, common goal-setting and a client-centred approach. The members of an interprofessional care team vary widely. For example, a physiotherapist working in a specialist pain management unit may work collaboratively with psychologists, psychiatrists, pain specialists, nurses, occupational therapists, pharmacists, dentists and social workers (Gordon et al. 2018); in a neurological rehabilitation facility managing people with stroke the health care team might include neurologists, neurosurgeons, rehabilitation specialists, occupational therapists, speech therapists, dietitians and nurses. Case study 27.1 provides a detailed example of an IPP model of care.

FUTURE DIRECTIONS

Perhaps one of the most likely progressions in the way physiotherapy services will be delivered in the future is in the field of telerehabilitation. This is a service provided to a client without direct face-to-face consultation, instead being carried out via a mobile, or other electronic device such as a laptop computer. This has obvious advantages for the client from an accessibility perspective with many populations potentially benefitting, for example, someone with a significant mobility

---

CASE STUDY 27.1   Interprofessional Models of Care

Ted is a 68-year-old man living with his wife in a two-bedroom home. While dressing in the morning he suffered a large cerebral vascular accident (CVA), or stroke, and was taken to the hospital by ambulance. After 10 days in hospital he was discharged to an inpatient rehabilitation facility. At this time, Ted was partly paralysed on his left arm and leg (hemiplegia), had difficulty speaking (dysphasia) and swallowing (dysphagia), as well as significant cognitive impairment including short-term memory loss and difficulty processing information. Additionally, he contracted COVID-19 while at the hospital. His wife was extremely upset and distressed at the situation, particularly as Ted was very fit and healthy prior to the stroke. They used to walk for over 60 minutes together daily and spent much time working in the garden together. He needed assistance getting in and out of bed and chair, and was unable to walk independently, even with a walking aid.

On the first day of his stay at the rehab facility, he was seen by the physiotherapist. They talked with Ted and his wife to understand their goals and concerns, then assessed Ted's ability to walk, get in and out of chairs and bed, balance and the strength of his limbs. Additionally, the physiotherapist listened to Ted's lungs and breathing patterns to determine any ongoing issues associated with his previous COVID-19 diagnosis that might impact on his ability to participate in his treatment. Following this, the physiotherapist met with the rest of Ted's health care team which included an occupational therapist, speech pathologist, dietician, medical officer, social worker, psychologist and nurse to discuss their assessment and collaboratively develop a management plan with both Ted and his wife involved. Planning involved refining the treatments each professional had developed, establishing a strategy to ensure they were timed during the day to maximise Ted's outcomes and not overly fatigue him, particularly given his ongoing recovery from COVID-19, and wherever possible, arrange co-treatment such as working on arm function during eating and drinking tasks, which would involve multiple health professions. A key challenge was that Ted got very fatigued due to his conditions and was only able to engage in therapy for 20 minutes at a time. Consequently, the health professionals had to prioritise what areas they would work on for any given day. This required each health professional to compromise their therapy to some degree. For example, the physiotherapist was unable to spend more than 10 minutes at a time working with Ted to improve his walking to ensure he had sufficient energy to work on his other functional and cognitive tasks. At times, this led to some conflict between the health professionals involved, and also caused some anguish for Ted's wife who felt he was not spending enough time working on his walking and mobility therapy. In order to help address these issues, regular team meetings were required, with the social worker in frequent communication with both Ted and his wife to keep them updated and provide feedback to the rest of the team.

disability, those living in remote regions, and indeed any client who would benefit from the convenience of being able to have a physiotherapy consultation during a lunchtime at work. There are obvious advantages in being able to have a face-to-face consultation, particularly when an assessment of physical movement is generally an important component of most physiotherapy consultations, along with manual therapy supplementing many management strategies. However, with an ever-increasing focus on education and exercise therapy as critical management strategies within the profession, along with improvements in remote video technology, the demand for telerehabilitation services is likely to increase over the next decade. The focus on telerehabilitation services greatly increased during the SARS-CoV-2 pandemic, which meant many physiotherapy practices were unable to conduct face-to-face consultations, and many clients were unable or unwilling to attend due to either quarantine restrictions or the increased risk of contracting COVID-19 associated with increased social activity. As a result of this, many electronic platforms were developed to improve accessibility, functionality and security issues associated with telerehabilitation in the community. There is increasing evidence to support the effectiveness of telerehabilitation as a modality (Seron et al. 2021; Van Egmond et al. 2018; Wang et al. 2021) and with more health insurers agreeing to fund these services, it would seem the growth of telerehabilitation is inevitable. It is, however, unlikely to ever completely replace the role of face-to-face services given the therapeutic value of physical touch, a greater ability to perform more complex assessments and the superior communication experience of a face-to-face interaction.

Virtual Reality

The field of virtual and augmented reality continues to expand in both physiotherapy practice and education. There is a huge range of potential applications across clinical populations and settings. Private health insurers in Australia have run trials to incorporate virtual reality into telerehabilitation services to improve the overall client experience, signalling their intention to endorse physiotherapists adopting this technology into practice. However, what remains to be seen is both the funding model the industry implements as well as the specific service delivery model physiotherapists will be required to use to attract insurer funding.

Another field that has embraced the use of virtual reality (VR) is the management of people who have experienced a neurological event such as stroke or brain injury. Key principles of rehabilitation exercises for people with neurological disorders is to maximise the frequency and number of repetitions, and to ensure the exercises are task oriented, for example shopping in a supermarket. VR facilitates all of these principles and provides a safe and accessible environment for people to work within. VR also provides the ability to easily alter the degree of difficulty of any exercise to ensure it is neither too easy nor too challenging, which also optimises treatment effectiveness. There is an increasing body of evidence for the use of VR when used in conjunction with usual care to improve the level of function for people with neurological disorders for both upper and lower limb activities as well as improved balance, all of which are critical outcomes to improve the quality of life for this population (Juras et al. 2019; Laver et al. 2018).

DRIVERS FOR CHANGE – EXPANDING THE SCOPE OF PRACTICE

There is growing international recognition that, to deliver sustainable health care into the future, new and innovative models of care need to be developed requiring a shift in traditional professional boundaries by changing current scopes of practice (Duckett et al. 2014; Somerville et al. 2018). This shift in boundaries includes both the development of **extended-scope physiotherapist (ESP)** roles, allowing health professions to take on roles previously undertaken by other professions, and the shifting of tasks from qualified physiotherapists to physiotherapy assistants.

An increasing aged population in Australia has contributed to medical services struggling to meet demand. Two examples of how this is influencing the health system are an increase in waiting times to see medical specialists and increasing demands on EDs. These two issues have been a key driver for the development of new roles for physiotherapists in Australia over the past 15 years. Physiotherapists have expanded their scope of practice to take on roles traditionally undertaken by the medical profession in order to cost-effectively improve productivity in an increasingly strained health care system. An example of an advanced- or extended-practice role is the use of physiotherapists in the ED. Physiotherapists in these roles are able to manage a cohort of patients presenting to hospital EDs without a doctor needing to assess them. Presentations suitable to be managed by a physiotherapist are most commonly minor trauma involving soft-tissue injuries, lower-back pain, uncomplicated bone fractures or vestibular disorders. Studies have consistently shown that people managed by a physiotherapist are seen faster and spend significantly less time in the hospital than if they had been seen by a doctor (Henderson et al. 2020; Sayer et al. 2017,). Physiotherapists have, additionally, expanded into roles that reduce waiting times for specialist outpatient appointments – for example, assessing people waiting to see an orthopaedic specialist due to hip, knee, shoulder or back problems and providing an appropriate management plan. Health services that have implemented these services have shown reductions in their waiting times to see a specialist (Samsson et al. 2020).

> **Pause *for* Reflection ...**
>
> Long COVID, or post-COVID syndrome, affects around 5% of people diagnosed with COVID-19 in Australia with ongoing symptoms after three months (Liu et al. 2021). While studies assessing the effectiveness of exercise on the outcomes of long COVID are yet to provide evidence of efficacy, World Physiotherapy and other professional bodies such as the Royal Australian College of General Practitioners are advising patients to undertake rehabilitation strategies that incorporate safe exercise and/or physical activity while closely monitoring any ongoing symptoms.
>
> * Considering that both physiotherapists and exercise physiologists deliver exercise and physical activity interventions, how do you think each would differ in their approach?
> * How could both professions work together? Consider the expertise both professions have in the fields of exercise and cardiorespiratory function.

SUMMARY

This chapter has provided a broad outline of the role of the physiotherapy profession within the Australian health care system.

* Physiotherapists play an important role in the delivery of health care services in Australia.
* There are many clinical fields in which physiotherapists work, including musculoskeletal, cardiorespiratory, neurological, paediatric, women's health, occupational health, community and palliative care.
* The roles of physiotherapists have evolved significantly in the 20th century, owing to factors such as the World

Wars, poliomyelitis, the introduction of evidence-based practice, the advent of primary-contact status and the increase in prevalence of chronic diseases.

* Physiotherapy accreditation and registration are overseen by the Australian Physiotherapy Council (APC) and the Australian Health Practitioner Regulation Agency.
* Physiotherapists work in many different health environments, including public, private and non-government organisations.
* Professional practice will continue to evolve through the increased use of telehealth-type services and VR.

REVIEW QUESTIONS

1. If you were asked by someone what a physiotherapist does, how would you answer? Consider not only the potential roles of a physiotherapist, but also the types of conditions and populations seen, as well as some strategies physiotherapists use to treat people.
2. Outline some of the key differences in the roles performed by a public and a private physiotherapist (in the same clinical field, e.g. musculoskeletal).
3. Physiotherapists are able to see people without the need of a referral from a doctor (referred to as 'primary-contact practitioners'). Think of three advantages and three disadvantages of having this status.
4. If the current trend of an increasing private health physiotherapy workforce continues, what changes in skills and knowledge will be required to be a successful physiotherapist?
5. Consider a patient who has had a severe stroke and is finding it difficult to perform their daily functions, such as walking and dressing. What potential benefits can you identify for incorporating telehealth and virtual reality into their physiotherapy management?

REFERENCES

Australian Government, 2019. 2019 physiotherapists. Australian Government, Canberra. https://hwd.health.gov.au/resources/publications/factsheet-alld-physiotherapists-2019.pdf.

Australian Government, 2021. *Rates for medical and allied health treatment.* Australian Government, Canberra. https://www.comcare.gov.au/service-providers/medical-allied-health/treatment-rates.

Australian Health Practitioner Regulation Agency (Ahpra), 2022. Approved programs of study. Ahpra, Melbourne. https://www.ahpra.gov.au/Accreditation/Approved-Programs-of-Study.aspx?ns=1.

Chipchase, L.S., Galley, P., Jull, G., et al. 2006. Looking back at 100 years of physiotherapy education in Australia. Aust J Physiother 52 (1), 3–7.

Duckett, S., Breadon, P., Farmer, J., 2014. Unlocking skills in hospitals: better jobs, more care. Grattan Institute, Melbourne.

Duckett, S., 2018. Expanding the breadth of Medicare: learning from Australia. Health Econ Policy Law 13 (3–4), 344–368.

Forster, A., 1969. Physiotherapy in Australia. Aust J Physiother 15 (3), 96–99.

Gordon, D.B., Watt-Watson, J., Hogans, B.B., 2018. Interprofessional pain education–with, from, and about competent, collaborative practice teams to transform pain care. Pain Reports 3 (3).

Gwynne-Jones, D.P., Gray, A.R., Hutton, L.R., 2018. Outcomes and factors influencing response to an individualized multidisciplinary chronic disease management program for hip and knee osteoarthritis. J Arthroplasty 33(9), 2780–2786.

Health Workforce Australia (HWA), 2014. Australia's health workforce series – physiotherapists in focus. HWA, Adelaide.

Henderson, J., Gallagher, R., Brown, P., et al., 2020. Emergency department after-hours primary-contact physiotherapy service reduces analgesia and orthopaedic referrals while improving treatment times. Aust Health Rev 44 (3), 485–492.

Jayakumar, P., Moore, M.L.G., Bozic, K.J., 2019. Team approach: A multidisciplinary approach to the management of hip and knee osteoarthritis. JBJS Reviews 7 (6), e10.

Juras G., Brachman A., Michalska J., et al., 2019. Standards of virtual reality application in balance training programs in clinical practice: a systematic review. Games Health J 8 (2), 101–11.

Laver, K.E., Lange, B., George, S., et al., 2018. Virtual reality for stroke rehabilitation. Stroke 49 (4), e160–1.

Liu, B., Jayasundara, D., Pye, V., et al., 2021. Whole of population-based cohort study of recovery time from COVID-19 in New South Wales Australia. Lancet Regional Health-Western Pacific 12, 100193.

McMeeken, J., 2017. Physiotherapy education–investment in our future. N Z J Physiother 45 (3), 105–106.

McMeeken, J., 2014. Celebrating a shared past, planning a shared future: physiotherapy in Australia and New Zealand. N Z J Physiother 42 (1), 1.

Mitchell, G., Senior, H., Foster, M., et al., 2017. The role of allied health in the management of complex conditions in a comprehensive primary care setting.

O'Leary, H., Smart, K.M., Moloney, N.A., et al., 2018. Pain sensitization associated with nonresponse after physiotherapy in people with knee osteoarthritis. Pain 159 (9), 1877–1886.

Orrock, P., Engel, R., Vaughan, B., 2020. Evidence of increasing demand for musculoskeletal health services in older Australians: a report on Medicare consultation data and the implications for health profession education. doi:10.21203/rs.3.rs-26889/v1.

Samsson, K.S., Grimmer, K., Larsson, M.E.H., et al., 2020. Effects on health and process outcomes of physiotherapist-led orthopaedic triage for patients with musculoskeletal disorders: a systematic review of comparative studies. BMC Musculoskeletal Disorders 21 (1), 1–20.

Sayer, J.M., Kinsella, R.M., Cary, B.A., et al., 2017. Advanced musculoskeletal physiotherapists are effective and safe in managing patients with acute low back pain presenting to emergency departments. Aust Health Rev 42 (3), 321–326.

Seron, P., Oliveros, M.J., Gutierrez-Arias, R., et al., 2021. Effectiveness of telerehabilitation in physical therapy: a rapid overview. Physical Therapy 101 (6), pzab053.

Somerville, L., Davis, A., Milne, S., et al., 2018. Exploration of an allied health workforce redesign model: quantifying the work of allied health assistants in a community workforce. Aust Health Rev 42 (4), 469–474. doi:10.1071/AH16266. PMID: 28738968.

Van Egmond, M.A., Van Der Schaaf, M., Vredeveld, T., et al., 2018. Effectiveness of physiotherapy with telerehabilitation in surgical patients: a systematic review and meta-analysis. Physiotherapy 104 (3), 277–298.

Wang, Q., Lee, R.L.T., Hunter, S., et al., 2021. The effectiveness of internet-based telerehabilitation among patients after total joint arthroplasty: an integrative review. Int J Nurs Stud 115, 103845.

World Physiotherapy, 2019. Policy statement: description of physical therapy. https://world.physio/policy/ps-descriptionPT.

Zwarenstein, M., Goldman, J., Reeves, S., 2009. Interprofessional collaboration: effects of practice-based interventions on professional practice and healthcare outcomes. Cochrane Database Syst Rev (3), CD000072.

FURTHER READING

Australian Health Practitioner Regulation Agency – codes and guidelines: www.physiotherapyboard.gov.au/Codes-Guidelines.aspx.

Australian Physiotherapy Association – NDIS resources: http://www.physiotherapy.asn.au/APAWCM/Resources/Clinician_resources/DisabilityNDIS/APAWCM/Advocacy/NDIS_Resources.aspx?hkey=f3d995ed-e314-48b0-b200-21216a125390.

Australian Physiotherapy Association – Australian standards for physiotherapy practices: http://www.physiotherapy.asn.au/DocumentsFolder/Resources_Private_Practice_Standards_for_physiotherapy_practices_2011.pdf.

Physiotherapy Board of Australia & Physiotherapy Board of New Zealand – Physiotherapy practice thresholds in Australia and Aotearoa New Zealand: https://www.physiotherapyboard.gov.au/documents/default.aspx?record=WD15%2f16750&dbid=AP&chksum=LWuk27uBUFj5MTUort6Qug%3d%3d.

ONLINE RESOURCES

Australian Physiotherapy Association (APA): http://www.physiotherapy.asn.au.

Centre for the Advancement of Interprofessional Education (CAIPE): https://caipe.org.uk.

Physiotherapy Board of Australia: http://www.physiotherapy-board.gov.au/.

World Physiotherapy – resources: https://world.physio/resources.

28

Speech Pathology and Audiology: Assessment and Intervention for Communication Impairment

Jane Bickford, Lisa Callahan, Giriraj Singh Shekhawat and Lauren Sullivan[a]

KEY LEARNING OUTCOMES

When you finish this chapter you should be able to:
- identify common communication difficulties that occur over the life-span, arising from speech, language and/or hearing difficulties, and the impact of communication impairments on everyday life
- identify some major clinical intervention activities undertaken by speech pathologists and audiologists
- contrast patterns of public and private service provision in speech pathology and audiology
- identify political, commercial and professional forces that have shaped current models of speech pathology and audiology services
- identify the purpose and impact of, and delivery models for, addressing communication impairment.

KEY TERMS AND ABBREVIATIONS

audiologist
auditory processing disorder (APD)
autism spectrum disorder (ASD)
biopsychosocial model
Child and Family Health Service (CaFHS)
communication access
communication impairment
complex communication needs
conductive hearing loss
developmental disabilities
dysphagia
ear, nose and throat (ENT) specialist

expressive communication impairments
Hearing Australia
International Classification of Functioning, Disability and Health (ICF)
interprofessional education and collaborative practice
intervention services
National Disability Insurance Agency (NDIA)
National Disability Insurance Scheme (NDIS)

noise-induced hearing loss
otitis media (OM)
presbycusis
professional development
receptive communication impairment
rubella
speech pathologist
Speech Pathology Australia
tinnitus
universal neonatal hearing screening (UNHS)

[a]We acknowledge the contributions of Chris Brebner and Christopher Lind to the chapter in the 4th edition of this book.

INTRODUCTION

This chapter outlines service delivery models for two allied health professions that together play key roles in assessing and alleviating **communication impairment** in today's Australian health care system. Despite commonality of purpose, the two professions – speech pathology and audiology – are practised in very different ways. The interplay of forces influencing current care models presented to the general public in speech pathology and audiology include:

- introduction of the National Disability Insurance Scheme (NDIS) for service provision to people with long-term needs related to disability
- the balance between service delivery and supply of devices/equipment
- the role of government in service delivery (Duckett 2014)
- the availability of services to various sectors of the Australian community (Tuohy 1999).

COMMUNICATION AND COMMUNICATION IMPAIRMENT

Communication is a basic human right (United Nations 1948) and is fundamental to how people relate to each other across their life-span. Babies begin to develop their communication skills from birth, but are exposed to the sounds of their parents' voices from as early as 25 weeks' gestation (Graven & Browne 2008). Their earliest reciprocal communication experiences start with development of eye contact with their caregiver. Infants play with imitating, taking turns and experimenting with sounds. These foundations of early communication facilitate interpersonal relationships, which shapes their social skills. These skills enable learning of spoken language, supporting later development of reading and writing. Children develop language and communication skills through their experiences and interactions with others, with the development of complex and flexible communication skills continuing well into adulthood (Owens 2019). As adults, we use communication skills to establish and maintain relationships as well as to plan, work and interact within our communities. Through communication we solve problems, converse with others, tell stories and argue points. Communication enables us to recall and share memories, to predict and look forwards and to reflect. It shapes our image of our self and of others. In fact, communication is a critical yet subtle human behaviour that facilitates participation in all aspects of life.

To communicate, spoken and/or written messages need to be formulated and understood. In this process, there are many points when communication can be compromised or interrupted, resulting in communication impairment (Damico et al. 2021). **Expressive communication impairments** occur when delivery of a message is disrupted. This can result from cognitive, intellectual, motor or physiological processes that are immature/delayed or impaired, impacting on intelligibility or meaning of a spoken message. **Receptive communication impairments** occur when understanding of another's message is disrupted. This may include impairments of hearing or decoding spoken or written language, which may impact on an individual's participation in everyday interaction.

Expressive and receptive impairments of speech, hearing, language and communication are often 'invisible' until the person who is affected by them interacts with others. They are more prevalent than is often realised.

The World Health Organization's **International Classification of Functioning, Disability and Health (ICF)** (World Health Organization (WHO) 2001) is a **biopsychosocial model** that has influenced allied health practice. The ICF provides a framework for the relationship between structure and function, activity and participation and has influenced understanding and treatment of communication disorders internationally. Historically, clinic-based intervention dominated speech pathology and audiology practices, but the ICF has increased awareness of the impact of communication disorders on everyday participation, bringing these services into the community. In addition to the social stigma related to communication disorders (McCormack et al. 2018), visible signs of communication difficulty such as facial palsy associated with neurological damage, or hearing aids worn to reduce the impact of hearing loss, may influence one's social identity. More recently, models of intervention based on patient- and family-centred care have become more frequent in both professions. This has changed the balance between clinically measured outcomes commonly addressing impairment and psychosocial assessment of everyday participation and quality of life. The World Health Organization (2010) also promotes the importance of **interprofessional education and**

collaborative practice to support people with complex health and social care needs. It provides a useful framework for health professionals such as **audiologists** and **speech pathologists** to work together across the continuum of care for individuals experiencing communication impairment. Interprofessional practice opportunities are being increasingly embedded via education pathways to ensure the future workforce of health professionals such as audiologists and speech pathologists have the knowledge and skills to work collaboratively (Moran et al. 2020).

Speech Pathology – Speech, Language and Swallowing

Difficulties understanding and/or producing speech are relatively common, and arise from developmental disabilities, acquired acute difficulties or degenerative neurological conditions. **Developmental disabilities** can have known or unknown causes, and may be of genetic origin. Developmental disabilities include disorders such as **autism spectrum disorder (ASD)**, intellectual disability and cerebral palsy. Acquired acute difficulties arise from traumatic brain injury (TBI) or cerebral vascular accident (CVA)/stroke, cancer and degenerative neurological conditions such as dementia or motor neurone disease. Speech pathologists also work with people experiencing swallowing problems or **dysphagia**. Dysphagia often occurs after stroke or brain injury, and can result in food or liquid entering the airways or lungs, causing respiratory problems and increasing health risks such as dehydration, and resulting in longer hospital stays (Reber et al. 2019). People with lifelong disabilities such as cerebral palsy may also experience dysphagia. In fact, dysphagia in children with developmental disorders has been estimated to be between 50% and 90% (Blair et al. 2019; Mayer & Zeiter 2021; Mayes & Zickgraf 2019; Speyer et al. 2019). In this population, dysphagia may be associated with inadequate nutrition and hydration, respiratory problems leading to increased morbidity, and increased choking risk. Dysphagia also co-occurs with dementia, with reports of 93% of dementia patients experiencing dysphagia and conservative estimates suggesting that 9–35% of the elderly population are affected (Abu-Ghanem et al. 2020).

Five per cent of Australians have some form of communication impairment (Australian Bureau of Statistics (ABS) 2015). It is also estimated that one million Australians have difficulty in swallowing by **Speech Pathology Australia**, the national peak body for speech pathologists (Speech Pathology Australia n.d.). Exact figures are difficult to establish owing to coexistence across disorders; for example, people with hearing impairment commonly also experience other communication impairments. Prevalence measures vary across ages and by area of difficulty; for example, 10% of preschool children have difficulty with speech (Skeat et al. 2013), 20% of 4-year-old children have difficulty with language skills (Australian Government 2013) and 25% of adults over 85 years have dementia (Speech Pathology Australia 2014a).

There are effective **intervention services** for communication and swallowing issues, and recent international studies demonstrate their clinical cost–benefit (Speech Pathology Australia 2014a). The need for early intervention for children with communication impairment is well established. Difficulties with speech, language and communication impact on children's social and emotional well-being and on acquisition of literacy skills, with children with communication impairments having a higher incidence of difficulty learning to read and write (Reilly et al. 2015; Snow 2021). These difficulties often continue to impact negatively on social and emotional well-being, educational and employment outcomes into adulthood (del Zoppo et al. 2015; Mustard 2008).

Case study 28.1 examines the management of complex health needs after surgery.

Audiology – Hearing and Related Disorders

Hearing loss impacts one in seven Australians (3.6 million people) and if left untreated can enhance the risk of other health problems such as memory loss and depression.

The overall prevalence of hearing loss in the Australian community has been reported to be as high as 16%–20% (Chia et al. 2007; Wilson et al. 1999). Further, the prevalence of hearing loss is substantially skewed, particularly by age and gender. Approximately 33% of the Australian population aged over 48 are reported to have some degree of age-related hearing loss, with significantly more men than women under 80 years of age experiencing this type of hearing loss (Gopinath et al. 2009).

The World Health Organization (WHO) released the *World report on hearing* in 2021, outlining that hearing loss is a considerable economic burden globally estimated to be costing over $980 billion annually in health

---

CASE STUDY 28.1   Complex Health Needs Managed Over Long Distances

Ron is 64 years old and lives alone in a large regional town. He is a former labourer having stopped owing to a back problem. Four months ago he had a laryngectomy (surgical removal of his larynx) and radiotherapy for advanced laryngeal cancer. The laryngectomy has resulted in him needing to breathe through a hole in his neck (stoma) and has affected his ability to talk and eat. Ron's treatment took place in the capital city (250 kilometres from his home), at a major hospital with a multidisciplinary team of specialist doctors, nurses and allied health professionals.

Since his laryngectomy, Ron has had difficulty adjusting to the changes to his life and he has avoided using his electronic communication device because of its synthetic sound. He also continues to travel to the city for specialist appointments. These visits are expensive for Ron and exacerbate his back pain. Recently, he had a surgical procedure so he can now use a voice prosthesis to help him talk. The voice prosthesis must be changed every few months by a speech pathologist.

To avoid Ron having to come to the city for his prosthesis to be changed, the hospital-based speech pathologist contacts the local speech pathologist in his regional town's health service. She finds out that this speech pathologist is a new graduate with no direct experience with laryngectomy management. This is a common scenario as there is often little local expertise with laryngectomy. She recommends that the speech pathologist completes an online study package to familiarise herself with voice rehabilitation after laryngectomy and then comes and spends a day with her to get some supervised practice with voice prosthesis management. The local speech pathologist arranges regular telehealth sessions with the hospital speech pathologist so she is supervised when she changes Ron's voice prosthesis for the first few times.

Initially, the local speech pathologist sees Ron weekly. She identifies that he is quite isolated and links him with a local community support group and some online support groups. These groups appear to help him with his communication proficiency and acceptance of his situation.

Case Study Questions

1. What issues does the local-based speech pathologist face in supporting Ron with his voice rehabilitation in his local community?
2. How might the hospital speech pathologist further support the local speech pathologist to support Ron?
3. Outline what other benefits Ron may experience from having his care needs being managed locally.
4. How have advances in digital technology assisted with the management of Ron's ongoing health and well-being needs?

---

care, education, loss of productivity and societal costs. An estimated (US) $1 trillion is lost each year due to collective failure to address hearing loss. Globally over 1.5 billion people currently live with some degree of hearing loss, and it is projected to be 2.5 billion by 2050. Hearing loss has far-reaching consequences, it adversely impacts speech and language acquisition, cognition, education, communication and listening, employment, social isolation and loneliness, relationships, mental health and overall quality of life. The annual cost of hearing loss in Australia is 33.3 billion dollars.

Children are also commonly affected by hearing loss. **Otitis media (OM)**, a condition affecting the middle ear (and thus causing a **conductive hearing loss**), is the most common cause of hearing loss in children, and has its highest prevalence among children up to the age of 6–7 years (Jervis-Bardy et al. 2014). OM is a fluctuating condition that typically results in mild–moderate hearing loss and, at worst, results in a moderate degree of hearing loss. The prevalence of childhood OM is influenced by the child's anatomy, exposure to infectious agents and access to primary health care. Rates of chronic middle ear infections among Indigenous children, particularly those who live in rural and remote Australia, are much higher than among urban non-Indigenous children, which is primarily due to social and environmental factors (Delacy et al. 2020). Hearing health is critical to quality of life, yet many children do not have access to the appropriate primary health care either through a general practitioner (GP) or a local audiologist.

Sensorineural (and most commonly, permanent) hearing loss occurs when the cochlea or hearing nerve is damaged or malformed. Between two and three babies in every thousand live births have a detectable level of sensorineural hearing loss in one or both ears (National Institute on Deafness and Other Communication Disorders 2015). In Australia, up to 12 babies in every 10,000 will have moderate or greater loss in both ears, and a further 23 will acquire hearing loss requiring hearing aids by the age of 17 years (Australian Hearing

2015). If left unmanaged, any type of hearing loss in childhood has the potential to impact on speech and language development, communication, learning and quality of life, and may result in lifelong disability.

While there are a number of known risk factors for permanent congenital hearing loss, including family history, ototoxic medications, craniofacial abnormalities and **rubella** or cytomegalovirus (CMV) infection in the baby, many children born with permanent hearing loss do not have these risk factors. Currently, although **Universal Neonatal Hearing Screening (UNHS)** protocols vary between states and territories, these programs report hearing screening of more than 95% of all live births in Australia (Leigh 2010). Since the introduction of newborn hearing screening programs in Australia, the average age for diagnosis of congenital hearing loss has dropped from 2.5 years to 3 months, meaning more children are able to access early-intervention services for hearing loss.

Early diagnosis by 3 months of age, and early intervention (often comprising a hearing-aid fitting and speech/language therapy program) by 6 months of age may potentially decrease or avoid some of the negative impacts of congenital hearing loss. Audiologists and speech pathologists work closely with families and other service providers such as the **Child and Family Health Service (CaFHS)** to implement evidence-based strategies supporting language and communication development.

Early-intervention programs for children with sensorineural hearing loss have different perspectives on sign language (such as Signed English or Auslan) and the use of visual speech cues (such as lip-reading and cued articulation). Signed English is a signed version of English where there is a one-to-one correspondence between the spoken or written word and the sign. Auslan (Australian sign language) is a unique language with its own grammar and syntax. The ideologies behind various early-intervention models of practice require that parents be supported in their selection of the services that best suit their child.

The most commonly occurring causes of adult-onset hearing loss are (a) **noise-induced hearing loss**, which largely affects adults working in industry, in the armed forces or in the music industry, results in permanent damage to the inner ear and is most commonly bilateral; and (b) age-related hearing loss (or **presbycusis**), which has its greatest effect on those over 55–60 years of age and is also a permanent bilateral condition.

Audiological practice may be divided according to its diagnostic and rehabilitative focus. By far the more common practice of the two in audiology today is rehabilitation, particularly the selection and provision of hearing aids to adults who have acquired hearing loss. Interventions direct clinical effort towards addressing the needs of the patient in their everyday communicative environment and by extension on the impact of the individual's hearing impairment on their family members. These patient- and family-centred care models emphasise functional clinical outcomes as the ultimate goals of hearing rehabilitation.

Audiologists also deal with hearing-related disorders such as **tinnitus** (ringing in the ears), **auditory processing disorders (APD)** (problems with the way individuals process what they hear) and some cases of vertigo (dizziness) arising from pathologies of the ear and/or along the pathways from the ear to the brainstem.

Pause _for_ Reflection ...

Together, speech pathologists and audiologists assess and treat communication impairment (as outlined in the text) and ultimately support the participation of the individual in everyday activities. As such, the work of audiologists and speech pathologists moves beyond impairment to consider issues of participation. In what ways may their clinical work be considered to fit within a biopsychosocial model of health?

Case study 28.2 examines the management of newborn hearing impairment.

EDUCATION, EMPLOYMENT AND REGISTRATION

Speech Pathology

Speech pathology is a university-level professional entry allied health qualification. There are currently 25 universities across Australia offering 22 undergraduate and 16 postgraduate degree programs. In 2021, 21 programs had full professional accreditation with Speech Pathology Australia. There are no registration requirements for speech pathologists, however, speech pathologists who are members of Speech Pathology Australia can apply for Certified Practising Speech Pathologist status.

There were over 11,000 members of Speech Pathology Australia in 2022 (Speech Pathology Australia n.d.).

CASE STUDY 28.2   Navigating Referral Pathways: Communication and the Case of Newborn Hearing Impairment

Anna is one of four paediatric audiologists at a community health service in metropolitan Adelaide who performs hearing assessments for babies who don't pass their newborn hearing screenings. These tests allow for early diagnosis of permanent hearing impairment and referral to other service providers to help manage the hearing loss, including **ear, nose and throat (ENT) specialists**, speech pathologists and audiologists who specialise in fitting hearing aids and cochlear implants.

Anna receives a referral from a community nurse to see 2-month-old Andrew, who did not pass his newborn hearing screenings in either ear. The referral documentation from the nurse states that Andrew's family has recently immigrated to Australia from Italy and speaks little English. Andrew was unwell for several weeks at birth and requires the ongoing use of an oxygen tank. The family was reported to have missed several earlier appointments because of difficulty arranging care for their two older children and arranging transport. Andrew's father is noted to be a native English speaker, while his mother speaks Mandarin, with limited English.

Andrew and both of his parents attend the hearing assessment appointment, where Andrew is diagnosed with a permanent, moderate degree of hearing loss in both ears. Anna makes a number of referrals for Andrew to an ear, nose and throat (ENT) specialist, a speech pathologist who specialises in early intervention for children with hearing loss, a social worker, a paediatrician and an audiologist who specialises in fitting hearing aids and cochlear implants to children. The speech pathologist contacts Anna the same day that the referral is received, to clarify some details about Andrew's background and to check how the family are managing following the diagnosis.

Case Study Questions

1. What are the positive aspects of communication in this case study?
2. What things will Anna need to consider when contacting the family to make a hearing assessment appointment for Andrew?
3. What are the important aspects of the style and content of communication between Anna and the service providers who help to manage hearing loss?
4. Early intervention for speech and language is a key principle in the management of permanent hearing loss in childhood. How might Anna, the social worker and the speech pathologist work together to help ensure a smooth transition for Andrew and his family into early intervention?

It is a young, feminised profession with nearly half of Speech Pathology Australia's practising membership in 2015 under 35 years of age and with less than 3% men (Speech Pathology Australia 2016).

Speech pathologists assess and treat people who have communication and swallowing impairments. These encompass speech, language, swallowing, voice, fluency (i.e. stuttering) and multimodal communication (i.e. using additional means of communicating such as sign language). They work with people across the life-span in a variety of private and public settings, including kindergartens, schools, aged-care facilities and hospitals, rehabilitation and mental health services, community health centres, maternal and child health services and private practices. Speech pathologists provide consultative, individual and group therapy; work in multidisciplinary teams; and provide home-based services and work in communities to build **communication access**.

Speech pathologists are employed in a range of sectors. Recent employment growth in the private sector now sees 62.5% of Speech Pathology Australia members working in private practice. Other sectors include government services (37.6%) and non-government organisations (5.3%). Nationally, speech pathologists predominantly work in urban areas, with only 4.5% of speech pathologists in rural locations (Speech Pathology Australia 2016). Speech pathologists often work part-time. In 2011, the average number of hours worked per week was 30.3 (Health Workforce Australia 2014).

There is an unmet need for speech pathology services in early childhood and school settings, aged-care and disability sectors, the juvenile justice system, and acute and subacute hospital and rehabilitation settings (Speech Pathology Australia 2016). Policy changes and new funding arrangements in disability, education, health and aged care, including the NDIS, Commonwealth home support packages and activity-based funding, influence speech pathology service delivery and practice. Technology enhancements are enabling innovations such as telepractice to meet service demands in regional locations (Speech Pathology Australia 2018).

Audiology

Audiology in its current form is a relatively young profession. Audiology commenced in Australia as professional training by the (then) Commonwealth Acoustics Laboratories for psychology graduates in the 1960s (Upfold 2008), and became a graduate diploma course in the mid 1970s and a Master's degree program in 1996. There are currently seven Australian university programs for audiology and a few more in the pipeline. The enrolment numbers of audiology students have grown in the past few years. Australian audiology graduates are required to demonstrate clinical competency in order to be eligible for membership of Audiology Australia on the basis of their having graduated from an accredited course and having met competency standards, which are assessed while on clinical placement during their study. Audiologists are not required to be registered in order to practise in Australia, nor do they need to be members of a professional body. Employment in Australia requires only eligibility for membership to Audiology Australia. However, for some time membership of the professional body has been required for the practitioner to undertake clinical activities on behalf of the federal government's Office of Hearing Services. More recently, membership has also been required in order to provide audiology services under the NDIS (see Chapter 12).

Much of the audiological practice we know today grew out of two important world events – the first inflicted on adults and the second arising among children. First, at the end of World War II, audiological services were offered to servicemen and servicewomen who had returned from their military service with hearing loss arising from chronic and acute noise exposure (Upfold 2008). In North America, veterans' medical institutions such as the Walter Reed Army Hospital published much early research in rehabilitative audiology, primarily on the outcomes of supplying hearing aids to veterans. Second, in the 1940s many of the currently used paediatric audiology practices were developed in response to the children affected by the rubella epidemics that occurred between 1939 and 1941 (Upfold 2008). It is of note that the incidence of hearing loss in newborns dropped largely as a result of the community health vaccination programs to prevent rubella (Gelfand 2009). Now, among children who have hearing loss, close to 50% of permanent sensorineural hearing losses occurring prior to 3 years of age are genetic in origin (Gorlin & Toriello 2013).

Diagnostic audiology services are undertaken primarily by public hospitals for inpatient or outpatient clients, commonly provided in conjunction with ENT, oncology, paediatric, geriatric or surgical referrals. More recent hospital-based audiological practices have included the assessment of newborns, leading to the UNHS programs around Australia that were established in 2000. Recent developments in the analysis of genetic sites of hearing disorders, and the instigation of the UNHS programs, have greatly increased the sensitivity of diagnosis and identification of the causes of hearing loss in young children (Shearer et al. 2013).

> **Pause *for* Reflection …**
> Both speech pathologists and audiologists must complete an accredited tertiary-level qualification in order to practise. There is growth in the availability of these degree programs available in Australia but there remains a critical shortage in the availability of both professions working in rural areas. In what ways may these workforce shortages impact people with communication impairment living in rural areas?

PRACTICE WITHIN THE AUSTRALIAN HEALTH CARE SYSTEM

This section highlights how funding models impact on service delivery to the Australian community for communication impairment. Although the issues outlined are often particular to speech pathology or audiology, the case studies and questions raise matters for consideration, and we encourage you to look behind the detail to the broader issues. In many cases these issues are pertinent to other areas of health practice and are influenced by the dynamics of government policy pertaining to health care funding (Tuohy 1999). However, the availability of speech pathology and audiology services for people with communication impairment is also influenced by the changing landscape of disability, education and social welfare policy-making.

Speech pathologists and audiologists share the goal of alleviating the impact of communication impairment via a number of service delivery models. Speech pathologists provide services in a range of settings (e.g. acute (public) hospital, community centre, home, school, etc.) and within a number of different structures (e.g. consultative, individual, small treatment group, group training and information sessions for clients and/or their communication partners).

In contrast, few private-practice audiologists work in interdisciplinary settings. Note that audiology is heavily reliant on technology for its practice in both diagnosis and intervention. The supply of hearing aids raises some of the most interesting and contentious issues in the conduct of health services in the Australian health system. The fundamental issue is one of equity of access to increasingly expensive and sophisticated hearing aids and devices. Two issues around the delivery and pricing of technology-driven services, addressed in previous editions of this book (Lind & Olsson 2012; Lind et al. 2016), remain central to models of service delivery among private-practice audiology clinics. The first involves aggregation of service and device costs, which typically results in offers of 'free' hearing tests where the cost of the test is actually built in to the cost of supplying a hearing device. The second involves the acceptance of direct and indirect inducements to favour the supply of a particular company's devices.

The majority of publicly funded audiology hearing-aid provision services today are available to eligible members of the general public through the federal government's hearing-aid voucher scheme provided by **Hearing Australia** or by registered providers in private clinics. As a result, Medicare rebates for these hearing services are of limited relevance. Those not eligible for government-funded services may seek relief from commercial hearing-aid costs via private health insurance. Private health insurers may fund a portion of the cost of an eligible hearing-aid fitting every 3–5 years. The federal government acknowledged the need for a substantial restructuring of Hearing Australia's services in its 2014 Budget, but at the time of writing no announcement on the nature of any change has been made.

ETHICAL CLINICAL PRACTICE IN A COMPLEX AND CHALLENGING ENVIRONMENT

Complexities and challenges face health care clinicians in all workplace environments (e.g. health care, education, disability) where demand and supply diverge, where distance impacts on service delivery, where vulnerable client groups (especially those with **complex communication needs**) are disadvantaged, where emerging technologies prompt clinicians to re-examine and change practice, where client issues are diverse, where chronic and long-term care and management are

required, where organisations are uncertain about funding levels, where program direction and organisational structure are changing and where there is increasing legislation and compliance required at federal and state/territory levels.

With particular reference to the supply of devices (e.g. hearing aids), the pressures to meet standards of accountability simultaneously to government, shareholders, employers and professional bodies have brought great tension to hearing health care service providers. The premise that the health provision model will operate as a free-market economy fails when the service and the device supplied to the client are sufficiently complex to prevent consumers from acting on the basis of informed choice in these purchases. Selection of devices is thus an 'expert' decision, and may sometimes mask incentive-driven practice which potentially limits client access to the full range of available devices.

The contemporary approach to problem-solving in ethical service delivery is to inform, educate and discuss with clinicians the integration of decision-making into everyday practice, how to view ethical dilemmas as they arise and what approaches clinicians can use to resolve and even anticipate such dilemmas (Audiology Australia 2014; Speech Pathology Australia 2020). In addition to a set of shared clinical values, each clinician brings a unique set of underlying perspectives and beliefs to each event. For newer graduates, it may be that these perspectives cannot clearly be articulated, but ethical enquiry allows clinicians to make explicit the decision-making processes they undertake.

THE IMPACT OF COVID-19 ON SPEECH PATHOLOGY AND AUDIOLOGICAL PRACTICE

In late 2019, a novel strain of coronavirus primarily affecting the respiratory system emerged (SARS-CoV-2). By early 2020, the situation had developed into a pandemic. With no immediate treatment strategy or vaccine available, social distancing measures were implemented to prevent the spread of the disease. The sudden lifestyle changes caused by this strategy, however, risked increasing levels of depression and reducing well-being in the general population. For many, this pandemic has disrupted social interactions, financial security and access to health care. Speech pathology and audiological services in Australia were impacted by multiple lockdowns and social restrictions across the country. Telepractice in speech pathology is endorsed by Speech Pathology Australia but was not widely implemented for both assessment and management services for people with communication and swallowing difficulties prior to the pandemic (Speech Pathology Australia 2014b). The greatest area of uptake was for providing specialist services living in rural and remote parts of Australia (Burns et al. 2017). The public health restrictions accelerated the adoption of telepractice for speech pathology services. The position statement for telepractice in speech pathology is currently under review.

In contrast, telepractice was used with limited success for the delivery of audiological services as neither clients nor the clinicians were ready for the same. The SARS-CoV-2 pandemic increased the use of telepractice in the audiology sector in Australia and worldwide. Audiology Australia is currently working with the Australian Digital Health Agency to craft recommendations of technical standards that would be appropriate for telehealth in Australia.

Various strategies have been engaged to ensure continuity of care for people with hearing loss. Some strategies have provided options for clients to self-test their hearing, through the use of purpose-built applications or the transport of audiological equipment to clients (Palmer 2021). Others have involved audiologists remotely assessing hearing and fitting hearing devices, either directly with the client or with support from a local health practitioner (Palmer 2021). Technology such as video otoscopes, video conferencing software and systems that allow for shared control of another computer or device have been instrumental in allowing audiology services to continue via telehealth (Palmer 2021). Interestingly, there has also been a significant increase in the amount of audiology appointments that focus on counselling and rehabilitation strategies outside of amplification, which may support more effective management of hearing loss and hearing disorders in the long term (HSP 2021). These strategies may have ongoing applications following the conclusion of the pandemic, particularly in ensuring timely access to audiology services for people in aged-care settings, rural and remote areas and those who are unable to leave their home to attend a clinic.

Another development arising from the pandemic for the speech pathology profession has been global consensus-building responses between practitioners to ensure optimal outcomes for patients and safety for clinicians. For example, an international consortium was established early in the pandemic using electronic communication to reach a consensus for the management and rehabilitation of communication and swallowing function in intensive care units (ICU) (Freeman-Sanderson et al. 2021).

THE NATIONAL DISABILITY INSURANCE SCHEME

In health service delivery for those eligible for government support, short-term funding responses have often been applied to long-term intervention needs for those with communication impairment. To address this, and to give people with disability a greater say in the services they receive, the *National Disability Insurance Scheme Act 2013* was passed into legislation, establishing the **National Disability Insurance Scheme** (NDIS) and the agency responsible for delivering the scheme, the **National Disability Insurance Agency** (NDIA).

As you may recall from Chapter 12, the NDIA was chartered to fund reasonable and necessary support to help participants (i.e. individuals with disability, their families and carers) to reach their goals, objectives and aspirations, and undertake activities that enable the participant's social and economic participation. The NDIS has resulted in a transition from block-funding of disability service provider organisations to individualised funding for participants in the NDIS. Access to the NDIS for children and adults under 65 years with a range of communication difficulties has had a significant impact on therapeutic service provision, with a proliferation of private practitioners providing services to these individuals.

Children with developmental difficulties and long-term intervention needs may also experience limitation on activity in other developmental areas such as gross motor or cognitive development. They will often require support relating to technology or therapeutic support aiming to reduce the impact of communication difficulties (e.g. direct intervention, provision of assistive technology such as electronic speech output devices, hearing aids or cochlear-implant speech processors for individuals with hearing impairment). They may also need support such as assistance with personal care, social skills development and technology intended to address other support needs (such as independent mobility) (Ncube et al. 2018; Woodgate et al. 2020).

In conjunction with the NDIS, the health and education sectors are expected to maintain provision of services and support to people with speech and/or hearing disabilities (Department of Human Services n.d.). Historically, access to services with a medical or educational focus for people with these disabilities has been limited. The best outcomes for people with speech language and/or hearing disabilities are achieved through coordinated person-centred services (Smith-Merry & Gillespie 2016; Smith-Merry et al. 2018). Implementation of the NDIS provides an opportunity to develop a set of principles and protocols to assist in determining roles and responsibilities across and between sectors (Smith-Merry et al. 2018). However, there are significant challenges in creating a consistent national approach.

Pause *for* Reflection ...

Tuohy (1999) discusses the factors influencing the availability of health services to people in need. Recent developments such as the introduction of the National Disability Insurance Scheme and the increased use of technology to deliver services via telehealth in response to the public health restrictions imposed by a pandemic have widened the availability of speech pathology and audiology services. How might these developments have advantaged or disadvantaged people with communication impairments living in Australia?

A FINAL WORD

Inequality of access to services has critical social consequences. Many people are not eligible for government support and cannot afford to attend for diagnosis and possible amelioration of the barriers they face to communication participation. This limited access to services impacts on the individuals themselves, and those who wish to communicate with them. There is current and clear evidence of the effects of changes to government regulation and funding models on the provision of speech and/or hearing services, particularly to low-income earners and others who are disenfranchised in the community. Changes in the profile and funding of service provision impacts on clinical governance, such as clinicians' access to **professional development**, with particular emphasis on the identification and provision of services that are more clinically complex. Thus there are potential risks for quality of service delivery. In response, professional bodies tend to step in to ensure that minimum practice standards are being met, via continuing professional development in some cases and by professional regulation in others (Tuohy 1999). It remains a balancing act to maintain and develop knowledge and skills across a workforce, while recruiting large numbers of professionals to meet increased demand.

SUMMARY

In this chapter we have outlined:

- the practice of two professions whose major focus is remediation of motor, sensory, cognitive and behavioural impairments influencing everyday communication: speech pathology and audiology
- the similarities and differences in their modes of practice, particularly in (a) the balance of diagnostic and intervention activities, (b) the emphasis on technological versus communication-based intervention, and (c) the government regulation applied to the two professions' activities
- some of the ethical issues in delivering care to clients, with particular focus on the National Disability Insurance Scheme (NDIS)
- the impact of federal government funding for speech pathology and audiology services via the NDIS.

REVIEW QUESTIONS

1. What impact on the relationship between the state, providers and the private system may flow from the roll-out of NDIS funding?
2. What is problematic about being allowed to diagnose clients' hearing loss as well as recommend and supply their hearing aids?
3. Discuss the issues raised in the Pause for Reflection boxes and the case studies in the light of arguments that health is a human right, not a commodity.
4. Compare and contrast the examples of Tuohy's (1999) interplay of regulatory/commercial/professional pressures model from within speech pathology

and audiology, with respect to their effects on client access and outcomes.

5. Discuss the types of speech pathology services that might be more likely to be provided in acute care versus community rehabilitation contexts. Why might there be a difference in the services provided in different contexts?

REFERENCES

Abu-Ghanem, S., Chen, S., Amin, M.R., 2020. Oropharyngeal dysphagia in the elderly: evaluation and prevalence. Curr Otorhinolaryngol Rep 8, 34–42.

Audiology Australia, 2014. Ethics guidelines. http://www.audiology.asn.au.

Australian Bureau of Statistics (ABS), 2015. Disability, ageing and carers, Australia: summary of findings, 2015. Cat. no. 4430.0. ABS, Canberra.

Australian Government, 2013. A snapshot of early childhood development in Australia 2012 – AEDI National Report. Australian Government, Canberra.

Australian Hearing, 2015. Hearing loss. Australian Hearing, North Ryde. https://www.hearing.com.au/category/about-hearing.

Blair, E., Langdon, K., McIntyre, S., et al., 2019. Survival and mortality in cerebral palsy: observations to the sixth decade from a data linkage study of a total population register and National Death Index. BMC Neurology, 19.

Burns, C.L., Ward, E.C., Hill, A.J., et al., 2017. Randomized controlled trial of a multisite speech pathology telepractice service providing swallowing and communication intervention to patients with head and neck cancer: evaluation of service outcomes. Head Neck 39 (5), 932–939. https://doi.org/10.1002/hed.24706.

Chia, E.M., Wang, J.J., Rochtchina, E., et al. 2007. Hearing impairment and health-related quality of life: the Blue Mountains Hearing Study. Ear Hear 28, 187–195.

Damico, J., Muller, N., Ball, M.J., 2021. The Handbook of Language and Speech Disorders. second ed. Wiley & Sons. pp. 1–8.

Delacy, J., Dune, T., MacDonald, J.J., 2020. The social determinants of otitis media in Aboriginal children in Australia: are we addressing the primary causes? A systematic content review. BMC Public Health 20 (1), 1–9.

del Zoppo, C., Sanchez, L., Lind, C., 2015. A long-term follow-up of children and adolescents referred for assessment of auditory processing disorder. Int J Audiol 54 (6), 368–375.

Department of Human Services, n.d. People with disability. Australian Government, Canberra. https://www.human-services.gov.au/individuals/people-disability.

Duckett, S., 2014. Is Medicare sustainable? and, Is the question helpful or not? Presentation to Grattan Institute AHHA roundtable, Canberra. https://grattan.edu.au/wp-content/uploads/2014/05/540_presentation_duckett_medicare_anniversary_140130.pdf.

Freeman-Sanderson, A., Ward, E.C., Miles, A., et al., 2021. A consensus statement for the management and rehabilitation of communication and swallowing function in the ICU: a global response to COVID-19. Arch Phys Med Rehabil 102 (5), 835–842. doi:10.1016/j.apmr.2020.10.11.

Gelfand, S.A., 2009. Essentials of Audiology, third ed. Thieme, New York.

Gopinath, B., Rochtchina, E., Wang, J.J., et al. 2009. Prevalence of age-related hearing loss in older adults: Blue Mountains Study. Arch Intern Med 169 (4), 415–418.

Gorlin, R.J., Toriello, H.V., 2013. Genetic hearing loss – a brief history. In: Toriello, H.V., Smith, S.D. (Eds), Hereditary Hearing Loss and its Syndromes, third ed. OUP, New York, pp. 1–3.

Graven, S.N., Browne, J.V. 2008. Auditory development in the fetus and infant, newborn and infant. Nursing Reviews 8(4), 187–193. https://doi.org/10.1053/j.nainr.2008.10.010.

Health Workforce Australia (HWA), 2014. Australia's Health Workforce Series: Speech Pathologists in Focus. HWA, Canberra.

Hearing Services Program (HSP), 2021. Annual program statistics (2017–21) Australian Government, Department of Health, Canberra. https://hearingservices.gov.au/wps/portal/hso/site/about/program_stats/.

Jervis-Bardy, J., Sanchez, L., Carney, A.S., 2014. Otitis media in Indigenous Australian children: review of epidemiology and risk factors. J Laryngol Otol 128 (Suppl.S1), S16–S27.

Leigh, G., 2010. Early identification of hearing loss in Australia: well begun is not all done! The 2010 Libby Harricks Memorial Oration. Conference paper, Sixth Australian National Deafness Sector Summit, Sydney, Australia. doi:10.13140/RG.2.1.2935.6002.

Lind, C., Olsson, C., 2012. Speech pathology and audiology: service delivery and technology in communication disorders. In: Willis, E., Reynolds, L., Keleher, H. (Eds), Working in the Australian Health Care System, second ed. Elsevier, London, pp. 291–304.

Lind, C., Olsson, C., Brebner, C., et al., 2016. Speech pathology and audiology: assessment and intervention for communication impairment. In: Willis, E., Reynolds, L., Keleher, H. (Eds.), Understanding the Australian Health

Care System, third ed. Elsevier Australia, Sydney, pp. 345–348.

Mayer, R., Zeiter, D., 2021. Nutrition and feeding for children with developmental disabilities, In: Wyllie, R., Hyams, J., Kay, M. (Eds), Pediatric Gastrointestinal and Liver Disease, sixth ed. Elsevier, pp. 1032–1038.e2. https://doi.org/10.1016/B978-0-323-67293-1.00092-X.

Mayes, S., Zickgraf, H., 2019. Atypical eating behaviours in children and adolescents with autism, ADHD, other disorders and typical development. Res Autism Spectr Disord 64, 76–83. doi.org/10.1016/j.rasd.2019.04.002.

McCormack, J., Baker, E., Crowe, K., 2018 The human right to communicate and our need to listen: learning from people with a history of childhood communication disorder. Int J of Speech-Language Pathology 20 (1), 142–151. doi:10.1080/17549507.2018.1397747.

Moran, M., Bickford, J., Barradell, S., et al., 2020. Embedding the International Classification of Functioning, Disability and Health in health professions curricula to enable Interprofessional Education and Collaborative Practice. J Med Educ Curric Dev 7, 1–8. https://doi.org/10.1177/2382120520933855.

Mustard, F., 2008. Early childhood development: the best start for all South Australians. Report commissioned for the Department of Education and Children's Services, South Australia. http://parliament.wa.gov.au/parliament%5Ccommit.nsf/(Evidence+Lookup+by+Com+ID)/042B5F88C1D95F8148257831003C11C1/$file/ef.aar08.aqton.Education.attachment.pdf.

National Disability Insurance Scheme Act 2013 (Cwlth), https://www.comlaw.gov.au/Details/C2013A00020.

National Institute on Deafness and Other Communication Disorders (NIDCD), 2015. Quick statistics. NIDCD, Bethesda, MD. https://www.nidcd.nih.gov/health/statistics/pages/quick.aspx.

Ncube, B.L., Perry, A., Weiss, J.A., 2018. The quality of life of children with severe developmental disabilities. J Int Disability Research 62 (3), 237–244. doi:10.1111/jir.1246.

Owens, R., 2019. Language Development: An Introduction, tenth ed. Pearson Education.

Palmer, C.V., 2021. Tele-audiology: ready or not. Seminars in Hearing 42 (2), 85–87.

Reber, E., Gomes, F., Dähn, I A., et al., 2019. Management of dehydration in patients suffering swallowing difficulties. J Clin Med 8 (11), 1923. https://doi.org/10.3390/jcm8111923.

Reilly, S., McKean, C., Morgan, A. et al. 2015. Identifying and managing common childhood language and speech impairments. BMJ: Br Med J (Online), 350. doi:10.1136/bmj.h2318.

Shearer, A.E., Hildebrand, M.S., Sloan, C.M., et al., 2013. Genetic diagnosis and gene discovery for hearing loss using massively parallel sequencing. In: Toriello, H.V., Smith, S.D. (Eds), Hereditary Hearing Loss and Its Syndromes, third ed. OUP, New York, pp. 91–97.

Skeat, J., Wake, M., Ukoumunne, O.C., et al. 2013. Who gets help for pre-school communication problems? Data from a prospective community study. Child Care Health Dev 40 (2), 215–222.

Smith-Merry, J., Gillespie, J., 2016. Flexible funding for effective, individualised, integrated care. 4th World Congress on Integrated Care (WCIC4). International Foundation for Integrated Care (IFIC), Wellington.

Smith-Merry, J., Hancock, N., Gilroy, J., et al., 2018. Mind the Gap: the National Disability Insurance Scheme and psychosocial disability. Final report: Stakeholder identified gaps and solutions.

Snow, P., 2021. SOLAR: The science of language and reading. Child Lang Teach Ther 37(3), 222–233. doi:10.1177/0265659020947817.

Speech Pathology Australia, 2014a. Submission to the inquiry into the prevalence of different types of speech, language and communication disorders and speech pathology services in Australia (submission 224). https://www.aph.gov.au/Parliamentary_Business/Committees/Senate/Community_Affairs/Speech_Pathology/Submissions.

Speech Pathology Australia, 2014b. Telepractice in speech pathology. Speech Pathology Australia, Melbourne.

Speech Pathology Australia, 2016. Understanding the landscape – a stimulus paper. Speech Pathology Australia, Melbourne.

Speech Pathology Australia, 2018. Clinical education in Australia: building a profession for the future. https://www.speechpathologyaustralia.org.au/SPAweb/Resources_For_Speech_Pathologists/.

Speech Pathology Australia, 2020. Code of ethics. https://speechpathologyaustralia.cld.bz/SPA-Code-of-ethics-July2020-HIGHRES.

Speech Pathology Australia, n.d. Swallowing Awareness Day. https://www.speechpathologyaustralia.org.au/SPAweb/whats_on/Swallowing_Awareness_Day/

Speech Pathology Australia, n.d. Find a certified practising member of Speech Pathology Australia. https://www.speechpathologyaustralia.org.au/SPAweb/Resources_for_the_Public/Find_a_Speech_Pathologist/SPAweb/Resources_for_the_Public/Find_a_Speech_Pathologist/All_Searches.aspx?hkey=0b04c883-80b2-43e7-9298-7e5db5c75197.

Speyer, R., Cordiere, R., Kim, J., et al., 2019. Prevalence of drooling, swallowing and feeding problems in CP across the lifespan: a systematic review and meta-analyses. Dev Med & Child Neuro 61 (11), 1249–1258.

Tuohy, C.J., 1999. Accidental Logics: The Dynamics of Change In the Health Care Arena in the United States, Britain, and Canada. Oxford University Press, New York.

United Nations (UN), 1948. Universal Declaration of Human Rights. http://www.un.org/en/udhrbook/pdf/udhr_booklet_en_web.pdf.

Upfold, L., 2008. A History of Australian Audiology. Phonak Australia, Sydney.

Wilson, D.H., Walsh, P.G., Sanchez, L., et al., 1999. The epidemiology of hearing impairment in an Australian adult population. Int J Epidemiol 28, 247–252.

Woodgate, R.L., Gonzalez, M., Demczuk, L., et al., 2020. How do peers promote social inclusion of children with disabilities? A mixed-methods systematic review. Disabil Rehabil 42 (18), 2553–2579. doi:10.1080/09638288.2018.1561955.

World Health Organization (WHO), 2001. International classification of functioning, disability and health: ICF. WHO, Geneva. http://www.who.int/iris/handle/10665/42407.

World Health Organization (WHO), 2010. Framework for action on interprofessional education and collaborative practice. WHO, Geneva. https://www.who.int/publications/i/item/framework-for-action-on-interprofessional-education-collaborative-practice.

World Health Organization (WHO), 2021. World report on hearing. WHO, Geneva.

FURTHER READING

Access Economics, 2006. Listen hear! The economic impact and cost of hearing loss in Australia, Access Economics. https://hearnet.org.au/wp-content/uploads/2015/10/ListenHearFinal.pdf.

Couzos, S., Metcalf, S., Murray, R., 2008. Ear health. In: Couzos, S., Murray, R. (Eds.), Aboriginal Primary Health Care: An Evidence-Based Approach, third ed. OUP, Melbourne, pp. 308–354.

ONLINE RESOURCES

Audiology Australia – National Competency Standards: https://audiology.asn.au/Advocacy/National_Competency_Standards.

Department of Health – Diagnostic audiology items: https://www.servicesaustralia.gov.au/diagnostic-audiology-items?context=20.

Department of Health Hearing Services Program: https://www.hearingservices.gov.au.

National Disability Insurance Scheme: http://www.ndis.gov.au/.

Speech Pathology Australia – Rebates and Funded Programs for Medicare and NDIS - https://www.speechpathologyaustralia.org.au/SPAweb/Resources_For_Speech_Pathologists/Professional_Resources/Rebates_and_Funded_Programs/SPAweb/Resources_for_Speech_Pathologists/Medicare/Rebates_and_Funded_Programs.aspx?hkey=3aebffdf-3dcd-45d2-a287-b8fa823911af.

Speech Pathology Australia – Scope of practice: https://www.speechpathologyaustralia.org.au/spaweb/About_Us/SPA_Documents/SPA_Documents.

29

The Social Work Profession in the Australian Health Care System

Joanne Travaglia, Angel Carrasco, Bobbi Henao Urrego

KEY LEARNING OUTCOMES

When you finish this chapter you should be able to:
- provide a brief outline of the history of social work in health care
- describe the purpose and roles of social work in health care
- discuss the impact of the social environment and context on health and well-being

- outline issues relating to the self-regulation of the social work profession
- discuss the main challenges for the social work profession in contemporary health care.

KEY TERMS AND ABBREVIATIONS

almoner
Australian Association of Social
   Workers (AASW)
equality
equity

International Association of
   Schools of Social Work
   (IASSW)
International Federation of
   Social Workers (IFSW)

quality of life
social determinants of health
   (SDH)
structural inequality

INTRODUCTION

Social workers within the Australian health care system have become one of the largest allied health workforces within health care (Australian National Skills Commission 2022). This has been predominantly due to changing government health care policies and funding that have focused on the social arrangements, legislation and structures that impact the experience and access of people to hospital care and other health services. These changes have also occurred due to the new legislative requirements of hospitals and health services to respond to child protection, guardianship, elder abuse, domestic and family violence, sexual assault, Aboriginal and Torres Strait Islander people's access to health, human rights legislation and human-social responses to disasters as indicated by the various disaster management Acts across Australia. This has occurred parallel to increasing evidence of the **social determinants of health (SDH)** and how health care systems, within themselves, mediate patient and community health outcomes.

SOCIAL WORK IN AUSTRALIA

Social work in Australia is a diverse profession with social workers employed in a broad range of settings and organisations including schools, government organisations, disability services, community legal services, universities and research centres, child and family welfare, community-based welfare organisations, the homeless sector, private practice, aged care, mental health, and health services including hospitals (Healy & Lonne 2010).

According to the Australian Government National Skills Commission (2022) there are currently 30,000 social workers employed in Australia. The workforce is 84% female and, on average, 42 years of age. The Australian Government reports that the future growth of social workers in the employment sector is very strong. Unlike nursing, medicine or psychology, social work is not a registered profession and is not included within the Australian Health Practitioner Regulation Agency (Ahpra) list of registered health professions. This remains an area of contention and debate within the profession and community at large (McCurdy et al. 2020). Social work is currently a self-regulated profession, with regulation managed by the **Australian Association of Social Workers** (**AASW**) (2022a).

The AASW sets entry, education and training requirements into the profession and provides ethical and practice standards frameworks for social work practice in Australia. Membership to the AASW is not mandatory to practise as a social worker in Australia, although a number of government organisations, including health services, have placed mandatory recruitment standards for social worker positions that require applicants to 'meet eligibility for membership to the AASW'. To meet eligibility requirements for membership to the AASW, a social worker must complete a general-entry university-level training program in social work at either the 4-year undergraduate Bachelor's or 2-year postgraduate Master's of Social Work course level. Although membership to the AASW is not mandatory for all social workers, mental health social workers wishing to become registered providers of Medicare and receive government subsidies for their private practice work with consumers/clients must be formally accredited by the AASW and meet AASW continuing professional development (CPD) requirements (Australian Association of Social Workers 2014).

THE ROLE OF THE SOCIAL WORKER

Social workers are involved in improving the well-being and **quality of life** of all people in society by utilising their knowledge and professional skills to connect people to the resources they require (social, psychological, economic and/or political) (Lawrence 2016). In this way, they assist people to attain the best possible level of well-being to achieve a fulfilling life. The **International Federation of Social Workers** (**IFSW**) and the **International Association of Schools of Social Work** (**IASSW**) endorsed the following definition of social work:

Social work is a practice-based profession and an academic discipline that promotes social change and

development, social cohesion, and the empowerment and liberation of people. Principles of social justice, human rights, collective responsibility, and respect for diversities are central to social work. Underpinned by theories of social work, social sciences, humanities and indigenous knowledges, social work engages people and structures to address life challenges and enhance wellbeing.

(International Federation of Social Workers (IFSW) 2022, n.p.)

The definition of the IFSW is extremely broad in nature, however, it captures the main purpose of the social work profession in addressing human well-being and responding to human need and suffering resulting from structural inequalities in society. '**Structural inequality**' refers to the way in which society is organised and structured and the way that resources, including access to health and health outcomes, are distributed differently across society benefitting some people more than others. This concept is discussed later in this chapter in relation to inequities in health and well-being (see **equity** and **equality** in the Glossary). The IFSW definition recognises that the conditions in which people are born, live, develop, thrive, become ill and die are, in turn, shaped by political, social and economic forces. The IFSW further states that social work '... is driven by the need to challenge and change those structural conditions that contribute to marginalization, social exclusion and oppression' (International Federation of Social Workers (IFSW) 2022, n.p.). The IFSW definition of social work has been adopted by the Australian Association of Social Workers and by many other social work associations internationally.

The purpose and aim of the social work profession set it apart from many other disciplines working in health care, which predominantly work from a biomedical and science-based evidence framework. Social work uses a range of interdisciplinary and transdisciplinary knowledges from a variety of sources such as social sciences, welfare policy, law, human behaviour, anthropology, economics, education, psychology, public health, sociology, psychiatry and politics, while valuing the co-constructed theory with service users and Indigenous knowledges. This broad knowledge base provides a rich and valuable context in which to better understand the person within the context of their environment and relationships. In this way, within health care, social workers are increasingly called upon to provide 'person-centred care' rather than 'patient care', which can at times be misunderstood by the multidisciplinary team (Innes et al. 2006). Case study 29.1 describes a complex scenario involving social work in a multidisciplinary context.

Pause *for* Reflection …

Based on your reading of the chapters on other professions in this book, do you think social workers should be registered? Why/why not?

THE HISTORY OF THE SOCIAL WORK PROFESSION IN AUSTRALIA

The social work profession has its antecedents in the English Poor Laws of the seventeenth century and later in the Charity Organisation Societies (COS) and settlement movements that originated in England, which influenced many English-speaking countries such as Australia, New Zealand and the United States (Noble & Nash 2012; Trattner 2007). The concept that governments have a role and function to assist people who were sick, had a disability or needed social assistance

---

CASE STUDY 29.1

Jane, in her mid 30s, presents to the emergency department, brought in by the Sheriff's office at the request of the NSW Trustee and Guardian (TAG) on the day she is evicted from her home. Her father's house is sold as part of his estate following his death meaning that her residence of the last 10 years is no longer her home. Under the TAG for many years, Jane becomes homeless as there are not enough funds in her account to find new accommodation. Jane is admitted by a medical officer to hospital as a 'social admission' to address her significant care needs and health issues directly associated with her current homelessness that otherwise could result in the increased likelihood of harm, injury or risk to life.

On admission to hospital, Jane weighs 280 kg. She has multiple co-morbidities including poor cardiac function, high blood pressure, diabetes and mental health diagnoses. This is compounded by a complex history of sexual abuse, children from the abusive relationship being removed into care, substance abuse and incarceration. She has very limited contact with her mother and no contact with her other family. Jane insists on only eating food from Uber eats while in hospital, which means her caloric intake is well above what is recommended for her medical co-morbidities. Soon after admission her condition deteriorates and it takes up to six staff for transfers and personal care. She also becomes doubly incontinent and requires further medical intervention.

Throughout Jane's year-long admission the multidisciplinary team attempt to discharge her to a number of short-term accommodation options with no success. Significant advocacy is required by the multidisciplinary team in attempts to get her onto the National Disability Insurance Scheme (NDIS). Jane is accepted by NDIS, and a behavioural specialist is called in to assist with a behavioural

management plan to complement the extensive multidisciplinary team, as Jane becomes increasingly abusive to staff and fluctuates in engagement with care. In attempts to remain in hospital, Jane tries to remove herself from the NDIS, with Hospital Executive and Ministry of Health teams working with the multidisciplinary team to ensure she is not disadvantaged in the community by not having access to services and supports.

Guardianship orders are sought and granted for decision-making on living arrangements and service provision. The multidisciplinary team works with TAG to address the Uber eats and contracts with Jane about ordering.

Jane loses over 120 kg throughout her hospital stay and at 366 days into her admission, following extensive preparations with all staff and service providers to ensure safe and successful transition to her new home, Jane is discharged to NDIS accommodation with police and ambulance escort. Despite 'successful' discharge (with no readmission to hospital), Jane is unhappy with the decisions that have been made and continues to abuse staff through telephone calls and text messages following discharge.

Case Study Questions

1. What aspects of the SDH do you recognise?
2. What is the role of the social worker in this scenario?
3. With so many complexities, what do you focus on in this case study?
4. What factors contribute to hospitals often seen within communities as the 'place of last resort'?
5. How do you think social workers can sustain themselves in a case that lasts a year in an acute hospital setting?

and support originated in the Poor Law of 1601. The Poor Law required local parishes to collect taxes from people in those parishes to be able to provide money to people who were not able to work due to sickness or inability to work, and to provide care for the increasing number of orphaned or destitute children that resulted from the movement from agrarian work to work in the cities (Chenowith & McAuliffe 2018).

The earliest welfare practitioners were the 'friendly visitors' in the early 1800s. The friendly visitors were predominantly women from wealthy families who were motivated by 'Christian' values of charity and benevolence (Bisman 2004). The friendly visitors visited poor families to better understand their circumstances and aimed to change those circumstances through the provision of material aid, and, through this practical assistance, to change the behaviours and motivation of those they visited. The friendly visitors became aware of the role, for example, of alcohol misuse, child abuse, domestic and family violence, unemployment, disability and sickness on general well-being and the person's ability to escape the cycle of poverty and improve their overall quality of life. It was through these charity organisations that modern social work originated in London in the 1890s as a response to the social impacts of the industrial revolution. The Charity Organisation Societies' friendly visitors often visited hospitals to assist the poor and destitute (Burnham 2016). These first female friendly visitors were employed by London hospitals as 'lady almoners' to assist patients in their transition from hospital to their homes by organising extended family resources, or other church parish supports such as food or childcare, and providing social support in the home (Bamford 2015).

The first hospital **almoner** was Mary Stewart, appointed at the Royal Free Hospital of Central London in 1895 (Cullen 2013). Mary Stewart, within her paid role as a hospital almoner, paved the way in the early developments of medical social work. Mary Stewart was selected for this role due to her experience helping others in her previous work at a COS, together with her local knowledge of the circumstances of inner-city London and of local community resources able to assist patients presenting at the Royal Free Hospital. Mary Stewart trained other women as almoners for other hospitals though an apprenticeship-type system (Cullen 2013). By 1913 medical authorities in Britain noted that the work of the hospital almoners greatly supported other

hospital staff, including doctors and nurses, in making the necessary arrangements to allow the patient to remain in hospital until their medical treatment was finalised, and then assisting in discharging patients home (Cullen 2013).

It was this early English hospital almoner model that was adopted in the early 1920s at the Melbourne Hospital following a visit by hospital board members and staff to St Thomas's Hospital, London. The first hospital almoner at Melbourne Hospital was Agnes McIntyre from St. Thomas's Hospital (Gleeson 2008). Agnes McIntyre established the first Australian training body for hospital almoners in Melbourne. This was a two-year certificate course in general social work by the Board of Social Studies, a training institute run by the Victorian Council for Social Training (O'Brien & Turner 1979). It was through this course that candidates could specialise in medical social work and undertake supervised practical work in hospitals with experienced medical social workers. From 1937 hospital almoner training was provided in Sydney, with the establishment of a similar training institute. Candidates from other Australian states interested in taking up the increasing new positions on offer within their state hospital systems for almoner positions, particularly as a response to the Great Depression of the 1930s, had to travel to Melbourne or Sydney to undertake this training. Training as a hospital almoner gave many of these women paid work opportunities within hospitals that were seen as 'reputable jobs' and were well regarded despite the challenges at the time of working under the authority of a heavily male and patriarchal medical system (Gleeson 2008).

The Catholic Bureau in Australia in the late 1920s offered scholarships to three Australian women – Norma Parker, Connie Moffit and Elaine Davidson – to undertake university-level training in social work in the USA (Parker 1979). These three women would be seen as the pioneers of professional social work in Australia. On their return to Australia these women would go on to establish social work departments in several hospitals in Melbourne and Sydney. Norma Parker established the first social work department in a public psychiatric hospital in Australia at Callan Park in Sydney (Foley 2007). Norma Parker and her colleagues were also influential in establishing social work education at Sydney University and Melbourne University in 1940, with Adelaide University following soon after in 1942. Norma Parker became the first president of the **Australian Association of**

Social Workers (**AASW**) in 1945 (Australian Association of Social Workers (AASW) 2020b).

THE PURPOSE AND ROLES OF SOCIAL WORKERS IN HEALTH CARE

Social workers in health care work across a range of different fields, inclusive of tertiary and primary health care as well as private practice, mental health, community health, justice health, drug and alcohol services, government and non-government sectors (Australian Association of Social Workers (AASW) 2015; Noble & Nash 2012). To help support and guide clinicians, the AASW established a number of scope of practice documents (Australian Association of Social Workers (AASW) 2022b), many related to social work health care practice. These documents sit alongside the AASW code of ethics and practice standards to assist and inform the practice of social workers across multiple fields of practice (Australian Association of Social Workers 2020).

Social work roles across the span of health care services use a variety of techniques and skills to be able to advocate and assist people's social and emotional functioning, well-being and quality of life within their systems. The skills that social workers bring to the table also means they are not only in front-facing consumer roles. There are roles in policy, planning and executive positions that enable social workers to influence structures and health outcomes for the broader community (Keefe & Jurkowski 2012).

All public and many private hospitals across the country employ social workers as part of the multidisciplinary team. In these settings social workers engage individuals, families and carers in discharge planning, identifying care needs and case management of patients with complexity including disability and socio-legal components (Cleak & Turczynski 2014). Social workers in hospital settings are skilled at psychosocial assessments, crisis intervention,

brief interventions and risk assessment, and 'maintain a dual focus in both assisting with and improving human wellbeing; and addressing any external issues that may be negatively affecting it, such as inequality, injustice and discrimination' (AASW 2020a, p. 3). Many also work across specialised areas of practice including oncology and palliative care, trauma, sexual assault and rehabilitation. There is a growing shift towards person-centred care within the health system, including working in co-designed systems and reviewing people's experiences to improve care and outcomes (Australian Commission for Safety and Quality in Healthcare 2022). This lens favours social workers' practice of responding to people's needs and focusing on quality of life, and acknowledges the role the social determinants play in people's outcomes.

There is scope for social work to play a pivotal role in preventive health care by working with individuals, families and carers to address basic needs and focus on health inequities. Tangible actions in preventive health care can lead to multigenerational benefits for health outcomes.

THE IMPACT OF THE SOCIAL ENVIRONMENT, CONTEXT AND HEALTH INEQUITIES ON HEALTH AND WELL-BEING

An understanding of the social dimensions of health and of health care is central to social work. The SDH are those economic and social conditions that influence the health of individuals, groups and communities. They are '… the circumstances in which people grow, live, work, and age, and the systems put in place to deal with illness. The conditions in which people live and die are, in turn, shaped by political, social, and economic forces' (Commission on Social Determinants of Health 2008, n.p.). The SDH are influenced by policy choices (Centers for Disease Control and Prevention 2021). This concept is further explained in Chapter 5, which describes public health in Australia.

Social determinants can be seen as either risk or protective factors that can either strengthen or damage the health of individuals, groups and communities. People from poorer social or economic circumstances are at greater risk of poor health than people from higher socio-economic circumstances, a difference which starts in childhood (with increased rates of childhood mortality, lower birth weight and increased risk of accidental death) and lasts the person's entire life (including increased risk of both chronic and other diseases) (Raphael 2011) and potentially across generations (Australian Institute of Health and Welfare (AIHW) 2020).

These factors result in inequities, some of which can be addressed by health care professionals (Marmot 2010; World Health Organization (WHO) 2016). Health inequities are the '... differences in health status or in the distribution of health resources between different population groups, arising from the social conditions in which people are born, grow, live, work and age. Health inequities are unfair and could be reduced by the right mix of government policies' (WHO 2018, n.p.). Inequities are differences which are 'not only unnecessary and avoidable but are also considered unfair and unjust' (Whitehead 1991, p. 219). 'Inequities in health systematically put people who are already socially disadvantaged (e.g. poor, female, and/or members of a disenfranchised racial, ethnic or religious group) at further disadvantage with respect to their health' (Braveman & Gruskin 2003, p. 254).

Social workers, we would argue, are in a unique position to help unpack the representation of health problems from the perspective of the SDH. By exploring the underlying premises of problems, including 'how "problems" are constituted within policies and policy proposals' (Bacchi 2016, p. 12) and shifting the focus away from shallow or reactive approaches to 'problem-solving', social workers can engage in an active process of '... disrupt[ing] modes of governing that install forms of marginalization and domination' (Bacchi, 2016, p. 12). Understanding Aboriginal and Torres Strait Islanders' health status from the perspective of colonisation and separation from country is a significant step away from considering health problems, like diabetes, solely from the perspective of a single individual's diet.

THE MAIN CHALLENGES FOR THE SOCIAL WORK PROFESSION IN CONTEMPORARY HEALTH CARE

Health social work brings unique challenges, based often in the context of working in a predominantly medical model (Auslander 2001). Australia's changing landscape of cultures means that social workers are faced with an ever-evolving learning platform. Dealing with the complexity of people's biopsychosocial histories and diversity of lived experience within social determinants means that no review or intervention is the same.

Coupled with this are other overlying political and policy measures that impact service delivery. Recent examples of this include voluntary assisted dying, now accessible in Victoria, South Australia, Queensland, Western Australia, Tasmania, and New South Wales; the Royal Commission into Violence, Abuse, Neglect and Exploitations of People with Disability (2022); the Royal Commission into Aged Care Quality and Safety (2021); and the Royal Commission into Institutional Responses to Child Sexual Abuse (2017).

Rural and remote workers face yet more challenges as they not only have the socio-political and health inequities that metro areas have but are faced with geographical implications (AIHW 2017). These not only impact waiting time for specialised treatment in many cases but also enhance challenges with social connectedness and psychosocial impacts should someone need to be relocated for care. On a clinician well-being level, there is also the added pressure of often being a sole clinician or a clinician with limited access to supervision and being regularly accessible to the community you live in due to the size of populations (Saltman et al. 2004).

The SARS-CoV-2 pandemic has brought with it a new diversity of challenge across health. Social work has pivoted in the pandemic, working on ways of engaging people during fear of the unknown. Early concerns about increased mental health needs and increases in domestic and family violence have been realised. Mental health and domestic violence have seen a significant increase across the country since the pandemic began (Pfitzner et al. 2022; Usher et al. 2021). The importance of social work in health has never been more valid and will well exceed the end of the pandemic. Hospital treatment and social isolation has changed with visiting restrictions and isolation for positive cases and close contacts being mandated in some settings. This has forced video conferences for interventions, viewings and counselling (Mishna et al. 2021). Access to technology has been a silver lining for the health industry in treating COVID-19, including allowing access to care for those normally homebound. While being inclusive for some, the increased use of telehealth has marginalised others, with poor access to technology or ageing and disability related health issues making these methods impossible to use. The use of telehealth has also brought other challenges, including safety for those in family and domestic violence situations where domestic violence screening is not as easily done due to inability to be aware of who is listening to a conversation or tracing calls (Australian Government Department of Health 2021).

Within health care, social workers are often working with many of the most vulnerable, marginalised and disenfranchised people of society. Links to social determinants can see many in this group with poorer health literacy levels, which we know can impact on people's health outcomes and decision-making (Nutbeam, 2000; Sørensen et al. 2012). Interventions in these circumstances may need to be more frequent or intensive to enable advocacy, understanding and clarification of information to ensure that people are informed and able to partake in decision-making where possible.

SUMMARY

Although one of the oldest allied health professions, social work has continued to change and adapt over the last century while remaining true to its core values and mission – that of improving the well-being and quality of life of all people in a society (Lawrence 2016). This has never been more evident than in the SARS-CoV-2 pandemic when it became clear that the most vulnerable individuals and groups in all societies (including the elderly, people with disabilities, people from lower socio-economic backgrounds and Indigenous peoples among other groups) were at greater risk, not only of the virus itself, but of the way in which governments, societies and health systems viewed, and at times directly discriminated against, them (Lee & Miller 2020; Lichtenstein 2021).

Challenges in health care will continue to be ever-changing and it is necessary that social workers remain contemporary in their planning and service delivery to address the community needs as things evolve. This will ensure that those principles of social justice and human rights stay at the forefront of the profession's contribution to society.

REVIEW QUESTIONS

1. What is the purpose of social work?
2. What are the critical issues in health care that social workers are involved in addressing?
3. What skills do social workers bring to health care?
4. Can you identify one or more of the fields of social work practice, the target groups with whom social workers might work?
5. What challenges might social workers face in these roles?

REFERENCES

Auslander, G., 2001. Social work in health care: what have we achieved? J Soc Work 1(2), 201–222. doi:10.1177/146801730100100206.

Australian Association of Social Workers (AASW), 2014. Practice standards for mental health social workers. AASW, Melbourne.

Australian Association of Social Workers (AASW), 2020. Australian Association of Social Workers Code of Ethics 2020. AASW, Melbourne.

Australian Association of Social Workers (AASW), 2015. Social work in health. AASW, Melbourne. https://www.aasw.asn.au/document/item/8306.

Australian Association of Social Workers (AASW), 2020a. Social work in hospitals. AASW, Melbourne. https://www.aasw.asn.au/document/item/8644.

Australian Association of Social Workers (AASW), 2020b. Social work milestones. AASW, Melbourne. https://www.aasw.asn.au/whoweare/aasw-milestones/milestones.

Australian Association of Social Workers (AASW), 2022a. Australian Association of Social Workers. AASW, Melbourne. https://www.aasw.asn.au/.

Australian Association of Social Workers (AASW), 2022b. The scope of social work practice. AASW, Melbourne. https://www.aasw.asn.au/practitioner-resources/the-scope-of-social-work-practice.

Australian Commission for Safety and Quality in Health Care, 2022. Person centred care. https://www.safetyandquality.gov.au/our-work/partnering-consumers/person-centred-care

Australian Government Department of Health, 2021. Violence, abuse and neglect and Covid-19. https://www.health.nsw.gov.au/Infectious/covid-19/Pages/violence-abuse-neglect.aspx#tele-1.

Australian Institute of Health and Welfare (AIHW), 2017. Rural and remote health. AIHW, Canberra.

Australian Institute of Health and Welfare (AIHW), 2020. Australia's health data insights 2020. AIHW, Canberra.

Australian National Skills Commission, 2022. Labour market insights social workers ANZSCO ID 2725. https://labour-marketinsights.gov.au/occupation-profile/social-workers?occupationCode=2725.

Bacchi, C., 2016. Problematizations in health policy: questioning how "problems" are constituted in policies. Sage Open 6(2), 1–16.

Bamford, T., 2015. A contemporary history of social work: learning from the past. Policy Press, Bristol.

Bisman, C., 2004. Social work values: the moral core of the profession. Br J Soc Work 34 (1), 109–123.

Braveman, P., Gruskin, S., 2003. Defining equity in health. J Epidemiol Community Health 57 (4), 254–258.

Burnham, D., 2016. The social worker speaks: a history of social workers through the twentieth century. Routledge, London.

Centers for Disease Control and Prevention, 2021. Social determinants of health: know what affects health. https://www.cdc.gov/socialdeterminants/index.htm

Chenowith, L., McAuliffe, D., 2018. The Road to Social Work and Human Services, fifth ed. Cengage Learning, Melbourne.

Cleak, H.M., Turczynski, M., 2014. Hospital social work in Australia: emerging trends or more of the same? Soc Work Health Care 53(3), 199–213.

Commission on Social Determinants of Health, 2008. Closing the gap in a generation: health equity through action on the social determinants of health: final report of the commission on social determinants of health. World Health Organization (WHO), Geneva.

Cullen, L.T., 2013. The first lady almoner: the appointment, position, and findings of Miss Mary Stewart at the Royal Free Hospital, 1895–99. J Hist Med Allied Sci 68 (4), 551–582.

Foley, M., 2007. The origins of mental health social work in Western Australia: a psychiatric 're-conception'. Studies in Western Australian History 25, 132–147.

Gleeson, D.J., 2008. Some new perspectives on early Australian social work. Aust Soc Work 61 (3), 207–225. doi:10.1080/03124070802233195.

Healy, K., Lonne, B., 2010. The Social Work and Human Services Workforce: Report from a National Study of Education, Training and Workforce Needs. Australian Learning and Teaching Council, Sydney.

Innes, A., Macpherson, S., McCabe, L., 2006. Promoting person-centred care at the front line. Joseph Rowntree Foundation, York.

International Federation of Social Workers (IFSW), 2022. Global definition of social work. https://www.ifsw.org/what-is-social-work/global-definition-of-social-work/.

Keefe, R., Jurkowski, E.T., 2012. Handbook for public health social work. Springer, New York.

Lawrence, R.J., 2016. Professional social work in Australia. ANU Press, Canberra.

Lee, H., Miller, V.J., 2020. The disproportionate impact of COVID-19 on minority groups: a social justice concern. J Gerontol Soc Work 63 (6–7), 580–584. doi:10.1080/01634372.2020.1777241.

Lichtenstein, B., 2021. From "Coffin Dodger" to "Boomer Remover": outbreaks of ageism in three countries with divergent approaches to coronavirus control. J Gerontol: Series B, 76 (4), e206–e212.

Marmot, M., 2010. Fair society, healthy lives: strategic review of health inequalities in England post 2010 (The Marmot Review). Institute of Health Equity, London.

McCurdy, S., Sreekumar, S., Mendes, P., 2020. Is there a case for the registration of social workers in Australia? Int Soc Work 63(1), 18–29.

Mishna, F., Milne, B., Sanders, J., et al., 2021. Social work practice during COVID-19: client needs and boundary challenges. Glob Soc Welf 1–8. doi:10.1007/s40609-021-00219-2.

Noble, C., Nash, M., 2012. Social work in Australia and New Zealand. In: Healy, L.M., Link, R.J. (Eds), Handbook of International Social Work: Human Rights, Development, and the Global Profession, pp. 377–382. OUP, Oxford.

Nutbeam, D., 2000. Health literacy as a public health goal: a challenge for contemporary health education and communication strategies into the 21st century. Health Promot Int 15(3), 259–267.

O'Brien, L., Turner, C., 1979. Hospital almoning: portrait of the first decade. Aust Soc Work 32(4), 7–12.

Parker, N., 1979. Early social work in retrospect. Aust Soc Work 32 (4), 13–20.

Pfitzner, N., Fitz-Gibbon, K., Meyer, S., 2022. Responding to women experiencing domestic and family violence during the COVID-19 pandemic: exploring experiences and impacts of remote service delivery in Australia. Child Fam Soc Work 27(1), 30–40.

Raphael, D., 2011. Poverty in childhood and adverse health outcomes in adulthood. Maturitas 69(1), 22–26. doi:10.1016/j.maturitas.2011.02.011.

Royal Commission into Aged Care Quality and Safety, 2021. Final report (volumes 1–5). Royal Commission into Aged Care Quality and Safety, Canberra.

Royal Commission into Institutional Responses to Child Sexual Abuse, 2017. Final report (volumes 1–17). Royal Commission into Institutional Responses to Child Sexual Abuse, Canberra.

Royal Commission into Violence, Abuse, Neglect and Exploitations of People with Disability, 2022. Royal Commission into Violence, Abuse, Neglect and Exploitations of People with Disability. https://disability.royalcommission.gov.au/

Saltman, J., Gumpert, J., Allen-Kelly, K., et al., 2004. Rural social work practice in the United States and Australia: a comparison. Int Soc Work 47(4), 515–531. doi:10.1177/0020872804046258.

Sørensen, K., Van den Broucke, S., Fullam, J., et al., 2012. Health literacy and public health: a systematic review and integration of definitions and models. BMC Public Health 12(1), 1–13.

Trattner, W.I., 2007. From poor law to welfare state: A history of social welfare in America (6th ed.). Simon and Schuster, New York.

Usher, K., Bradbury Jones, C., Bhullar, N., et al., 2021. COVID-19 and family violence: is this a perfect storm? Int J Ment Health Nurs 30 (4), 1022–1032.

Whitehead, M., 1991. The concepts and principles of equity and health. Health Promot Int 6 (3), 217–228.

World Health Organization (WHO), 2016. Action on social determinants of health. http://www.who.int/social_determinants/action_sdh/en/.

World Health Organization (WHO), 2018. Health inequities and their causes. https://www.who.int/news-room/facts-in-pictures/detail/health-inequities-and-their-causes.

FURTHER READING

Alston, M., McCurdy, S., McKinnon., 2018. Social Work. Fields of Practice, third ed. Oxford University Press, Melbourne.

Chenowith, L., McAuliffe, D., 2018. The Road to Social Work and Human Services, fifth ed. Cengage Learning, Melbourne.

Joubert, L., Hampson, R., Acuto, R., et al., 2022. Resilience and adaptability of social workers in health care settings during COVID-19 in Australia. Soc Work Health Care 1–19.

OTHER RESOURCES

Australian Association of Social Workers: https://www.aasw.asn.au/.

Fronek, P. (Host). (2014, February 18). Hospital social work: In conversation with Shelley Craig and Barbara Muskat [Episode 65]. Podsocs. Podcast, Griffith University. http://www.podsocs.com/podcast/hospital-social-work/.

International Federation of Social Workers: https://www.ifsw.org/.

Wilkinson, R.G., Marmot, M., World Health Organization Regional Office for Europe (1998). The Solid Facts: Social Determinants of Health. WHO Regional Office for Europe, Copenhagen. https://apps.who.int/iris/handle/10665/108082.

GLOSSARY

A

ableist or ableism Discrimination against people living with disability. The 'ableist' world-view is that able-bodied are the norm in society, and that people living with disability must strive to become that norm. The ableist view holds that disability is a mistake or tragedy rather than a simple consequence of human diversity, akin to ethnicity, sexual orientation or gender.

Aboriginal and Torres Strait Islander Australia's First Peoples.

Aboriginal Community Controlled Health Organisation (ACCHO) A primary care service that provides culturally responsive holistic and comprehensive care and is operated by the local Aboriginal community.

acceptability Social and cultural factors that influence a client's preference for a service (Levesque et al. 2013).

access The degree of 'fit' between the characteristics of providers and health services and the ability of the clients (potential access) (Penchansky & Thomas 1981).

activities of daily living (ADLs) The things we normally do most often daily to live, including activities such as eating, bathing, dressing, grooming, work, homemaking and leisure.

activity-based funding (ABF) A hospital funding system whereby hospitals are paid on the basis of the volume of services provided and the cost of that service. See also casemix.

acute care Care provided for patients, usually in hospitals, for the period when they are very ill.

advanced practice A state of professional maturity in which the individual demonstrates a level of integrated knowledge, skill and competence that challenges the accepted boundaries of practice (McGee & Castledine 2003).

adverse events A harmful event that occurs because a person has received care in a hospital or from a health professional.

affordability Financial and time costs related to using the service (Levesque et al. 2013).

allopathy A philosophy of medicine that cures with opposites. The action of the pharmaceutical drug is the direct opposite to the effects of the illness, e.g. codeine phosphate, the primary effect of which is to cause constipation, used to treat diarrhoea.

almoner The earliest term for a person undertaking the activities associated with social work.

Alzheimer's disease The most common form of dementia, affecting up to 70% of all people with dementia. Alzheimer's disease damages the brain, resulting in impaired memory, thinking and behaviour.

ambulance services Out-of-hospital health services providing a range of emergency, urgent and non-urgent clinical care, patient transport and retrieval services.

approachability Identifying that a service exists, that it can be used and can change a client's health status (Levesque et al., 2013).

appropriateness The fit between a client's health care needs and the timeliness and care spent trying to provide the correct treatment and care (Levesque et al., 2013).

audiologist A health-care professional with postgraduate training in hearing sciences and human communications who tests, diagnoses, and manages hearing loss, tinnitus, and balance problems across the life-span.

auditory processing disorder (APD) A problem with the way an individual processes what they hear.

Australian Health Practitioner Regulation Agency (Ahpra) The government agency which manages the registration and renewal processes for health practitioners on behalf of 15 national health bodies.

authority required (streamlined) benefit A medicine which is included on the Schedule of Pharmaceutical Benefits only when specific patient criteria are fulfilled, and which requires a number to appear on the prescription as confirmation.

authority required benefit A medicine which is included on the Schedule of Pharmaceutical Benefits only when specific patient criteria are fulfilled, and approval given by Services Australia or the Department of Veterans Affairs prior to the medicines being dispensed.

autonomy of practice Capacity to work without interference from any other group in terms of what is done and the resources used.

availability and accommodation The existence and geographical location of a service and appropriately skilled personnel that can potentially be reached by clients (Levesque et al. 2013).

B

benefits Financial payments made to a sick person such as an injured worker, or to health care and other providers on behalf of the sick or injured person. These may include health care, income replacement, lump sums or other payments subject to the provisions of the workers' compensation legislation.

bioequivalent Demonstration that one brand behaves in a similar manner to another brand in relation to the concentration of the medicine in the blood at different times after a patient takes a dose.

biomedical model An approach that sees injury and recovery from an entirely physiological perspective.

biopsychosocial model An approach to health care that sees illness and health as the interaction between the biological, the psychological and the social.

bipartisan agreement An agreement involving two parties finding enough common ground to support core principles of health reforms.

blame game Tactic whereby different levels of government shift blame to each other for problems within the health system.

block-funded Refers to non-individualised funds whereby consumers purchase goods or services directly from a service provider, rather than a portable package of funds given to an individual to choose services.

bulk-billing Where the health practitioner accepts the government fee as full payment for a service, meaning the patient does not contribute to the cost of the service.

bureaucracy The organisation of government departments into many divisions.

C

casemix 'Casemix funding for hospitals [uses] diagnosis-related groups (DRGs) which organise patients' conditions into similar clinical categories with similar costs' (Braithwaite & Hindle 1998, p. 558).

cause-based systems In the context of workers' compensation, a system where benefits are only provided if the injury or illness is attributed to conditions of the workplace.

claim An application for injury compensation made by an injured person to a compensation authority, sometimes through a third-party insurer.

claims management organisation The organisation responsible for managing workers' compensation claims on behalf of the system regulator. In some jurisdictions this is the regulator and in others this is a private sector insurer.

claims manager The professional responsible for managing a compensation claim, including reviewing and approving payments for health care and rehabilitation expenses.

client-centred practice An 'approach to service that incorporates respect for and partnership with clients as active participants in the therapy process' (Schell et al. 2014, p. 1230).

close the gap Australian government policy which focused on improving the well-being of Indigenous Australians. Also a policy directive of the World Health Organization.

closing the gap A policy that aims to improve the lives of First Peoples by eliminating the gap in health and social outcomes between Indigenous and non-Indigenous Australians.

Closing the Gap (CTG) PBS co-payment program A scheme designed to improve access to medicines by First Nations Australians through provision of additional subsidies under the PBs.

code of conduct Good medical/health care practice (the code) describes what is expected of all health professionals registered to practise in Australia. It sets out the principles that characterise good practice and makes explicit the standards of ethical and professional conduct expected of the health professional by their professional peers and the community.

colonisation The act of assuming control over a people and/or place through means such as conflict, treaty, dispossession or settlement.

Commonwealth Ombudsman A government agency that assists members of the public with disputes.

communication access Activities aimed at creating a world where people who have speech and hearing difficulties are able to communicate successfully with everyone.

communication impairment Umbrella term covering all limitations in expressive and/or receptive communication, and arising in speech, language, literacy, voice, fluency and/or social communication (Speech Pathology Australia 2014).

community control The local community having control of issues that directly affect their community. Implicit in this definition is the clear statement that Aboriginal people must determine and control the pace, shape and manner of change and decision-making at local, regional, state and national levels.

community paramedicine A model of care which expands the scope of practice of paramedics to include the delivery of primary health care, substitution and/or coordination of care.

community pharmacy A pharmacy business which is owned by pharmacist(s), operates within a single store, and normally has a retail component and a dispensary.

Community Pharmacy Agreement (CPA) An agreement between the Australian Government and the Pharmacy Guild of Australia. It provides funding to around 5400 community pharmacies for dispensing PBS medicines and providing pharmacy services and to pharmaceutical wholesalers.

complex communication needs People with complex communication needs have communication problems associated with a wide range of physical, sensory, cognitive and environmental causes which restrict/limit their ability to participate independently in society. Hearing loss affecting the outer ear and/or middle ear and thus limiting the conduction of sound to the inner ear (or cochlea). Most commonly conducive hearing losses are amenable to medical or surgical intervention.

compulsory health insurance Where there is a legislated requirement for residents to have health insurance. Australia's Medicare program is an example of a compulsory health insurance scheme.

concession card The Commonwealth Government offers a series of concession cards to target population groups such as aged-care pensioners, low-income household and recipients of certain welfare payments. Concession cardholders are entitled to additional financial support for some health care services and products such as pharmaceuticals.

concessional beneficiaries Patients who hold a Medicare card and receive an Australian pension or other welfare-eligible benefit or are ex-service men and women.

conductive hearing loss Hearing loss caused by a blockage in the middle or outer ear which halts the transmission of sound waves to the inner ear.

constructivist learning Encouraging students to use active techniques (experiments, real-world problem-solving) to create more knowledge and then to reflect on and talk about what they are doing and how their understanding is changing.

consultant pharmacist A pharmacist who has done additional training and is accredited to perform home medicine reviews and residential medication management reviews.

consumer A term used to refer to a person who receives health services, such as a person with lived experiences of mental disorder and of using mental health services, or a person who may use any pharmacy products and/or services.

contextual learning Learning that takes place when teachers are able to present information in a way from which students are able to construct meaning based on their own experiences.

continuity of midwifery care (CoC) A maternity service model in which women receive continuity of care from a known midwife throughout pregnancy, during birth and across the early parenting journey (usually to 6 weeks postpartum).

co-payment Amount that the patient pays towards the cost of a PBS-subsidised medicine.

corporatised To be subject to corporate ownership or control. In medicine, medical practices are increasingly being bought out by organisations that then re-employ the doctors to work in their clinics for a salary.

cost-shifting   A practice whereby one level of government seeks to shift responsibility of health care delivery (and funding) to another level of government. For example, if state governments reduce clinics offered by public hospital, patients may seek care at federally-funded general practices.

COVID-19   The disease caused by infectious SARS-CoV-2 virus.

cultural competence   A diversity of definitions exist – one defines cultural competence as 'the ability of systems to provide care to patients with diverse values, beliefs and behaviours, including tailoring delivery to meet patients' social, cultural and linguistic needs' (Betancourt et al., 2002, p. v).

cultural safety   Both a philosophy and way of working that is mindful of cultural difference, defined by the NZ Nursing Council as the effective care 'of a person or family from another culture, and is determined by that person or family. Culture includes, but is not restricted to, age or generation; gender; sexual orientation; occupation and socioeconomic status; ethnic origin or migrant experience; religious or spiritual belief; and disability.' (Nursing Council of New Zealand 2011).

customer   Someone who, regardless of whether the visit is for health- or medicine-related reasons, interacts with a community pharmacy or service provider with the intention of purchasing products and/or using the service.

D

day hospital   A hospital providing services for patients who then return home or to another facility at night.

deinstitutionalisation   The process of moving long-term residents from institutional (hospital) care into the community.

dementia   A chronic and progressive condition characterised by memory loss and other cognitive deficits.

dental decay/dental caries   Disease of the teeth.

dental prosthetists   Dental prosthetists provide assessment, treatment, management and provision of removable dentures and mouth-guards used for sporting activities. With additional education and a written referral from a dentist, they also provide various types of splints, sleep apnoea devices, anti-snoring devices, immediate dentures and additions to existing dentures.

dental therapists (DT)   Dental therapists provide oral health assessment, diagnosis, treatment, management and preventive services for children, adolescents and young adults (and, with additional education, for all adults) within a preventive philosophy. They provide fillings and tooth removal, additional oral care, and oral health education and promotion for individuals and communities. Dental therapists are autonomous practitioners who work in collaborative and referral relationships with dentists.

dentate   Refers to individuals with teeth (as opposed to 'edentulous').

dentist   Dentists practise all parts of dentistry, including assessment, diagnosis, treatment, management and preventive services for patients of all ages.

developmental disabilities   Developmental physical, sensory, cognitive or psychological problems that are generally severe and chronic and impact on everyday life.

Diagnosis Related Groups (DRG)   A patient classification scheme that provides a means of relating the numbers and types of patients treated in a hospital to the resources required by the hospital (AIHW 2001, p. 148). Usually measured through length of stay and resource allocation.

dietitian   An expert in human nutrition and dietetics with tertiary qualifications in both nutrition education/promotion and medical nutrition therapy.

disability   A social construct that results from barriers experienced in the environment in which a person lives and interacts and is not inherent within the person. It reflects the interaction between features of a person's body and features of the society or environment in which he or she engages.

disability-based systems   In the context of workers' compensation, a system where compensation is provided to people with work disability regardless of cause (Lippel & Lötters 2013).

diversity   An understanding that each individual is unique and recognising our individual differences. These can be along the dimensions of race, ethnicity, gender, sexual orientation, socio-economic status, age, physical abilities, religious beliefs, political beliefs or other ideologies (Associated Students of the University of Oregon 1999).

dysphagia   A neuromuscular condition which causes difficulties in swallowing.

E

economic rationalism   A term used to describe a range of economic policies which aim to reduce the extent of government intervention in the economy and to increase reliance on markets to direct economic activity. Some policies which are associated with economic rationalism include outsourcing, reducing government spending, privatisation and deregulation.

edentulous   Refers to individuals without teeth (as opposed to 'dentate').

effectiveness   In health, this refers to care that results in positive outcomes.

efficiency   'The relationship between the cost of various inputs and the output produced' (National Health Ministers' Benchmarking Commonwealth of Australia 1996, p. 21).

Efficient Funding of Chemotherapy   PBS program funding costs associated with chemotherapy.

electronic health record (EHR)   A system where health information about individuals or populations is compiled electronically over time.

emergency departments (EDs)   Units in hospitals that provide 24-hour emergency care for serious illnesses and injuries.

enrolled nurse (EN)   A second-level nurse who provides nursing care under the direct or indirect supervision of a registered nurse, and must hold enrolled nursing registration with the Nursing and Midwifery Board of Australia. This group is also known as a Division 2 nurse in the State of Victoria.

equality   A measure of sameness, that is, whether or not all people within a society are given the same resources, including for example health services, irrespective of their needs.

equity   Refers to the justice or fairness in the distribution of resources (such as health services), including supplying, for example, more or different services to those in greater need.

evidence-based medicine (EBM)   An approach to medicine holding that all clinical practice should be based on evidence from randomised control trials to ensure treatment effectiveness and efficacy.

evidence-based practice   The incorporation of the best research evidence to inform clinical treatment decisions and patient values.

expressive communication impairments Reduced ability to convey spoken, gestural/ sign language or written information.

extended care paramedic (ECP) Paramedic specialist with the knowledge, skills and expanded scope of practice to provide high-level care for patients with non-emergency health care needs.

extended scope of practice Health professional whose scope of practice adopts knowledge, skills and abilities that traditionally belong in the expert domain of another profession (e.g. nurse practitioners).

F

Family Tax Benefit Part A (FTB(A)) Eligibility for FTB(A) is based on a means test on family income, and is adjusted for the number and age of children in the family. Eligible families receive a financial benefit from the government and are also eligible for the lower Extended Medicare Safety Net (EMSN) threshold.

fee-for-service A payment model where services are unbundled and paid for separately. In health care, it gives an incentive for physicians to provide more treatments because payment is dependent on the quantity of care, rather than quality of care.

feminisation of care A theory which suggests the majority of unpaid care of people with a mental illness, the elderly or those with a disability is done by women.

financial protection Health insurance offers financial protection from the potentially high cost of health care when sick.

First Nations Peoples The original peoples of this continent – Aboriginal and Torres Strait Islander people.

food insecurity Whenever people do not at all times have physical, social and economic access to sufficient, safe and nutritious food (Gallegos et al. 2017).

formal services Services provided by government and non-government services wherein care is delivered by trained staff.

G

gap fee The difference between what is charged by the doctor, hospital or health professional for the service and what the client receives in reimbursements by Medicare or a private insurer.

gate-keeper A service provider who controls access to higher levels of medical care. Patients require a referral from their GP to gain access to other parts of the health care system such as specialist consultations, pathology, diagnostic imaging and prescription medicine. It is one of the roles GPs play in the Australian health care system (as well as in many other countries).

general patients Individuals and families who are not eligible for a concession card.

general practice The name given in various nations, such as the United Kingdom, India, Australia, New Zealand and South Africa, to the services provided by general practitioners. In some nations, such as the USA, similar services may be described as family medicine or primary care.

general practitioner (GP) A doctor who is qualified in general medical practice. GPs are often the first point of contact for someone, of any age, who feels sick or has a health concern. They treat a wide range of medical conditions and health issues.

generic brand A brand of a medicine which is produced after the patent on that medicine has expired, and which is an alternative to the originator brand.

generic substitution Replacement of one brand of a medicine by another which is considered to be brand equivalent.

geographical classification system The use of physical location data that can be used to inform policy and/or resource allocation (McGrail & Humphreys 2009).

H

health care financing The system that characterises the way revenue to pay for health care is sourced, for example, through taxation, health insurance or out-of-pocket costs.

health care system An organised plan of health services. The term is usually used to refer to the system or program by which health care is made available to the population and financed by government, private enterprise, or both (WHO 2007).

health care system performance Includes the three dimensions of accessibility, quality and efficiency. Together these determine the extent to which the achievable in health care can be attained. Health system performance refers to how far health systems achieve each of these goals relative to the country's overall context (WHO 2007).

health equity The rights of people to have equitable access to services on the basis of need, and the resources, capacities and power they need to act upon the circumstances of their lives that determine their health (Keleher & MacDougall 2015).

health financing Refers to how financial resources are mobilised, allocated and used to ensure that the health system can adequately cover the collective health needs of every person (WHO 2007).

health gap Describes the inequities between population groups that may happen because of circumstances related to where they live, or their socio-economic status.

health security The existence of strong and resilient public health systems that can prevent, detect and respond to infectious disease threats, wherever they occur in the world (WHO 2007).

health system Consists of all organisations, people and actions whose primary intent is to promote, restore or maintain health. This includes efforts to influence determinants of health as well as more direct health-improving activities (WHO 2007).

health workforce shortages Shortages of skilled health care workers.

Hearing Australia The national body providing hearing services to people eligible under the Australian Government Hearing Services Program.

highly specialised drugs (HSD) Medicines provided on the PBS which, due to either their clinical use or other special features, have restrictions on where they can be prescribed or supplied.

holistic An approach to healing which recognises a person as a unique totality; mind, body and spirit.

home medicines review (HMR) A service for persons living in their own home. It involves collaboration between a GP and a pharmacist to review the medication management needs of a resident.

horizontal equity When people with the same needs have the access to the same resources (Starfield 2011).

human rights model A model for addressing disability or disadvantage to go beyond legal requirements to policy and practices.

I

iatrogenic A term referring to further illness conditions that result from medical treatment. For example, when older people are hospitalised for treatment, they may become disoriented, fall, acquire infection or be afflicted by drug interactions.

impairment Any loss or abnormality of psychological, physiological or anatomical structure or function.

Independent Health and Aged Care Pricing Authority (IHACPA) Government agency responsible for calculating the national efficient price of hospital episodes. The agency was formerly known as the Independent Hospital Pricing Authority (IHPA).

Indigenous In Australia, 'Indigenous' with a capital 'I' denotes First Nations Peoples.

Indigenous Australians' Health Programme (IAHP) A program that aims to improve the health of Indigenous people, improve access to comprehensive culturally responsive primary health care and support primary health care services to improve the way they operate to better cater for Aboriginal and Torres Strait Islander peoples.

individualised funding A portable package of funds allocated to a particular individual that facilitates their control over how they purchase support for their needs.

inpatient A patient receiving treatment as an admitted patient in a hospital, generally staying in hospital on an overnight basis or longer.

institutional mix An assessment of what institutions are involved in an issue.

integration of care This involves services working together to meet care needs to improve access and equity and ensure all consumer needs are met. This may involve joint service planning.

intensive care paramedic (ICP) Paramedic specialist with the knowledge, skills and expanded scope of practice to provide high-level emergency care for acutely ill and injured patients.

interprofessional education and collaborative practice Where two or more health and/or social care professionals work together to provide person-centred care. Students training to be a health or social care professional are provided collaborative learning opportunities with students from other health or social care disciplines to provide person-centred care.

interprofessional education/practice (IPE/IPP) 'An intervention where the members of more than one health or social care profession, or both, learn interactively together, for the explicit purpose of improving interprofessional collaboration or the health/well being of patients/clients, or

both' (Reeves et al. 2013, p. 2). This interaction allows for two or more health professionals to learn from, with and about each other as part of ongoing professional development, improved collaboration and the quality care provided to patients or clients (Health Workforce Australia 2013).

intersectoral collaboration Work across sectors such as health, education, justice, sport and recreation, and agriculture, to achieve an outcome that a single sector could not achieve alone.

intervention services Services that target development of specific skills (e.g. speech pathology services for children with delayed speech or language, audiology services for adults with hearing loss or tinnitus or applied behaviour analysis therapy for autism spectrum disorders).

K

knowledges The knowledge and belief systems of a particular cultural group.

L

life expectancy The average number of years that a newborn would be expected to live if they are subject to the age-specific mortality rate during a given period.

lived experience A person's unique experiences of and insights about mental ill-health and recovery.

M

mainstream General term for Western biomedical health care; usually denotes majority or dominant government-controlled services.

market pressure In the context of health care, the pressure experienced by providers to keep their fees low because patients are looking for the best deal.

market-driven health care system a private system where the services are run by private providers, and citizens pay for their own health care.

MBS benefit The total benefit patients will receive from Medicare for their claim. It comprises the Medicare rebate as well as the EMSN amount.

MBS fee A fee set by government for each service listed on the MBS. It forms the basis for calculating the amount of money that patients are entitled to receive if they make a claim.

medical dominance A situation where the profession of medicine has the majority of the power over health care decisions,

including over the work of other health professionals.

medical model A model that sees normal human conditions such as childbirth, ageing or disability as requiring medical intervention. Disability is viewed as a problem of the person, directly caused by disease, trauma, or other health condition, which therefore requires sustained medical care provided in the form of individual treatment by professionals. In the medical model, management of the disability is aimed at a 'cure'.

medical nutrition therapy The specific nutritional management of a range of health conditions and associated symptoms involving the application of current nutrition practice.

medical rationing defined Implicitly or explicitly allowing people to go without beneficial health care services' (Emanuel et al., 2018, p. 29). Also known as 'health care rationing'.

Medicare The Australian public health insurance scheme.

Medicare Benefits Schedule (MBS) Health care services subsidised by the Australian government.

Medicare levy A 2% additional income tax paid by most income earners, although there are exemptions for those on low incomes and people who are not entitled to Medicare benefits (e.g. some classes of visa holders).

Medicare rebate The part of the Medicare benefit that is determined by the MBS fee. For most out-of-hospital services, the Medicare rebate is equal to 85% of the MBS fee. For most primary care services, the Medicare rebate is equal to 100% of the MBS fee.

medication reconciliation A systematic process to obtain an accurate and complete list of all medications at transitions of care.

medicines Chemical or biological substances which are used to prevent and/or treat health conditions.

mental disorder The experience of living with a mental health condition.

minor ailment A medical condition which may be managed without necessarily accessing medical services.

mixed system A system of health care or education that has both public (and free) services as well as services that can be purchased.

mobile-driven health service delivery Health service delivery utilising the functionality of mobile devices to collect, share, record and deliver health data or services.

modalities   Distinct areas of complementary and alternative health practice, e.g. naturopathy, massage.

moral hazard   An economic term referring to a lack of incentive to protect oneself against risk or make cost-efficient choices because others will pay for the consequences; in healthcare it refers to the additional healthcare patients may receive because it is paid for by insurance.

morbidity   Illness, disease.

mortality   Deaths. The mortality rate is a measure of the number of deaths in a given population.

N

national competency standards   Benchmark skills and knowledge set by accrediting agencies.

National Disability Insurance Scheme (NDIS)   A scheme for provision of support services to people with disabilities where people are given a budget to purchase the services that they require.

national health insurance (NHI) model   Model using private-sector providers, but payment comes from a government-run insurance program that every citizen pays into.

National Medicines Policy (NMP)   A national framework for the provision of medicines in Australia which covers appropriate access and quality.

National Registration and Accreditation Scheme (NRAS)   A 2012 government initiative to establish national boards for the purpose of regulating registered health professionals' practice in a competent and ethical manner in order to protect the health and safety of the public.

neoliberalism   A new (Mazurek Melnyk et al. 2017) look at liberal political policy that argues that the economy is best controlled by the private sector rather than by governments.

new public health   An explicitly social and political approach to health development that emphasises knowledge to action on the social determinants of health, intersectoral action to support health, healthy public policy, environments for health, sustainable development and equity in health (Keleher & MacDougall 2015).

new public management (NMP)   The principles of the market are applied to public institutions and as a consequence to the working conditions of those employed in these institutions (Cairney 2002).

noise-induced hearing loss   Hearing loss affecting the inner ear (i.e., cochlear or auditory nerve) as a result of either long-term exposure to high levels of noise or exposure to explosive noise such as rifle fire. NIHL most commonly arises from occupational noise exposure but also may arise from the use of personal amplification systems.

non-government organisation (NGO)   A private organisation that is independent of the government.

not-for-profit (NFP)   An organisation whose operations provides services to community (e.g. childcare, art centre, neighbourhood associations, sports clubs, aged care) and do so without making a profit for its membership or shareholders.

nurse practitioner (NP)   A registered nurse whose registration has been endorsed by the Nursing and Midwifery Board of Australia as a nurse practitioner under Section 95 of the National Law, and holding a Master's level qualification. Nurses in this group can apply to have access to the PBS by the Commonwealth Health Minister.

Nursing and Midwifery Board of Australia (NMBA)   The legally constituted body in Australia charged with the regulation of nursing and midwifery professional practice with an aim to protect the public through ensuring nurses and midwives demonstrate acceptable standards of practice.

nutritionist   An expert in human nutrition, usually with tertiary qualifications in nutrition education/promotion.

O

obesity epidemic   A term used to illustrate the increase in severity and rapid expansion of the prevalence of obesity in many nations globally, including Australia.

obesogenic environment   A term that includes all features of the environment in which people live out their lives which can contribute to obesity for both individuals and whole populations. This includes the built, physical, food and social environment which encourages overconsumption, unhealthy food choices, sedentary behaviour and reduced physical activity.

occupation   The day-to-day activities of life.

occupational engagement   The 'performance of occupations as the result of choice, motivation, and meaning within a supportive context and environment' (American Occupational Therapy Association (AOTA) 2014, p. S42).

occupational justice   'Access to and participation in the full range of meaningful and enriching occupations afforded to others, including opportunities for social inclusion and the resources to participate in occupations to satisfy personal, health and societal needs' (AOTA 2014, p. S35).

occupational rehabilitation   Rehabilitation activities focused on returning an injured person to the workplace, rather than treating the underlying health condition.

old public health   A social movement of the 19th century that worked to improve living conditions through the development of physical infrastructure, including water, sanitation and housing, as well as policy and legislation to support and drive change (Keleher & MacDougall 2015).

oral health therapy practitioners   A practitioner qualified as a dental therapist and dental hygienist.

originator brand   The brand of a medicine which is first made available for patient use, usually while a patent is in operation.

out-of-hospital service   A health care service delivered outside of the hospital setting, such as when visiting a medical specialist or GP for the regular review of a chronic health condition.

out-of-pocket (OOP) cost   The difference between what is charged by the doctor, hospital or health professional for the service and what the client receives in reimbursements by Medicare or a private insurer. Also known as a co-payment or gap payment.

outpatient   A patient receiving treatment where they are not required to be admitted to a hospital bed, such as when visiting a medical specialist for the regular review of a chronic health condition or accessing an emergency department for short-term treatment.

P

Paramedicine Board of Australia (PBA) One of the 15 health professional boards established under the Health Practitioner Regulation National Law (the National Law) to regulate paramedics in Australia under the National Registration and Accreditation Scheme (the National Scheme).

patent A legally enforceable right for a device, substance, process or method which gives the owner or inventor exclusive commercial rights for a specified period of time.

patient A person who interacts with a specific health provider for health or medicine-related reasons.

payment for performance (P4P) Payment closely linked to activity-based funding model, where health care systems are paid for the amount of throughput, rather than outcomes.

peer worker A person with lived experiences of recovery who is employed to support others' recovery.

periodontal disease Disease of the gums and supporting structures of the teeth.

personal recovery Individually determined recovery, which is about leading a meaningful and fulfilling life whether or not the effects of a mental health condition are present.

person-centred approach An approach, service philosophy and range of processes that aims to discover and act on what is important to a person. It involves continual listening and learning, focusing on what is important to someone now and in the future, and acting on this in consultation with their family and their friends. The individual and their aspirations and goals are at the centre of decision-making.

Pharmaceutical Benefits Advisory Committee (PBAC) An independent expert body appointed by the Australian Government who recommends new medicines for inclusion on the PBS.

Pharmaceutical Benefits Scheme (PBS) A scheme designed to provide necessary subsidised medicines to Australians at a cost that individuals and the community can afford.

pharmaceutical reform Revision of PBS arrangements to include delivery of additional medicines as well as supply of PBS funded medicine on discharge from public hospitals.

Pharmaceutical Society of Australia The peak national professional pharmacy organisation representing Australia's 28,000 pharmacists working in all sectors and across all locations.

Pharmacy Guild of Australia The national peak body representing the owners of Australia's 5400 community pharmacies.

population ageing The increase in median age of proportion of the older person population over time. This is due to the decrease in fertility rates and increased life expectancy.

population strategy A strategy that attempts to control the incidence of the determinants of health, and thus to shift the distribution of exposure across the whole population.

practice nurse A registered or enrolled nurse employed in a general practice setting (not a registered group, like the nurse practitioner, but so named because they work in general practice).

presbycusis Bilateral (and most commonly) sensorineural hearing impairment that occurs as people age.

presumptive rules In the context of workers' compensation, in specified occupations, certain conditions are automatically assumed to be work-related (e.g. silicosis in coal miners).

prevention paradox Interventions that achieve large overall health gains for whole populations as opposed to those that offer small advantages to individuals at high risk. In other words, preventing small risks in large populations leads to greater health outcomes than avoiding large risks in a smaller number of high-risk individuals.

price elasticity A measure of how responsive demand for a good or service is when the price changes. Specifically, price elasticity tells us by what percentage the quantity demanded will decrease for a 1% increase in price.

primary care (or primary medical care) A narrower scope of definition than primary health care and refers to general practice or family doctor services delivered to individuals.

primary contact practices People who are able to make contact with a service without a referral from a GP.

primary health care (PHC) 'a whole-of-society approach to health that aims at ensuring the highest possible level of health and well-being and their equitable distribution by focusing on people's needs and as early as possible along the continuum from health promotion and disease prevention to treatment, rehabilitation and palliative care, and as close as feasible to people's everyday environment' (WHO and UNICEF 2018)

private for-profit Where an organisation operates a service or product that is sold for a profit.

private health insurance (PHI) Health insurance that is provided by industry rather than government-run insurance.

private health insurance (PHI) model A term referring to health insurance plans marketed by the private health insurance industry, as opposed to government-run insurance programs. It is characterised by employment-based or individual purchase of private health insurance financed by individual and employer contributions. It allows the insuree to be treated in a private or public hospital as a private patient; it also provides cover for services not covered by national or social health insurance.

private health insurance rebate A means-tested contribution through the taxation system to individuals and families towards the cost of private health insurance.

private hospital Hospital owned by a for-profit or not-for-private entity, with services paid for by patient themselves, insurance companies, or agreements with governments.

private prescriptions Prescriptions for medicines which are not eligible for subsidy under the PBS.

privatisation The transfer of previously public services or products to the private sector.

proceduralist A physician or surgeon who is skilled at diagnostic or therapeutic procedures, or whose work consists largely of carrying out such procedures, e.g. an endoscopist.

productivity '[T]he relationship between the mix of inputs and outputs' (NHMBWG 1996, p. 34).

professional development Ongoing education and training taken by professionals to increase and extend their skill and knowledge.

professional monopoly A situation where a profession controls a particular service.

programmatic assessment An approach in which routine information about the learner's competence and progress is continually collected, analysed and, where needed, complemented with purposively collected additional assessment information, with the intent to both maximally inform the learner and their mentor and allow for high-stakes decisions at the end of a training phase.

prophylactically Where therapy is used to prevent an illness or disease, e.g. giving a patient antibiotics to prevent an infection.

protected title A designated professional title which is protected by law. Making claims of and acting as a registered health professional when not registered is an offence under National Law.

provider fee The fee charged by a provider for their health care service.

public dental services Dental services funded by governments and provided to eligible people through public and community sector agencies.

public health insurance A type of health insurance that is financed through taxation and other sources of government revenue; in a US context, a program run by US federal, state or local governments in which people have some or all of their health care costs paid for by the government (Medicare or Medicaid).

public health nutrition A branch of nutrition practice with a focus on promoting good health and the primary prevention of disease at the population level utilising policy, research and interventions which highlight healthy eating.

public health system The system of health care delivered by the State.

public–private partnership (PPP) 'An arrangement where the private sector supplies assets and services that traditionally have been provided by the government. In addition to private execution and financing of public investment, PPPs have two other important characteristics: there is an emphasis on service provision, as well as investment, by the private sector; and significant risk is transferred from the government to the private sector' (World Bank 2014, pp. 17–18) although governments are usually required to pay back the funds used to provide the service.

public–private partnerships (PPPs) 'An arrangement where the private sector supplies assets and services that traditionally

have been provided by the government. In addition to private execution and financing of public investment, PPPs have two other important characteristics: there is an emphasis on service provision, as well as investment, by the private sector; and significant risk is transferred from the government to the private sector' (World Bank 2014, pp. 17–18) although governments are usually required to pay back the funds used to provide the service.

Q

quality of life An individual's perception of their position in life in the context of the culture and value systems in which they live and in relation to their goals, expectations, standards and concerns' (WHO 2012, p. 8).

quality use of medicines (QUM) One of the four tenants of Australia's National Medicine Policy and means the safe, efficacious, judicious and appropriate use of medicines.

quality-adjusted life-year (QALY) A value, measured in years, that takes into account both the quality and quantity of life and is a measure of the benefit to a patient that results from taking a new medicine or treatment.

R

ramping When an ambulance presents to an emergency department and no bed is available, forcing the patient to remain under the care of ambulance personnel.

receptive communication impairment Reduced ability to understand another person's communication (spoken, gestured/signed or written).

reciprocal health care agreement (RHCA) A formal written agreement with another country which allows access to the PBS and Medicare for their citizens while visiting Australia, and some health care benefits to Australians when they are visiting the other country.

reference pricing Setting the price of a PBS medicine by comparing it with the price of the other brands (originator and/or generic) of that medicine or the cost paid for the medicine in other countries.

reflective learning A way of allowing students to step back from their learning experience to help them develop critical thinking skills and improve on future performance by analysing their experience.

registered nurse (RN) A nurse with a minimum 3-year training certificate and postgraduate qualifications who must be registered with the Nursing and Midwifery Board of Australia. A registered nurse works without supervision and is accountable for providing nursing care. This group is also known as a Division 1 nurse in the state of Victoria.

regulation The act of being regulated, which means being subject to laws, principles or rules that control or govern.

regulator The government authority responsible for oversight and management of the workers' compensation system.

Repatriation Pharmaceutical Benefits Scheme (RPBS) A scheme designed to provide subsidised medicines and wound care items to ex-service men and women.

repeats Additional supplies of a medicine which are allowed on a prescription and which can be provided to a patient after the initial prescription supply has been used.

residential aged-care facility (RACF) A home for older people who can no longer live at home and need ongoing help with everyday tasks or health care

residential medication management review (RMMR) A service for permanent residents of a residential aged-care facility (RACF). It involves collaboration between a GP and a pharmacist to review the medication management needs of a resident.

residential services Government-regulated facilities that house and provide long-term medical and social care to frail elderly people. These facilities also offer short-term respite care.

resilience (of the health system) The capacity of health actors, institutions and populations to prepare for and effectively respond to crises; maintain core functions when a crisis hits; and, informed by lessons learned during the crisis, reorganise if conditions require it. Health systems are resilient if they protect human life and produce good health outcomes for all during a crisis and in its aftermath.

restricted benefit A medicine which is included on the Schedule of Pharmaceutical Benefits only when specific patient criteria are fulfilled but which does not require a number to appear on the prescription as confirmation.

restrictive practices any practice or intervention that has the effect of restricting the rights or freedom of movement of a person with disability' (NDIS Act (2013) (Cwlth) Section 9). There are five restrictive practices that are subject to regulation and oversight by the NDIS Commission: chemical, mechanical, physical, environmental and seclusion.

rubella A virus (also known as German measles) that can cause birth defects or death of an unborn fetus if contracted during pregnancy. Sensorineural (inner ear) hearing loss in a newborn baby is a common consequence of maternal rubella.

S

safeguarding Those rules that are in place to protect vulnerable persons from harm, abuse, neglect or exploitation.

Safety Net scheme A scheme under the PBS and Medicare which provides additional financial assistance to families with high medicines or health costs.

SARS-CoV-2 pandemic Worldwide spread of infectious SARS-CoV-2 virus that causes COVID-19 disease.

Schedule of Pharmaceutical Benefits The list of medicines which have been approved for government subsidy under the PBS.

school dental services A government service providing free general dental care to eligible school-aged children.

scope of practice The boundaries of practice for a health profession.

secondary care Health care that is provided by a specialist upon referral from a primary health provider.

section 100 Medicines available on the PBS but distributed under alternative arrangements such as via public or private hospitals.

self-determination The ability or right to make one's own decisions without interference from others.

self-regulate The capacity of individuals, organisations or professions to rule or govern themselves without outside interference.

sentinel event A serious event in a hospital or health care setting that results in the death of a patient or major physical harm (Australian Commission for Safety and Quality in Health Care 2017).

social care Care by public organisations and private companies for people in society who need special help in order to live comfortably (e.g. aged care and disability services).

social contract An agreement between the individual and the state over what the state will provide for the citizen, e.g. financial support when sick.

social determinants of health (SDH) The economic and/or social conditions that influence the health of individuals, groups and communities.

social health insurance A scheme initiated by the government to serve as a source of revenue for health financing to decrease the out-of-pocket burden on the people

social model of disability A model that sees 'disability' as a socially created problem and not an attribute of an individual, but rather a complex collection of conditions, many of which are created by the social environment. Effective management requires social action and it is the collective responsibility of society to make the environmental modifications necessary to facilitate full participation of people living with impairment in all areas of life. From this perspective, equal access for someone living with impairment/disability is a human rights issue.

social model of health A model oriented to a holistic understanding of a client, patient or resident. This model promotes social participation and self-fulfillment despite the effects of disease and impairment.

speech pathologist (SP) Tertiary qualified professional who works with people with communication and/or swallowing difficulties.

Speech Pathology Australia The national peak body for the speech pathology profession in Australia.

spinal cord injury A disruption of the nervous tissue in the spinal cord, generally following trauma, which impairs sensation or movement control.

stigma A feeling of being devalued when you have experienced a mental disorder, live with disability or belong to a stigmatised group, because of negative stereotypes; can be due to mental disorder, race, culture, gender or sexual preferences.

structural balance The balance of influence across key categories including, in the case of health care, the balance across the State, the medical profession and private finance.

structural inequality Inequality that is facilitated by a society's institutions (including health care, the police, education, etc.), which advantage some groups in a society and not others.

surge workforce A workforce model which utilises a range of options to meet increased staffing to address service demand. Flexible options include recruiting enrolled students, the newly retired or those who had a period of time away from recent practice, and overseas registered practitioners.

systematic literature review (SLR) A highly structured literature review that deals with a particular research question.

T

targeted public health Targeted public health approaches are those focused on particular population groups – those at higher risk for contracting a communicable disease, for example.

tertiary care Care for more complex and/or acute conditions requiring intensive support and treatment, usually provided in hospitals.

the State The government, the opposition, the public service, the military and the legal system of judges, publicly employed lawyers and the police.

theory An intellectual tool for understanding a situation.

Therapeutic Goods Administration (TGA) The Australian Government Department responsible for the regulation of medicines.

tinnitus The experience of buzzing or ringing in the ears. In most cases, the cause is unknown.

traditional Denoting practices that have historically been undertaken by First Nations Peoples since before colonisation.

transdisciplinary Approaches that require team members to share roles and systematically cross discipline boundaries. Primarily to pool and integrate the expertise of team members so that efficient and comprehensive assessment and intervention may be provided. Professionals from different disciplines teach, learn and work together to accomplish a common set of intervention goals for an individual. The role differentiation between disciplines is defined by the needs of the situation rather than by discipline-specific characteristics.

U

universal approaches Universal approaches to public health are those available to everyone at no cost or very little cost, such as immunisation, maternal and child health and cancer screening programs.

universal health coverage (UHC) Universal health coverage means that all people have access to the health services they need, when and where they need them, without financial hardship. It includes the full range of essential health services, from health promotion to prevention, treatment, rehabilitation, and palliative care.

unlicensed health worker A person who performs care duties under supervision but is not granted a licence under formal registration, e.g. nursing registration. This group is trained to provide care or other duties either through further education sector or in-house training at their place of work. They do not have the right to use the title of the profession.

unrestricted benefits Medicines provided via the PBS where there are no restrictions applied to therapeutic use.

utilisation The act of accessing health care (also *realised* access) (Penchansky & Thomas 1981).

V

vertical equity Situation where people with more needs are provided with more resources (Starfield 2011).

W

welfare health care system The provision of services for the whole population and highlight the ability of the health system to reach the entire population with the available healthcare services.

welfare state A system where the government provides for the welfare (education, health, unemployment, etc.) of its citizens.

woman-centred care In midwifery, the woman is at the centre of her care and the midwife has a relationship with the woman who has a relationship with the baby. In this relationship, each woman is seen as an individual with different needs, values and cultural beliefs.

work disability The inability to participate in employment due to a health condition, such as an injury or illness.

work disability duration The amount of time taken away from work due to injury or ill health.

World Physiotherapy The global body that represents the profession of physiotherapy.

REFERENCES

American Occupational Therapy Association (AOTA), 2014. Occupational therapy practice framework: domain and process, third ed. Am J Occup Ther 68 (Suppl. 1), S1–S51.

Associated Students of the University of Oregon, 1999. Summer Diversity Initiative: definition of diversity. http://gladstone.uoregon.edu/~asuomca/diversityinit/definition.html.

Australian Commission for Safety and Quality in Health Care (ACSQHC), 2017. Australian safety and quality framework for health care: putting the framework into action. ACSQHC, Sydney. https://www.safetyandquality.gov.au/wp-content/uploads/2011/01/ASQFHC-Guide-Healthcare-team.pdf.

Australian Institute of Health and Welfare (AIHW), 2001. National health data dictionary. Version 10. Cat. no. HWI 30. AIHW, Canberra.

Betancourt, J.R., Green, A.R., Carrillo, J.E., 2002. Cultural competence in health care: emerging frameworks and practical approaches. The Commonwealth Fund, New York. http://www.commonwealthfund.org/usr_doc/betancourt_culturalcompetence_576.pdf.

Braithwaite J, Hindle D, 1998. Casemix funding in Australia. Med J Aust 168 (11), 558–60.

Cairney, P., 2002. New public management and the Thatcher healthcare legacy: enough of the theory, what about the implementation? Br J Polit Int Relat 4 (3), 375–398.

Emanuel, E., Schmidt, H., Steinmetz, A., 2018. Rationing and resource allocation in healthcare: essential readings. OUP, New York.

Gallegos, D., Booth, S., Cleve, S., et al., 2017. Food insecurity in Australian households from charity to entitlement. In: Germov, J., Williams, L. (Eds.), A Sociology of Food and Nutrition, fourth ed. OUP, Melbourne, Chapter 4.

Health Workforce Australia (HWA), 2013. Health professionals prescribing pathway (HPPP) project, final report. HWA, Adelaide.

Keleher, H., MacDougall, C. (Eds.), 2015. Glossary. In: Understanding Health, fourth ed. OUP, Melbourne.

Levesque, J.F., Harris, M.F., et al., 2013. Patient-centred access to health care: conceptualising access at the interface of health systems and populations. Int J Equity Health 12 (18), 1475–9276.

Lippel K, Lötters F., 2013. Public insurance systems: a comparison of cause-based and disability-based income support systems. In: Loisel, P., Anema, J.R., Handbook of Work Disability. Springer, New York, pp. 183–202. doi:10.1007/978-1-4614-6214-9_12.

Mazurek Melnyk, B., Fineout-Overholt, E., Giggleman, M., et al., 2017. A test of the ARCC C model improves implementation of evidence-based practice, healthcare culture, and patient outcomes. Worldviews Evid Based Nurs 14 (1), 5–9.

McGee, P., Castledine, G., 2003. Advanced Nursing Practice, second ed. Blackwell Science, Oxford.

McGrail, M.R., Humphreys, J.S., 2009. Geographical classifications to guide rural health policy in Australia. Aust New Zealand Health Policy 6, 28.doi:10.1186/1743-8462-6-28.

National Health Ministers' Benchmarking Working Group (NHMBWG), 1996. First national report on health sector performance indicators: public hospitals – the state of play. AIHW, Canberra. https://www.aihw.gov.au/getmedia/a6bff00a-d7d8-45d6-8dd0-42ace859d4b8/fnrhspi-c00.pdf.aspx.

NDIS Act (2013) (Cwlth) Section 9.

Nursing Council of New Zealand, 2011. http://pro.health-mentoronline.com/assets/Uploads/refract/pdf/Nursing_Council_cultural-safety11.pdf.

Penchansky, R., Thomas, J.W., 1981. The concept of access: definition and relationship to consumer satisfaction. Med Care 19 (2), 127–140.

Reeves, S., Perrier, L., Goldman, J., et al., 2013. Interprofessional education: effects on professional practice and healthcare outcomes (update). Cochrane Database Syst. Rev. (3), CD002213.

Schell, B., Gillen, G., Scaffa, M. (Eds.), 2014. Willard and Spackman's Occupational Therapy, twelfth ed. Lippincott Williams & Wilkins, Philadelphia, p. 1230.

Speech Pathology Australia, 2014. Communication impairment in Australia. http://www. speechpathologyaustralia. org.au/library/2013Factsheets/Factsheet_Communication_Impairment_in_Australia.pdf.

Starfield, B., 2011. The hidden inequity in health care. Int J Equity Health 10 (1), 15.

World Bank, 2014. 2014. Public–private partnerships: reference guide. Version 2.0. World Bank Group, Washington, DC. http://documents.worldbank.org/curated/en/2014/01/20182310/. public-private-partnerships-reference-guide-version-20/.

World Health Organization, 2007. Everybody's business – strengthening health systems to improve health outcomes: WHO's framework for action. World Health Organization. https://apps.who.int/iris/handle/10665/43918.

World Health Organization (WHO), 2012. Programme on mental health WHOQOL user manual. Division of Mental Health and Prevention of Substance Abuse World Health Organization. WHO, Geneva.

World Health Organization (WHO) and United Nations Children's Fund (UNICEF), 2018. A vision for primary health care in the 21st century: towards universal health coverage and the Sustainable Development Goals. World Health Organization.

ABBREVIATIONS

AASW	Australian Association of Social Workers
ABF	activity-based funding
ABS	Australian Bureau of Statistics
ACAT	Aged Care Assessment Team
ACCHO	Aboriginal Community Controlled Health Organisation
ACCHS	Aboriginal Community Controlled Health Services
ACHSM	Australasian College of Health Service Management
ACM	Australian College of Midwives
ACSQHC	Australian Commission on Safety and Quality in Health Care
ADG	Australian Dietary Guidelines
ADHA	Australian Digital Health Agency
AEP	Accredited Exercise Physiologist
AES	Accredited Exercise Scientist
AHP	allied health professional
AHPA	Allied Health Professions Australia
Ahpra	Australian Health Practitioner Regulation Agency
AHRC	Australian Human Rights Commission
AIDS	acquired immune deficiency syndrome
AIHW	Australian Institute of Health and Welfare
AMA	Australian Medical Association
AMC	Australian Medical Council
ANMAC	Australian Nursing and Midwifery Accreditation Council
AOD	alcohol and other drug
AOTA	American Occupational Therapy Association
APA	Australian Physiotherapy Association
APAC	Australian Psychology Accreditation Council
APC	Australian Physiotherapy Council
APD	Accredited Practising Dietitian
AQF	Australian Qualifications Framework
ARIA	Accessibility/Remoteness Index of Australia
ARN	Access Relative to Need
ASD	autism spectrum disorder
ASGC-RA	Australian Standard Geographic Classification – Remoteness Areas
CaFHS	Child and Family Health Service
CAM	complementary and alternative medicine
CAN	Australian College of Nursing
CAPHIA	Council of Academic Public Health Institutions Australia
CDM	Chronic Disease Management
CHP	Community Health Program
CHS	community health service
CHSP	Commonwealth Home Support Program
CLP Scheme	Cleft Lip and Palate Scheme
CMHS	Community Mental Health Services
CNA	comprehensive needs assessment
CNC	clinical nurse consultant
CNS	clinical nurse specialist

COAG	Council of Australian Governments
CPD	continuing professional development
CS	caesarean section
CSIRO	Commonwealth Scientific and Industrial Research Organisation
DA	Dietitians Australia
DAA	Dietitians Association of Australia
DAP	daily accommodation payment
DE	developmental educator
DEAI	Developmental Educators Australia Incorporated
DH	dental hygienist
DRG	Diagnosis Related Groups
DT	dental therapist
DVA	Department of Veterans' Affairs
EBM	evidence-based medicine
ECHO	Extension for Community Healthcare Outcomes
ED	emergency department
EHO	environmental health officer
EHR	electronic health record
EMSN	Extended Medicare Safety Net
ENT	ear, nose and throat specialist
ESP	extended-scope physiotherapist
ESSA	Exercise & Sports Science Australia
GDP	gross domestic product
GFC	global financial crisis
GP	general practice/general practitioner
GPMP	general practitioner management plan
HAC	hospital-acquired condition
HACC	Home and Community Care
HAI	hospital-acquired infection
HCH	Health Care Home
HCP	home care package
HIV	human immunodeficiency virus
HSS	health system strengthening
IASSW	International Association of Schools of Social Work
ICER	incremental cost-effectiveness ratio
ICF	International Classification of Functioning, Disability and Health
ICN	International Council of Nurses
IEO	Index of Education and Occupation
IER	Index of Economic Resources
IFSW	International Federation of Social Workers
IHPA	Independent Hospital Pricing Authority
IMA	independent medical assessment
IPE	interprofessional education
IPP	interprofessional practice
IRSAD	Index of Relative Socio-economic Advantage and Disadvantage
IRSD	Index of Relative Socio-economic Disadvantage
LGO	Local Government Organisation
LHN	Local Hospital Network

MBS	Medicare Benefits Schedule	**PCMH**	Patient Centred Medical Home
MDGs	Millennium Development Goals	**PCO**	primary care organisation
MDT	multidisciplinary team	**PCP**	primary-contact practitioners
MGP	midwifery group practice	**PCW**	personal care worker
MHCC	Mental Health Coordinating Council	**PHAA**	Public Health Association of Australia
MHR	My Health Record	**PHC**	primary health care
MMM	Modified Monash Model	**PHDB**	Private Hospital Data Bureau
MPH	Master of Public Health	**PHI**	private health insurance
NACCHO	National Aboriginal Community Controlled Health Organisation	**PHIDU**	Public Health Information Development Unit
		PHN	Primary Health Network
NASRHP	National Alliance of Self Regulating Health Professionals	**PHRSG**	Primary Health Reform Steering Group
		PII	professional indemnity insurance
NBN	National Broadband Network	**PPP**	public–private partnership
NCD	non-communicable disease	**PSA**	patient services assistant
NDIA	National Disability Insurance Agency	**QCPP**	Quality Care in Pharmacy Program
NDIS	National Disability Insurance Scheme	**RACMA**	Royal Australasian College of Medical Administrators
NFP	not-for-profit		
NGO	non-government organisation	**RAD**	refundable accommodation deposit
NHMRC	National Health and Medical Research Council	**RCT**	randomised controlled trial
NHPA	National Health Priority Area	**RMO**	resident medical officer
NHRA	National Health Reform Agreement	**RMO**	registered medical officer
NICM	National Institute of Complementary Medicine	**RNutr**	registered nutritionist
NMBA	Nursing and Midwifery Board of Australia	**RRMA**	rural, remote and metropolitan areas
NMHC	National Mental Health Commission	**RTW**	return to work
NMP	National Medicines Policy	**SDG**	Sustainable Development Goals
NPM	new public management	**SEIFA**	Socio-Economic Indexes for Areas
NPY	Ngaanyatjarra, Pitjantjatjara and Yankunytjatjara	**SLR**	systematic literature review
NPYWC	Ngaanyatjarra, Pitjantjatjara, Yankunytjatjara Women's Council	**SP**	speech pathologist
		SPA	Speech Pathology Australia
NRHA	National Rural Health Alliance	**SRHS**	small rural health services
NSA	Nutrition Society of Australia	**TAFE**	Technical and Further Education
NSQHS	National Safety and Quality Health Service	**TCA**	team care arrangements
OECD	Organisation for Economic Co-operation and Development	**TMO**	trainee medical officer
		UHC	universal health coverage
OHT	oral health therapist	**UK**	United Kingdom
OM	otitis media	**UN**	United Nations
OT	occupational therapist	**UNHS**	universal neonatal hearing screening
OTA	Occupational Therapy Australia	**VBHC**	value-based health care
OTBA	Occupational Therapy Board of Australia	**VET**	Vocational Education and Training
PBA	Physiotherapy Board of Australia	**WFOT**	World Federation of Occupational Therapists
PBS	Pharmaceutical Benefits Scheme	**WHO**	World Health Organization
PCEHR	Personally Controlled Electronic Health Record	**WPR**	What's the problem represented to be?

INDEX

A

AASW. *see* Australian Association of Social Workers
ABF. *see* activity-based funding
ableist, 142
Aboriginal and Torres Strait Islander people
    ageing in, 93, 93f
    health workforce, 203–204
    mental disorder in, 126
    oral health and, 176–177
Aboriginal Community Controlled Dental Services, 181t
Aboriginal Community Controlled Health Organisation
    (ACCHO), 69
Aboriginal Community Controlled Health Services (ACCHS), 115, 117
    funding for, 120–121, 120b, 121b
    key features of, 120f
    pioneering, perspectives from, 118–119b
    role of, in dealing with the COVID-19, 121–122
Aboriginal Liaison Officers (ALOs), 115
Aboriginal Medical Service (AMS), 117–118, 118–119b
ABS. *see* Australian Bureau of Statistics
ACATs. *see* Aged Care Assessment Teams
acceptability, 102
access, in rural health, 102, 103f
Access all areas: new solutions for GP shortages in rural Australia, 167
Access Relative to Need (ARN), 104–106
Accessibility/Remoteness Index of Australia (ARIA), 107
ACCHO. *see* Aboriginal Community Controlled Health Organisation
ACCHS. *see* Aboriginal Community Controlled Health Services
Accidental Logics, 4
accommodation, 102
accreditation, 242
    in health workforce, 207
Accredited Exercise Physiologist (AEP), 214–215
    career pathways for, 216
    clinical reasoning and the modes of practice of, 216–217, 217f
    multidisciplinary practice, 219–221, 220–221b, 221b
    professional standards of, 215
Accredited Exercise Scientists (AES), 214–215
Accredited Practising Dietitians (APDs), 226
ACECQA. *see* Australian Children's Education and Care Quality Authority
ACHSM. *see* Australasian College of Health Service Management
acquired immune deficiency syndrome (AIDS), prevention of, 61b
ACSQHC. *see* Australian Commission on Safety and Quality in
    Health Care
activities of daily living (ADLs), 138–139
    clinical exercise physiology and, 215
activity-based funding (ABF), 3, 26, 49
acute care, 9–10
ADGs. *see* Australian Dietary Guidelines
ADLs. *see* activities of daily living
administrative school, 239
advanced practice, 208

adverse events, 3
AEP. *see* Accredited Exercise Physiologist
AES. *see* Accredited Exercise Scientists
affordability, 102
Aged Care Act (1997), 95
Aged Care Assessment Teams (ACATs), 64–65b, 95–96
aged-care, 89–99
    of Aboriginal and Torres Strait Islander, 93, 93f
    case study on, 98b
    community care in, 96–97
    context of, 90
    cultural diversity in, 92, 92b
    future trends and directions of, 97
    history, 90, 90b
    legislative and funding environment in, 93–95, 94f, 95f
    population ageing in, 91–92, 91b, 91f, 92f
    residential aged care and oral health, 177b
    residential care in, 95–96
    Royal Commission into Aged Care, 95
    summary on, 97–98
ageing, non-communicable diseases and, 50
AHMAC. *see* Australian Health Ministers' Advisory Council
AHPRA. *see* Australian Health Practitioner Regulation Agency
AHRC. *see* Australian Human Rights Commission
AIDS. *see* acquired immune deficiency syndrome
AIHW. *see* Australian Institute of Health and Welfare
ailments, minor, 306–307, 307b
Akeyulerre Healing Centre, 116
alcohol and other drug (AOD), 204
allied health professionals (AHPs), 204
Allied Health Professions Australia (AHPA), 208
allied health services, utilisation of, trends in, 74f
allopathy, 165
Alma-Ata and Astana Declaration, 66–67
almoner, 339
ALOs. *see* Aboriginal Liaison Officers
Alzheimer's disease, 283
AMA. *see* Australian Medical Association
ambulance services, 294
    funding of, 296
American Occupational Therapy Association (AOTA), 282–283
AMS. *see* Aboriginal Medical Service
APDs. *see* Accredited Practising Dietitians
applications, for digital health, 195–197, 196b
approachability, 102
appropriateness, 102
APRA. *see* Australian Prudential Regulation Authority
AQF. *see* Australian Qualifications Framework
ARIA. *see* Accessibility/Remoteness Index of Australia
ARN. *see* Access Relative to Need
ASGC-RA. *see* Australian Standard Geographical Classification-
    Remoteness Areas

ASPPH. *see* Association of Schools and Programs of Public Health
assessment, treatment *versus,* workers' compensation, 155–156
Association of Schools and Programs of Public Health
    (ASPPH), 55, 56b
asylum seekers, oral health services for, 181t
audiologists, 324–325
audiology, 323–335, 332b
    communication impairment and, 324–327
    with education, employment and registration, 329, 329b
    ethics and clinical practice, 330
    hearing and related disorders, 325–327, 327b
    NDIS, 331–332
    practice within, 329–330
auditory processing disorders (APD), 327
Australasian College of Health Service Management
    (ACHSM), 239–241
Australia
    complementary and alternative medicine in, 163–174, 164b
        case study on, 165–166b
        changes in, 168
        common features of, 164
        Commonwealth Ombudsman and, complaint to, 170
        consumer confidence in, 165–166
        with conventional medicine, 164
        education and training in, 168–171
        history of, 164–167
        marginalisation of, 167
        natural therapies, 169
        practitioners, 167
        primary contact practices, 168, 168t
        private health insurance policy, 169
        private health insurance rebates, 168–170
        problems of evidence for, 170–171
        recognised components for, 168
        use of, 164–165
    dietetics in, 226–227
        case study on, 229b
        clinical, 227–228
        community-based, 228
        food and nutrition policy, 231–232
        interprofessional collaboration in, 228–229
        interprofessional practice in, 228–229
        multidisciplinary care in, 229b
        private practice, 228
    disability professionals in, 143–146, 144b
    medical profession in, 248–257
        case study of, 253–254b
        employment in, 254–255
        future of, 255
        medical workforce in, 254
        modern medical professional, 251–253, 251b, 252b
        public view of, 255
        remuneration in, 254–255
    midwifery in, 258–270
        case study of, 267b
        continuity of care, 265
        education, 261–262, 262b

Australia *(Continued)*
        funding and cost in, 266, 266b
        midwife and, 260–261
        regulation, 260–261
        scope of practice, 260–261
    nursing in, 271–281
        interprofessional issues, nursing-medical boundary,
            275–277, 277b
        as licensed profession, 272–273
        regulation and qualifications of, 272t
        scope of, 275
        staffing and patient safety, 277–278
        workforce, 273–275, 273t, 274f, 274t, 275b
    physiotherapy in, 313–322
        AHPRA and, 314
        APA, 314
        APC, 314–315
        case study of, 318b
        current status of, 315
        drivers for change - expanding the scope of practice,
            319–320, 320b
        history of, 314
        IPC and role, 317–318
        NGOs and physiotherapists, 315
        private health, working in, 316–317, 317b
        public health, working in, 315–316
        registration pathway and requirements, 314
        relevant professional and regulatory bodies, 314–315, 315b
    primary health care in, 64–78
        case study on, 64–65b
        community health and community-based services in, 70
        current state of, 71–73, 72f, 73b
        definition of, 65–66, 66b
        dental services in, 70–71
        general practice in, 68
        importance of, 66–67
        Indigenous services in, 68–69, 69f
        private allied health and pharmacy services in, 69, 74f
        reform agenda and future of, 73–75
        spending on, 68f
        system of, 67–71, 67f
        utilisation of, trends in, 73f
    private health care sector in, 34–36
    private hospitals in, 34–36, 35b, 35f
    public health in, 55–63, 56b
        definition of, 56
        funding of, 59
        libertarian to egalitarian, 61–62
        messaging, during COVID-19 pandemic, 62b
        'old' and 'new,' 56–58
        pathways into, 57
        responsibilities for, 60–61
        targeted, 59
        workforce, 57–58, 58b
    social work in, 336–337
    workers' compensation system in, 150–162
        benefits or payments, 153

Australia *(Continued)*
        case study on, 151b, 152t
        claims management, 155
        employment with, 158
        health care provider engagement in, 156–157
        interaction with health care system, 154–157
        process, 153–154
        regulator, 152–153, 152t
        during SARS-CoV-2 pandemic, 158–159
        system impact on worker health and well-being, 157
        system structure and operation, 152–153
        with treatment and assessment, 155–156
        work and health, 150
Australian aged-care system, 90
Australian Association of Social Workers (AASW), 208, 336–337,
        339–340
Australian Bureau of Statistics (ABS), 7, 239–240
Australian Children's Education and Care Quality Authority
        (ACECQA), 232
Australian College of Midwives (ACM), 262
Australian College of Nursing (ACN), 208
Australian Commission on Safety and Quality in Health Care
        (ACSQHC), 6, 242, 252, 308
Australian Dental Council (ADC), 187
Australian Dietary Guidelines (ADGs), 230
Australian Digital Health Agency (ADHA), 192
Australian health care system, 1–13
        in 21st century, 4
        case study on, 5b
        health service managers in, 237–247
                core competencies of, 240–241, 241b
                COVID-19 and, 243–245, 244b, 245b
                equity of care and, 242–243, 243b
                management and, 239–245, 240b
                quality and safety of care and, 241–242, 242b
        new public management in, 5–6
        philosophies, practices and pandemics driving change in, 5
        professionals in, thinking about, 2–10, 3b
        reform in, questions about, 8
        SARS-CoV-2 on, impact of, 6–7, 7–8b, 7b
        social work profession in, 336–344
                case study on, 338b
                challenges for, 341–342
                health inequities and, 340–341
                history of, 338–340, 340b
                social environment and, 340–341
Australian Health Ministers' Advisory Council (AHMAC), 130
Australian Health Practitioner Regulation Agency (AHPRA), 3, 169,
        202–203, 227, 249, 260–261, 272, 292–293
        occupational therapy and, 286–287
        physiotherapy and, 314
Australian Hearing, 326–327
Australian Human Rights Commission (AHRC), 122
Australian Institute of Health and Welfare (AIHW), 6, 35, 71–72,
        104, 139, 167, 217, 259
Australian Medical Association (AMA), 5b, 208, 276, 316–317
Australian Medical Council (AMC), 207, 249

Australian Nursing and Midwifery Accreditation Council
        (ANMAC), 207, 273
Australian Occupational Therapy Journal, 287
Australian Physiotherapy Association (APA), 208, 314
Australian Physiotherapy Council (APC), 314–315
Australian Prudential Regulation Authority (APRA), 31–32
Australian Psychology Accreditation Council (APAC), 207
Australian Qualifications Framework (AQF), 168
Australian Standard Geographical Classification-Remoteness Areas
        (ASGC-RA), 107, 107t
Australia's health 2018, 167
authority, 238
authority benefits, 82–83
authority required (streamlined) benefits, 82–83, 83t
autism spectrum disorder (ASD), 325
autonomy of practice, 3, 252
availability, 102
Ayurvedic medicine, 169

B
Bacchi, Carol, 8, 9t
benefits
        Child Dental Benefits Scheme, 177
        by workers' compensation, 153
Better Access, 131
Better Oral Health in Residential Care program, 177b
Beveridge model, 44
bioequivalent, 85
biomedical model, 151
biopsychosocial model
        mental disorder and, 126
        in speech pathology and audiology, 324–325
        workers' compensation, 151
bipartisan agreement, 50
birthing, maternity care and, 267
Bismarck model, 44–45
blame game, 25–26
block-funded, 145
'Blue Zones' project, 101
body of knowledge, monopoly of, notion of, 253
building blocks, of health system, 43, 43f, 47f
bulk-billing, 19, 19f, 255

C
CAAC. *see* Central Australian Aboriginal Congress
caesarean section (CS) rate, 260
CAM. *see* complementary and alternative medicine
Canada, workers' compensation in, 157
CAPHIA. *see* Council of Academic Public Health Institutions
        Australia
cardiologist-supervised stress test, 218
care
        aged-care, 89–99
                of Aboriginal and Torres Strait Islander, 93, 93f
                case study on, 98b
                community care in, 96–97
                context of, 90

care *(Continued)*
    cultural diversity in, 92, 92b
    future trends and directions of, 97
    history, 90, 90b
    legislative and funding environment in, 93–95, 94f, 95f
    population ageing in, 91–92, 91b, 91f, 92f
    residential aged care and oral health, 177b
    residential care in, 95–96
    Royal Commission into Aged Care, 95
    summary on, 97–98
  maternity, 259–260
  multidisciplinary, in dietetics and nutrition, 229b
  shared, 264–265t
case management, workers' compensation and, 155
case study
  complementary and alternative medicine, 165–166b
  dietetics, 229b
  digital health, 195b, 196b
  disability, 139, 140b, 141b
  health workforce, 210–211b
  medical profession, 253–254b
  midwifery, 267b
  nutrition, 229b
  occupational theory, 289b
  oral health, 177b, 180b, 185b
  Pharmaceutical Benefits Scheme (PBS), 86b
  pharmacists, 310b
  physiotherapy, 318b
  primary health care, 64–65b
  private health insurance (PHI), 32–33b
  social work, 338b
  speech pathology, 326b
  workers' compensation, 151b, 152t
casemix funding, 3, 26
cause-based systems, 151–152
CDM. *see* Chronic Disease Management
Central Australian Aboriginal Congress (CAAC), 117–118, 118–119b
charge nurse. *see* nurse managers
Child and Family Health Service (CaFHS), 327
Child Dental Benefits Schedule, 181t
Child Dental Benefits Scheme, 177
Chinese medicine, 164
CHP. *see* Community Health Program
Chronic Dental Disease Program, 177
Chronic Disease Dental Scheme, 26
Chronic Disease Management (CDM), 215–216, 317
chronic diseases
  mobile applications to screen, 197b
  population ageing and, 91
CHS. *see* community health services
CHSP. *see* Commonwealth Home Support Program
claims, 152–153
claims management, workers' compensation and, 155
claims management organisation, 153
claims manager, 155
Cleft Lip and Palate (CLP) Scheme, 181t

client-centred practice, 287–288
clinical dietetics, 227–228
clinical exercise physiology, 214–224
  Accredited Exercise Physiologist (AEP), 214–215
    career pathways for, 216
    clinical reasoning and the modes of practice of, 216–217, 217f
    multidisciplinary practice, 219–221, 220–221b, 221b
    professional standards of, 215
  client assessment and, 217f, 218–219, 219f
  efficacy of, 218, 218b
  exercise paradox, 218
  goals of, 215
  historical perspective of, 215–216
  leading causes of morbidity and mortality and, 217–218
  regulation of, 215–216
Clinical Framework for the Delivery of Health Services, 155–156, 156b
clinical governance, 241–242
clinical nurse consultant (CNC), 208
clinical nurse specialist (CNS), 208
Close the Gap Report, 122
Closing the Gap, 84, 122
CMHs. *see* community mental health services
CNA. *see* comprehensive needs assessment
code of conduct, 251–252
colonisation, Indigenous health systems, 115, 115f
combined care, 264–265t
Commonwealth Acoustics Laboratories (CAL), 329
Commonwealth funding, 204
Commonwealth Home Support Program (CHSP), 93–94, 96, 97
Commonwealth Ombudsman, 170
Commonwealth Scientific and Industrial Research Organisation (CSIRO), 230
Commonwealth Seniors Health Card, 21t, 23
communication
  access, 328
  complex communication needs, 330
  impairment, 324–327
  with speech pathology and audiology, 324–327
community care
  aged care, 96–97
  in health workforce, 205
Community Health Program (CHP), 70
community health services (CHS), 70
community mental health, 128
community mental health services (CMHs), 131
community mental health teams, 205–206
community paramedicine, 298
community pharmacy, 306–308
Community Pharmacy Agreement (CPA), 303–304
community-based dietetics and nutrition, 228
Comparative Performance Monitoring report, 153b
compensation, workers'
  benefits or payments, 153
  in Canada, 157
  case study on, 151b, 152t
  claims management, 155
  employment with, 158

compensation, workers' *(Continued)*
  health care provider engagement in, 156–157
  interaction with health care system, 154–157
  process, 153–154
  regulator, 152–153, 152t
  during SARS-CoV-2 pandemic, 158–159
  system, in Australia, 151–154
  system impact on worker health and well-being, 157
  system structure and operation, 152–153
  with treatment and assessment, 155–156
  work and health, 150
complementary and alternative medicine (CAM), 163–174, 164b
  case study on, 165–166b
  changes in, 168
  common features of, 164
  Commonwealth Ombudsman and, complaint to, 170
  consumer confidence in, 165–166
  with conventional medicine, 164
  education and training in, 168–171
  in healthcare workforce, 202–203
  history of, 164–167
  marginalisation of, 167
  natural therapies, 169
  practitioners, 167
  primary contact practices, 168, 168t
  private health insurance policy, 169
  private health insurance rebates, 168–170
  problems of evidence for, 170–171
  recognised components for, 168
  use of, 164–165
complex communication needs, 330
compounding, medicine, 306
comprehensive needs assessment (CNA), 71
compulsory health insurance, 15
concession card, 19, 21t, 22t
concessional beneficiaries, 82
conductive hearing loss, 326
constructivist, 250
consultant pharmacist, 308–309
consumer, 306
  confidence, in CAM, 165–166
  in health care systems, role of, 50–51
contextual learning, 250
continuing professional development (CPD), 169, 250–251, 286–287, 314
continuity of midwifery care, 265
co-payment, 82
corporatised, 254–255
costs, in midwifery, 266, 266b
cost-shifting behaviours, 25–26
Council of Academic Public Health Institutions Australia (CAPHIA), 57
COVID-19
  CAM and, 165–166b
  in health care systems, 51
  health service managers and, 243–245, 244b, 245b
  impact of, 6, 7–8b, 7b
  impact on speech pathology, 330–331
  public health messaging during, 62b
  role of ACCHSs in, 121–122

CPD. *see* continuing professional development
cream skimming, 37
CSIRO. *see* Commonwealth Scientific and Industrial Research Organisation
CTG. *see* Closing the Gap
cultural competence, Indigenous health system and, 122–123
cultural diversity, ageing and, 92, 92b
cultural safety, Indigenous health system and, 122–123
customers, 306–307

D

DA. *see* Dietitians Australia
DALYs. *see* disability-adjusted life years
Davidson, Elaine, 339–340
day hospitals, 34
DEAI. *see* Developmental Educators Australia Incorporated
Deeble, John, 15
deinstitutionalisation, 128
dementias, 90
Dental Board of Australia, 185–186
dental decay/dental caries, 176
dental hygienist, 183
dental prosthetists, 183
dental relocation and infrastructure program, 181t
dental services, 70–71, 175–190
  dental decay, 176
  dental hygienists, 184–185
  dental prosthetists, 184
  expenditure, 179f
  funding, 178–182, 181t
  Medicare in, 181b
  practitioners, 182–183t, 182–187, 184t
  private health, 178–179
  public health, 179–182
dental therapists, 183, 184–185
Dental Training Expanding Rural Placements (DTERP), 181t
dentate, 176
dentists, 184–185
Department of Veterans' Affairs (DVA), 21, 70–71, 204
DEs. *see* developmental educators
development, professional, CPD, 286–287, 314
developmental educators (DEs), 143, 144b
Developmental Educators Australia Incorporated (DEAI), 143
Diagnosis Related Groups (DRG), 3, 26
dietary advice, in Australia, 230–232
dietetics, 225–236
  in Australia, 226–227
  case study on, 229b
  clinical, 227–228
  community-based, 228
  food and nutrition policy, 231–232
  interprofessional collaboration in, 228–229
  interprofessional practice in, 228–229
  multidisciplinary care in, 229b
  private practice, 228
dietitian, 226, 229–230
Dietitians Association of Australia (DAA), 207
Dietitians Australia (DA), 226, 228

digital divide, 197
digital health, 191–192, 192b
  applications, 195–197, 196b
  case study, 195b, 196b
  digital divide, 197
  electronic health records, 192–194, 193f, 194b, 195t
  in Indigenous health context, 198, 198b
  in rural and remote Australia, 197–198
Digital Inclusion Index, 191
digital tertiary hospital, case study on, 195b
disability
  health care of, responsibility for, 145–146, 145b
  NDIA, 331
  NDIS, 288, 331
  profession, changes in, 144–145
  professionals, in Australia, 143–146, 144b
  support and health systems for, 138–149
    case study on, 139, 140b, 141b
    concepts of, 141–143, 142b
    skills and knowledge, 142–143, 143b
disability-adjusted life years (DALYs), clinical exercise physiology
    and, 217
disability-based systems, 151–152
discrimination, in mental disorder, 128
disease
  CDM, 317
  Chronic Dental Disease Program, 177
  non-communicable, 226
  oral cancer, 176
  oral health, population and, 176–177
  periodontal, 176
DRG. see Diagnosis Related Groups
DVA. see Department of Veterans' Affairs
dysphagia, 325

E
ear, nose and throat (ENT) specialist, 328b
EBM. see evidence-based medicine
EBP. see evidence-based practice
ECHO. see Extension for Community Healthcare Outcomes
ecological paradigm, 232
economic rationalism, 4, 5, 252
ECP. see extended care paramedic
ED. see emergency department
edentulous individuals, 176
education
  in CAM, 168–171
  in health workforce, 207
  medical, in Australia, 249–250t, 249–251
  midwifery, 261–262, 262b
  occupational therapy and, 286
  in speech pathology and audiology, 327–329
educators, developmental, 143, 144b
effectiveness, in health care system, 4
efficiency, in health care system, 4
Efficient Funding of Chemotherapy program, 84, 85
egalitarian, libertarian to, 61–62
EHOs. see environmental health officers

EHRs. see electronic health records
electronic health records (EHRs), 50–51, 192–194, 193f, 194b, 195t
emergency department (ED), 297, 316
  for healthcare workforce, 206
  mental health and, 132, 132–133b
employment, 254–255
  for nutritionists and dietitians, 229–230
  in paramedicine, 298, 298–299b
  in speech pathology and audiology, 327–329
  with workers' compensation, 158
EMSN. see Extended Medicare Safety Net
endorsed midwife, 261
Enhanced Primary Care (EPC), 181t, 317
enrolled nurse (EN), 272, 272t
environmental health officers (EHOs), 61
epidemic, obesity as, 228, 233
equality, 101f, 337
equity, 337
  in health care system, 4
  horizontal, 101–102
  in rural health, 101–102, 101f
  vertical, 101–102
ESSA. see Exercise & Sports Science Australia
evidence-based medicine (EBM), 10, 170
evidence-based practice (EBP), 252
  in AEP practice, 215
'Examining alternative therapy claims,' 168–169
Exercise & Sports Science Australia (ESSA), 214
exercise paradox, 218
exercise physiology, clinical, 214–224
  Accredited Exercise Physiologist (AEP), 214–215
    career pathways for, 216
    clinical reasoning and the modes of practice of,
      216–217, 217f
    multidisciplinary practice, 219–221, 220–221b, 221b
    professional standards of, 215
  client assessment and, 217f, 218–219, 219f
  efficacy of, 218, 218b
  exercise paradox, 218
  goals of, 215
  historical perspective of, 215–216
  leading causes of morbidity and mortality and, 217–218
  regulation of, 215–216
expressive communication impairments, 324
extended care paramedic (ECP), 298
Extended Medicare Safety Net (EMSN), 22
extended scope of practice, 209
extended-scope physiotherapist (ESP), 319
Extension for Community Healthcare Outcomes (ECHO), 109

F
family, oral health for low-income/working-poor, 180b
Family Tax Benefit Part A (FTB(A)), 23
Fayol, Henri, 239
federal responsibilities, for public and population health, 60
fee-for-service, 254–255
  payments, 204
Fifth National Mental Health and Suicide Prevention Plan, 129

financial protection, 15
First National Plan, 129
First Nations People, 114
Follett, Mary Parker, 239
food
    insecurity, 233, 233b
    labelling, 230
    policy, in Australia, 231–232
    system, sustainability and health, 232
formal services, 96
for-profit sector, 2
Freidson, Eliot, 2
friendly visitors, 339
funding
    activity-based, 3
    in aged care, 93–95, 94f, 95f
    of ambulance services, 296
    block-funded, 145
    dental services, 178–182, 181t
    individualised, 141
    of Medicare, 4
    of Medicare benefits schedule, 20
    in midwifery, 266, 266b
    of public health, 59
    source of, 17

G

gap fee, 254–255
GDP. *see* gross domestic product
general patients, 82
general practice, 65, 68
general practice, funding of, 4
general practitioner management plans (GPMPs), 228
general practitioner obstetrician care, 264–265t
general practitioners (GPs), 4, 68, 141, 167, 180–181, 228, 276
generic brands, 85
generic substitution, 85
Geographical classification systems, 107
GFC. *see* global financial crisis
global financial crisis (GFC), 6
good health financing system, 43
governance, in health care systems, 43, 51
government, 2
    CAM and, 167
    non-government organisations (NGOs), 315
GPMPs. *see* general practitioner management plans
GPs. *see* general practitioners
Gratton Institute, 167
gross domestic product (GDP), 16
Gurriny Yealamucka Health Service, 121–122

H

HACC. *see* Home and Community Care
Hawke Labor Government, 70
HCH. *see* Health Care Home
HCPs. *see* home care packages

health
    definition of, 142
    digital, 191–192, 192b
        applications, 195–197, 196b
        case study, 195b, 196b
        digital divide, 197
        electronic health records, 192–194, 193f, 194b, 195t
        in Indigenous health context, 198, 198b
        in rural and remote Australia, 197–198
    oral, 175–190
        case study, 177b, 180b, 185b
        dental service expenditure, 179f
        funding, 178–182
        Indigenous Australians, 177–178, 185b
        Medicare in, 181b
        models of care, 185–186
        population oral health and disease, 176–177
        practitioners, 182–183t, 182–187, 184t, 187b
        service delivery system, 177–187
        therapists, 184–185
        therapy practice, debates around, 186–187
        therapy practitioners, 184–185
    social model of, 228
health care, 41–42
Health Care Card, 21t
health care financing, 15, 16–23, 16f, 17b, 17f, 18f
health care funding, in health workforce, 204–205
Health Care Home (HCH), 50
health care provider, workers' compensation and, 156–157
health care system, 1–13
    in 21st century, 4
    case study on, 5b
    health service managers in, 237–247
        core competencies of, 240–241, 241b
        COVID-19 and, 243–245, 244b, 245b
        equity of care and, 242–243, 243b
        management and, 239–245, 240b
        quality and safety of care and, 241–242, 242b
    Indigenous, 114–124
        Aboriginal Community Controlled Health Services (ACCHS), 115, 117
        controlled health systems and services today, 116–122, 117b, 118–119b, 119b, 120f
        as oldest health care systems and services in the world, 115–116, 115f, 116b
        where to, 122–123
    international, 41–54
        driving factors for, 45–46, 46b, 48b
        future directions and challenges for, 50–51, 51b
        key concepts of, definition of, 41–42, 42b
        models or typologies of, 44–45, 45b, 46f
        organisation, functions and goals of, 42–44, 43f, 44b
    new public management in, 5–6
    paramedicine, 292–302
        case study on, 298–299b
        current and future employment opportunities, 298

health care system *(Continued)*
   demographics, 294–295, 295b, 296b
   future of, 297–298, 298b
   National Registration and Accreditation Scheme
      (NRAS), 292–294
   occupational hazards, 297, 297b
   working life, 296, 296t, 297t
  for people living with disability, 138–149
   case study on, 139, 140b, 141b
   concepts of, 141–143, 142b
   profession, 144–145
   professionals, 143–146, 144b
   responsibility for, 145–146, 145b
   skills and knowledge, 142–143, 143b
  pharmacists in, 303–312
   case study, 310b
   funding, 303–304
   with hospital pharmacy, 308
   in medical centres, 309
   medicine and, 304–305, 304b, 305b
   minor ailments, management of, 306–307
   non-supply roles, 309–310
   payments for triage role, 307
   Professional Practice Standards, 306–307
   QCPP, 305
   RACFs and, 309
   role of, 305–309
   towards prescribing, 309–310
   workplace, 303–304, 304t
  philosophies, practices and pandemics driving change in, 5
  professionals in, thinking about, 2–10, 3b
  reform in, questions about, 8
  SARS-CoV-2 on, impact of, 6–7, 7–8b, 7b
  social work in, 336–344
   case study on, 338b
   challenges for, 341–342
   health inequities and, 340–341
   history of, 338–340, 340b
   social environment and, 340–341
  social workers in, 340
  Tuohy's theory of, 4
  workers' compensation interaction with, 154–157
health care system performance, 42b, 46–50, 48t, 49b
health equity, 58–59, 242
health financing, 42b
health gap, 59
health inequality, 101
health inequity
  in rural health, 101
  on social workers, 340–341
health insurance
  NDIS, 331
  private, 168–169
Health Practitioner Regulation National Law Act, 260–261
health practitioners, Health Practitioner Regulation National Law
   Act, 286–287
health professionals, registered and employed in Australia, 273t

health records, electronic, 192–194, 193f, 194b, 195t
health sector, 41–42
health security, 42b
health service delivery system, 41–42
health service managers, 237–247
  core competencies of, 240–241, 241b
  COVID-19 and, 243–245, 244b, 245b
  equity of care and, 242–243, 243b
  management and, 239–245, 240b
   leadership and, 238–239, 238b, 239b, 239t
   organisations and, 237–238, 238b
  quality and safety of care and, 241–242, 242b
health services organisations, 41–42
health spending flows, 67f
Health Star Rating System (HSR), 231–232
health system, 41–42., 73 *see also* health care system
health system strengthening (HSS), driving factors for, 45–46, 48b
Health Training Package, 168
health workforce, 201–213
  advanced practice in, 208–209, 209b
  case study in, 210–211b
  emerging trends and issues in, 209–210
  extended scope of practice in, 208–209, 209b
  governance and regulation of, 207–208
   education and accreditation, 207
   professional associations, 208, 208b
   registration, 207
  organisation of, 204–206
   health care funding, 204–205
   primary and community care, 205
   secondary referral services, 205–206
   tertiary referral services, 206, 206b
  overview of, 202–204
  registered practitioners, 202–203t
  shortages, 90
  size and distribution of, 202–204, 204f
  specialisation in, 208–209, 209b
Health Workforce Australia, 315
Healthcare Clinical Information System Providers, 193
hearing
  conductive hearing loss, 326
  disorders, related, 325–327
  noise-induced hearing loss, 327
  UNHS, 327
Highly Specialised Drugs (HSD), 84–85
high-risk strategy, 58
HIV. *see* human immunodeficiency virus
holistic view, 164
Home and Community Care (HACC), 96, 97
home care packages (HCPs), 93–94, 96
home medicines review (HMR), 308–309
homoeopathy, 168t, 170
horizontal equity, 101–102
hospitals
  pharmacy, 308
  private, 34–36, 35b, 35f
  public, 23–27

Howard Liberal-Coalition Government, 31
HSD. *see* Highly Specialised Drugs
HSR. *see* Health Star Rating System
HSS. *see* health system strengthening
human immunodeficiency virus (HIV), prevention of, 61b
human rights, 284–285
    model, 141

I

IAHP. *see* Indigenous Australians' Health Programme
IASSW. *see* International Association of Schools of Social Work
iatrogenic nature, 156
ICER. *see* incremental cost-effectiveness ratio
IFSW. *see* International Federation of Social Workers
IHACPA. *see* Independent Health and Aged Care Pricing Authority
IHI. *see* Institute for Health Innovation
IHPA. *see* Independent Hospital Pricing Authority
IMAs. *see* independent medical assessments
impairment
    communication, 324–327
    disability and, 138–139
income, oral health for low-income/working-poor family, 180b
incremental cost-effectiveness ratio (ICER), 82
incremental test protocols, 218
Independent Health and Aged Care Pricing Authority (IHACPA), 26
Independent Hospital Pricing Authority (IHPA), 3
independent medical assessments (IMAs), 156
Indigenous Australians
    oral health, 177–178, 185b
        in Aboriginal community, 176–177, 185b
Indigenous Australians' Health Programme (IAHP), 15, 69
Indigenous health context, digital health in, 198, 198b
Indigenous health systems and services, 114–124
    Aboriginal Community Controlled Health Services
        (ACCHS), 115, 117
        funding for, 120–121, 120b, 121b
        key features of, 120f
        pioneering, perspectives from, 118–119b
        role of, in dealing with the COVID-19, 121–122
    controlled health systems and services today, 116–122, 117b,
        118–119b, 119b, 120f
    as oldest health care systems and services in the world, 115–116,
        115f, 116b
    where to, 122–123
Indigenous medicine, 168t
Indigenous services, 68–69, 69f
individualised funding, 141
inequality, structural, 337
injury management, workers' compensation and, 155
inpatients, 85–86
    Medicare services for, 19
Institute for Health Innovation (IHI), 242
institutional mix, 5b
insurance
    model, 151
    private health, 30–40, 45, 168–169
        case study on, 32–33b

insurance *(Continued)*
        environment, contemporary, 31–34, 34b
        history of, 30–34
        policy, 169
        rebates, 15, 31, 169, 181t
integration of care, 97
integrative medicine, 167
intensive care paramedic (ICP), 298–299b
intentional self-harm, prevalence of, 127
International Association of Schools of Social Work
        (IASSW), 337
International Council of Nurses (ICN), 271–272
International Federation of Social Workers (IFSW), 337
international health care systems, 41–54
    driving factors for, 45–46, 46b, 48b
    future directions and challenges for, 50–51, 51b
    key concepts of, definition of, 41–42, 42b
    models or typologies of, 44–45, 45b, 46f
    organisation, functions and goals of, 42–44, 43f, 44b
interprofessional collaboration, in dietetics and nutrition, 228–229
interprofessional education (IPE), 8–9
interprofessional models of care, 318b
interprofessional practice (IPP), 8–9
    in dietetics and nutrition, 228–229
    role of physiotherapy, 317–318
intersectoral collaboration, 59
intervention, communication with intervention services, 327
intervention services, 325
IPE. *see* interprofessional education
IPP. *see* interprofessional practice

K

Kambu Health, 118–119b
Keating Labor Government, 31
KICA. *see* Kimberley Indigenous Cognitive Assessment
Kimberley Indigenous Cognitive Assessment (KICA), 93
Koori Growing Old Well, 93

L

labelling, food, 230
leadership, 238–239, 239t
    in health care systems, 43, 51
legislation, aged care, 93–95
LGOs. *see* local government organisations
LHNs. *see* Local Hospital Networks
liberation, 101f
libertarian, to egalitarian, 61–62
licensed profession, nursing as, 272–273
life expectancies, 90
Lifetime Health Cover Loading, 31
lived experience workforce, 130–131, 131b
local government organisations (LGOs), 228
local government responsibilities, for public and population
        health, 60–61, 60–61b
Local Hospital Networks (LHNs), 26, 71
low income, oral health and, 180b
Low Income Health Care Card, 21t

M

management, 238–239, 239t
  claims, workers' compensation and, 155
  functions of, 239
  of minor ailments, pharmacists, 306–307, 307b
market, 3
market pressures, 22
market-driven health care systems, 44
market-driven system, 4
Master of Public Health (MPH), 57
maternity care
  birthing and cultural care, 267
  future of, 267–268
  models of, 264–265t, 264–265
  mortality rates, 259, 259f, 260f
  during SARS-COV-2 pandemic, 266–267
  services, reform of, 262–264, 263f
    national strategic approach to, 262
    woman-centred care, 263–264, 263f
MBS. *see* Medicare Benefits Schedule
McIntyre, Agnes, 339
MDGs. *see* Millennium Development Goals
medical dominance, 3
medical education, in Australia, 249–250t, 249–251
Medical Leadership and Management curriculum, in RACMA, 241
medical model, 141
medical nutrition therapy, 226
medical practitioner, 248–249
medical profession
  in Australia, 248–257
  case study of, 253–254b
  future of, 255
  public view of, 255
medical professional, modern, 251–253, 251b, 252b
  autonomy of practice, concept of, 252
  body of knowledge, monopoly of, notion of, 253
  price setting, notion of, 252
  self-regulation, notion of, 252
  strong service ethic, 253, 253b
medical rationing, 243
medical workforce, in Australia, 254
  employment and remuneration, 254–255
  under-serviced groups, 254
Medicare
  in Australia, program of, 15
  extended Medicare safety net entitlements and, 24–25b, 24t
  funding of, 4
  public health sector and, 14–29
  rebate, 24–25b
  rebates, during COVID-19, 75
  role of, 2
  subsidised services, for mental health, 131–132
Medicare Australia Chronic Disease Management (CDM), 215–216
Medicare Benefits Schedule (MBS), 15, 18–21, 19f, 20b, 20f, 23b, 196, 276, 307
  benefits, 19
  entitlements of, 22t

Medicare Benefits Schedule *(Continued)*
  exercise physiology practice and, 216
  fee, 18
Medicare Chronic Disease Dental Scheme, 181t
Medicare levy, 17
Medicare Levy Surcharge, 31
Medicare Rebate Freeze, 5b
Medicare Teen Dental Program, 181t
medicine
  Ayurvedic, 169
  Chinese, 164
  complementary and alternative, 164b
    in Australia, 163–174
    changes in, 168
    common features of, 164
    Commonwealth Ombudsman and, complaint to, 170
    consumer confidence in, 165–166
    with conventional medicine, 164
    education and training in, 168–171
    marginalisation of, 167
    natural therapies, 169
    practitioners, 167
    primary contact practices, 168, 168t
    private health insurance policy, 169
    private health insurance rebates, 168–170
    problems of evidence for, 170–171
    recognised components for, 168
    use of, 164–165
  compounding, 306
  dispensing of, 305–306
  home medicines review (HMR), 308–309
  Indigenous, 168t
  integrative, 167
  NMP, 304
  nutritional, 168t
  pharmacists and, 304–305, 304b, 305b
  QUM, 308
  vaccination, 307–308, 308b
  Western herbal, 168t
  WHO and, 304
mental disorder, 126
  costs of, 127–128, 128b
  prevalence of, 126, 126b
  stigma and discrimination on, 128
mental health, 125–137
  consumer movement, 128–129
  defined, 125
  deinstitutionalisation and, 128, 128b
  emergency departments and, 132, 132–133b
  Mental Health Acute Assessment Team, 132
  reform, 129–130
  service system, 131–132
  social determinants of health and, 126
  suicide and, 126–128, 127t
  well-being and, 125–126
Mental Health Coordinating Council (MHCC), 126–127
Mental Health Intervention Team, 132

Menzies Coalition Government, 31
MHCC. *see* Mental Health Coordinating Council
microeconomic reform, 5
midwifery
    in Australia, 258–270
    case study of, 267b
    continuity of care, 265
    education, 261–262, 262b
    funding and cost in, 266, 266b
    midwife and, 260–261
    regulation, 260–261
    scope of practice, 260–261
midwifery group practice (MGP), 266
midwifery group practice caseload care, 264–265t
Millennium Development Goals (MDGs), 43–44
minor ailments, 306–307
mixed system, 4
MMM. *see* Modified Monash Model
mobile-driven health service delivery, 196
modalities, CAM and, 164
modern medical professional, 251–253, 251b, 252b
    autonomy of practice, concept of, 252
    body of knowledge, monopoly of, notion of, 253
    price setting, notion of, 252
    self-regulation, notion of, 252
    strong service ethic, 253, 253b
Modified Monash Model (MMM), 107, 107t
Moffit, Connie, 339–340
moral hazard, 37
mortality rates, 259, 259f, 260f
MPH. *see* Master of Public Health
multidisciplinary care, in dietetics and nutrition, 229b
multidisciplinary rehabilitation, 219–220
multidisciplinary team (MDT), 206
My Health Record (MHR), 193, 194f

N

NACCHO. *see* National Aboriginal Community Controlled Health
        Organisation
NASRHP. *see* National Alliance of Self Regulating Health Professions
National Aboriginal Community Controlled Health Organisation
        (NACCHO), 69, 119
National Advisory Committee on Dental Health (NACDH), 180
National Alliance of Self Regulating Health Professions
        (NASRHP), 215
National Broadband Network (NBN), 195–196
national competency standards, 226
National Competition Policy, 178
National Disability Insurance Agency (NDIA), 140, 331
National Disability Insurance Scheme (NDIS), 15, 131, 204, 285, 288,
        331–332
National Disability Insurance Scheme (NDIS) Act, 139–140, 142b
National E-Health Strategy, 167
National E-Health Transition Authority (NEHTA), 192
National Framework for Recovery-oriented Mental Health
        Services, 130–131
National Health Act 1953, 31, 84

National Health and Medical Research Council (NHMRC), 168–169
National health insurance (NHI), 45
National health model, 44
National Health Priority Areas (NHPAs), 139
National Health Reform Agreement (NHRA), 15, 26–27
National Health Strategy, 178
National Health Workforce Taskforce, 168b
National Institute of Complementary Medicine (NICM), 166
National Medicines Policy (NMP), 80, 304
National Mental Health Commission (NMHC), 128, 129
National Mental Health Policy, 129
National Mental Health Strategy, 129
National Partnership Agreement oral health implementation, 181t
National Registration and Accreditation Scheme
        (NRAS), 3, 292–294
National Rural Health Alliance (NRHA), 208
National Safety and Quality Health Service (NSQHS), 242, 252
National Study of Mental Health and Wellbeing, 126
National Weighted Activity Unit (NWAU), 26–27
naturopathy, 168t
NCDs. *see* non-communicable diseases
NDIA. *see* National Disability Insurance Agency
NDIS. *see* National Disability Insurance Scheme
NDIS Quality and Safeguards Commission, 146
needs, complex communication, 330
neoliberalism, 4, 252
new public health, 56–58
new public management (NPM), 4, 5–6
Ngaanyatjarra, Pitjantjatjara, Yankunytjatjara Women's Council
        (NPYWC), 116
Ngangkari, 116
Ngangkari Program, 116, 116b
NGOs. *see* non-government organisations
NHI. *see* National health insurance
NHMC. *see* National Mental Health Commission
NHMRC. *see* National Health and Medical Research Council
NHPAs. *see* National Health Priority Areas
NHRA. *see* National Health Reform Agreement
NICM. *see* National Institute of Complementary Medicine
NMP. *see* National Medicines Policy
noise-induced hearing loss, 327
non-communicable diseases (NCDs), 66, 226
    ageing and, 50
non-government organisations (NGOs), 204
    Indigenous health system and, 122
    physiotherapists and, 315
not-for-profit (NFP), 95–96, 205
NPM. *see* new public management
NPYWC. *see* Ngaanyatjarra, Pitjantjatjara, Yankunytjatjara Women's
        Council
NRAS. *see* National Registration and Accreditation Scheme
NSA. *see* Nutrition Society of Australia
NSQHS. *see* National Safety and Quality Health Service
nurse managers, 240
nurse practitioner (NP), 272, 272t
nurse supervisor. *see* nurse managers
nurse unit manager. *see* nurse managers

nursing, in Australia, 271–281
  interprofessional issues, nursing-medical boundary, 275–277, 277b
  as licensed profession, 272–273
  regulation and qualifications of, 272t
  scope of, 275
  staffing and patient safety, 277–278
  workforce, 273–275, 273t, 274f, 274t, 275b
Nursing and Midwifery Board of Australia (NMBA), 260–261, 272
nursing-medical boundary, interprofessional issues, 275–277, 277b
nutrition, 225–236
  in Australia, 226–227
  case study on, 229b
  community-based, 228
  interprofessional collaboration in, 228–229
  interprofessional practice in, 228–229
  issues in, 232–233
  multidisciplinary care in, 229b
  obesity and, 232–233
  policy, in Australia, 231–232
  private practice, 228
Nutrition Society of Australia (NSA), 227
nutritional medicine, 168t
nutritionist, 226
  in Australia, 227, 227b
  employment for, other areas of, 229–230
NWAU. see National Weighted Activity Unit

O

obesity
  as epidemic, 228, 233
  nutrition and, 232–233
obesogenic environment, 233
occupation
  defined, 282–283
  occupational engagement and, 282–283, 283b
  well-being and impact of, 284, 284b
occupational engagement, 282–283
occupational hazards, in paramedicine, 297, 297b
occupational justice, 284–285, 285b
occupational rehabilitation, 150
occupational theory
  case study, 289b
    well-being, impact of occupation, 284, 284b
  education and, 286–287
  occupational justice, 284–285, 285b
  occupational science, 284
  occupational therapy practice, 287–288
  organisation of, 286–287
  as therapy, 285–286
occupational therapist (OT), 282
occupational therapy, 282–291, 283b
Occupational Therapy Australia (OTA), 286–287
Occupational Therapy Board of Australia (OTBA), 286–287
OECD. see Organisation for Economic Co-operation and Development
old public health, 56–58
opiate crisis, collaborating to manage, 306

oral cancer, 176
oral health, 175–190
  case study, 177b, 180b, 185b
  dental service expenditure, 179f
  funding, 178–182
  Indigenous Australians, 177–178, 185b
  Medicare in, 181b
  models of care, 185–186
  population oral health and disease, 176–177
  practitioners, 182–183t, 182–187, 184t
  service delivery system, 177–187
  therapists, 184–185
  therapy practice, debates around, 186–187
  therapy practitioners, 184–185
Oral Health Therapist (OHT) Graduate Year Program, 181t
Organisation for Economic Co-operation and Development (OECD), 46–47, 48t, 74, 91, 260
organisations, definition of, 238
originator brand, 85
otitis media (OM), 326
out-of-hospital services, 18
out-of-pocket (OOP) costs, 15
  financial protection from, 21–23, 21t
out-of-pocket model, 45
outpatients, 85–86

P

P4P. see payment for performance
pandemics, in health care systems, 51
paramedic regulation, 292–293
paramedicine, 292–302
  case study on, 298–299b
  current and future employment opportunities, 298
  demographics, 294–295, 295b, 296b
  future of, 297–298, 298b
  National Registration and Accreditation Scheme (NRAS), 292–294
  occupational hazards, 297, 297b
  working life, 296, 296t, 297t
Paramedicine Board of Australia (PBA), 293
paramedics
  moving beyond urgent care, 297–298, 298b
  regulated, responsibilities of, 293–294
Parker, Norma, 339–340
patent, 85
pathology, speech, 323–335, 332b
  case studies, 326b
  communication impairment and, 324–327
  COVID-19 on, 330–331
  education, employment and registration, 327–328
  ethics and clinical practice, 330
  NDIS, 331–332
  practice within, 329–330
patient, 306
Patient Centered Medical Home (PCMH), 50
patient safety, 277–278
patient services assistant (PSA), 210–211b
payment for performance (P4P), 49

payments
   for triage role, pharmacists, 307
   by workers' compensation, 153
PBA. *see* Paramedicine Board of Australia
PBAC. *see* Pharmaceutical Benefits Advisory Committee
PBS. *see* Pharmaceutical Benefits Scheme
PCMH. *see* Patient Centered Medical Home
PCOs. *see* Primary Care Organisations
peer workers, 130–131
penicillin, discovery of, 80
Pensioner Concession Card, 21t
periodontal disease, 176
personal care workers (PCWs), 272–273, 277–278
personal recovery, 130
Personally Controlled Electronic Health Record (PCEHR),
   192, 193f
person-centred approach, 143
PH. *see* private health insurance
PHAA. *see* Public Health Association of Australia
Pharmaceutical Benefits Act, 80–81
Pharmaceutical Benefits Advisory Committee (PBAC), 80–82
Pharmaceutical Benefits Scheme (PBS), 2, 15, 22t, 25, 79–88, 261,
   276, 303–304
  case study on, 86b
  Closing the Gap, 84
  costs of, managing, 85–86
  definition of, 80–83, 80b
  development of, 80–81, 81b
  eligible for, 81
  future challenges of, 86
  medicines in, 81
    affordability of, 82, 82t
    in hospital setting, 85–86, 86b
    prescribing, 82–83, 83t
    pricing of, 82
    with special arrangements, 84–85, 84t
  safety net, 83–84
pharmaceutical reform, 85–86
Pharmaceutical Society of Australia, 306–307
pharmacists, 303–312
  case study, 310b
  funding, 303–304
  with hospital pharmacy, 308
  in medical centres, 309
  medicine and, 304–305, 304b, 305b
  minor ailments, management of, 306–307
  non-supply roles, 309–310
  payments for triage role, 307
  Professional Practice Standards, 306–307
  QCPP, 305
  RACFs and, 309
  role of, 305–309
  towards prescribing, 309–310
  workplace, 303–304, 304t
Pharmacy Guild of Australia, 309
pharmacy services, 69
PHC. *see* primary health care

PHDB. *see* Private Hospital Data Bureau
PHI. *see* private health insurance
PHIDU. *see* Public Health Information Development Unit
PHNs. *see* Primary Health Networks
PHRSG. *see* Primary Health Reform Steering Group
physiotherapy, 313–322
  AHPRA and, 314
  APA, 314
  APC, 314–315
  case study of, 318b
  current status of, 315
  drivers for change - expanding the scope of practice,
    319–320, 320b
  history of, 314
  IPC and role, 317–318
  NGOs and physiotherapists, 315
  private health, working in, 316–317, 317b
  public health, working in, 315–316
  registration pathway and requirements, 314
  relevant professional and regulatory bodies, 314–315, 315b
Physiotherapy Board of Australia (PBA), 314–315
Pika Wiya Health Service Aboriginal Corporation, 118–119b
Pinel, Philippe, 285–286
Pinel a la Salpêtrière, 286f
Poisons and Therapeutic Goods Act 1996 (NSW), 305
policy
  food and nutrition, 231–232
  National Competition Policy, 178
  NMP, 304
Poor Laws and the Workhouse system, 90
population
  ageing, 91–92, 91b, 91f
  oral health and disease, 176–177
population health, 58–59, 58b
  health equity in, 58–59
  issues of, 61
  responsibilities for, 60–61
    federal, 60
    local government, 60–61, 60–61b
    state and territory government, 60
  social determinants of health in, 59
population strategy, 58
Position Statement on Human Rights, 284–285
PPPs. *see* public-private partnerships
practice nurse, 276
practitioners
  CAM, 167
  dental and oral health, 182–183t, 184t
  medical, 248–249
  oral health therapy practitioners, 184–185
  registered, 202–203t
Pre-National Health Reform Arrangements, 25–26
presbycusis, 327
prescriptions require review, 305–306
presumptive rules, 158–159
prevention paradox, 58
price setting, notion of, 252

primary care, 65
    in health workforce, 205
Primary Care Organisations (PCOs), 71, 71b
primary contact practices, CAM, 168, 168t
primary health care (PHC), in Australia, 64–78, 104–106,
        105f, 106b, 117
    case study on, 64–65b
    community health and community-based services in, 70
    current state of, 71–73, 72f, 73b
    definition of, 65–66, 66b
    dental services in, 70–71
    general practice in, 68
    importance of, 66–67
    Indigenous services in, 68–69, 69f
    private allied health and pharmacy services in, 69, 74f
    reform agenda and future of, 73–75
    spending on, 68f
    system of, 67–71, 67f
    utilisation of, trends in, 73f
Primary Health Networks (PHNs), 71, 104, 193
Primary Health Reform Steering Group (PHRSG), 73–74
primary-contact practitioners (PCPs), 316
primary-contact status, 314
prisoners, oral health services for, 181t
private allied health, 69
private for-profit sector, 3
private health
    dental services, 178–179
    physiotherapy and working in, 316–317, 317b
private health care sector, 34–36
    private hospitals in, 34–36, 35b, 35f
private health insurance (PHI), 30–40, 45, 168–169
    case study on, 32–33b
    environment, contemporary, 31–34, 34b
    history of, 30–34
    policy, 169
    rebates, 15, 31, 169, 181t
Private Hospital Data Bureau (PHDB), 35
private hospitals, 30
    in Australia, 34–36, 35b, 35f
    ownership of, 35–36
    SARS-CoV-2 pandemic and, 36–37
private insurance model, 4
private midwifery care, 264–265t
private obstetrician care, 264–265t
private prescriptions, 82
privatisation, 31–32, 37
proceduralists, 255
productivity, in health care system, 5
Productivity Commission, 127, 129–130, 139
professional, modern medical, 251–253, 251b, 252b
professional associations, in health workforce, 208, 208b
professional bodies, physiotherapy, 318b
professional development, 332
professional identity, 294, 294b
professional indemnity insurance (PII), 261–262
professional monopoly, 2–3

professional practice standards, pharmacists, 306–307
programmatic assessment, 250
protected title, 293
provider, health care, workers' compensation and, 156–157
provider fees, 23
public dental services, for adults, 180
public health, in Australia, 55–63, 56b
    definition of, 56
    dental services, 179–182
    funding of, 59
    libertarian to egalitarian, 61–62
    messaging, during COVID-19 pandemic, 62b
    nutrition, 226–227
    'old' and 'new,' 56–58
    pathways into, 57
    physiotherapy and working in, 316–317, 317b
    responsibilities for, 60–61
        federal, 60
        local government, 60–61, 60–61b
        state and territory government, 60
    targeted, 59
    workforce, 57–58, 58b
Public Health Association of Australia (PHAA), 59
Public Health Information Development Unit (PHIDU), 104
public health insurance, 15–16, 42b
public health sector, Medicare and, 14–29
public hospital high risk maternity care, 264–265t
public hospital maternity care, 264–265t
public hospitals, 23–27
public view, of medical profession, 255
public-contracted service delivery model, 4
public-integrated model, 4
public-private health space, tensions in, 37–38, 38b
public-private partnerships (PPPs), 5–6, 36–38

Q
QALYs. see quality-adjusted life-years
quality, Australian Commission on Safety and Quality in Health
        Care, 252
Quality Care in Pharmacy Program (QCPP), 305
quality of life, social workers and, 337
quality use of medicines (QUM), 80, 308
quality-adjusted life-years (QALYs), 82
QUM. see quality use of medicines

R
racism, Indigenous health system and, 122–123
RACMA. see Royal Australasian College of Medical
        Administrators
RADs. see refundable accommodation deposits
ramping, 297
randomised controlled trials (RCTs), 170
RCTs. see randomised controlled trials
realised access. see utilisation
receptive communication impairments, 324
reciprocal health care agreements (RHCA), 81

recovery-oriented mental health services, 130–131, 132–133b
    National Framework for Recovery-oriented Mental Health Services, 130–131
    personal recovery, 130
Redfern Aboriginal Medical Service, 118
reference pricing, 82
reflective learners, 250
refundable accommodation deposits (RADs), 93–94, 96
registered medical officers (RMOs), 250
registered nurse (RN), 272, 272t
registered nutritionist (RNutr), 227
registered practitioners, 202–203t
registration
    in health workforce, 207
    physiotherapy, registration pathway, 314
    in speech pathology and audiology, 327–329
regulation, 3
    Health Practitioner Regulation National Law Act, 286–287
    physiotherapy, regulatory bodies, 314–315, 315b
regulator, workers' compensation, 152–153, 152t
rehabilitation services, 206
remote area maternity care, 264–265t
remuneration, 254–255
Repatriation Pharmaceutical Benefits Scheme (RPBS), 80–81
repeats, 81
research, funding of, CAM and, 166–167
resident medical officers (RMOs), 206
residential aged-care facilities (RACFs), 272–273, 278b, 309
    reducing sedative prescribing in, 309
residential care
    aged care with, 95–96, 96t, 177b
    Better Oral Health in Residential Care program, 177b
residential medication management reviews (RMMRs), 308–309
residential services, 91, 131
resilience, of health system, 42b
restricted benefit, 82, 83t
restrictive practices, for people living with disability, 141
return to work (RTW), 150, 151
RHCA. *see* reciprocal health care agreements
rights, human rights, 284–285
Robert-Fleury, T., 285–286, 286f
Rose, Geoffrey, 58
Royal Australasian College of Medical Administrators (RACMA), 240–241
Royal Commission into Aged Care, 95
Royal Institute for Deaf and Blind Children (RIDBC) Teleschool, case study, 196b
RPBS. *see* Repatriation Pharmaceutical Benefits Scheme
RRMA. *see* rural, remote, and metropolitan area
RTW. *see* return to work
rubella, 327
rural, remote, and metropolitan area (RRMA), 107
rural and remote Australia, digital health in, 197–198
rural health, 100–113
    access in, 102, 103f
    access relative to need, 104–106, 105f, 106b
    determinants of health in, 102–103, 103b
    equity in, 101–102, 101f

rural health (*Continued*)
    geographical classification system, 107, 107t
    health service utilisation in, 103f, 106, 106b
    health status and behaviours in, 104, 104b
    inequitable health outcomes in, 107–110
    minimum health service provision in, 106
    models of health care in, 108–109, 109b
    service funding in, 109–110
    workforce initiatives in, 108

S

Safe Havens, 132
Safe Work Australia website, 153b
safeguarding, for people living with disability, 141
safety, Australian Commission on Safety and Quality in Health Care, 252
Safety Net scheme, 83–84
SARS-CoV-2 pandemic
    exercise physiology and, 217–218
    health inequity, 102
    impact of, 2, 6–7, 7–8b, 7b
    maternity care during, 266–267
    private hospitals and, 36–37
    social work profession and, 341–342
    workers' compensation during, 158–159
Schedule of Pharmaceutical Benefits, 81
school dental services, 179
school of scientific management, 239
science, occupational science, 284
scope of practice, 208–209
Scotton, Richard, 15
SDGs. *see* Sustainable Development Goals
SDH. *see* social determinants of health
secondary care, 205
secondary referral services, in health workforce, 205–206
section 100 programs, 84
SEIFA. *see* Socio-Economic Indexes for Areas
self-determination, 141
    Indigenous health system and, 117
self-regulation, 3, 252
sentinel events, 3, 35
services
    ambulance, 294
        funding of, 296
    dental
        dental decay, 176
        dental hygienists, 184–185
        dental prosthetists, 184
        expenditure, 179f
        funding, 178–182, 181t
        practitioners, 182–183t, 182–187, 184t
        private health, 178–179
        public health, 179–182
    intervention, 325
shared care, 264–265t
single intensity tests, 218
Six Minute Walk Test, 218
SLR. *see* systematic literature review
small rural health services (SRHS), 110

social care, 239
social contract, 152
social determinants of health (SDH)
    Indigenous health system and, 122
    mental health and, 126
    in public health, 59
    in social work, 340–341
    workers' compensation and, 151b, 158
social environment, of social workers, 340–341
social health insurance, 42b
social insurance model, 44–45
social model of health, 141, 228
social work, 336–344
    case study on, 338b
    challenges for, 341–342
    health inequities and, 340–341
    history of, 338–340, 340b
    social environment and, 340–341
social worker
    purpose of, 340
    role of, 337–338, 338b
Socio-Economic Indexes for Areas (SEIFA), 102–103, 103b
specialised mental health facilities, 131–132
speech pathologist (SP), 289
speech pathology, 323–335, 332b
    case studies, 326b
    communication impairment and, 324–327
    COVID-19 on, 330–331
    education, employment and registration, 327–328
    ethics and clinical practice, 330
    NDIS, 331–332
    practice within, 329–330
    speech, language and swallowing, 325
    speech pathologists, 324–325
Speech Pathology Australia (SPA), 207, 325
spinal cord injury, 288
SRHS. see Small rural health services
staffing, nurse, 277–278
stakeholder feedback, in price-setting processes, 27
state and territory government responsibilities, for public and
        population health, 60
stewardship, 42–43
Stewart, Mary, 339
stigma, in mental disorder, 128
Strengthening Medicare package, 22
streptomycin, discovery of, 80
strong service ethic, 253, 253b
Stronger Futures in the Northern Territory, 181t
structural balance, 4
structural inequality, 337
structural power, 5b
suicidality, 126–128
suicide, 126–128
    costs of, 127–128, 128b
    mental health support services and, 127t
    prevalence of, 127
surge workforce, 298

Survey of Disability, Ageing and Carers, 139
Sustainable Development Goals (SDGs), 43–44, 66
swallowing, speech pathology, 325
systematic literature review (SLR), 10

T
TAFE. see Technical and Further Education
targeted public health, 59
taxes, for Medicare, 17
Taylor, Frederick Winslow, 239
TCAs. see team care arrangements
team care arrangements (TCAs), 228, 317
team midwifery care, 264–265t
Technical and Further Education (TAFE), 145, 207
technology, in health care systems, role of, 50–51
telehealth
    digital health and, 195–196
    social work and, 341–342
tertiary referral services, in health workforce, 206, 206b
TGA. see Therapeutic Goods Administration
the State, 2, 3
theory, 4
Therapeutic Goods Act, 305
Therapeutic Goods Administration (TGA), 81–82
therapists
    dental, 184–185
    oral health, 185
    WFOT, 284–285
therapy
    medical nutrition, 226
    occupational theory as, 285–286
    occupational therapy practice, 287–288
    oral health, 185, 186–187
tinnitus, 327
Torres Strait Islander people
    ageing in, 93, 93f
    health workforce, 203–204
    mental disorder in, 126
    oral health and, 176–177
Traditional Healers of Central Australia: Ngangkari, 116
trainee medical officers (TMOs), 250
training
    in CAM, 168–171
    Health Training Package, 168
transdisciplinary approach, 143–146
treatment, assessment *versus,* workers' compensation, 155–156
triage role, payments for, 307
Tuohy's theory, of health care systems change, 4

U
UHC. see universal health coverage
UN. see United Nations
under-serviced groups, 254
United Nations (UN)
    Sustainable Development, 101
    Universal Declaration of Human Rights, 284–285
    WFOT and, 284–285, 287

universal approaches, to public health, 59
Universal Declaration of Human Rights, 284–285
universal health coverage (UHC), 15, 42b, 43–44, 66
universal neonatal hearing screening (UNHS), 327
unlicensed health workers, 272
unrestricted benefits, 82
utilisation, 102

V

vaccination, 307–308, 308b
value-based health care (VBHC), 210
vertical equity, 101–102
Veterans' Affairs programs, 181t
Victorian Government Food Act 1984, 60
virtual reality, physiotherapy, 319
Virtual Rural Generalist Service (VRGS), 109b
Vocational Education and Training (VET), 183–184, 205–206
Voluntary Dental Graduate Year Program, 181t
VRGS. *see* Virtual Rural Generalist Service

W

Waminda Balaang healing framework, 267b
welfare state, 4
welfare-based health care systems, 42b, 44
wellness, well-being influenced by occupation, 284, 284b
Western herbal medicine, 168t
What's the problem represented to be (WPR), 8, 9t
WHO. *see* World Health Organization
Willis, Karen, 32–33b
Woman-Centred Care, 262, 263f
work disability, 151
    duration, 154
WorkCover, 317
workers' compensation
    benefits or payments, 153
    in Canada, 157
    case study on, 151b, 152t
    claims management, 155
    employment with, 158
    health care provider engagement in, 156–157
    interaction with health care system, 154–157
    process, 153–154
    regulator, 152–153, 152t
    during SARS-CoV-2 pandemic, 158–159
    system, in Australia, 151–154
    system impact on worker health and well-being, 157

workers' compensation *(Continued)*
    system structure and operation, 152–153
    with treatment and assessment, 155–156
    work and health, 150
*Workers' Compensation and Injury Management Amendment
        (COVID-19 Response) Act 2020,* 159
workforce
    challenges, in health care systems, 51
    medical, in Australia, 254
        employment and remuneration, 254–255
        under-serviced groups, 254
    nursing, 273–275, 273t, 274f, 274t, 275b
workforce, health, 201–213
    advanced practice in, 208–209, 209b
    case study in, 210–211b
    emerging trends and issues in, 209–210
    extended scope of practice in, 208–209, 209b
    governance and regulation of, 207–208
        education and accreditation, 207
        professional associations, 208, 208b
        registration, 207
    oral health for low-income/working-poor, 180b
    organisation of, 204–206
        health care funding, 204–205
        primary and community care, 205
        secondary referral services, 205–206
        tertiary referral services, 206, 206b
    overview of, 202–204
    registered practitioners, 202–203t
    size and distribution of, 202–204, 204f
    specialisation in, 208–209, 209b
workplace, pharmacists, 303–304, 304t
World Federation of Occupational Therapists (WFOT),
        284–285, 287
World Health Organization (WHO), 9–10, 16, 41–42, 65, 186
    health and, 142
    ICF, 324–325
    International Classification of Function, Disability and Health
        (WHO-ICF), 158
    medicines and, 304
    mental health definition, 125
    WFOT and, 284–285, 287
World Physiotherapy, 313
World War I (1914-1918), 286, 314
World War II (1939-1945), 165, 286, 314, 329
WPR. *see* What's the problem represented to be